KU-028-819

GP Companion

THE CONSULTATIVE PROCESS

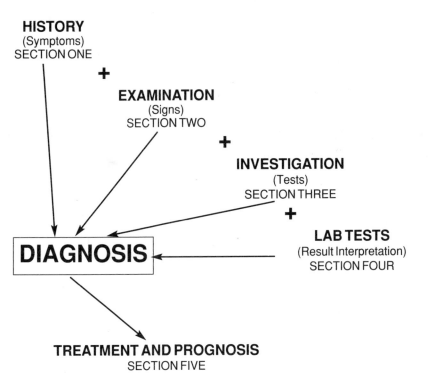

HISTORY
(Symptoms)
SECTION ONE

+

EXAMINATION
(Signs)
SECTION TWO

+

INVESTIGATION
(Tests)
SECTION THREE

+

LAB TESTS
(Result Interpretation)
SECTION FOUR

DIAGNOSIS

TREATMENT AND PROGNOSIS
SECTION FIVE

THIS PROCESS OCCURS IN EVERY CONSULTATION

Author Warwick J. Carter MB BS FRACGP

Editor Joe Ridge MRPharmS

Electronic Composition Sue Feather

Published by Euromed Communications Ltd
The Old Surgery
Liphook Road
Haslemere
Surrey GU27 1NL

Telephone:01428 656665
Fax: 01428 656643
email: euromed@pavilion.co.uk

Printed by Iberian Print Group

ISBN 1 899015 35 3

Supported by an educational grant from Eli Lilly and Company Limited

Contents copyright© 2002 by Warwick J Carter. All rights reserved. No portion of this publication may be reproduced in any form or by any means (electronic, mechanical or otherwise) including photocopying, recording or any information storage and retrieval system, without the prior written authorisation of the copyright holder.

NB: Clinical decisions are the responsibility of the individual practitioner. Although every effort has been made in compiling and checking the information given in this publication to ensure that it is accurate, the author, the publisher and their servants or agents shall not be responsible for the continued currency of the information, or for any errors, omissions or inaccuracies in this publication whether arising from negligence or otherwise howsoever, or for any consequences arising therefrom.

GP COMPANION

PREFACE

More than two million copies of this book have now been distributed in over 85 countries and ten languages (Chinese, English, Flemish, French, German, Italian, Korean, Polish, Spanish and Turkish). This book has been written by an Australian general practitioner, primarily for general practitioners, but surveys have found that a very wide range of doctors find it useful. Medical students, hospital interns, and specialists who require information outside their area of immediate expertise, all find the GP COMPANION invaluable.

The traditional text book deals with each disease separately. The GP COMPANION deals with a disease in the way that the doctor first sees it. A patient does not come to the doctor and immediately give a diagnosis, but complains of various symptoms, and the doctor notes different signs.

Doctors need to know the possible causes of these symptoms and signs, and the GP COMPANION can supply this information in the most concise way possible.

The logical steps of the normal consultation are shown in the diagram on page i, and the GP Companion is designed to assist the doctor at every stage, without the necessity of delving into large text books that are arranged as though the diagnosis is already known.

Every year, hundreds of alterations and additions are made to the text, particularly in those sections relating to pathology and treatment, to keep it as up to date as possible.

Hundreds of thousands of doctors around the world are now using the GP COMPANION as routinely as a prescription pad or pathology request form. I trust that you too will find it useful.

Dr. Warwick Carter
FRACGP
Brisbane, Australia

CONTENTS Page

HOW TO USE THIS BOOK

You want to know:	You already know:	See Section:
Diagnosis	Symptoms	One
	Clinical signs	Two
	Pathology results	Four
Pathology tests to perform	Suspected diagnosis	Three
Differential diagnosis		Three
Clinical signs		Three
Physiology of disease		Three
Reference interval of test	Pathology test result	Four
Physiology of pathology test	Pathology test	Four
Indications for performing test		Four
Explanation of clinical sign	Clinical sign	Two
Physiology of clinical sign		Two
Treatment	Diagnosis	Five
Prognosis		Five
Details about syndrome	Syndrome name	Six
Syndrome name	Symptoms	One
Definition of pathology term	Pathology term	Appendices
Prescription notation	Drug	Appendices
Meaning of abbreviation	Abbreviation	Introduction

ABBREVIATIONS

+	positive
++	very positive / exaggerated
−	negative
A.	artery
AB	abnormal
abdo.	abdomen
ACTH	adrenocorticotrophic hormone
ACP	acid phosphatase
AIDS	acquired immune deficiency disorder
ALP	alkaline phosphatase
ALT	alanine amino transferase
alt.	alternate / alternative
Ant-AChR	anti-acetylcholine receptor antibody
APTT	activated partial thromboplastin time
ASOT	antistreptolysin O titre
AST	aspartate amino transferase
AV	atrioventricular / arteriovenous
B.	blood
Ba	barium
BP	blood pressure
BSP	bromsulfophthalein retention test
BUN	blood urea nitrogen
Ca	calcium
CA	carbohydrate (cancer) antigen
cap.	capsule
CASA	cancer associated serum antigen
CAT	computerised axial tomography
CEA	carcinoembryonic antigen
CHF	congestive heart failure
CK	creatine kinase
Cl	chloride / chlorine
cm	centimetre
CNS	central nervous system
CO	carbon monoxide
COAD	chronic obstructive airways disease
Comm.	Comment
Comp.	Compound
cps	cycles per second
C-RP	C reactive protein
CSF	cerebrospinal fluid
CT	computerised tomography
CVA	cerebrovascular accident
d	day
DC	direct current
DD	differential diagnosis
DES	description
ECG	electrocardiograph
EEG	electroencephalogram
ELISA	enzyme linked immunosorbent assay
EMG	electromyogram
ERCP	endoscopic retrograde cholecysto-pancreatography
ESR	erythrocyte sedimentation rate
Exp.	explanation
FANA	fluorescent antinuclear antibodies
FBC	full blood count
Fe	iron
fL	femtolitre
f/r	failure rate
FSH	follicle stimulating hormone
FT	falling titre

FTA	fluorescent treponema antibody
FTI	free thyroxine index
GnRH	gonadotrophin releasing hormone
G6PD	glucose-6-phosphate dehydrogenase
GPI	general paralysis of insane
GTT	glucose tolerance test
h	hour
H	high
Hb	haemoglobin
HbF	fetal haemoglobin
HCG	human chorionic gonadotrophin
HCl	hydrochloric acid
Hg	mercury
HIAA	hydroxyindole acetic acid
HIV	human immunodeficiency virus
HLA	human leucocyte associated antigen
HMMA	4-hydroxy-3-methoxy mandelic acid
HPF	high powered field
Ig	immunoglobulin
IM	intramuscular
IMI	intramuscular injection
incl.	including
Ind.	indication
insuf.	insufficient
Int.	Interpretation
IU	international unit(s)
IV	intravenous
IVI	intravenous injection
IVP	intravenous pyelogram
J	joule
JVP	jugular venous pressure
K	potassium
KAu	King-Armstrong units
kg	kilogram
kJ	kilojoule
kPa	kilopascal
kph	kilometres per hour
L	left / litre / low
LCR	ligase chain reaction
LDH	lactic dehydrogenase
LE	lupus erythematosus
LFT	liver function tests
LH	luteinising hormone
LIF	left iliac fossa
m	metre
MAOI	monoamine oxidase inhibitor
M/C/S	microscopy, culture and sensitivity
MCV	mean corpuscular volume
mEq	milliequivalent
mg	milligram
MI	myocardial infarct
min	minute
mL	millilitre
mm	millimetre
mmol	millimol
mOsm	milliosmole
MRI	magnetic resonance imaging
MS	multiple sclerosis
N	normal
ng	nanogram
nmol	nanomol
no.	number
NSAID	nonsteroidal anti-inflammatory drug
NSU	non-specific urethritis

O	oxygen
P	phosphorus / plasma
PAN	polyarteritis nodosa
pCO$_2$	partial pressure of carbon dioxide
PCR	polymerase chain reaction
PCV	packed cell volume
pg	picogram
pH	acidity
Phys.	physiology
PKU	phenylketonuria
pmol	picomol
pO$_2$	partial pressure of oxygen
post	posterior
pr	per rectum / rectally
prn	as required
R	right
RAST	radioallergosorbent test
RBC	red blood cell
RCC	red cell count
req.	required
RI	reference interval
RIF	right iliac fossa
RT	rising titre
RUQ	right upper quadrant
S	serum
SC	subcutaneous
SCI	subcutaneous injection
sec	second
SG	specific gravity
SGGT	serum gamma-glutamyl transpeptidase
SI	système internationale
SLE	systemic lupus erythematosus
SSRI	selective serotonin reuptake inhibitor
stat	statim / at once
syn.	syndrome
T4	protein bound thyroxine
TB	tuberculosis
TENS	transcutaneous electrical nerve stimulation
TIA	transient ischaemic attack
Treat.	treatment
TSH	thyroid stimulating hormone
U	urine / unit
μmol	micromol
μg	microgram
μL	microlitre
URTI	upper respiratory tract infection
us.	usually / usual
VD	venereal disease
VH	very high
vit.	vitamin
VL	very low
VMA	vanillylmandelic acid / HMMA
vol.	volume
VPRL	volume of packed red cells
WBC	white blood cells
WCC	white cell count
WR	Wassermann reaction

TEST SUBSTANCES
Methods of obtaining samples for testing.

Amniotic Fluid
Obtained by puncturing the uterus via the abdominal wall with a large gauge needle (amniocentesis) after the fifteenth week of pregnancy, and drawing off a small amount of amniotic fluid. Experience, asepsis and extreme care are essential. Usually done under ultrasound control.

Blood
For most purposes, blood should be taken before breakfast, and with the patient seated, to avoid interference from food, and variations arising from the body position and time of day.
Venous blood is used except for : blood gases (taken from radial or femoral artery); glucose tolerance tests and thromboplastin time (capillary blood from finger tip used).

Haemolysis may interfere with results and can be prevented by : mixing blood gently with additives, not quickly; using disposable equipment; puncturing dry skin; avoiding aspiration and pressure; removing needle before expressing blood from syringe; using plasma instead of serum; separating cells within one hour; avoiding freezing and heating sample in transport. Despite these precautions, a slow or difficult blood flow may still cause haemolysis.
Blood should be taken with tourniquet released if possible, and should not be taken from a limb receiving an intravenous infusion.

Blood should be stored and transported in glass or plastic tubes that may have anticoagulants or other preservatives and stabilisers added, as listed in the table below:-

Tests	Additive	Volume required
Biochemistry (urea, electrolytes, urate, glucose, most enzymes)	Lithium heparinate	10mL
Blood sugar	Sodium fluoride	1mL
Bleeding studies (prothrombin time etc.)	Sodium citrate	5mL
Haematology (Hb, FBC*, ESR etc.)	EDTA	2.5 - 5mL
Serology (Ig, antibodies, blood group)	Nil (clotted blood)	10mL
Blood gases (O_2, CO_2)	Heparin (minimal amount)	#

* Plus two slide films.   # Transported in syringe in which it is taken or tube with no head space.
All additives are incorporated by gentle but thorough mixing by inversion.

Inaccurate blood test results may be due to errors in collection technique, transportation or processing, as listed in the table below:-

Cause	Consequences
Prolonged venous stasis during collection caused by cuff being left up around arm	High serum calcium and protein
Sample left unrefrigerated or frozen (haemolysed) Should be stored at 4°C	Low hormones High potassium and enzymes
Exertion prior to or during sampling	High enzymes
Pollution and dilution by intravenous fluids running into sample limb	Electrolytes altered. Other results low
Fasting and non-fasting samples	Fasting overnight for glucose, triglycerides, insulin and hormones
Timing of sample	Electrolytes, hormones, glucose etc. vary at different times of day
Drugs	Many drugs may affect results

Cerebrospinal Fluid (CSF)
Obtained by puncturing the dura mater of the spinal cord with a long broad gauge needle, and allowing the CSF to drip into a sterile container. This is normally done in the lumbar region. Any pressure reading should be taken before allowing CSF to escape. 2.5 to 5 mL is usually sufficient. If more is removed, a sterile normal saline solution should be introduced to replace the CSF lost.
There are many complications associated with this procedure, and the physician should be familiar with these before proceeding.

Exudate
Use a sterile swab to touch only infected area. Place swab in Stuart's transport medium or other specific medium (eg. for Chlamydia or Trichomonas) until examined. Do not refrigerate.
Smears are made by rolling another swab on a glass slide, and should be fixed immediately. Smears should always be sent with swabs to the investigating laboratory.

Faeces
A specimen of faeces is passed into a clean pan, and then using a sterile spatula, is collected into a sterile container for examination. For parasites, three specimens on alternate days required. Liquid faeces should be checked within 30 minutes to detect motile trophozites. Formed faeces may be stored at 4°C.

Gastric Fluid
Obtained directly during fibreoptic gastroscopy, or by passing a tube into the stomach via the mouth or nose with the patient sitting up. The sample should be taken several hours after any food.

Marrow, Bone
Performed under scrupulous asepsis. The sternum, just below the sterno-manubrial junction; or the posterior iliac crest; are the usual sites. After surgical preparation of the area, the skin and subcutaneous tissues are infiltrated with local anaesthetic. A needle with an obturator is then used to pierce the skin and bore through bone into the marrow cavity. A specimen is aspirated into a sterile syringe.

Nasopharyngeal Secretions
> 5 years - Gargle 5 to 10 mL of normal saline for one minute, then expectorate fluid into sterile jar
< 5 years - Fine bore catheter passed through nostril to posterior nasopharynx, and secretions are aspirated into a syringe attached to the end of the catheter. After catheter withdrawn, aspirate 5 mL sterile saline into catheter and syringe. Then flush contents of syringe into a sterile container.

Semen
Collected after masturbation in a clean container. Should be examined immediately after collection. Entire volume of ejaculate should be collected. Do not cool. Transport at 37°C.

Sputum
For bacteriology, patient is instructed to brush teeth and rinse mouth with water. Patient then coughs directly into a sterile container. The assistance of a physiotherapist may be needed to induce proper coughing. Sputum for cytology should be collected in 50% aqueous alcohol.

Synovial Fluid
A large gauge needle is placed carefully into a major joint cavity using a totally aseptic technique, and along the appropriate parenteral approach for that joint. Local anaesthetics may be used in the tissues outside the joint capsule. 2 to 5 mL of synovial fluid are drawn out of the joint for investigation. Knee joint most commonly used for synovial tap.

Urine
A mid-stream specimen of urine is caught in a sterile container. In the female, the labia should be held apart to give a good stream. The specimen should be kept cool until examined. 20 mL is usually sufficient, but more may be required for hydrometry to determine the specific gravity.

Worms
Whole worms from anus or other area are placed in normal saline, refrigerated and sent to the laboratory within 24 hours. If longer storage is required, fix specimen in 10% formalin. Worm segments must be handled very carefully (use instruments and gloves). Rest in tap water for 30 minutes, then fix in 10% formalin. Pinworm and Taenia may be detected by placing sticky tape across the perineal area at night, and removing it in the morning before washing or defaecation, then sending sticky tape to laboratory for microscopic examination.

DEFINITIONS

The definitions of common terms used in investigative procedures:

Agglutination Test: Agglutination of cells or particles results from an antigen (particle)-antibody (added substance) reaction. Clumping of the cells or particles is visible to the naked eye. Tanned red cells, collodion or polystyrene particles that have been coated with antigen, may be used. Test detects presence of antibody in a test substance.

Biochemistry: The study of the chemical substances that enable life to proceed. In practice, the measurement of the elements, salts, acids, alkalis, enzymes etc. in a selected fluid or tissue.

Complement Fixation Test: Lysis of sensitised sheep red blood cells indicates that complement remains in a solution consisting of complement, specific antigen and an unknown serum. If a specific antibody to the antigen is present in the serum, complement is absorbed and lysis prevented. Thus lack of cell lysis is a positive result.

Cytology: The study of cells and tissue. In practice, the macroscopic and microscopic examination of tissue to enable its nature to be determined.

Electrolytes: Salts in a serum solution separate into elemental ions, and can be individually identified and quantified. Bicarbonate, phosphate and chloride anions balance cations of sodium, potassium, calcium etc.

ELISA: Enzyme linked immunosorbent assay. Test for types of hepatitis, HIV, Herpes simplex and other antibodies.

Haematology: The study of the function and nature of blood. In practice, the investigation of the cellular elements in blood, and the physical characteristics of blood.

Histology: The study of microscopic anatomy. In practice, the diagnosis of disease by microscopic examination of affected tissue.

HLA Antigens: Human leucocyte associated (HLA) antigens exist on the surface of most cells, but are easily found on leucocytes. They are specific to the individual and are responsible for the rejection of heterogeneous tissue grafts. They can be detected by a standardised serological test. Specific antigen groups have been found in association with certain diseases, and thus HLA antigens have become a diagnostic tool. HLA-B27 is the antigen that is of greatest use at present.

Immunology: The study of biological immunity and related phenomena. In practice, the detection of specific antibodies against diseases (eg: hepatitis B) and allergens, and the study of immunoglobulins.

MRI: Magnetic resonance imaging (also known as NMRI – nuclear magnetic resonance imaging). While in a high intensity magnetic field, a radio-frequency signal is applied to the body to excite hydrogen nuclei to a higher energy state and cause them to gyrate in phase. When the field is removed, reversion to the equilibrium state result in the emission of radiation which can be detected and measured. A computer is used to generate a cross-sectional image of the area being examined (similar to a CT scan), including details of soft tissue as well as bone.

PET: Positron emission tomography. Oxygen[15], fluorine[18] or similar are taken into the body, and the resultant intermittent annihilation of positrons causes the emission of X-ray photons that can be measured by tomographic apparatus similar to that of a CT scanner. Used mainly for cerebrovascular disease diagnosis.

Plasma: The yellow fluid portion of blood in which cells are suspended. Produced from blood by sedimentation or centrifugation. Plasma will clot, and produce a clear fluid known as serum.

Reference Interval: Abnormal may be normal. The graph below demonstrates why, with reference intervals covering only 95% of normal subjects, the more tests that are done, the more likely it will be that at least one result will be outside the normal range.

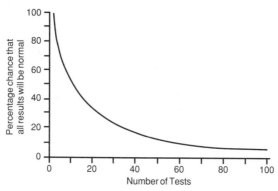

Serum: The study of the fluid base in which the cellular elements of blood are suspended. Serum consists of water, proteins, metabolites, catabolites, lipids, hormones, salts, enzymes and ions.

Titre: An expression of the strength of a volumetric solution. The greatest dilution at which a process that occurs readily can proceed.

RESPIRATORY FUNCTION TESTS

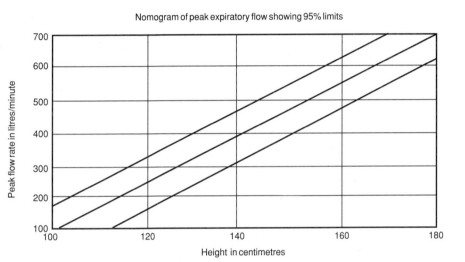

Nomogram of peak expiratory flow showing 95% limits

Spirogram of lung volumes

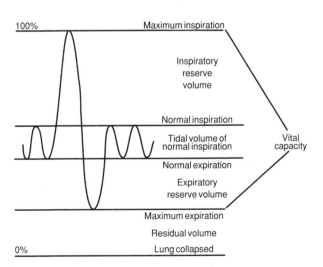

CARDIAC CYCLE

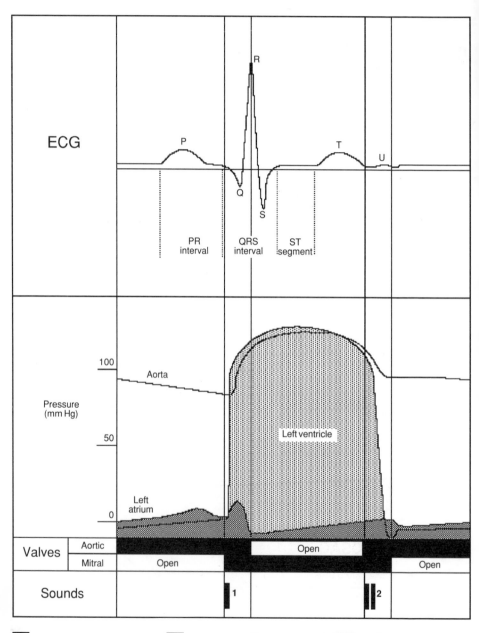

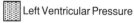

PRESCRIPTION NOTATION

Abbreviations used in prescription writing.
The use of these abbreviations is diminishing and is not encouraged.

Abbrev.	Latin/Greek origin	Meaning	Abbrev.	Latin/Greek origin	Meaning
aa	ana	of each	oculent	ocullentum	eye ointment
ac	ante cibum	before food	o alt hor	omnibus alternis horis	every other hour
ah	alternis horis	every other hour			
altern d	alterno die	every other day	od	omni dei	every day
ap	ant prandium	before dinner	oh	omni hora	every hour
aq	aqua	water	om	omni mane	every morning
aur	auris	the ear	on	omni nocte	every night
aur dextr	auris dextrae	to right ear	paa	parti affectae applicandus	apply to affected part
aur laev	auris laevae	to left ear			
bd	bis die	twice a day	p aeq	partes aequales	equal parts
bds	bis die sumendum	strictly twice a day	pc	post cibum	after food
bid	bis in die	twice in a day	pig	pigmentum	paint
c	cum	with	po	per os	by mouth
cib	cibus	food	ppa	phiala prius agitata	shake bottle before taking
coch	cochleare	spoonful			
collyr	collyrium	eye lotion	pr	per rectum	rectally
d	dies	a day	prn	pro re nata	when necessary
deglut	deglutiatur	let it be swallowed	pulv	pulvis	powder
dieb altern	diebus alternis	every other day	q3h	quaque 3 hora	every 3 hours
dol urg	dolore urgente	when pain is severe	q6h	quaque 6 hora	every 6 hours
dolent part	dolenti parti	to affected part	qd	quater die	four times a day
ex aq	ex aqua	with water	qds	quater die sumendum	strictly four times a day
ex lac	ex lactis	with milk			
gtt	guttae	drops	qid	quater in die	four times in a day
hac noct	hac nocte	tonight	qh	quaque hora	every hour
haust	haustus	draught	qqh	quaque quarta hora	every fourth hour
hd	hora decubitus	at bedtime	qs	quantum sufficiat / satis	sufficient quantity
hn	hac nocte	tonight			
hs	hora somni	at bedtime	rpt	repetatur	repeat
ic	inter cibus	between meals	sig	signa	label
in p aeq	in partes aequales	in equal parts	sos	si optus sit	if necessary
m	mane	morning	stat	statim	immediately
md	more dicto	as directed	syr	syrupus	syrup
mdu	more dicto utendus	use as directed	tdd	ter de die	three times a day
m et v	mane et vespere	morning and evening	tid	ter in die	three times in a day
mist	mistura	mixture	tds	ter die sumendum	strictly three times a day
mitt	mitte	send / dispense	ung	unguentum	ointment
n	nocte	at night	ut dict	ut dictum	as directed

OBSTETRIC DATES CALCULATOR

Day last period started PLUS 7 days = Expected day of confinement
Month last period started PLUS 9 months = Expected month of confinement

PAEDIATRIC DOSAGE GUIDE

FOR CHILDREN OVER 2 YEARS OF AGE:-

$$\text{PAEDIATRIC DOSE} = \frac{\text{Age in years} \times \text{Adult dose}}{\text{Age in years} + 12}$$

FOR CHILDREN UNDER 2 YEARS OF AGE:-

$$\text{PAEDIATRIC DOSE} = \frac{\text{Age in months} \times \text{Adult Dose}}{150}$$

SECTION ONE
SYMPTOMS

SYMPTOMS TO DIAGNOSIS

SYMPTOM: The consciousness of a disturbance in a bodily function.

Butterworths Medical Dictionary

FORMAT

Presenting Symptom (Alternate Name)
Explanation of terminology

SYMPTOM OR OTHER GROUP OF SYMPTOMS

Diagnoses that may present with this symptom [alternate name of diagnosis] (other symptoms of each diagnosis, or a discussion of the diagnosis)

See also Symptom of Similar Significance

Alternate Name

See Presenting Symptom

Please note: many syndromes are characterised by their association with particular organs, diseases, activities or even ethnic groups. These are listed in this section under the particular organ, disease, activity or ethnic groups (eg. cancer-associated syndromes).

Abdominal Colic

Severe, spasmodic, remitting abdominal pain
Gastroenteritis (diarrhoea, vomiting)
Food poisoning
Constipation
Gastric cancer
Peptic ulceration (epigastric, eased by antacids)
Small bowel obstruction (eg. postsurgical, stricture, hernia)
Large bowel obstruction (eg. volvulus, diverticulitis)
Intussusception (child, red currant jelly faeces)
Small or large intestinal neoplasm or tumour
Uterine colic (eg. missed abortion, period pain)

See also Abdominal pain

Abdominal Distension

(Abdominal Bloating)
Giardial intestinal infection
Irritable bowel syn. (pain, irregular bowel habits)
Severe constipation
Nervous swallowing of air
Depression (poor sleep, loss of interest)
Eating disorders (eg. anorexia nervosa)
Ileus (nausea, pain, silent abdomen)
Premenstrual syndrome
Peritonitis (pain, fever)
Intestinal obstruction (pain, borborygmi)
Sigmoid volvulus (colic)
Ascites (shifting dullness)
Denervation syn. (diarrhoea, oesophageal surgery)
Gaseous drinks and fermentable foods (eg. legumes, grains)
Hormone replacement therapy

See also Ascites

Abdominal Noise

See Borborygmi

Abdominal Pain

Common causes of pain in various regions of the abdomen
A   Right Upper Quadrant : Acute cholecystitis, biliary colic, hepatitis, pneumonia
B   Epigastrium : Peptic ulcer, gastritis, pancreatitis, Crohn's disease, heart disease
C   Left Upper Quadrant : Splenomegaly (? cause), irritable bowel syndrome, basal pneumonia.
D   Right Loin : Ureteric colic, pyelonephritis, duodenal ulcer.
E   Periumbilical : Early appendicitis, small bowel obstruction, perforated peptic ulcer, ruptured aortic aneurysm, mesenteric artery occlusion, Crohn's disease, Meckel's diverticulitis.
F   Left Loin : Ureteric colic, diverticulitis, irritable bowel syndrome, pyelonephritis.
G   Right Iliac Fossa : Appendicitis, mesenteric adenitis, ureteric colic, unruptured ectopic pregnancy, ovarian cysts, Meckel's diverticulitis, salpingitis, inguinal and femoral hernia, testicular torsion

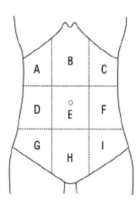

H   Hypogastrium : Large bowel obstruction, ruptured ectopic pregnancy, cystitis, uterine cramps, endometriosis, pelvic inflammatory disease.
I   Left Iliac Fossa : Gastroenteritis, colonic carcinoma, ureteric colic, diverticulitis, unruptured ectopic pregnancy, ovarian cysts, ulcerative colitis, constipation, salpingitis, inguinal or femoral hernia, testicular torsion

CARDIOVASCULAR

Aortic aneurysm (pulsatile mass, shock)
Haemolytic anaemia (jaundice, malaise, pallor)
Sickle cell anaemia (jaundice, fever, negroid)
Thalassaemia major (hepatosplenomegaly, lethargy, jaundice)
Rheumatic fever (arthralgia, chorea, fever)
Mesenteric artery occlusion (nausea, melaena, diarrhoea)
Subacute bacterial endocarditis (fever, malaise, arthralgia)

GASTROINTESTINAL

Gastritis (anorexia, haematemesis, nausea)
Peptic ulcer (us. epigastric, tender, nausea)
Irritable bowel syn. (dyspepsia, varied bowel habits)
Crohn's disease (us. epigastric, tender, nausea)
Small intestine tumours (melaena, anorexia, nausea)
Meckel's diverticulum (melaena, anorexia, nausea)
Gut obstruction (colic, vomiting, constipation)
Ileus (precipitating factor, distension, vomiting)
Appendicitis (us. RIF, anorexia, nausea)
Diverticulitis (us. LIF, diarrhoea and constipation, melaena)
Coeliac disease (anaemia, underweight)
Ulcerative colitis (diarrhoea, fever, weight loss)
Intussusception (child, brief attacks)
Infantile colic (4 to 16 weeks of age)
Constipation (cause should be determined)
Pseudomembranous colitis (diarrhoea)

HEPATOBILIARY-PANCREATIC

Hepatitis (us. RUQ, jaundice, nausea)

Cirrhosis (us. RUQ, fatigue, nausea)
Cholecystitis (us. RUQ, nausea, jaundice)
Biliary colic (intermittent, tender, shock)
Pancreatic carcinoma (symptoms vary with site)
Pancreatitis (nausea, tender, shock)

GENITOURINARY

Testicular torsion (tender testicle, nausea, <40 years)
Endometriosis (dysmenorrhoea, dyspareunia)
Salpingitis (cramps, fever, leucorrhoea)
Ectopic pregnancy (abnormal vaginal bleeding)
Abortion (vaginal bleeding, hypogastric cramps)
Cystitis (dysuria, frequency, hypogastric pain)
Pyelonephritis (loin pain, nausea, headache)
Renal and ureteric colic (nausea, haematuria)
Nephrotic syn. (proteinuria, oedema)
Pelvic inflammatory disease (vaginal discharge, dysuria)

INFECTIONS

Protozoal or metazoal intestinal infections
Tuberculosis (symptoms vary with organs involved)
Mumps pancreatitis (tender and swollen parotid glands)
Viral, bacterial and toxic enteritis
Typhoid fever and other salmonelloses
Brucellosis (fever, fatigue, arthralgia)
Leptospirosis (fever, myalgia, nausea)
Actinomycosis (fever, colic, sinuses in skin)
Infectious mononucleosis (adenitis, fever)
Septicaemia (fever, tachycardia, malaise)
Bilharzia (diarrhoea, urticaria, fever)

SYNDROMES (see SYNDROMES SECTION 6)

Afferent loop syn. (relief by vomiting, steatorrhoea)
Budd-Chiari syn. (hepatomegaly, ascites)
Carcinoid syn. (cramps, flush, neck oedema, facial oedema)
Dumping syn. (epigastric, postprandial)
Fitz-Hugh-Curtis syn. (vaginal discharge, perihepatitis)
Henoch-Schoenlein syn. (purpura, excess bleeds)

OTHER

Muscular strain
Peritonitis (acutely tender, ileus)
Adhesions (colic)
Intestinal spasm (intermittent)
Mesenteric adenitis (nausea, anorexia, fever)
Polyarteritis nodosa (nodules, rash, arthritis)
Depression (insomnia, changed mood)
Addison's disease (fatigue, pigmentation)
Hypoparathyroidism (tetany, wheeze, stridor)
Phaeochromocytoma (headache, hypertension, sweating)
Porphyria (nausea, tachycardia, changed bowel habits)
Pleurisy (rapid, shallow respiration)
Basal pneumonia (cough, short of breath)
Splenomegaly (determine cause)
Inguinal or femoral hernia
Vertebral lesions and nerve root compression
Muscular strains
Nerve entrapment syndromes
Diabetic ketosis and hypoglycaemia
Anaphylaxis

Emotional (daytime only, often child)
Drugs (eg. NSAIDs)

See also Groin Pain; Loin Pain ; Pelvic Pain
SIGNS SECTION 2: Abdominal Rigidity

Abortion, Recurrent

Cervical incompetence
Uterine fibroids
Pelvic inflammatory disease (pelvic pain)
Gonorrhoea (vaginal discharge)
Other pelvic or uterine infections
Corpus luteum deficiency
Immunological factors
Congenital uterine abnormalities
Hereditary congenital fetal abnormalities
Intrauterine adhesions
Retroverted uterus
Diabetes mellitus
Hypothyroidism
Hyperthyroidism
Chronic maternal disease
Antiphospholipid syn.
Autoimmune disease (eg. SLE)
Polycystic ovaries
Coeliac disease
Parental chromosomal translocation
Smoking

Acne

Acne vulgaris (common form)
Papular acne (inflamed papules)
Comedonal acne (less inflammation)
Cystic acne (inflamed nodules, scarring)
Steroid acne (secondary to steroid therapy)
Acne medicamentosa (due to drugs or cosmetics)
Acne mechanica (due to friction from straps, etc.)
Rosacea (telangiectasia, central face papules)
Chloracne (contact with oils and chemicals)
Pseudofolliculitis barbae (ingrown hair)
Acne keloidalis (keloid scar from traumatised acne)
Pituitary tumour

SYNDROMES (see SYNDROMES SECTION 6)

Adrenogenital syn. (amenorrhoea, rough skin)
Cushing's syn. (ecchymoses, obese, hirsute)
Premenstrual tension syn. (mastalgia, headache)

Acromegaly
See Head, Large

Adenitis and Lymphadenopathy
Inflamed and enlarged lymph nodes

INFECTIONS

Localised spread of viral or bacterial infection (superficial infective site, tenderness, erythema, fever)

Septicaemia (fever, malaise, major organ infection)
Tuberculosis [scrofula] (cough, haemoptysis, pustular lymph nodes)
AIDS or primary HIV infection
Actinomycosis (discharging sinuses, painless)
Cytomegalovirus (fever, arthralgia, hepatomegaly)
Filariasis (fever, oedema, orchitis)
Toxoplasmosis (varied symptoms)
Trypanosomiasis (apathy, neurological signs)
Measles (rash, cough, coryza)
Cat scratch disease (primary lesion, suppuration)
Infectious mononucleosis (fever, malaise, splenomegaly)
Brucellosis (fever, confusion, fatigue)
Tularaemia (papule inoculation, fever, nausea)
Plague (fever, headache, muscle aches)
Syphilis (rash, varied tertiary symptoms)
Mesenteric lymphadenitis (abdominal pain, fever, nausea)
Lymphogranuloma venereum (inguinal nodes)
Gonorrhoea (urethral discharge, dysuria)

SYNDROMES (see SYNDROMES SECTION 6)

AIDS (splenomegaly, fever, cachexia, skin lesions)
Chronic fatigue syn. (weakness, fever)
Felty's syn. (splenomegaly, migratory arthritis)
Heerfordt's syn. (uveitis, sarcoidosis)
Idiopathic lymphadenopathy syn. (homosexual)
Kawasaki syn. (rash, fever)
Letterer-Siwe syn. (fever, rash, infant)
Mikulicz syn. (parotitis)
Sicca syn. (dry mouth, dry eyes)
Uveoparotid syn. (uveitis, facial paralysis)

OTHER

Eczema
Haemolytic anaemia
Rheumatoid arthritis (joint pain)
SLE
Leukaemia, chronic (pallor, malaise)
Hand-Schuller-Christian disease (eczema, infections)
Sarcoidosis (splenomegaly, skin lesions)
Hodgkin's disease (fever, fatigue, pruritus)
Thyrotoxicosis (sweating, heat intolerance)
Immunisation
Serum sickness
Lymphomas
Metastatic carcinoma
Lyme disease (myalgia, rash)
Branchial cyst and other developmental remnants may be confused with glands
Drugs (eg. phenytoin)

See also SIGNS SECTION 2: Splenomegaly
See also INVESTIGATION SECTION 3: Adenitis

Adrenal Abnormalities

Schmidt's syn. (hypothyroidism, adrenal insufficiency)
Waterhouse-Friderichsen syn. (prostration, petechiae, purpura)

Agnosia

Sensory suppression

Parietal lobe lesions (astereognosis, personality changes)

Gerstmann syn. (agraphia, unable to calculate)

Agraphia

Inability to write

Cerebrovascular accident (hemiparesis, neurological signs)
Cerebral disease (eg.Gerstmann's syndrome) (R to L disorientation, agnosia, constructional disorders)
Psychiatric disturbances
Tremors or muscular weakness from any cause
Dyslexia
Visual problems

Albinism

See Skin, Depigmented

Alcoholism

Amnestic syn. (amnesia, thiamine deficit)
Organic brain syn. (multiple psychiatric changes)
Episodic dyscontrol syn. (abusive, sex crimes)
Pseudo-Cushing's syn. (hypercorticalism)
Wernicke-Korsakoff syn. (ataxia, mental deterioration)

Aldosteronism

Conn's syn. (weak, hypertensive)

Alopecia

Loss of hair

Male pattern baldness (genetic)
Idiopathic (thinning of hair, either sex)
Areata (patchy)
Telogen effluvium (diffuse, after stress)
Iron or zinc deficiency
Hypopituitarism
Postmenopause
Rapid weight loss
Protein deficiency (eg. malnutrition, vegetarian)
Postpartum (diffuse loss)
SLE (butterfly rash, arthritis, nephritis)
Addison's disease (groin and axilla only)
Myxoedema (fatigue, dry skin, cold intolerance)
Hypervitaminosis A (anorexia, weight loss, rashes)
Trichotillomania (recurrent trauma)
Syphilis (variable symptoms)
Diabetes mellitus (polydipsia, polyuria)
Renal failure
Thyrotoxicosis (sweating, heat intolerance)
Shock or stress (eg. bereavement, surgery)
Testosterone secreting tumour
Dubowitz syn. (reduced growth, ptosis)
Fröhlich's syn. (thin skin, low libido, obese)
Hallermann-Streiff syn. (dwarf, cataracts)
Langer-Giedion syn. (bullous nose, exostoses)
Loose Anagen syn. (see SYNDROMES SECTION 6)
Drugs (eg. cancer therapy, anticoagulants, vitamin A, lithium, beta-blockers, oral contraceptives)

Amaurosis Fugax

Intermittent fleeting blindness
Vascular insufficiency of retina or optic nerve
Carotid artery disease (bruit, other cerebral signs)
Migraine (headache not necessarily present)
Epilepsy (seizures not necessarily obvious)
Other seizures
Hypotension (faint, lightheaded)
Giant cell arteritis (temple pain, high ESR)

See also Blindness, Partial or Total

Amenorrhoea and Oligomenorrhoea

Cessation of menstrual periods, failure of menarche, infrequent menstruation

PRIMARY

Hypothalamic disease (debility, neurological signs)
Pituitary tumours (growth anomalies)
Ovarian disease
Genital malformations
Androgenic tumours (virilism)

SECONDARY

Menopause
Pregnancy
Lactation
Emotional, psychiatric and constitutional causes
Ovarian tumours
Cushing's disease (central obesity, hirsute, striae)
Addison's disease (pigmentation, fatigue, nausea)
Pituitary tumour
Myxoedema (fatigue, cold intolerance, dry skin)
Hyperprolactinaemia (galactorrhoea)
Hyperthyroidism (sweating, nervous, heat intolerance)
Weight loss to below 75% of ideal
Strenuous exercise
Drugs and hormone therapy (eg. oral contraceptives)

SYNDROMES (see SYNDROMES SECTION 6)

Adrenogenital syn. (acne, rough skin, hirsute)
Asherman's syn. (infertile, post curette)
Chiari-Frommel syn. (post lactation)
Cushing's syn. (moon face, striae, hirsute)
Sheehan's syn. (postpartum haemorrhage, no lactation)
Stein-Leventhal syn. (polycystic ovaries, obesity, hirsute)
Turner's syn. (genital and breast hypoplasia)

See also INVESTIGATION SECTION 3: Amenorrhoea, Secondary

Amnesia

Total or partial loss of memory
Epilepsy (convulsions, faint, paroxysmal)
Cerebrovascular accident (headaches, confusion, weak)
Cerebral haemorrhage
Transient global amnesia
Hysteria
Cerebral trauma
Menopause (flushes, sweating, menstrual changes)
Post-traumatic stress syn. (nightmares, depression)
Hypothermia (shiver, confusion, arrhythmias)

Cerebral tumours (headache, nausea, neurological signs)
Viral encephalitis
Meningitis (cerebral irritation)
Hydrocephalus (papilloedema)
Wernicke's encephalopathy
Alzheimer's disease (irrational)
Anoxia and hypoxia
Psychiatric disorders (eg. fugue states)
Hypoglycaemia (see PATHOLOGY SECTION 4)
Hyponatraemia (see PATHOLOGY SECTION 4)
Alcohol and other drugs

See also Memory Disturbance

Anaemia

See Pallor
See also PATHOLOGY SECTION 4: Haemoglobin, Blood

Anaesthesia

Loss of pain sensation
Cerebrovascular accident (weak, headache, confusion)
Transient ischaemic attack (brief, confusion, drop attack)
Diabetes mellitus (peripheral, pruritus, polyuria)
Embolism (pain, weak, cold)
Syringomyelia (other senses intact, weak)
Vertebral disc herniation (back pain)
Posterolateral sclerosis (paraesthesiae, weak)
Polyneuritis (weak, tenderness, wasting)
Leprosy (macular rash, peripheral)
Brown-Sequard syn. (hemisection of cord)
Refsum's syn. (distal sensorimotor polyneuropathy)
Psychiatric disorders (glove and stocking distribution)
Drugs and poisons

Anal Atresia

Johanson-Blizzard syn. (nasal anomalies, deaf)

Anal Itch

See Pruritus Ani and Proctitis

Anal Pain

Haemorrhoids (bleeding, pruritus, discharge)
Fissure-in-ano (bleeding, constipation)
Perianal abscess (tender lump)
Fistula-in-ano (discharge, pruritus)
Pruritus ani (itch, rash)
Crohn's disease (fissure, abdominal pain, diarrhoea)
Proctalgia fugax (fleeting, severe)
Zoonotic intestinal infections
Lymphogranuloma venereum (ulcer, adenitis)

Angina

See Abdominal Pain ; Chest Pain ; Throat Pain

Anhidrosis

See Sweating, Lack of

Anorexia
Loss of appetite

INFECTIONS
Hepatitis (nausea, jaundice)
Subacute bacterial endocarditis (fever, malaise, arthralgia)
Tuberculosis (productive cough, weight loss, fatigue)
Brucellosis (fever, fatigue, arthralgia)
Many other bacterial and viral infections

GASTROINTESTINAL
Oral/dental disease
Gastritis (pain, nausea, haematemesis)
Appendicitis (RIF pain, nausea, fever)
Stomach carcinoma (fullness, nausea, heartburn)
Crohn's disease (diarrhoea, flatus, pain)
Cirrhosis (fatigue, nausea, RUQ pain)
Intestinal ischaemia
Pancreatitis (pain, nausea)
Zollinger-Ellison syn. (recurrent peptic ulcers)
Hepatic metastases
Small bowel obstruction (colic)
Other gastrointestinal disorders

OTHER
Rheumatic fever (chorea, arthralgia, fever, rash)
Depression (insomnia, loss of interest)
Anorexia nervosa (young woman)
Dementia
Cardiovascular disease (eg. congestive cardiac failure)
Malignancy of any type
Hypopituitarism
Uraemia (fatigue, thirst, headache)
Pernicious anaemia (dyspepsia, sore tongue)
Leukaemia (malaise, arthralgia, fever)
Beriberi (oedema, leg cramps, paraesthesiae)
Hypervitaminosis A (hair loss, rash)
SLE (rash, malaise, arthritis)
Glomerulonephritis (oliguria, headache, oedema)
Addisonian crisis (fatigue, nausea, diarrhoea)
Diabetic acidosis (polyuria, nausea, fatigue)
Hyperparathyroidism (polyuria, polydipsia, bone pain)
Chronic pain
Social isolation
Fadism
Alcoholism
Smoking
Drugs (eg. digitalis, diuretics, amphetamines, narcotics)

See also Weight Loss; Failure to Thrive

Anorgasmia
See Orgasm, Lack of

Anosmia
Loss of the sense of smell
Nasal infections (discharge, fever, headache)
Myxoedema (fatigue, dry skin, cold intolerance)
Frontal lobe tumour (amnesia, fits, aphasia)
Brain abscess (preceding infection, neurological changes)
Fracture of skull involving olfactory plate
Kellmann's syn. (hypogonadism)
Drugs (eg. phenol, chromium)

Anuria
See Oliguria and Anuria

Anxiety
Neuroses (phobias, hyperventilation, headaches)
Depression (insomnia, phobias)
Alcoholism (dependence, delirium tremens)
Reaction to stress or environment
Postpartum depression
Menopause (flush, amenorrhoea, sweating)
Cardiac disease
Chronic renal disease
Phaeochromocytoma (hypertension)
Pulmonary oedema
Pulmonary embolism

See also Psychiatric Disturbance Associated Syndromes

Aphasia and Dysarthria
Loss of the power of speech, or difficulty in speaking
Cerebrovascular accident (confusion, neurological changes)
Transient ischaemic attack (brief, confusion, drop attack)
Cerebral tumour (headaches, nausea, amnesia)
Multiple sclerosis (diverse neurological anomalies)
Sydenham's chorea (involuntary jerks, weak)
Myasthenia gravis (weak, diplopia, ptosis)
Myxoedema (fatigue, cold intolerance, dry skin)
Phaeochromocytoma (hypertension, sweating, headache)
Motor neurone disease (weak, myalgia)
Moebius's syn. (ptosis, fixed facies)
Shy-Drager syn. (tremor, vertigo)
Guillain-Barré syn. (weak, dysphagia)
Alcohol and other drugs

Appetite, Excess
See Hunger, Excess

Appetite Loss
See Anorexia

Arm Pain
Angina pectoris (chest pain, worse with exercise)
Myocardial infarct (chest pain, shock)
Claudication (intermittent, alopecia, wasting)
Embolism (numbness, cold, weakness)
Causalgia (trauma history, skin changes)
Sickle cell anaemia (fever, abdominal pain, jaundice)
Multiple myeloma (bone pain, malaise, anaemia)

Osteoarthritis, rheumatoid arthritis or fibrositis
Tenosynovitis or bursitis (eg. tennis elbow)
Fibromyositis (fatigue, stiffness)
Polymyalgia rheumatica (pain, stiffness)
Repetitive strain injury (controversial)
Other musculoskeletal disorders
Multiple myeloma (fever, bone pain)
Spinal dysfunction
Pancoast's tumour
Bone neoplasm
Osteomyelitis
Septic arthritis (hot, red joint)
Polyneuritis (weakness, anaesthesia, wasting)
Gas gangrene (wound, oedema, tachycardia)
Trauma

SYNDROMES (see SYNDROMES SECTION 6)

Cervical rib syn. (hand weak, paraesthesiae)
Eosinophilia-myalgia syn. (cough, arthralgia)
Fibrositis syn. (tender, stiff muscles)
Guyton's canal syn. (ulnar nerve lesion)
Occupational overuse syn. (burning pain)
Carpal tunnel syn. (tingling radiating from wrist)
Thoracic outlet syn. (see SYNDROMES SECTION 6)
Painful arc syn. (shoulder movement pain)
Pancoast's syn. (Horner's syn., lung cancer)
Pronator syn. (median nerve lesion)
Rotator cuff syn. (shoulder pain)
Scapulocostal syn. (neck and scapular pain)
Seckel syn. (elbow and hip dislocation)
Subclavian steal syn. (cerebral symptoms)

See also Arthritis and Arthralgia; Hand Pain; Shoulder Pain; Wrist Pain

Arthritis and Arthralgia
Joint inflammation and pain

INFECTIONS

Septic arthritis (fever, swelling, erythema)
Osteomyelitis (fever, tenderness, swelling)
Tuberculosis (tenderness, swelling)
Syphilis (swelling, other system disease)
Cytomegalovirus (adenitis, fever, hepatomegaly)
Brucellosis (fever, fatigue, headache)
Mumps (large parotids, fever)
Viraemias (fever, malaise)
Rubella (rash, adenitis)
Hepatitis B (fever, anorexia, rash)
Postdysenteric (migratory, chronic)
Melioidosis (cough, chest pain)
Gonorrhoea (penile or vaginal discharge, skin lesions)
Subacute bacterial endocarditis (anorexia, fever, malaise)
Epidemic polyarthralgia (rash, muscle ache)
Lyme disease (fever, myalgia, rash)

BONE AND JOINT DISEASE

Rheumatoid arthritis (nodules, malaise)
Ankylosing spondylitis (back pain, uveitis)
Osteoarthritis (stiffness, no systemic disease)
Chondrocalcinosis (swelling)

Osgood-Schlatter's disease (tender tibial tuberosity)
Henoch-Schoenlein purpura (rash, child)
Acromegaly (joint enlargement, visual loss, headaches)
Osteogenesis imperfecta (blue sclera)
Synovial chondromatosis
Pigmented villonodular synovitis
Haemarthrosis (trauma)
Tumours
Trauma

SYNDROMES (see SYNDROMES SECTION 6)

AIDS (fever, adenitis, rash)
Behcet's syn. (uveitis, mouth and genital ulcers)
Chronic fatigue syn. (weakness, fever)
Felty's syn. (fever, migratory arthritis, splenomegaly)
Fibrositis syn. (stiff, muscle pain)
Hunter's syn. (gross facies, cardiac anomalies)
Hurler's syn. (dwarf, retarded, gross facies)
Jaccoud's syn. (rheumatoid-like changes)
Lesch-Nyhan syn. (retarded, gout, mutilation)
Marfan's syn. (hypermobile joints, kyphoscoliosis)
Post-polio syn. (fatigue, myalgia, weakness)
Reiter's syn. (urethritis, conjunctivitis)
Shoulder-Hand syn. (scapulo-humeral periarthritis)
Sjögren's syn. (dry eyes and mucous membranes)
Sweet's syn. (skin plaques, fever)

OTHER

Gout (often hallux, severe pain, erythema & swelling)
Bursitis (tender, fluctuant swelling)
Frozen shoulder (limited movement, tender)
Psoriasis (rash, nail changes)
Pseudogout (red, swollen)
Neurogenic (eg. diabetes, tabes dorsalis, cord injury)
Malignancy (any type)
Rheumatic fever (migratory arthritis, nodules, rash)
Leukaemia (fever, malaise, anorexia)
SLE (rash, anorexia, malaise)
Scleroderma (Raynaud's phenomenon, gut symptoms)
Dermatomyositis (proximal weakness, rash)
Ulcerative colitis (mouth ulcers, diarrhoea)
Hypothyroidism (dry skin, mental changes)
Sarcoidosis (fever, erythema nodosum)
Hypoparathyroidism (tetany, stridor)
Polyarteritis nodosa (fever, tachycardia, skin disorder)
Serum sickness (headache, fever, rash)
Amyloidosis
Haemochromatosis (skin pigmentation)
Whipple's disease (symmetrical large joints, small bowel disease)
Hyperparathyroidism (polyuria, polydipsia, nausea)

See also Arm Pain; Hand Pain; Joint, Swollen; Knee Pain; Leg Pain; Polyarthritis; Shoulder Pain; Erythema, Joint

Ascites
Excess peritoneal fluid
Cirrhosis (jaundice, nausea, RUQ pain)
Hepatoma (cachexia, anorexia, asthenia)
Lymphoma (hepatomegaly, cachexia)
Other gastrointestinal malignancies
Bilharzia (diarrhoea, urticaria, fever)

Congestive cardiac failure (dyspnoea, oedema, cough)
Chronic renal failure (nausea, pruritus, lethargy)
Hepatitis (jaundice, hepatomegaly, malaise)
Pericarditis (chest pain, friction rub)
Pancreatitis (abdominal pain, diarrhoea)
Protein losing enteropathy
Malnutrition (cachexia)
Hepatic vein obstruction (hepatomegaly)
Hypothyroidism (fatigue, cold intolerance, dry skin)
Tuberculosis
Trypanosomiasis (myocarditis, anaemia)

SYNDROMES (see SYNDROMES SECTION 6)

Budd-Chiari syn. (abdominal pain, hepatomegaly)
Meig's syn. (ovarian fibroma, hydrothorax)
Nephrotic syn. (oedema, proteinuria, anorexia, striae, hypertension)
Asthenia

See also Fatigue, Abnormal
See also INVESTIGATIONS SECTION 3: Ascites

Asthenia

See Fatigue, Abnormal

Ataxia

See SIGNS SECTION 2: Ataxia

Athetosis

Involuntary, slow, writhing movements
Infantile cerebral palsy
Hemiplegia from any cause
Cerebrovascular accident (aphasia, headache, confusion)
Wilson's disease (copper poisoning)
Lesch-Nyhan syn. (see SYNDROMES SECTION 6)
Juvenile Huntington's chorea
Dystonic juvenile movement disorders
Louis-Bar syn. (telangiectasia of face and flexures)

Aura

A premonition or sensation preceding a paroxysmal disorder
Epilepsy (twitching, loss of consciousness)
Anaphylaxis (oedema, itch, rash)
Migraine (headache, visual disturbances)
Transient ischaemic attack (various CNS symptoms)

Baby, Floppy

See Floppy Baby

Back and Vertebral Pain

MUSCULOSKELETAL

Disc lesions (radiating pain)
Scoliosis
Sciatica (leg pain)
Osteomalacia
Paget's disease (headaches, skull enlargement)
Osteomyelitis (malaise, tenderness, fever)
Spondylolisthesis
Fibrositis or myositis
Vertebral fractures
Spinal stenosis (paraesthesia worse with walking, relieved by rest)
Gout (rubor, calor, oedema)
Rheumatoid arthritis (extension from small joints)
Tuberculosis (miliary form)
Scheuermann's disease
Ankylosing spondylitis (limited movement, uveitis)
Osteoarthritis (radiating pain, eg. sciatica)
Trauma or strain to muscles or ligaments
Discitis (often child, mild symptoms)
Hip disorders (eg. osteoarthritis, avascular necrosis)
Osteoporosis (pathological fractures)
Metastatic carcinoma (eg. prostate, breast)
Iliolumbar syn. (iliac crest pain)
Piriformis syn. (sciatica)
Posterior facet syn. (leg pain)
Scapulocostal syn. (neck and arm pain)

GENITOURINARY

Salpingitis (hypogastric tenderness, leucorrhoea, dyspareunia)
Endometriosis (cyclical, abnormal vaginal bleeding)
Torted ovarian cyst (abdominal tenderness)
Pregnancy (amenorrhoea, breast fullness)
Dysmenorrhoea (cyclical)
Uterine prolapse
Other gynaecological infections and tumours
Pyelonephritis (nausea, headache, fever)
Prostatitis (dysuria, frequency, discharge)
Renal and ureteric colic (nausea, haematuria)

OTHER

Peptic ulceration (epigastric tenderness, nausea)
Pancreatitis (epigastric pain, nausea, shock)
Menopause (flushing, amenorrhoea)
Multiple myeloma (malaise, anaemia, weight loss)
Cushing's syn. (central obesity, hirsute, plethora, ecchymoses)
Acromegaly (coarse facies, psychiatric changes)
Aortic aneurysm (check distal pulses)
Vascular insufficiency
Guillain-Barré syn. (weak, dysphagia)
Ulcerative colitis (changed bowel habits)
Crohn's disease (diarrhoea, abdominal mass)
Psychogenic causes (widespread pain, inappropriate responses to examination)
Bacterial and viral infections (eg. meningitis, influenza, brucellosis)
Hyperparathyroidism (polyuria, polydipsia, nausea)
Steele-Richardson-Olszewski syn. (axial rigidity, dementia)
Syphilis (varied symptoms)
Postural

See also Scoliosis; Arthritis and Arthralgia

Bad Breath

See Halitosis

Balance, Disturbed

Vestibulitis (inner ear dysfunction)
Blocked eustachian tube (nasal congestion)
Hypotension (faints)
Parkinson's disease (abnormal gait, tremor)
Cerebrovascular accident (paralysis, dysarthria)
Cerebellar disease
Frontal lobe tumour (personality changes)
Dementia (inappropriate responses)
Hypothyroidism (constipated, weak)
Drugs (eg. sedatives, tranquillizers)

See also Vertigo

Baldness

See Alopecia

Ballism

See Chorea

Behavioural Problems

*See Mental Retardation; Overactive; Psychiatric
Disturbance Associated Syndromes; Swearing,
Uncontrolled; Violence*

Black Spots in Visual Field

See Vision, Black Spots in Field of

Black Spots on Skin

See Pigmentation of Skin, Excess

Blackout

See Syncope

Bleeding

*See Bleeding, Excessive; Bruising, Excess; Epistaxis;
Haematemesis; Haematuria and Red Urine;
Haemoptysis; Melaena and Rectal Bleeding; Purpura
and Petechiae; Vaginal and Uterine Bleeding, Abnormal*

Bleeding, Excessive

Thrombocytopenia (bruising, purpura)
Aplastic anaemia (lassitude, pallor, purpura)
Haemophilia and other blood factor deficiencies
Disseminated intravascular coagulation
Hypovitaminosis K
Scurvy (inflamed and bleeding gums)
Drugs (eg. warfarin, heparin, aspirin)

*See also Bruising, Excess; Epistaxis; Haematemesis;
Haematuria and Red Urine; Haemoptysis; Melaena and
Rectal Bleeding; Purpura and Petechiae*

Blindness, Partial or Total

Vision loss

Welding flash burn (pain, red)
Conjunctival ulcer or trauma
Migraine (headache, photophobia, nausea)
Cataract (gradual, opaque lens) (see separate entry)
Glaucoma (rapid, pain)
Diabetes mellitus (polyuria, polydipsia)
Cerebrovascular accident (confusion, paralysis)
Transient ischaemic attack (brief, variable)
Temporal arteritis (headache, jaw claudication, malaise)
Retinal detachment (sudden, unilateral)
Optic neuritis (eg. in multiple sclerosis)
Senile macular degeneration (gradual, elderly)
Head trauma (eg. optic canal haematoma)
Malignant hypertension (sudden, unilateral)
Acute chorioretinitis
Optic nerve compression
Keratitis (pain, red eye)
Uveitis (pain, photophobia)
Thyrotoxicosis (gradual onset, painless)
Vitreous haemorrhage (sudden, flashes)
Retinal vascular disease (eg. thrombosis)
Cerebral abscess (preceding infection, headache)
Cerebral tumour (neurological signs, headache)
Acute glomerulonephritis
Carotid artery disease (transient, bruit)
Anaphylaxis
Poisoning (eg. methanol, quinine) (sudden, bilateral)

SYNDROMES (see SYNDROMES SECTION 6)

Behcet's syn. (arthritis, mouth ulcers)
Down's syn. (typical facies, mental retardation)
Hurler's syn. (corneal clouding, dwarf, arthralgia)
Lissencephaly syn. (seizures, corneal opacity)
Lowe's syn. (retarded, cataracts, epicanthal folds)
Marfan's syn. (lens dislocation, kyphoscoliosis)
Nelson's syn. (postadrenalectomy, field defects)
Pseudoexfoliation syn. (glaucoma)
Stargardt's syn. (adolescent, inherited)
Vogt-Koyanagi-Harada syn. (uveitis, vertigo)
Von Hippel-Lindau syn. (retinal hamartoma)

*See also Hemianopia; Vision, Blurred; Amaurosis Fugax
See also symptoms listed under Eye*

Blisters

See Rash, Bullous

Bloating, Abdominal

See Abdominal Distension

Blood

See Bleeding, Excessive; Bruising, Excess; Pallor

Blue Skin

See Cyanosis, Central; Cyanosis, Peripheral

Blurred Vision
See Vision, Blurred

Bone
See Arm Pain; Arthritis and Arthralgia; Back and Vertebral Pain; Fractures, Pathological; Leg Pain; Scoliosis

Bone Mass or Tumour
Osteoma (small, painful)
Sarcoma (pain, swelling, hot)
Other bone neoplasms
Chrondromas
Metastatic carcinoma (eg. breast, prostate)
Osteitis fibrosa (painless, sexual precocity)
Bone cysts
Subperiosteal haematoma (trauma history)
Healed or recent fracture

Bone Pain
See Arthritis and Arthralgia; Arm Pain; Leg Pain

Borborygmi
Excessively noisy bowel peristalsis
Gut obstruction (pain, constipation, vomiting)
Gastroenteritis (diarrhoea, nausea, pain)
Excess swallowed air (rapid eating, nervous swallowing)
Aerated drinks

Bowel
See symptoms listed under Intestine

Bradycardia
See SIGNS SECTION 2: Bradycardia

Bradykinesia
Abnormally slow movement
Parkinson's disease (tremor, rigidity, disturbed balance)
Cerebrovascular accident (mental changes, paralysis)
Cerebellar disease (disturbed balance)
Hypothyroidism (constipation, dry skin, bradycardia)
Arthritis (joint pain)
Frontal lobe tumour (personality changes, disturbed balance)
Depression (early waking, loss of interest)
Dementia (mental changes)
Drugs (eg. sedatives, tranquillizers)

Brain
See Memory Disturbance; Mental Retardation; Neurological Symptoms; Psychiatric Disturbance Associated Syndromes; Syncope

Breast, Abnormal
See Breast, Atrophic or Atresic; Breast Lump; Breast Pain; Gynaecomastia; Lactation, Failure of; Discharge, Nipple, and Galactorrhoea

Breast, Atrophic or Atresic
Adrenogenital syn. (acne, hirsute, amenorrhoea)
Menopausal syn. (menstrual changes, flushes)
Turner's syn. (genital hypoplasia, amenorrhoea)

Breast Enlargement
See Gynaecomastia

Breast Lump
Breast carcinoma (pain, erythema, firm, fixed)
Hormonal dysplasia (fluctuating, cyclical pain)
Fibroadenoma (asymptomatic)
Mastitis (hot, tender, erythema)
Blocked milk duct during lactation
Cysts
Fat necrosis or fibrosis after trauma

See also Gynaecomastia

Breast Pain
Breast carcinoma (lump, erythema, firm, fixed)
Hormonal dysplasia (fluctuating, cyclical, lump)
Mastitis (erythema, fever, tender, hot)
Abscess (tender mass, erythema, often lactating)
Dysmenorrhoea (pelvic fullness and pain)
Pregnancy (breast fullness, amenorrhoea)
Trauma
Menopausal syn. (flushes, menstrual changes)
Premenstrual tension syn. (headache, irritable)

Breath, Bad
See Halitosis

Breathing, Abnormal
See Cough; Cyanosis, Central; Cyanosis, Peripheral; Dyspnoea; Haemoptysis; Orthopnoea; Wheeze

Breathing, Difficult
See Dyspnoea; Orthopnoea; Stridor; Wheeze

Bronchospasm
See Wheeze

Bruising, Excess

Thrombocytopenia (bleeding time increased)
Idiopathic purpura
Hereditary disorders of coagulation (eg.haemophilia, von Willebrand's, Christmas disease)
Bone marrow suppression
Ionising radiation (eg. X-rays, gamma rays)
Systemic viral infections
Leukaemia (abnormal white cell count)
Typhus (fever, malaise)
Subacute bacterial endocarditis
Insect and snake bites
Following massive blood transfusions
Renal failure
Hepatic failure
Polycythaemia vera
Scurvy (inflamed and bleeding gums)
Cushing's syn. (moon face, obese, amenorrhoea)
AIDS (splenomegaly, fever, cachexia)
Defibrination syn. (see SYNDROMES SECTION 6)
Painful bruising syn. (female, paraesthesiae)
Drugs (eg. steroids, arsenic, quinine, aspirin, warfarin, chlorothiazide)

See also Bleeding, Excessive; Ecchymosis

Bruxism

Excessive grinding of teeth
Habit
Sleep disorder or nightmares
Myofascial syn. (face pain, trismus)
Psychiatric disturbances
Subnormal mentality

Buccal

See symptoms listed under Mouth

Bulimia

See Hunger, Excess

Bullae

See Rash, Bullous

Burping, Excessive

Passage of gas by mouth
Rapid eating or passage of gaseous foods
Nervous air swallowing
Reflux oesophagitis (waterbrash, heartburn)
Hiatus hernia (epigastric discomfort, waterbrash)
Peptic ulcer (epigastric pain and tenderness)

Cachexia

See Weight Loss; Malabsorption
See also SIGNS SECTION 2: Cachexia

Cancer Associated Syndromes

AIDS (splenomegaly, adenitis, skin lesions)
Bloom syn. (Jewish, photosensitive, small at birth)
Dysplastic naevus syn. (multiple moles)
Pancoast syn. (shoulder, arm and chest pain, Horner syn.)
Tumour lysis syn. (ileus, cardiac arrhythmias, renal failure)
Turcot syn. (brain tumours, polyposis coli)
Werner syn. (multiple endocrine neoplasia)

See also SYNDROMES SECTION 6

Cardiac Associated Syndromes

Barlow syn. (mitral valve prolapse)
Carcinoid syn. (flush, abdominal cramps, diarrhoea)
Carney complex (atrial myxoma, mucosal pigmentation)
Conradi-Hunermann syn. (ventricular septal defect, patent ductus arteriosus)
Down's syn. (typical facies, mental retardation)
Dressler's syn. (post infarct, pericarditis)
Edwards' syn. (micrognathia, rocker-bottom feet)
Eisenmenger's syn. (patent ductus arteriosus, pulmonary hypertension)
Ellis-van Crevald syn. (atrial and ventricular septal defects)
Fallot's trilogy, tetralogy and pentalogy
Hunter syn. (gross facies, hepatomegaly, arthritis)
Hurler syn. (dwarf, arthralgia, gross facies)
Hypoplastic left heart syn. (neonate, cyanosis)
Jaccoud syn. (rheumatic heart disease)
Kartagener syn. (dextrocardia, sinusitis)
Leopard syn. (multiple spots, abnormal ECG)
Lown-Ganong-Levine syn. (atrial arrhythmia)
Marfan syn. (aortic & mitral valve lesions)
Maroteaux-Lamy syn. (bone dysplasia, cataracts)
Morquio syn. (bone dysplasia, cataracts)
Noonan syn. (short, webbed neck, pulmonary stenosis)
Patau syn. (polydactyly, cleft lip)
Patent ductus arteriosus (machinery murmur)
Pickwickian syn. (cardiac failure, obese, cyanosis)
Pompe syn. (abnormal ECG, hypotonia)
Rubenstein-Taybi syn. (patent ductus arteriosus, hypoplastic maxilla)
Sick sinus syn. (variable heart rate, syncope)
Toxic shock syn. (cardiac failure, diarrhoea)
Turner syn. (amenorrhoea, genital hypoplasia)
Waterhouse-Friderichsen syn. (prostration, petechiae)
Wolff-Parkinson-White syn. (paroxysmal arrhythmia)

Cat Cry

Cri-du-chat syn. (mental retardation, ocular hypertelorism)

Cataract

Senile cataract due to age
Genetic and chromosomal causes (eg. Down's syn., Patau's syn., X-linked recessive disorders)

Alport's disease (nepropathy, deaf)
Rubella *in utero*
Diabetes mellitus (polyuria, polydipsia)
Hypocalcaemia (tetany)
Infantile hypoxia
Starvation and malnutrition
Radiation (ultraviolet, x-ray, infrared)
Uveitis (inflammation)
Retrolental fibroplasia

SYNDROMES (see SYNDROMES SECTION 6)

Conrad syn. (deaf, limb contractures)
Hallerman-Streiff syn. (face anomalies, dwarf)
Lowe's syn. (retarded, epicanthal folds)
Maroteaux-Lamy syn. (bone dysplasia, cardiac lesions)
Morquio syn. (bone dysplasia, deaf)
Schiei syn. (recurrent respiratory infections, kyphosis)
Sly syn. (recurrent respiratory infections, kyphosis)

OTHER

Drugs (eg. glucocorticoids, phenothiazines, heavy metals)

See also Blindness, Partial or Total
See also SIGNS SECTION 2: Lens Opacity

Catarrh

See Rhinitis and Rhinorrhoea

Chest

See Chest Pain; Cough; Dyspepsia; Dysphagia;
Dyspnoea; Wheeze

Chest Pain

Common causes of pain in various regions of the chest

A   Myocardial ischaemia, angina, thyroiditis, tracheitis.
B   Myocardial ischaemia, angina, Pancoast syn.
C   Myocardial ischaemia, pneumothorax, Tietze's syn., Pancoast syn.
D   Myocardial ischaemia, angina, pulmonary embolus, pericarditis, reflux oesophagitis, oesophageal foreign body, pneumo mediastinum.
E   Myocardial ischaemia, angina, pneumothorax, Tietze syn., Pancoast syn.
F   Cholecystitis, pneumonia, pleurisy, vertebral neuralgia, pancreatitis, Tietze syn., slipping rib syn.
G   Myocardial ischaemia, dissecting aneurysm, reflux oesophagitis, hiatus hernia, oesophageal carcinoma, oesophageal foreign body, pulmonary embolus, pericarditis.
H   Splenic injury or inflammation, pneumonia, pleurisy, pericarditis, vertebral.

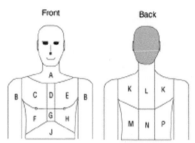

Front   Back

J   Myocardial ischaemia, dissecting aneurysm, xiphoid syn., peptic ulcer, pancreatitis.
See Abdominal Pain.

K   Vertebral neuralgia, muscular strain.
L   Myocardial ischaemia, thoracic spinal dysfunction, whiplash injury.
M   Thoracic spinal dysfunction, peptic ulcer, pyelonephritis, splenic inflammation.
N   Dissecting aneurysm, pericarditis, Scheuermann's disease, ankylosing spondylitis, peptic ulcer.
P   Thoracic spinal dysfunction, pyelonephritis, peptic ulcer, cholecystitis, pancreatitis.

CARDIAC

Pericarditis (worse supine, friction rub)
Myocardial infarct (shock, arrhythmias, pressure-like ache)
Angina pectoris (radiates, sudden, exertion related)
Pericardial effusion (dyspnoea, dysphagia)
Aortic aneurysm (symptoms vary with site)
Congenital heart disease (dyspnoea, fatigue, cyanosis)
Myocarditis (dyspnoea, vertigo, asthenia)
Anaemia (pallor, fatigue, dyspnoea)
Mitral valve prolapse (midsystolic click, late systolic murmur)

PULMONARY

Pleurisy (inspiratory pain and friction rub)
Pneumonia (cough, fever, foul sputum)
Bronchiectasis (dyspnoea, haemoptysis, recurrent infection)
Pulmonary thromboembolism (cough, dyspnoea, haemoptysis)
Pneumothorax (sudden dyspnoea)
Pneumo mediastinum (sudden substernal pain)
Tracheitis (cough, fever)
Hyperventilation (tetany)
Other pulmonary diseases and infections

GASTROINTESTINAL

Oesophagitis (burning pain, dysphagia, waterbrash)
Indigestion (burping, food excess)
Oesophageal carcinoma (dysphagia, weight loss)
Oesophageal foreign body
Hiatus hernia (heartburn, worse recumbent)
Cardiospasm (dysphagia, bloating)
Peptic ulcer (nausea, epigastric tenderness)
Cholecystitis (RUQ tender, nausea, jaundice)

Pancreatitis (sudden, nausea, shock, abdomen tender)
Dysphagia (see separate entry)

MUSCULOSKELETAL

Trauma, superficial infections and viral myalgia
Vertebral arthritis (back pain and tenderness)
Vertebral malignancy

SYNDROMES (see SYNDROMES SECTION 6)

Boerhaave's syn. (ruptured oesophagus)
Bornholm syn. (see SYNDROMES SECTION 6)
Chinese restaurant syn. (face pain, nausea)
Intermediate coronary syn. (variable angina)
Irukandji syn. (jellyfish sting, pulmonary oedema, severe pain)
Meig's syn. (hydrothorax, ascites)
Mendelson's syn. (pneumonitis, bronchospasm)
Pancoast's syn. (arm pain, lung cancer)
Slipping rib syn. (lower chest pain)
Tietze's syn. (costochrondral pain and tenderness)
Xiphoid syn. (sternal pain, nausea)

OTHER

Cardiac neuroses and other emotional disorders
Herpes zoster (shingles) (unilateral, radicular, rash)
Thoracic malignancy
Sarcoidosis
Hypothyroidism (dry skin, myalgia, cold intolerance)
Melioidosis (cough, skin abscesses)
Mediastinal and thymic tumours

See also Heartburn; Breast Pain; Dyspepsia

Child Abuse

Polle syn. (Münchausen's syn. by proxy)
Psychiatric disturbances.

Chloasma

See Pigmentation of Skin, Excess

Cholestasis

See Jaundice

Chorea and Ballism

Continual, nonrepetitive, purposeless limb jerks
Rheumatic fever (arthralgia, rash, fever)
Huntington's chorea (hereditary, mental deterioration)
Sydenham's chorea (weakness, aphasia)
Hyperthyroidism (tachycardia, sweating)
Chorea gravidarum (pregnancy or oral contraceptives)
SLE
Senility
Polycythaemia rubra vera
Lesch-Nyhan syn. (retarded, gout, mutilation)
Carbon monoxide poisoning
Drugs (eg. phenytoin, amphetamines, phenothiazines, oral contraceptives)

Claudication

See Leg Pain

Cleft Lip and/or Palate

Idiopathic
Dandy-Walker syn. (craniomegaly, nystagmus, vomiting)
Lip-pit syn. (lower lip involved)
Meckel syn. (polydactyly, cystic kidneys)
Oto-palatal-digital syn. (deaf, syndactyly)
Patau's syn. (polydactyly, cardiac anomalies)
Pierre-Robin syn. (micrognathia)
Wolf-Hirschhorn syn. (mental retardation, nose abnormal)

See also Facial Anomaly Associated Syndromes

Clumsiness

CRANIAL

Alcohol intake
Epilepsy (absences, convulsions)
Migraine (pain, visual disturbances, photophobia)
Parkinson's disease (tremor, dysarthria, stiff gait)
Cerebrovascular accident (paralysis, speech defect)
Transient ischaemic attack (brief, weak, headache)
Alzheimer's disease (elderly, dementia)
Cerebral space occupying lesion (eg. tumour, haemorrhage)
Multiple sclerosis (bizarre neurological signs)
Birth trauma
Hydrocephalus
Chorea (see separate entry)

OTHER

Myxoedema (cold intolerance, dry skin, fatigue)
Cervical myelopathy
Spinal cord tumour or compression
Motor neurone disease (incoordination, paralysis)
Peripheral neuropathy
Muscular dystrophy
Myopathies
Gerstmann-Straussler-Scheinker syn.

Cold Intolerance

Unable to tolerate cold climatic conditions normally
Hypothyroidism (tired, weight gain)
Pulmonary embolism (sweating, anxious)
Malnutrition

Colic

See Abdominal Pain

Coma

Unrousable loss of consciousness

CEREBRAL

Head injuries and other severe trauma
Cerebrovascular accident (paralysis, neurological changes)

Cerebral haematoma
Epilepsy (convulsions, auras, headaches)
CNS infections (fever, convulsions)
CNS tumours (neurological changes)
Degenerative CNS disease
Increased intracranial pressure
Brain abscess
Hysteria (conversion reaction)

ENDOCRINE

Diabetes mellitus (vomiting, dehydrated, tachycardia)
Hypothyroidism (dry skin, alopecia, anaemia)
Hypoglycaemia (flaccid, cold, sweating)
Addisonian crisis (vomiting, diarrhoea, pigmentation)

OTHER

Hypotension or shock (eg. myocardial infarct, haemorrhage)
Uraemia (oliguria, vomiting, fetid breath)
Hepatic coma (tremor, hyperreflexia, hyperventilation)
Electrolyte imbalance (eg. diuretics, IV therapy)
Anaphylaxis (shock, convulsions, dilated pupils)
Severe systemic infection (eg. cholera, septicaemia)
AIDS (rash, adenitis, fever)
Eclampsia (pregnant, hypertension, convulsions)
Porphyria (tachycardia, sweating, convulsions)
Hypothermia (pale, bradycardia)
Heat stroke (vomiting, convulsions)
Dehydration from any cause
Anoxia or hypoxia
Respiratory failure
Cardiac failure (dyspnoea, peripheral oedema)
Hypertensive encephalopathy
Hypothyroidism
Malaria
Cardiac arrhythmia or arrest
Severe dehydration
Typhoid fever
Waterhouse-Friderichsen syn.
Carbon monoxide poisoning (flushed)
Drug overdosage (eg. alcohol, barbiturates)
Poisons (ingested, snake bite, insect bite, spider bite, etc.)

See also Syncope

Confusion

Cerebrovascular accident (paralysis, anaesthesia, aphasia)
Dementia (eg. Alzheimer's disease)
Cerebral space occupying lesion
Encephalitis (headache, fever)
Uraemia (fatigue, headache, pruritus)
Schizophrenia (personality changes, hallucinations)
Depression (insomnia, anxiety)
Other psychiatric disorders
Postictal
Head injuries and other CNS diseases
Postsurgery/anaesthesia
Altered environment
Myocardial infarct (arrhythmias, chest pain, dyspnoea)
Pulmonary embolism (chest pain, haemoptysis, dyspnoea)
Visceral embolism (abdominal pain)

Cardiac failure and arrhythmias
Viral or bacterial meningitis
Septicaemia (fever)
Liver failure (jaundice)
Thyrotoxicosis (sweating, proptosis, tachycardia)
Myxoedema (cold, bradycardia, lethargy)
Anaemia (pallor)
Brucellosis (fever, fatigue, myalgia)
Hypercalcaemia (nausea, constipation)
Chronic fatigue syn. (weak, no exercise tolerance)
Post-traumatic stress syn. (nightmares, phobia)
Organic brain syndrome (sensory confusion, mood changes)
Alcohol
Drugs (eg. sedatives, narcotics, steroids, digoxin, antidepressants)

See also Psychiatric Disturbance Associated Syndromes

Conjunctivitis

See Eye Pain; Eye, Inflamed or Red

Constipation

Physical inactivity and low residue diet
Dehydration (nausea, thirst, weakness)
Piles (pain, rectal bleeding, pruritus ani)
Fissure-in-ano (pain, anal bleeding)
Colonic or rectal tumour (melaena)
Gut obstruction (vomiting, pain)
Diverticulitis (alternating diarrhoea, LIF pain)
Neurogenic colonic disease
Hirschsprung's disease (chronic impaction, abdomen distended)
Pregnancy (amenorrhoea, breast fullness)
Hypothyroidism (growth reduced, dry skin)
Typhoid fever (alt. diarrhoea, fever, abdominal pain)
Ulcerative colitis (changed bowel habits)
Rectal prolapse
Perineal descent syn.
Hypercalcaemia (chronic form)
Electrolyte disturbances
Diabetes (polyuria, polydipsia, nausea)
Porphyria (abdominal pain, vomiting)
Irritable bowel syn. (abdominal pain, bloated, alt. diarrhoea)
Lightwood's syn. (weight loss, vomiting, child)
Depression (insomnia, lack of interest)
Neuroses and other psychiatric disorders
Drugs (eg. codeine, antacids, anticonvulsants, antidepressants, diuretics, iron)

See also symptoms listed under Intestine.

Convulsions (Fits, Seizures)

CEREBRAL

Epilepsy (blackouts, paroxysmal, amnesia)
Hysteria (erratic, precipitating cause)
Cerebrovascular accident (neurological signs, aphasia)

TYPES AND PERIODICITIES OF HEADACHES

Tension Headache

Periodicity — M T W T F S S (Day)

Periodicity — J F M A M J J (Month)

Migraine

Periodicity — J F M A M J J (Month)

Cluster Headache

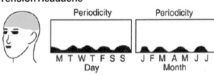

Periodicity — M T W T F S S (Day)

Cerebral tumour (headache, nausea, neurological signs)
Subdural haematoma (trauma, vomiting, pupil changes)
Migraine (headache, vomiting, visual disturbance)
Meningitis (fever, vomiting, neck stiffness)
Encephalitis (fever, nausea, sore throat)
Tuberosclerosis
Craniostenosis
Raised intracranial pressure from other causes
Syncope

SYNDROMES (see SYNDROMES SECTION 6)

Behcet syn. (uveitis, arthritis, mouth ulcers)
Catatonic syn. (hypertonia)
Creutzfeldt-Jakob syn. (dementia, paralysis)
Fragile X syn. (subnormal intelligence, overactive, facial dysmorphism)
Gilles de la Tourette syn. [Tourette syn.] (foul language)
Landau-Kleffner syn. (acquired aphasia)
Leigh syn. (encephalopathy)
Lennox-Gastaut syn. (mental retardation)
Lissencephaly syn. (hypotonia, jaundice)
Organic brain syn. (psychiatric changes)
Rett's syn. (female, autistic, hyperventilation)
Richner-Hanhart syn. (uveitis, keratoderma)
Sandifer syn. (reflux oesophagitis)
Stokes-Adams syn. (syncope, bradycardia)
Sturge-Weber syn. (port wine stain, mental retardation)

OTHER

Severe bacterial, viral, rickettsial or protozoal infections (eg. toxoplasma, cytomegalovirus)
Fever from any cause (common in children)
Hypertension (essential or secondary)
Electrolyte disturbances
Shock (hypovolaemia)
Hypoglycaemia (?insulin overdose)
Anoxia (physical or pathological causes)

Severe trauma (coma, paralysis, pupil signs)
Dehydration (from dehydration or water deprivation)
Menke's disease (low serum copper, kinky hair)
SLE (butterfly rash, arthritis)
Hypothyroidism and cretinism
Chromosomal abnormalities (often severe and prolonged)
Hypoparathyroidism (tetany, wheeze, stridor)
Eclampsia (pregnancy, hypertension)
Uraemia (fatigue, headache, pruritus)
Tetany (hyperventilation, hypocalcaemia, tetanic hand)
Behavioural problem
Breath holding (child)
Tetanus (rigid jaw, muscle spasms, trauma)
Porphyria (tachycardia, sweating, vomiting)
Niemann-Pick disease (mental retardation, hepatosplenomegaly)
Rabies (animal bite, hydrophobia, paraesthesia)
Drugs (eg.strychnine, atropine, cyanide, nicotine)

Cough

RESPIRATORY TRACT

Coryza (rhinitis, sore throat, malaise)
Influenza (fever, myalgia, headache)
Sinusitis (face pain, catarrh)
Rhinitis (allergic or vasomotor)
Postnasal drip (pharyngitis, halitosis)
Q fever and other rickettsioses
Pertussis (infant, coryza, anaemia)
Other respiratory tract bacterial and viral infections
Laryngeal tumour or oedema (dyspnoea, dysphagia, hoarseness)
Laryngeal foreign body (stridor, hoarseness, gagging)

PULMONARY

Bronchitis (sputum, rhonchi, fever)
Pneumonia (fever, pain, foul sputum)
Tuberculosis (malaise, fever, haemoptysis)
Bronchiectasis (purulent sputum, haemoptysis, rales)
Bronchial foreign body (wheeze, history)
Bronchogenic carcinoma (wheeze, haemoptysis, malaise)
Pulmonary oedema (crepitations, dyspnoea)
Asthma (expiratory wheeze, dyspnoea)
Hyperreactive airways disease (allergy-like symptoms)
Alveolitis (arthralgia, dry cough)
Silicosis (history, chronic respiratory infections)
Asbestosis (occupational exposure)
Pulmonary abscess
Pleurisy (pain, friction rub)
Allergic alveolitis (eg. farmer's lung, bird fancier's lung)
Emphysema (wheeze, dyspnoea, barrel chest)
Sarcoidosis (dyspnoea, malaise)
Pulmonary thromboembolism (pain, dyspnoea, haemoptysis)
Cystic fibrosis (steatorrhoea, viscid sputum)
Anthrax (dyspnoea, headache, animal contact)
Legionnaire's disease (influenza-like, diarrhoea)
Tularaemia (tick bite)
Brucellosis (fever, sweating, headache)
Hydatid disease (abdominal mass)
Plague

Psittacosis (fever, epistaxis, myalgia, bird contact)
Smoking (active or passive)
Inhaled irritants

SYNDROMES (see SYNDROMES SECTION 6)
Eosinophilia-myalgia syn. (arthralgia)
Goodpasture syn. (haemoptysis, dyspnoea, anaemia)
Kartagener syn. (dextrocardia, sinusitis)
Loeffler syn. (wheeze, fever, pulmonary eosinophilia)
Louis-Bar syn. (telangiectasia of face and flexures)

OTHER
Congestive cardiac failure (dyspnoea, fatigue, orthopnoea)
Mitral valve disease (dyspnoea, atrial fibrillation)
Otitis media (ear pain and discharge, fever)
Diaphragmatic irritation (eg. abscess, peritonitis)
Gastro-oesophageal reflux (burping, nonproductive cough, chest pain)
Aortic aneurysm (bruit, pain)
Pericarditis (cardiac failure, pain)
Goitre
Measles (rash, conjunctivitis, coryza)
Ascariasis (urticaria, haemoptysis, colic)
Histoplasmosis and other pulmonary mycotic infections
Melioidosis (chest pain, skin abscesses)
Actinomycosis (fever, dyspnoea, malaise)
External auditory canal stimulation (eg. excess wax, foreign body)
Anaphylaxis
Psychogenic
Drugs (eg. beta-blockers, ACE inhibitors)

See also Haemoptysis; Wheeze

Cramps, Muscular
Nocturnal and idiopathic
Pregnancy
Post exercise
Proctalgia fugax (relieved by bearing down)
Repetitive strain injury
L5-S1 compression
Liver cirrhosis
Hyperventilation (tetany)
Hypocalcaemia (tetany)
Salt loss from diarrhoea or renal disease
Cholera (diarrhoea, vomiting)
Tetanus (generalised muscle spasms)
Hypothyroidism (fatigue, dry skin, constipation)
Motor neurone disease
Drugs (eg. diuretics, phenothiazines, strychnine)

See also Myoclonus

Croup
See Stridor

Cyanosis, Central
Blue skin and mucous membranes

INFANT
Transposition of great arteries

Pulmonary atresia
Tricuspid atresia
Ebstein's anomaly
Pulmonary vein anomalies
Fallot's tetralogy
Ventricular anomalies

SYNDROMES (see SYNDROMES SECTION 6)
Eisenmenger's syndrome
Fallot's trilogy, tetralogy and pentalogy
Grey baby syn. (cardiovascular collapse, chloramphenicol use)
Hypoplastic left heart syn. (neonate, cardiac failure)
Pickwickian syn. (obese, cardiac failure)
Respiratory distress syn., adult (dyspnoea, hypoxia)
Waterhouse-Friderichsen syn. (prostration, petechiae)

OTHER
Intracardiac shunts and other arteriovenous fistulae
Anaemia (physical or pathological causes)
Pneumonia (productive cough, foul sputum)
Respiratory failure
Bronchiectasis (foul sputum, chest pain)
Emphysema (wheeze, barrel chest)
Chronic lung disease (eg. emphysema, chronic bronchitis)
Polycythaemia rubra vera (malaise, headache, itch)
Acute major pulmonary embolus (chest pain)
Alveolitis (dry cough, arthralgia)

See also Cyanosis, Peripheral

Cyanosis, Peripheral
Blueness of cooler body parts
Cold environment (hypothermia)
Raynaud's disease (intermittent, symmetrical, female)
Buerger's disease (pain, smoker, male)
Circulatory disturbances (eg. acrocyanosis, thrombosis)
Severe bacterial or viral infections
Mitral stenosis (atrial fibrillation, dyspnoea)
Pulmonary stenosis (dyspnoea, angina, oedema)
Cardiac failure (dyspnoea, oedema, cough)

See also Cyanosis, Central

Dandruff
See Scalp, Scaly

Deafness
Hearing loss
Sensorineural (Rinne +, poor speech discrimination)
Otitis media [glue ear] (pain, fever, bulging tympanum)
Upper respiratory tract infection
Barotrauma (flying or diving)
Perforated tympanum (infective or traumatic causes)
Otosclerosis (tinnitus, Rinne –, paracousis)
Cholesteatoma (foul smell, white debris)
Menière's disease (tinnitus, vertigo)
Impacted cerumen or foreign body
Paget's disease (bone pain)
Exostoses
Temporal bone fracture

Eighth [acoustic] nerve tumour (unilateral deafness)
Ossicular fracture or dislocation
Otic tumours
Cerebral space occupying lesions
Osteogenesis imperfecta (blue sclera, fragile bone)
Hypothyroidism (dry skin, myalgia, neuritis)
Senile deafness
Generalised infections (eg. measles, mumps, meningitis)
Multiple sclerosis (bizarre neurological signs)
Prenatal causes (eg. rubella, cytomegalovirus, toxoplasmosis)
Postnatal jaundice
Congenital and hereditary causes
Drugs (eg. salicylates, beta-blockers, quinine, cisplatin, aminoglycosides)

SYNDROMES (see SYNDROMES SECTION 6)

Alport syn. (glomerulonephritis, cataract, otitis)
Cogan syn. (tinnitus, vertigo)
Conrad syn. (cataracts, deformed limbs)
Hunter syn. (arthralgia, gross facies)
Jervell-Lange-Nielsen syn. (syncope)
Johanson-Blizzard syn. (anal atresia, retarded)
Maroteaux-Lamy syn. (bone dysplasia, cataracts)
Morquio's syn. (bone dysplasia, cataracts)
Oto-palatal-digital syn. (cleft palate, syndactyly)
Pendred syn. (congenital, goitre at puberty)
Treacher-Collins syn. (face abnormal)
Usher syn. (retinitis pigmentosa)
Waardenburg-Klein syn. (confluent eyebrows)

Death, Imminent
Ichabod syndrome (see SYNDROMES SECTION 6)

Death, Sudden, Unexpected

Coronary heart disease
Hypertrophic cardiac myopathy
Congenital coronary artery anomalies
Myocarditis
Pericarditis
Aortic stenosis
Cerebrovascular accident
Ruptured cerebral aneurysm
Ruptured aortic aneurysm
Sickle cell anaemia
Marfan's syn. (arachnodactyly, tall and thin)
Sudden infant death syn.
Brugada syn. (SE Asian, male)

Déjà Vu

Feeling of intense familiarity
Epilepsy (convulsions, amnesia, absences)
Emotional trauma or stress
Psychiatric disorders
Cerebrovascular accident (neurological changes)

Dementia

Alzheimer's disease
Cerebrovascular disease (eg. stroke)
Senile dementia

Cerebral trauma (eg. subdural haematoma)
Cerebral abscess or tumour
Meningitis (nuchal rigidity)
Encephalitis (fever, malaise)
Parkinson's diseased (advanced stages only)
Hypothyroidism (constipation, fatigue, dry skin)
Hepatic failure
Neurosyphilis (Argyll-Robertson pupils)
Pernicious anaemia (lethargy, sore tongue)
Pellagra (anaemia, rash, diarrhoea)
Metastatic carcinoma
Uraemia
Hypercalcaemia
Hypopituitarism
Hydrocephalus
Subacute sclerosing panencephalitis
Anoxia
Creutzfeldt-Jakob disease
Hyperuricaemia
Vitamin B deficiency
Poisons (eg. glue sniffing, organophosphates)
Drugs (eg. bromides, alcohol, barbiturates, amphetamines)

SYNDROMES (see SYNDROMES SECTION 6)

AIDS
Wernicke-Korsakoff syn. (alcohol dependent)
Cushing syn. (obese, striae, moon face)
Punchdrunk syn.

Depigmentation of Skin
See Skin, Depigmented

Depression

Stress and environment (anxiety, agitation, anger)
Elderly (insomnia, irritable, confused)
Endogenous depression (insomnia, phobias)
Hypoparathyroidism (tetany, wheeze)
Hyperparathyroidism (polyuria, polydipsia, bone pain)
Postpartum depression
Cerebral tumours (dementia, psychoses)
Parkinsonism (tremor, rigidity)
Multiple sclerosis (variable CNS symptoms)
Cerebrovascular disease
Hyperthyroidism (weak, weight loss, sweating)
Hypothyroidism (dry skin, myalgia, asthenia)
Addison's disease (weak, anorexia, nausea)
Pernicious anaemia (dyspepsia, sore tongue, pallor)
Rheumatoid arthritis
SLE (facial rash, arthritis)
Electrolyte disturbances
Menopause (amenorrhoea, flushing, tension)
Cushing syn. (central obesity, plethora)
Chronic fatigue syn. (tired, poor exercise tolerance)
Post-traumatic stress syn. (phobia, nightmares, confusion)
Pellagra (red skin and tongue, diarrhoea)
Infectious diseases (eg. hepatitis, influenza)
Drugs (eg. cortisone, methyldopa, propranolol, reserpine, oral contraceptives)

See also Psychiatric Disturbance Associated Syndromes

Dermatitis

See Skin Lesion Associated Syndromes
See also symptoms listed under Rash; Skin Disorders

Diaphoresis

See Sweating, Excessive and Abnormal

Diarrhoea

GASTROINTESTINAL

Food poisoning (toxin or infection – see below)
Lactose intolerance
Faecal impaction with overflow
Allergy (eg. milk, eggs)
Diverticulitis (LIF pain, colic, tender)
Irritable bowel syn. (abdominal pain, bowel habit changes, colic)
Appendicitis (RIF pain and guarding)
Crohn's disease (pain, anorexia, flatus)
Ulcerative colitis (bloody faeces, colic, fever)
Colonic or rectal carcinoma (melaena, pain)
Dietary anomalies and marasmus
Pancreatic insufficiency or tumours
Sprue (foul faeces, weight loss)
Inflamed perirectal tissues
Ischaemic bowel disease (abdominal pain)
Intussusception (bloody diarrhoea, child)
Postvagotomy
Small bowel resection
Cirrhosis (fatigue, nausea, RUQ pain)
Pseudomembranous colitis
Anal sex

INFECTIONS

Viral enteritis or food poisoning
Bacterial enteritis (eg. typhoid, other salmonelloses, shigellosis, yersinia)
Clostridium difficile infection (chronic, severe, post antibiotic)
Amoebiasis (abdominal cramps, tenesmus, foul stools)
Septicaemia (fever, malaise)
Tuberculosis, intestinal
Histoplasmosis
Meningitis (headache, neck stiffness, fever)
Urinary tract infections (dysuria, frequency)
Melioidosis (cough, chest pain, sores)
Cholera (liquid and odourless stools, vomiting)
Giardiasis (foul stools, flatulence, cramps)
Bilharzia (urticaria, abdominal pain, fever)
Other metazoal and protozoal infections

SYNDROMES (see SYNDROMES SECTION 6)

AIDS (fever, adenitis, rash)
Carcinoid syn. (flush, abdominal cramps, oedema)
Cori syn. (glycogen storage disease)
Denervation syn. (bloated, oesophageal surgery)
Dumping syn. (postgastrectomy, postprandial)
Gay bowel syn. (homosexual, tenesmus)
Haemolytic-uraemic syn. (haematuria, thrombocytopenia)
Nezelof syn. (infant, fever, rashes)
Toxic shock syn. (nausea, fever, hypotension)
von Gierke syn. (hypoglycaemia, hepatosplenomegaly)
Weil syn. (leptospirosis)
Zollinger-Ellison syn. (recurrent peptic ulcers)
Other malabsorption syndromes and enteropathies

OTHER

Anaphylaxis
Psychogenic (psychiatric changes, depression)
Neuropathies (eg. tabes dorsalis)
Hyperthyroidism (weakness, sweating, weight loss)
Pernicious anaemia (glossitis)
Vitamin B deficiency
Folate deficiency
Diabetes (polyuria, weakness, neuropathy)
Addison's disease (skin pigmentation)
Carcinoid tumour (sweating, abdominal pain)
Pellagra (depression, red skin and tongue)
Uraemia (fatigue, headache, anaemia)
Adrenal insufficiency (fatigue, nausea, headache)
Ciguatera poisoning (paraesthesiae)
Laxative abuse
Alcoholism
Antibiotics and other drugs (eg. antacids, methyldopa, propranolol, theophylline, indomethacin, antibiotics, colchicine, digoxin, quinidine)

See also Tenesmus; Melaena and Rectal Bleeding

Diplopia
Double vision
Paralytic squint due to 3rd, 4th or 6th cranial nerve palsy (limited movement of one eye)
Cerebrovascular accident (neurological changes)
Concussion (trauma, headache, nausea)
Orbital trauma
Migraine (nausea, headache, photophobia)
Botulism (dry mouth, dysphagia, paralysis)
Cerebral tumours (headache, neurological signs)
Myasthenia gravis (weakness, ptosis)
Thyroid diseases
Multiple sclerosis (weakness, abnormal sensation)
Gradenigo syn. (headache, facial pain)
Wernicke-Korsakoff syn. (ataxia, demented)

See also Optic Paralysis

Discharge, Ear
See Ear Discharge

Discharge, Nasal
See Rhinitis and Rhinorrhoea

Discharge, Nipple
See Nipple Discharge

Discharge, Otic
See Ear Discharge

Discharge, Urethral
See Urethral Discharge

Discharge, Vaginal
See Vagina, Discharge, Excessive

Dizziness
See Vertigo

Double Vision
See Diplopia

Drop Attack
Sudden brief loss of consciousness without warning

CARDIOVASCULAR

Atrioventricular conduction block
Ventricular tachycardia
Atrial fibrillation onset
Carotid sinus syncope
Aortic or mitral stenosis (bruit)
Pulmonary embolism (chest pain, dyspnoea)
Severe pulmonary hypertension
Atrial myxoma
Postural hypotension
Micturition syncope
Subclavian steal syn. (arm claudication)
Vasovagal syn. (bradycardia, recurrent)

OTHER

Severe chronic obstructive airways disease (cough)
Transient ischaemic attack
Epileptic seizure (incontinence)
Hypoglycaemia
Psychological attention seeking
Drugs (eg. glyceryl trinitrate, antihypertensives)

See also Syncope (Faint)

Dry Eye
See Eye, Dry; Mucous Membranes, Dry

Dry Mouth (Xerostomia)
See Mouth, Dry; Mucous membranes, Dry

Dry Mucous Membranes
See Mucous Membranes, Dry

Dry Skin (Xeroderma)
See Icthyosis; Skin, Dry

Dry Vagina
See Vagina, Dry

Dwarfism
See Growth, Reduced

Dysarthria
See Aphasia and Dysarthria

Dysgeusia
See Taste, Abnormal

Dyskinesia
See SIGNS SECTION 2: Dyskinesia, Tardive

Dysmenorrhoea
Painful menstruation
Functional [no organic cause] (80% of cases)
Menopausal syn. (flushes, 45-55 years old)
Salpingitis (leucorrhoea, dyspareunia, fever)
Adenomyosis (dyspareunia, abdominal pain)
Endometriosis (abdominal pain, infertility)
Gynaecological tumours (abnormal bleeding)
Uterine adhesions (postoperative or postinfection)
Pelvic congestion syn.
Uterine prolapse
Retroverted uterus
Hypercontractile uterus
Cervical stenosis (may be iatrogenic)
Congenital abnormalities
Imperforate hymen
Uterine polyps
Fibromyomata
Anaphylaxis
Intrauterine contraceptive device

Dyspareunia
Painful sexual intercourse

SUPERFICIAL

Bartholin's cyst
Psychological and psychiatric (vaginismus)
Decreased vaginal secretions (eg. thyroid, pituitary or
adrenal disease)
Vulvovaginitis (eg. herpes, allergy)
Rigid hymen
Vulval trauma
Episiotomy scar or other surgery

DEEP

Endometriosis (dysmenorrhoea, abnormal bleeding)
Ectopic pregnancy (abdominal pain and tenderness)
Uterine fibroids (pelvic mass)
Pelvic inflammatory disease (vaginal discharge)
Ovarian tumours and cysts

MIXED

Gynaecological infections (eg. thrush, trichomoniasis)
Gynaecological tumours (pain, abnormal bleeding)

Inflamed periuterine tissues (eg. pelvic abscess, peritonitis, diverticulitis)
Uterine prolapse (backache)
Cystitis or urethritis (dysuria, frequency)
Menopause (amenorrhoea, depression, flushes)

Dyspepsia
Abdominal pain made worse by meals
Peptic ulcer (epigastric pain, burping, nocturnal)
Irritable bowel syn. (abdominal pain, bowel habit changes)
Psychological (secondary to stress)
Gastritis (anorexia, nausea, malaise)
Duodenitis
Oesophagitis (dysphagia, waterbrash)
Cholelithiasis
Pancreatitis (sweating, nausea, abdominal tenderness)
Gastric carcinoma
Food allergy and drug intolerance (eg. NSAIDs)

See also Chest Pain; Dysphagia

Dysphagia
Difficulty in swallowing

GASTROINTESTINAL
Carcinoma of oesophagus or pharynx (pain, regurgitation, wasting)
Achalasia (dysergia, regurgitation, pain)
Stricture (regurgitation, dehydration)
Hiatus hernia (pain, reflux, waterbrash)
Oesophageal diverticulae (halitosis, foul taste, regurgitation)
Buccal or oesophageal candidiasis (white plaques)
Oesophageal spasm
Oesophageal peptic ulcer
Pharyngeal pouch
Vincent's and Ludwig's angina
Tongue oedema (eg. allergy)
Epiglottitis (fever, pain)
Oesophageal herpes
Foreign body (regurgitation, pain)

RESPIRATORY TRACT
Quinsy (fever, pain, trismus)
Laryngeal tumour (hoarse, cough, dyspnoea)
Pharyngeal abscess (dyspnoea, fever, pain)
Syndromes (see SYNDROMES SECTION 6)
Boerhaave syn. (ruptured oesophagus)
Guillain-Barré syn. (paralysis, polyneuritis)
Moebius syn. (ophthalmoplegia, fixed facies)
Plummer-Vinson syn. (oesophageal web, splenomegaly)
Riley-Day syn. (Jewish, no lacrimation)
Sjögren's syn. (dry eyes and mouth)
Steele-Richardson-Olszewski syn. (axial rigidity, dementia)

OTHER
Cervical masses (eg. lymph nodes, ectopic thymus)
Cerebrovascular accident
Transient ischaemic attack (brief, headache)
Bulbar palsy (tongue twitch, drooling, dysarthria)
Multiple sclerosis (various neurological symptoms)
SLE
Polymyositis

Chagas' disease
Iron deficiency anaemia (pallor, fatigue, dyspnoea)
Goitre (thyroid enlargement from any cause)
Thyrotoxicosis (sweating, headache)
Head injury
Parkinson's disease (tremor, rigidity)
Tetanus (muscle spasms, trauma)
Botulism (dry mouth, diplopia, paralysis)
Motor neurone disease (weak, myalgia)
Pericardial effusion (dyspnoea, ache)
Aortic aneurysm (dyspnoea, hoarse, pain)
Scleroderma (arthritis, Raynaud's phenomenon)
Dermatomyositis (proximal weakness, rash)
Myasthenia gravis (diplopia, ptosis)
Cervical osteoarthritis
Globus hystericus (psychogenic, common)
Lead poisoning
Radiotherapy

See also Mucous Membranes, Dry; Odynophagia

Dyspnoea
Shortness of breath

RESPIRATORY TRACT
Pharyngeal abscess (dysphagia, fever, pain)
Laryngeal tumour or oedema (hoarse, cough, dysphagia)
Obstructive sleep apnoea (snoring)
Severe rhinitis

PULMONARY
Asthma (expiratory wheeze, cough)
Pneumothorax (pain, sudden onset)
Pneumonia (cough, fever, pain, expectoration)
Bronchiolitis (child, wheeze, cough)
Croup (child, characteristic cough)
Chronic obstructive airways disease
Bronchiectasis (pain, malaise, haemoptysis)
Pressure on larynx from abscess, haematoma, neoplasm, etc.
Emphysema with bronchitis (wheeze, cough, barrel chest)
Atelectasis (cyanosis, fever, sudden onset)
Anthrax (animal contact, cough, congestion)
Sarcoidosis (cough, malaise)
Thromboembolism (pain, cough, haemoptysis)
Pleural effusion (pain)
Allergic alveolitis (cough, fever)
Histiocytosis X (smoker, young male)
Hydatid disease (abdominal mass)
Pulmonary haemorrhage
Pulmonary embolus

CARDIOVASCULAR
Myocardial infarct (pain, pallor, nausea)
Congestive cardiac failure (paroxysmal nocturnal dyspnoea)
Mitral stenosis (fatigue, paroxysmal and nocturnal)
Congenital heart disease (fatigue, cyanosis)
Pericardial effusion (dysphagia, ache)
Myocarditis (asthenia, pain, nausea)
Aortic aneurysm (pain, dysphagia, hoarse)
Hypotension (faint, vertigo, pallor)

Anaemia (pallor, fatigue, palpitations)
Cerebrovascular accident
Pulmonary hypertension
Cardiac arrhythmias

SYNDROMES (see SYNDROMES SECTION 6)

Eosinophilia-myalgia syn. (cough, arthralgia)
Fallot's tetralogy (cyanosis, cardiac lesions)
Goodpasture syn. (haemoptysis, anaemia, cough)
Guillain-Barré syn. (muscle weakness)
Hamman-Rich syn. (interstitial fibrosis)
Irukandji syn. (jellyfish sting, severe pain, tachycardia)
Pickwickian syn. (obese, cardiac lesions)
Potter syn. (neonate, renal agenesis, micrognathia)
Respiratory distress syn., neonate and adult (hypoxia, tachypnoea)
Shock syn. (pallor, hypotension, oliguria)

OTHER

Exertion or emotion (hyperventilation)
Hypoparathyroidism (tetany, wheeze, stridor)
Mediastinal tumour (substernal pain)
Gastro-oesophageal reflux (burping)
Kyphoscoliosis
Acidosis
Neuromuscular disorders
Hyperthyroidism (fatigue, sweating, weight loss)
Poliomyelitis (fever, paralysis)
Psychogenic causes
Carbon monoxide poisoning
Electrolyte imbalance (eg. hyper- or hypokalaemia)
Rib fracture or other trauma
Obesity

See also Orthopnoea; Stridor; Wheeze

Dystonia

See SIGNS SECTION 2: Hypertonicity or Hypotonia

Dysuria

Painful micturition

Cystitis (hypogastric pain, frequency)
Prostatitis (perineal pain, frequency, discharge)
Gonorrhoea (discharge, frequency)
Pelvic inflammatory disease (vaginal discharge, abdominal pain)
Nonspecific urethritis (discharge)
Pyelonephritis (loin pain, fever, proteinuria)
Cystocele (vaginal bulge, frequency, urgency)

SYNDROMES (see SYNDROMES SECTION 6)

Fitz-Hugh-Curtis syn. (vaginal discharge, perihepatitis)
Urethral syn. (urinary frequency, sterile urine)
Reiter syndrome (conjunctivitis, arthritis)

See also Strangury

Ear

See Deafness; Earache; Ear Discharge; Ear, Smelly; Tinnitus

Earache

Otitis externa (discharge, itch)
Otitis media (deaf, discharge, fever)
Mastoiditis (bone tenderness, discharge, fever)
Impacted cerumen (deaf)
Sinusitis (face ache, foul catarrh)
Coryza (nasal discharge, sore throat)
Furunculosis (boil in canal)
Dental caries
Glue ear (deaf, dull tympanum)
Perichondritis (pinna pain)
Malignancy of ear, tonsil, mouth or pharynx
Eustachian tube dysfunction
Cholesteatoma
Temporal arteritis (tender temples)
Parotitis (tender parotid gland)
Foreign body in ear
Trauma (eg. diving, high altitudes)
C2-3 vertebral lesions
Lesions of cranial nerves 5, 9 or 10
referred pain (eg: impacted molars, temporomandibular joint disorders, tongue malignancy, tonsillitis)

SYNDROMES (see SYNDROMES SECTION6)

Costen's syn. (tinnitus, deaf)
Gradenigo's syn. (facial pain, diplopia)
Hand-Schuller-Christian syn. (diabetes insipidus)
Louis-Bar syn. (telangiectasia of face and flexures)
Ramsay Hunt syn. (blistering rash)

See also Ear Discharge

Ear Discharge (Otorrhoea)

Trauma (i.e. direct injury or skull fracture - CSF)
Cerumen
Foreign body in canal
Acute otitis externa (pain)
Otitis media with ruptured tympanum
Other infections
Epithelial debris
Perichondritis
Otic tumours
Skin disorders (eg. eczema)

Ear Pain

See Earache

Ear, Smelly

Otitis media (ruptured tympanum with discharge)
Cholesteatoma (purulent discharge, deaf)
Fungal infection of ear canal

Ecchymosis

Bruise, purpuric macules

Thrombocytopenia (low blood platelets)
Coagulation defects (congenital or acquired)
Meningococcal infection
Septicaemia

Subacute bacterial endocarditis
Rickettsial diseases (eg. typhus, Rocky Mountain spotted fever)
Allergic vasculitis (arthralgia, myalgia)
Purpura fulminans (skin infarcts)
Scurvy (bleeding gums)
Basal skull fracture (mastoid ecchymosis)
Local trauma
Drug hypersensitivity

See also Bruising, Excess

Eczema
See Skin Lesion Associated Syndromes

Ejaculation, Premature
Anxiety
Unreasonable expectations
Emotional disorders
Very rarely organic

Ejaculation, Retarded
Diabetes mellitus (polyuria, polydipsia)
Hypogonadism
Hyperprolactinaemia
Spinal cord tumours, trauma or disease
Parkinson's disease (tremor, rigidity)
Cerebrovascular accident
Cerebral tumour, trauma or abscess
Genitourinary developmental defects
Urethral stricture, fistula or diverticulum
Prostatic disease
Aortic aneurysm
Surgical sympathectomy
Pelvic trauma or tumour

Ejaculation, Retrograde
Psychological stress
Prostatectomy
Pelvic surgery or trauma
Spinal cord trauma or tumour
Diabetes mellitus (polyuria, polydipsia)
Congenital abnormalities
Idiopathic
Drugs (eg. clonidine, bethanidine, guanethidine, methyldopa, phenothiazines, thiazides)

Energy, Lack of
See Fatigue, Abnormal

Enophthalmos
See SIGNS SECTION 2: Enophthalmos

Enuresis
Involuntary urinary incontinence
Urinary tract infections (dysuria, hypogastric discomfort, female)

Lifestyle stress (eg. family break-up, maternal separation, hospital admission, moving home)
Social pressures (eg. poverty, overcrowding, lack of privacy)
Excessively strict toilet training
Mental retardation
Congenitally small bladder
Diabetes mellitus (polydipsia, polyuria)
Diabetes insipidus
Renal insufficiency
Epilepsy
Spina bifida
Other neurological disorders
Familial

Epilepsy
See Convulsions
See also symptoms listed under Neurological Symptoms

Epistaxis
Nose bleed
Hypertension (headache, tinnitus, fatigue)
Nasal infection (rhinitis, fever, halitosis)
Nasal drying (crusting, ulceration)
Nasal tumours and polyps (rhinorrhoea, obstruction, pain)
Trauma (bruising, pain)
Foreign body in nose
High altitude
Rheumatic fever (chorea, arthralgia, fever, rash)
Haemorrhagic diseases (petechiae, bruising, bleeding)
Leukaemia (tired, malaise)
Measles (rash, coryza, photophobia)
Idiopathic thrombocytopenia (petechiae, ecchymoses)
Atrophic rhinitis
Arteriosclerosis
Squamous cell carcinoma
Adenocarcinoma
Rendu-Osler-Weber disease (hereditary haemorrhagic telangiectasia)
Blood factor deficits (eg. haemophilia, Christmas disease)
Psittacosis (cough, fever, myalgia)
Defibrination syn. (excess bleeding generally)
Drugs (eg. aspirin, steroid nasal sprays, heparin, warfarin)

See also Bleeding, Excessive

Erythema
Redness of skin
Dermatological
Contact dermatitis (oedema, vesciculation, crusting)
Dermatitis, stasis (pruritus, oedema, ulceration)
Dermatitis, exfoliative (pruritus, scaling, malaise)
Photodermatitis [sunburn](pain, oedema, vesciculation)
Rosacea (facial, exacerbated by vasodilation)
Psoriasis (plaque, scaling, nail changes, pruritus)
Seborrhoeic dermatitis (dry, scaling)
Acne (pimples; cysts; face, back and shoulders)
Urticaria (pruritus, wheals, oedema, malaise)

Eczema (scaling)
Intertrigo (pruritus, stinging, skin folds)
Erysipelas (oedema, hot pain, malaise)
Cellulitis (hot, diffuse, deep)
Mycosis fungoides
Tinea (pruritus, ring form, scaling)

SYNDROMES (see SYNDROMES SECTION 6)
Red man syn. (vancomycin infusion)
Rothmund-Thomson syn. (skin atrophy, pigmentation)
Sézary syn. (pruritus)
Stevens-Johnson syn. (conjunctivitis, stomatitis)

OTHER
Flush
Burn (eg. sunburn, scald)
Viral infections (eg. measles, rubella)
Allergic reaction
Scarlet fever (circumoral pallor, malaise)
Cirrhosis (palmar erythema, hepatic signs)
Erythema nodosum (nodules, female, painful rash)
Erythema multiforme (target lesions, extensor surfaces)
Lyme disease (fever, nausea, abdominal pain)
Pellagra (red tongue, diarrhoea, abdominal pain)
Discoid lupus erythematosus (plaques, scaling, telangiectasia)
Bilharzia (pruritus, diarrhoea or haematuria)
Diseases specific to area of erythema (eg. gout, mastitis, arthritis)
Alcohol excess

See also Facial Erythema; Flush; Port Wine Stain; Skin Lesion Associated Syndromes

Erythema, Joint
Red skin over joint
Cellulitis (tender, pain, heat)
Septic arthritis (pain, swelling, heat)
Gout (exquisite tenderness, swollen)
Pseudogout (tender, swollen)
Calcific periarthritis
Reiter syn. (conjunctivitis, urethritis, arthritis)
Acute osteoarthritis (pain, poor movement)
Palindromic rheumatoid arthritis (acute pain)
Erythema nodosum (rash)
Rheumatic fever

Exomphalos
Protrusion of gut into umbilical cord
Idiopathic
Beckwith syn. (macroglossia, neonate)

Exophthalmos
See SIGNS SECTION 2: Exophthalmos

Eye
See Amaurosis Fugax; Blindness, Partial or Total; Cataract; Diplopia; Eye Discharge; Eye, Dry; Eye,

Inflamed or Red; Eye Pain; Eye, Watery; Eyelids, Abnormal; Eyelid Disease; Flashes, Visual; Hemianopia; Iris Abnormality Associated Syndromes; Lacrimation, Abnormal; Microphthalmia; Optic Paralysis; Photophobia; Ptosis; Squint; Vision, Black Spots in Field of; Vision, Blurred; Xerophthalmia

Eye Discharge
Bacterial conjunctivitis (purulent, red, pain)
Viral conjunctivitis (serous, red, slight pain)
Allergic conjunctivitis (mucoid, red, itch)
Herpetic ulcer (serous, severe pain, photophobia)
Foreign body (serous, irritation, severe pain)
Arc damage (serous, red, severe pain)
Iritis (serous, depressed vision, pain)
Acute glaucoma (serous, severe pain, poor vision)
Scleritis (serous, severe pain, partial redness)

See also Eye, Watery

Eye Pain
Ophthalmic
Iritis (red, sluggish pupil, blurred vision)
Glaucoma (blurred vision, small pupil)
Conjunctivitis (red, discharge, photophobia)
Scleritis (red, photophobia, serous discharge)
Arc or UV damage (red, photophobia)
Herpetic conjunctivitis (photophobia, serous discharge)
Foreign body (history, sensation)
Keratitis and corneal ulcer (discharge, blurred vision)

OTHER
Sinusitis (fever, catarrh, rhinorrhoea)
Ankylosing spondylitis (back pain, arthritis)
Cluster headache (sudden, unilateral, lacrimation)
Migraine (headache, photophobia, nausea)
Ramsay Hunt syn. (blistering rash)
Ulcerative colitis (diarrhoea, rectal blood)
Hyperthyroidism (sweaty, fatigue, exophthalmos)
Yellow fever (generalised pain, jaundice, fever)
Syphilis (varied symptoms)
Sjögren's syn. (dry mouth, dysphagia)
Reiter's syn. (urethritis, arthritis)
Leptospirosis (fever, myalgia)

See also Photophobia

Eye, Black Spots in Visual Field
See Vision, Black Spots in Field of

Eye, Dry (Xerophthalmia)
Vitamin A deficiency (dry skin, loss of night vision, corneal ulcers)
Primary biliary cirrhosis (pruritus, dry mouth, cholestasis)
Rheumatoid arthritis (joint pain and swelling)
Idiopathic keratoconjunctivitis sicca (skin eczema)
Diabetes mellitus (polydipsia, polyuria)
Viral conjunctivitis (chronic)
Erythema multiforme

Mucus pemphigoid
Trachoma
Sjögren's syn. (dry mouth, dysphagia)
Other autoimmune disorders
Dry eye syn. (see SYNDROMES SECTION 6)
Facial nerve paresis
Riley-Day syn. (see SYNDROMES SECTION 6)
Trauma
Irradiation damage
Drugs (eg. antihypertensives, psychotherapeutics, sympathomimetics)

Eye, Inflamed or Red

Bacterial or viral conjunctivitis (diffuse injection, discharge, pain)
Iritis (circumcorneal injection, pain, blurred vision)
Glaucoma (pain, blurred vision)
Corneal trauma or foreign body (discharge, blurred vision, pain)
Allergic conjunctivitis (itch, watering, oedema, slight pain)
Keratitis (corneal ulcer, pain, discharge)
Acute glaucoma (severe pain, photophobia)
Trachoma (pain, discharge, lymphoid hypertrophy)
Cluster headaches (lacrimation, unilateral)
Leptospirosis (fever, myalgia)
Chemical irritation (eg. pool chlorine)
Excess alcohol
Drug abuse (eg. cocaine)

SYNDROMES (see SYNDROMES SECTION 6)

Louis-Bar syn. (mental deterioration, telangiectasia)
Reiter syn. (urethritis, arthritis)
Stevens-Johnson syn. (erythema, stomatitis)
Tolosa-Hunt syn. (ptosis, unilateral ophthalmoplegia)
Toxic shock syn. (fever, diarrhoea, vomiting)
Behcet's syn. (arthritis, genital and mouth ulcers)
Heerfordt's syn. (sarcoiditis, adenitis)
Richner-Hanhart syn. (tyrosinaemia)
Rieger syn. (iris dysgenesis, small teeth)
Uveoparotid syn. (parotid hypertrophy, facial paralysis)
Vogt-Koyangi-Harada syn. (vertigo, blind)

See also symptoms listed under Eye

Eye, Red
See Eye, Inflamed or Red

Eye, Watery

EXCESS TEAR PRODUCTION

Trauma and emotion
Infections (inflammation, pus)
Foreign bodies (pain, inflammation)
Dendritic ulcers
Congenital glaucoma
Congenital cataract
Iritis (pain, inflammation)
Entropion (infolding of lower lid)
Trichiasis (ingrown eye lash)

OBSTRUCTED TEAR DRAINAGE

Congenital tear duct obstruction
Trauma to medial canthus
Ectropion (everted lower lid)
Proptosis
Foreign body in tear duct
Radiation
Dacryocystitis
Sinusitis (pain, fever)

Eyelid Disease

Stye (tender red swelling)
Chalazion (Meibomian gland infection)
Blepharitis (generalised inflammation of lid margins)
Entropion (inward rolling of lower lid)
Ectropion (outward rolling of lower lid)
Allergic dermatitis (swollen excoriated lids)
Ptosis (see separate entry)
Thyrotoxicosis (upper lid retraction)
Trigeminal neuralgia (blepharospasm)
Myokymia (twitching with fatigue)
Basal and squamous cell carcinomas of lid
Keratoacanthoma (central core, rapid growth)
Trichiasis (ingrowing eye lash)
Xanthelasma (fatty deposit)
Dermatocholasis (senile skin folds)
Lagophthalmos (Bell's palsy, proptosis)
Floppy eyelid syn.

See also Eyelids, Abnormal

Eyelid Oedema
See Oedema, Eyelid

Eyelid, Drooping
See Ptosis; Eyelids, Abnormal

Eyelids, Abnormal

Coffin-Lowry syn. (antimongoloid eye slant)
Floppy eyelid syn.
Neu-Lexova syn. (absent eyelids, facial anomalies)
Treacher-Collins syn. (notched lower lid, face anomalies)
Williams' syn. (prominent epicanthal folds)

See also Eyelid Disease

Facial Anomaly Associated Syndromes

Apert syn. (exophthalmos, syndactyly)
Bloom syn. (malar hypoplasia, Jewish)
Cri-du-chat syn. (cat cry, ocular hypertelorism)
Coffin-Lowry syn. (prominent lips, coarse facies)
Coffin-Siris syn. (coarse features, hypoplastic toe nails)
Crouzon syn. (disproportion, exophthalmos, squint)
Cushing syn. (central obesity, hirsute)
Down syn. (mental retardation, mongoloid facies)
Fetal alcohol syn. (hirsute, reduced growth)
Fragile X syn. (subnormal intelligence, overactive, large testes)

Hallermann-Streiff syn. (dwarf, cataracts)
Hunter syn. (gross facies, arthralgia, hepatomegaly)
Hurler syn. (dwarfism, gross facies, arthralgia)
Johanson-Blizzard syn. (aplastic alae nasi)
Lip-pit syn. (cleft palate)
Lowe syn. (epicanthal folds, cataracts)
Miller-Dieker syn. (small body, lissencephaly)
Moebius syn. (ptosis, ophthalmoplegia, fixed facies)
Neu-Lexova syn. (hypoplastic nose, oedema)
Oto-palatal-digital syn. (deaf, cleft palate)
Parkinsonism (fixed facies, tremor, rigidity)
Potter syn. (epicanthal folds, renal agenesis)
Proteus syn. (gross disfigurement)
Ramsay Hunt syn. (shingles)
Rubenstein-Taybi syn. (hypoplastic maxilla, cardiac anomalies)
Sanfilippo syn. (hypertrichosis, mental retardation)
Seckel syn. (hip and elbow dislocation)
Smith-Lemli-Opitz syn. (narrow forehead, nose abnormal)
Smith-Magenis syn. (brachycephaly, hoarse)
Soto syn. (developmental delay, accelerated childhood growth)
Stewart-Morgagni-Morel syn. (hyperostosis frontalis)
Sturge-Weber syn. (port wine stain, convulsions)
Treacher-Collins syn. (multiple abnormalities)
Uveoparotid syn. (uveitis, facial paralysis)
Waardenburg-Klein syn. (deaf, broad nose)
Williams syn. (prominent lips, pendular cheeks)
Wolf-Hirschhorn syn. (mental retardation)

See also Acne; Cleft Lip and/or Palate; Facial Erythema; Facial Pain

Facial Erythema

Excessively red face
Vasomotor instability (eg. flushing)
Rosacea
Seborrhoeic dermatitis
Superior vena caval syn. (see SYNDROMES SECTION 6)
Perioral dermatitis
Contact dermatitis
Atopic dermatitis (pruritic)
Psoriasis (scaling)
Excess topical steroid use
Sunburn
Light sensitivity
SLE (butterfly pattern rash)
Erysipelas
Dermatomyositis
Acne vulgaris
Sarcoidosis
Essential telangiectasia
Slapped cheek syn. (see SYNDROMES SECTION 6)
Birthmarks (eg. port wine stain)
Carcinoid syn. (see SYNDROMES SECTION 6)

See also Facial Anomaly Associated Syndromes

Facial Pain

Sinusitis (nasal discharge, fever, toothache)
Facial tissue infections (eg. cellulitis, anthrax, lupus)

Herpes simplex infection
Dental disease (eg. dental abscess, periodontal disease, pericoronitis, alveolar osteitis)
Oral mucosal ulcers
Sialitis (tender salivary glands)
Stomatitis (see separate entry)
Migraine (nausea, unilateral, photophobia)
Cluster headache (paroxysmal, unilateral)
Temporomandibular joint disorders
Trigeminal neuralgia (severe, sudden intermittent)
Muscle spasms
Temporal arteritis
Tumours of sinuses, nose and facial nerves
Buccal candidiasis (white patches)
Trauma (eg. fractures)

SYNDROMES (see SYNDROMES SECTION 6)

Carotodynia syn. (tender carotid bulb)
Chinese restaurant syn. (nausea, chest pain)
Gradenigo'syn. (headache, diplopia)
Ramsay Hunt syn. (blistering rash)

See also Earache; Eye Pain; Facial Anomaly Associated Syndromes; Headache

Facial Weakness

Bell's palsy (unilateral, temporary)
Cerebrovascular disease (other neurological defects common)
Cerebral neoplasm
Multiple sclerosis
Motor neurone disease (bilateral)
Parkinson's disease (tremor, gait abnormal)
Parotid tumours (unilateral)
Brain stem encephalitis
Sarcoidosis
Poliomyelitis
Herpes zoster infection (vesicular rash, pain)
Mumps
Other serious viral infections
Tetanus (pain, paralysis)
Lyme disease
Brucellosis
Other serious bacterial infections
Myasthenia gravis
Guillain-Barré syn.
Muscular dystrophies
Trauma
Emotional and psychogenic

Faeces, Abnormal

See Constipation; Diarrhoea; Incontinence of Faeces; Melaena and Rectal Bleeding

Failure to Thrive

Child under 2 years, below 3rd percentile
Starvation (neglected, deprived or abused)
Chronic urinary infection (proteinuria)
Other chronic or recurrent infections
Gut infestations (eg. giardia, roundworms, tapeworms)

Genetic (familial)
Chromosomal (Down's syn., Turner's syn.)
Lead or mercury poisoning
Pyloric stenosis (projectile vomiting, 95% male)
Hypervitaminosis D (nausea, constipation, tremor)
Congenital heart disease (cyanosis, murmur)
Aminoacidosis (eg. phenylketonuria)
Cystinosis
Glycogen storage disease
Cerebral palsy and other CNS disease
Cystic fibrosis (steatorrhoea, respiratory disease)
Coeliac disease
Food allergies and intolerances
Achondroplasia
Renal dysplasia or obstruction
Rickets (weakness, leg pains)
Hypothyroidism (dry, yellow, cold skin)
Hypopituitarism (weak, hair loss)
Diabetes mellitus (polyuria, polydipsia)
Iron deficiency anaemia
Hypoparathyroidism
Adrenocortical insufficiency
Chronic osteomyelitis
Chronic septic arthritis
De Lange syn. (microcephaly, dwarf, mental retardation)
Fallot's tetralogy (cardiac lesions, cyanosis)
Fanconi syn.
Nezelof syn. (diarrhoea, infections, rashes)
Russel-Silver syn. (precocious puberty)
von Gierke syn. (hypoglycaemia, diarrhoea)

*See also Cachexia; Growth, Reduced; Malabsorption;
Weight Loss*

Faint
See Syncope; Drop Attack

Fall
Unexpected fall, particularly in the elderly
Sensory impairment (eg. poor vision)
Proprioceptive disturbances
Vestibular disease (dizzy)
Pernicious anaemia (sore tongue)
Cerebrovascular insufficiency (arteriosclerosis)
Transient ischaemic attacks (brief, headache)
Parkinson's disease (tremor, rigidity)
Cervical myelopathy
Dementia (eg. Alzheimer's disease)
Depression (poor sleep pattern)
Anxiety
Arthritis (joint pain, poor joint function)
Contractures
Muscle weakness (see separate entry)
Foot drop
Postural hypotension (vertigo)
Congestive cardiac failure (dyspnoea)
Malnutrition
Alcohol excess
Drugs (eg. sedatives, psychotropics, antihypertensives)
See also Drop Attack; Syncope (Faint)

Familiarity
See Déjà Vu

Fat
See Obesity

Fatigue, Abnormal (Asthenia)

GENERAL
Acute or chronic viral, bacterial or zoonotic infection
Chronic allergy reaction
Chronic illness of any type
Chronic pain
Connective tissue diseases (eg. rheumatoid arthritis,
SLE, scleroderma)
Dietary insufficiency
Excess physical or mental activity
Heavy metal poisoning (eg. lead, mercury, arsenic)
Malignancy of any organ
Oversleeping
Sedentary lifestyle
Shift work
Sleep apnoea (snoring)
Sleep deprivation

CARDIOVASCULAR
Agranulocytosis (fever, sore throat)
Anaemia (pallor, palpitations, dyspnoea)
Cardiac failure (dyspnoea, cough, orthopnoea)
Congenital heart disease (dyspnoea, cyanosis)
Cor pulmonale (cough, dyspnoea, oedema)
Endocarditis (fever, arthralgia, malaise)
Leukaemia (anorexia, arthralgia, fever)
Mitral stenosis (paroxysmal nocturnal dyspnoea)
Myocarditis (vertigo, dyspnoea, nausea)
Subacute bacterial endocarditis (fever, arthralgia)
Thalassaemia major or minor

METABOLIC
Avitaminosis
Diabetes mellitus (polyuria, polydipsia, blurred vision)
Electrolyte disturbances
Endocrine disorders (eg. hypopituitarism, acromegaly,
Addison's disease)
Hyperparathyroidism (polyuria, polydipsia, nausea)
Malnutrition
Menopause (sweating, irritability)
Metabolic disorders (eg. phenylketonuria, Fanconi syn.,
cystic fibrosis)
Hypothyroidism (constipation, hoarse, dry skin)
Obesity
Thyrotoxicosis (sweating, weight loss, heat intolerance)

SYNDROMES (see SYNDROMES SECTION 6)
AIDS (splenomegaly, adenitis, skin lesions)
Chronic fatigue syn. (postviral, poor exercise tolerance)
Cushing syn. (moon face, obese, striae)
Myelodysplastic syn. (anaemia)
Post-polio syn. (myalgia, arthralgia, weakness)
Sick building syn.

OTHER

Brucellosis (fever, headache, arthralgia)
Cerebrovascular accident (neurological signs)
Cirrhosis (anaemia, nausea, RUQ pain)
Head injury
Hepatitis (jaundice, nausea, fever)
Hepatoma (cachexia, ascites)
Hodgkin's disease (adenitis, pruritus, fever)
Hookworm (dyspnoea, diarrhoea, dermatitis)
Malabsorption syndromes
Multiple myeloma (bone pain, anaemia, weight loss)
Multiple sclerosis
Myasthenia gravis (ptosis, diplopia)
Myelofibrosis (splenomegaly)
Osteomalacia and rickets (bone weakness)
Parkinson's disease (tremor, abnormal gait)
Polycythaemia vera (weakness, headache, pruritus)
Polymyalgia rheumatica (muscle pain)
Polyneuritis (limb pain, anaesthesia)
Rheumatic fever (arthralgia, rash, corea)
Rickettsioses (muscle pain, rash, malaise)
Temporal arteritis (occipital headaches, jaw claudication)
Trypanosomiasis (fever, headache, neurological signs)
Tuberculosis
Ulcerative colitis (diarrhoea)
Uraemia (hypertension, anaemia, headache)
Recreational drugs (eg. marijuana, cocaine)
Excess caffeine
Alcohol abuse
Drugs (eg. antihistamines, sedatives, analgesics, beta-blockers)

Fear

See Phobia

Feet

See Foot Anomaly Associated Syndromes

Fever (Pyrexia)

INFECTIONS

Bacterial, viral, rickettsial and protozoal infections
Disseminated mycoses
Bacterial endocarditis (arthralgia, fatigue)
Tuberculosis (cough, sputum, weight loss)
Toxoplasmosis (adenitis, malaise, rash)
Hepatitis (jaundice, malaise, nausea)
Brucellosis (headache, arthralgia, malaise)
Abscess in any tissue, organ or teeth(eg.
phenylketonuria)

SYNDROMES (see SYNDROMES SECTION 6)

AIDS (splenomegaly, adenitis, skin lesions)
Chronic fatigue syn. (poor exercise tolerance)
Felty's syn. (polyarthritis, splenomegaly)
Kawasaki syn. (infant, rash, red feet and hands)
Letterer-Siwe syn. (infant, wasting, rash)
Loeffler's syn. (wheeze, cough)

Nezelof syn. (infant, diarrhoea, infections)
Neuroleptic malignant syn. (tranquillizer use)
Riley-Day syn. (Jewish, no lacrimation, sweating)
Stevens-Johnson syn. (conjunctivitis, erythema)
Sweet's syn. (neutrophilia, painful skin plaques)
Toxic shock syn. (vomiting, diarrhoea, hypotension)
Uveoparotid syn. (uveitis, parotid hypertrophy)
Vogt-Koyangi-Harada syn. (blind, uveitis)
Wiskott-Aldrich syn. (eczema, thrombocytopenia)

OTHER

Rheumatic fever (rash, chorea, arthralgia, nodules)
Haemolytic or sickle cell anaemia (jaundice)
Agranulocytosis (sore throat, malaise)
Leukaemias (malaise, arthralgia, pallor)
Hodgkin's disease (adenitis, pruritus, fatigue)
Thyrotoxicosis (sweats, palpitations)
Neoplasms (many types, but not all)
Gastrointestinal inflammations (eg. gastritis, appendicitis, Crohn's disease)
Chronic hepatic disease (eg. cirrhosis)
Pulmonary embolism (chest pain, dyspnoea, cough)
Temporal arteritis (temple pain and tenderness)
Vasculitis
Lymphomas
Phaeochromocytoma (hypertension)
Whipple's disease (intestinal lipodystrophy)
Hypothalamic lesions
Serum sickness
Rheumatoid arthritis
SLE (facial rash)
Polymyositis
Other autoimmune diseases (eg. scleroderma)
Sarcoidosis (skin lesions, cough, malaise)
Familial Mediterranean fever (Middle East ethnicity)
Drugs (e.g. methyldopa, amphetamines, cocaine, LSD)

Finger

*See Hand Anomaly Associated Syndromes; Hand Pain;
Polydactyly; Syndactyly*

Fits

See Convulsions

Flashes, Visual

Migraine (headache, photophobia, nausea)
Vitreous haemorrhage
Posterior vitreous detachment

Flatulence

Passing of gas per rectum
Aerophagia (eg. with terror or rapid eating)
Gaseous foods (eg. carbonated drinks)
Fermentation
Crohn's disease (diarrhoea, pain, anorexia)
Diverticulitis (alt. diarrhoea & constipation, pain)
Bacterial or protozoal bowel infections

Floppy Baby

Generalised muscle hypotonia in infancy

Viral or bacterial infection
Cerebral palsy (ataxia)
Starvation/Malnutrition
Werdig-Hoffman disease (familial, progressive, muscular dystrophy)
Myasthenic syndromes
Glycogen storage disease
Duchenne muscular dystrophy
Congenital muscular dystrophy
Intellectual deficits
Aminoaciduria
Osteogenesis imperfecta (fracture bones easily)
Rickets
Other neuromuscular diseases

SYNDROMES (see SYNDROMES SECTION 6)

Down syn. (typical facies, protruding tongue)
Ehlers-Danlos syn.
Marfan's syn.
Malabsorption syn.
Prader-Willi syn.

See also Paralysis and Muscular Weakness
See also symptoms listed under Neurological Symptoms

Fluid, Excess

See Ascites; Oedema

Flush

Thyrotoxicosis (sweating, tachycardia, heat intolerance)
Hormonal therapy
Menopausal syn. (menstrual changes, 45-55 years)
Anaphylaxis
Cushing's syn. (striae, obese)
Emotional states
Phaeochromocytoma (hypertension)
Pituitary disease
Carcinoid syn. (palpitations, bronchospasm, diarrhoea)
Stokes-Adams syn. (syncope, bradycardia)
Superior vena cava syn. (head and neck oedema)
Dengue fever (headache)
Alcohol

See also Erythema; Sweating, Excessive and Abnormal

Foot Anomaly Associated Syndromes

Edwards syn. (rocker-bottom feet, micrognathia)
Leriche syn. (cold feet, claudication, impotence)
Morton syn. (abnormal shaped foot)
Proteus syn. (gross disfigurement)
Rubenstein-Taybi syn. (broad toes)
Tarsal tunnel syn. (posterior tibial nerve lesion)

See also Foot Pain; Leg Pain; Syndactyly

Foot Pain

Osteoarthritis or rheumatoid arthritis
Diabetic neuropathy
Infection (eg. cellulitis, septic arthritis, TB)
Gout (often first metatarsophalangeal joint)
Ligamentous or muscular strain
Synovitis
Corn or callus
Plantar wart (verrucae)
Bunion
Bursitis (swollen)
Tendinitis
Tendoachilles trauma
Plantar fasciitis (under heel, tender)
Peripheral vasculitis
Erythema nodosum (rash, myalgia)
Alcoholic neuropathy
Pernicious anaemia (smooth sore tongue, paraesthesiae)
Arteriosclerosis (claudication, pallor)
Raynaud's phenomenon
Sudeck's dystrophy
Paget's disease (bone pain, kyphosis, large head)
Osteosarcoma
Morton's neuroma (between metatarsals and toes)
March or stress fracture (forefoot)
Hallux valgus
Fifth toe varus
Hammer or mallet toe
Epidermoid cyst (sole)
Dupuytren's (Ledderhose's) contracture
Ingrown nail with or without paronychia
Onychogryphosis
Nerve entrapment syndromes
Kohler's disease (navicular osteochondritis)
Exostoses
'Stone' bruise
Anterior impingement syn. (ankle, anterior)
Posterior impingement syn. (ankle, posterior)
Marfan's syn.
Tarsal tunnel syn.
Phlebitis

See also Arthritis and Arthralgia; Foot Anomaly Associated Syndromes; Leg Pain

Formication

Sensation of insects crawling on skin

Neurological sensory disorders
Psychiatric syndromes
Drugs

Fractures, Pathological

Bone fractures occurring with minimal trauma

Osteoporosis (female, elderly)
Milkman's syn. (pseudo-fractures, osteomalacia)
Riley-Day syn. (Jewish, no lacrimation)
Osteogenesis imperfecta (blue sclera)

Frequency of Micturition

See Polyuria and Pollakiuria

Frigidity
Lack of libido
Menopause (flushes, menstrual irregularities)
Hormone therapy (eg. oral contraceptives)
Psychological and psychiatric disturbances
Postnatal period
Fatigue and anxiety
Pituitary tumour
Drugs (eg. hypotensives, tranquillizers)

See also Libido, Reduced; Orgasm, Lack of

Gait, Abnormal
See SIGNS SECTION 2: Gait, Abnormal

Galactorrhoea
See Nipple Discharge

Gassy Urine
See Pneumaturia

Genital Ulcer
Herpes infection (pain)
Syphilis (painless)
Chancroid (painful)
Lymphogranuloma venereum
Behcet's syn. (uveitis, convulsions, arthritis)
Donovanosis (granuloma inguinale)
Drug eruption
Scabies
Malignancy
Pyoderma
Trauma

Giant (Gigantism)
See Growth and Height, Excessive; Head, Large

Giddiness
See Vertigo

Gingivitis
See Stomatitis and Gingivitis

Glands
See Adenitis and Lymphadenopathy; Salivary Gland Pain and/or Swelling

Glossitis
Sore mouth
Vitamin B deficiency
Denture problems
Candidiasis (white plaque)
Lichen planus

Hypothyroidism (fatigue, dry skin)
Pernicious anaemia
Iron deficiency
Diabetes mellitus (thirst, polyuria, tiredness)
Folate deficiency
Other anaemias
Oesophageal reflux (waterbrash, retrosternal pain)
Menopause (hot flushes, irregular menstruation)
Systemic infection
Chemical irritation
Psychogenic
Drug side effect

See also Mouth, Dry

Goitre
Thyroid gland enlargement
Simple endemic goitre (asymptomatic)
Thyrotoxicosis (weak, sweaty, weight loss)
Thyroid carcinoma (painless, normal function)
Thyroid cysts and nodules
Hypothyroidism (dry skin, myalgia, psychoses)
Iodine deficiency (diffuse, painless)
Hashimoto's thyroiditis
De Quervain's thyroiditis (painful)
Grave's disease
Laryngeal tumours and sacs
Cervical lymphadenitis
Drugs (eg. Interferon, lithium, amiodarone)

Groin Lump
Inguinal hernia (male, may be reducible)
Femoral hernia (usually female, may be reducible)
Inflamed or scarred lymph node
Femoral artery aneurysm (pulsatile, non-tender)
Psoas abscess (tender)
Lipoma or hydrocele of cord
Undescended testicle (empty scrotum)
Saphena varx (varicose vein)
Lymphoma

See also SIGNS SECTION 2: Abdominal Mass

Groin Pain
Strained ligament or tendon
Testicular torsion or infection
Osteoarthritis of hip
Osteitis pubis
Ovarian tumours
Endometriosis (cyclical, menorrhagia)
Abdominal abscess (tender, fever)
Inguinal hernia (above inguinal ligament)
Femoral hernia (below inguinal ligament)
Obturator hernia (female, hip kept flexed)
Nerve root entrapment
Neuralgia
Prostatitis

See also Abdominal Pain; Pelvic Pain

Growth and Height, Excessive (Gigantism)

Familial or genetic
Physiological growth advance
Precocious puberty
Pituitary disease (eg. acromegaly)
Cerebral space occupying lesions
Pituitary or gonadal tumours (continuing rapid growth)
Diabetes mellitus (polyuria, polydipsia, lethargy)
Pubertal hypogonadism (tall, small testes, high voice)
XYY syn. (male, violent)
Growth hormone excess
Hyperthyroidism
Congenital adrenal hyperplasia (continuing rapid growth)
Gonadotrophin producing hepatoblastoma
Marfan's syn. (long limbs, tall and thin)
Homocystinuria (thin, mental retardation)
Soto syn.
Klinefelter's syn.

See also Head, Large; Obesity

Growth, Reduced (Dwarfism)

Familial or genetic (chromosomal abnormality)
Nutrition (eg. kwashiorkor, marasmus)
Bone disease (eg. rickets)
Renal disease(eg. chronic renal failure, nephritis)
Metabolic disease (eg. cystic fibrosis, Fanconi's syn.)
Psychiatric disorders (eg. anorexia nervosa)
Hypothyroidism (mental retardation, dry skin)
Hypopituitarism (fatigue, hair loss, impotence)
Congenital or chronic heart disease
Hypergonadism (sexual precocity)
Asthma (expiratory wheeze, dyspnoea, cough)
Crohn's disease (irregular bowel habits, abdominal pain)
Coeliac disease (malnutrition)
Zinc deficiency (hypogonadism, dermatitis)
Chronic diseases of other major organs
Drugs

SYNDROMES (see SYNDROMES SECTION 6)

Bassen-Kornzweig syn. (ataxia, malabsorption)
Bloom syn. (Jewish, photosensitive skin)
CHARGE syn. (coloboma of iris/retina, congenital heart disease, choanal atresia)
Cori syn. (glycogen storage disorder)
De Lange syn. (mental retardation, hirsute, microcephaly)
Down syn. (mental retardation, typical facies)
Dubowitz syn. (ptosis, mental retardation)
Fetal alcohol syn. (hirsute, mental retardation)
Hallermann-Streiff syn. (cataracts, face anomalies)
Hurler syn. (gross facies, arthralgia)
Maroteaux-Lamy syn. (bone dysplasia, cataracts)
Mauriac syn. (obese, diabetes, hepatomegaly)
Miller-Dieker syn. (face abnormal, lissencephaly)
Morquio syn. (bone dysplasia, cataracts)
Noonan syn. (webbed neck, shield chest)
Rothmund-Thomson syn.(erythema, skin atrophy)
Russel-Silver syn. (asymmetry, precocious puberty)
Scheie syn. (recurrent respiratory infections, kyphosis)
Sly syn. (recurrent respiratory infections, kyphosis)
Seckel syn. (hip and elbow dislocation)

Turner's syn. (amenorrhoea, genital hypoplasia, scant hair)
von Gierke syn. (hypoglycaemia, diarrhoea)
Wolf-Hirschhorn syn. (mental retardation)

See also Failure to Thrive

Gum Pain

See Stomatitis and Gingivitis

Gut

See symptoms listed under Intestine

Gynaecological Pain

See Pelvic Pain

Gynaecology

See Amenorrhoea and Oligomenorrhoea; Breast, Atrophic or Atresic; Breast Pain; Dysmenorrhoea; Genital Ulcer; Gynaecomastia; Infertility; Lactation, Failure of; Menorrhagia; Mucous Membranes, Dry; Pregnancy Associated Syndromes; Puberty, Delayed; Puberty, Early; Vaginal and Uterine Bleeding, Abnormal

Gynaecomastia

Breast enlargement, male
Old age
Puberty (male and female)
Thyrotoxicosis (sweaty, fatigue, weight loss)
Hepatic disease (eg. cirrhosis)
Adrenal tumours
Testicular tumours
Drugs (eg. cimetidine, ketaconazole, oestrogens, spironolactone, alkylating cytotoxics, anabolics)

Haematemesis

Vomiting blood
Peptic ulceration of stomach or oesophagus (epigastric pain, nausea)
Oesophageal varices (splenomegaly, cirrhosis)
Gastritis (pain, anorexia, nausea)
Oesophageal or stomach carcinoma (fullness, nausea, pain)
Cirrhosis (fatigue, anorexia, nausea)
Mallory-Weiss syn. (excess vomiting, forceful vomits)
Yellow fever (jaundice, muscle pain, purpura)
Portal hypertension gastropathy
Leiomyoma
Lymphoma
Vascular malformation
Osler's disease
Oesophageal or stomach foreign body
Drugs (eg. NSAIDs, warfarin)

See also Bleeding, Excessive

Haematuria and Red Urine
Urinary blood

BLOOD IN URINE
Urinary tract infections of any type
Glomerulonephritis (oliguria, oedema, headache)
Cytomegalovirus (jaundice, neonate, purpura)
Renal and ureteric stones (severe pain, nausea)
Blackwater fever (severe form of malaria)
Bilharzia (urticaria, frequency, fever)
Renal tuberculosis
Bladder tumours (hypogastric pain)
Analgesic nephropathy (history of compound analgesics)
Haemoglobinuria
Acute renal failure (oliguria, nausea)
Haemophilia (melaena, excessive bleeding, ecchymoses)
Renal or bladder trauma
Polycystic kidneys
Extremely vigorous exercise
Alport syn. (deaf)
Goodpasture syn. (haemoptysis)
Haemolytic-uraemic syn. (anaemia, thrombocytopenia)
Henoch-Schoenlein syn. (purpura, abdominal pain)

NONBLOOD CAUSES
Porphyria (urine turns red when left standing)
Phenolphthalein and vegetable dyes (eg. fava beans, beetroot)
Heavy urate concentration (pink)\par Drugs (eg. warfarin, heparin, pyridium, aspirin, cyclophosphamide, carbidopa, phenindione, metronidazole)

See also Bleeding, Excessive; Renal Disease Associated Syndromes.
See also PATHOLOGY SECTION 4: Haematuria

Haemoptysis
Coughing blood
Bronchitis (cough, fever)
Bronchiectasis (purulent sputum, cough, rales)
Pneumonia (dyspnoea, chest pain, cough)
Lung abscess (purulent sputum, fever, malaise)
Tuberculosis (cough, malaise, fever)
Bronchial carcinoma (wheeze, cough, malaise)
Pulmonary thromboembolism (pain, cough, dyspnoea)
Cystic fibrosis (failure to thrive, lung infections)
Laryngeal tumour (dyspnoea, hoarse, pain)
Pulmonary oedema (crepitations, dyspnoea)
Mitral stenosis
Bleeding diatheses (easy bruising)
Coagulopathy
Chest trauma
Aspergilloma
Ascariasis (cough, colic, fever)
Hookworm (pruritus, diarrhoea, fatigue)
Melioidosis (chest pain, cough, skin lesions)
Foreign body in respiratory tract

SYNDROMES (see SYNDROMES SECTION 6)
Behcet's syn.
Goodpasture's syn. (dyspnoea, haematuria, anaemia, cough)

Henoch-Schoenlein syn. (purpura, abdominal pain)
See also Cough

Haemorrhage
See Bleeding, Excessive; Epistaxis; Haematemesis; Haemoptysis; Melaena and Rectal Bleeding; Vaginal and Uterine Bleeding, Abnormal

Haemorrhoids (Piles)
Constipation
Constipation
Straining (eg. heavy lifting, excess coughing)
Pregnancy
Portal hypertension (hepatomegaly)
Congenital
Obesity

Hair Loss and Thinning
See Alopecia

Hair, Excess (Hypertrichosis)
See Hirsutism and Hypertrichosis

Halitosis
Bad breath
Smoking
Chronic nasal and sinus infections
Dental caries (pain, discolouration)
Gum infections and poor oral hygiene
Tonsillitis (pain, fever)
Systemic infections (fever)
Lung infections and abscesses (cough, fever)
Peritonitis (pain, rigid abdomen)
Appendicitis (RIF pain, anorexia, nausea)
Gastro-oesophageal reflux (retrosternal pain, waterbrash)
Pharyngeal diverticulum
Other gastrointestinal diseases
Renal failure (ammonia smell)
Diabetes (acetone smell)
Fetor hepaticus of advanced liver disease
Stomatitis (see separate entry)
Xerostomia (see Mouth, Dry entry)
Periodontal disease (sore gums)
Oral or laryngeal carcinoma
Ozaena (chronic rhinitis)
Tuberculosis (cough, malaise, haemoptysis)
Syphilis (diverse symptoms)
Lung carcinoma (cachexia, cough)
Ketoacidosis (nausea, fatigue)
Agranulocytosis (chills, fever, sore throat)
Bronchiectasis (purulent sputum, cough, haemoptysis)
Salivary gland dysfunction (eg. Sjögren syn.)
Quinsy (severe throat pain, fever)
Vincent's angina (gums painful and bleeding)
Hiatus hernia (burping, heartburn)
Pyloric stenosis (gastric fullness, nausea)
Gastric carcinoma (epigastric pain, dyspepsia)

Gastrointestinal infections
Leukaemia (malaise, anorexia, fever, pallor)
Dehydration (poor skin turgor, dry mucous membranes)
Oesophageal diverticula (dysphagia, regurgitation)
Drugs (eg. lithium, griseofulvin, penicillamine)

Hallucinations

Schizophrenia (withdrawn, delusions, loss of ego)
Affective disorders
Other organic mental states
Metabolic encephalopathy
Encephalitis (fever, malaise, neck stiffness)
Epilepsy (auras, abscences, convulsions)
Delerium tremens
Alcohol dependence withdrawal
Posthypnotic
Charles Bonnet syn. (elderly, affective disorder)
Iatrogenic (eg. psychoactive drugs)
Drugs (eg. LSD, heroin, marijuana, amphetamines)

Halos, Visual

Cataracts (cloudy cornea)
Glaucoma (subacute angle closure type)
Allergic conjunctivitis
Conjunctival oedema
Corneal disease
Contact lenses

Hand Anomaly Associated Syndromes

Apert syn. (syndactyly, frontal bossing)
Coffin-Lowry syn. (tapered fingers)
Cronkhite syn. (pigmented hands and feet)
Down syn. (typical facies, single palmar crease)
Ellis-van Crevald syn. (polydactyly, short limbs)
Hurler syn. (claw hand, dwarf, arthralgia)
Jaccoud syn. (rheumatoid changes)
Klumpke syn. (limp wrist, neonate)
Marfan syn. (arachnodactyly, kyphoscoliosis)
Oto-palatal-digital syn. (cleft palate)
Patau syn. (polydactyly, cardiac anomalies)
Proteus syn. (gross disfigurement)
Shoulder-Hand syn. (hand atrophy, pain)

*See also Arthritis and Arthralgia; Arm Pain; Hand Pain;
Polydactyly; Syndactyly
See also SIGNS SECTION 2: Nail Changes*

Hand Pain

Raynaud's disease (cyanosis, rubor, pallor)
Polycythaemia vera (fingers, fatigue, pruritus)
Neuralgia (sharp, radiating pain)
Rheumatoid arthritis (poor function, nodes)
Pyogenic arthritis (hot, swollen joints)
Cellulitis (fever, erythema, oedema)
Osteoarthritis (stiffness, reduced function)
Tenosynovitis (swelling, impaired function)
Repetitive strain injury (controversial)
De Quervain's tenovaginitis (tender radial styloid)
Kienbock's disease (lunate pain, impaired grip)

Trauma and fractures (eg. scaphoid fracture)
Hypothyroidism (causes carpal tunnel syn.)

SYNDROMES (see SYNDROMES SECTION 6)

Carpal tunnel syn. (weakness, tingling, wrist radiation)
Occupational overuse syn. (burning pain)
Raynaud's phenomenon (pallor, cyanosis, oedema of
fingers)
Shoulder-Hand syn. (arthritis, atrophy)

*See also Arm Pain; Hand Anomaly Associated
Syndromes; Arthritis and Arthralgia; Wrist Pain*

Hand Wasting

Carpal tunnel syn.
Rheumatoid arthritis
Median or ulnar nerve neuropathy
Ulnar nerve trauma (elbow or palm)
Ulnar nerve entrapment
Severe arthritis causing nerve entrapment
Cervical rib or band
Vertebral trauma or arthritis
Spinal tumour or cancer
Syringomyelia
Spinal vascular lesions
Spinal muscular atrophy
Spondylosis
Sympathetic dystrophy
Motor neurone disease
Poliomyelitis
Neurofibromas (eg. von Recklinghausen's disease)
Secondary carcinoma (eg. lung, breast)
Irradiation of brachial plexus
Brachial plexus neuritis
Amyloidosis
Hypothyroidism
Pronator syn.
Myopathy of Gower
Inclusion body myositis
Dystrophia myotonica

Head

*See Facial Anomaly Associated Syndromes; Facial Pain;
Facial Weakness; Head, Large; Microcephaly
See also symptoms listed under Brain*

Headache

GENERAL

Bacterial, viral, rickettsial and protozoal infections of any
organ but particularly CNS
Fever of any cause
Ocular disorders (eg. refraction error, glaucoma)
Dental causes (eg. root abscess)
Muscular spasm (stress, occipital or temporal)
Trauma
Fatigue (acute or chronic)
Drugs (eg. methyldopa)

INFECTIONS
Sinusitis (frontal, fever, rhinorrhoea, face ache)
Mastoiditis (tender mastoid, earache)
Meningitis (fever, neck stiffness, confusion)
Otitis media (fever, ear pain)
Encephalitis (fever, malaise, neck stiffness)
Brucellosis (fever, arthralgia, fatigue)
Cerebral abscess (preceding infection, neurological signs)
Syphilis (varied symptoms)
Dengue fever (retro-orbital pain)

CENTRAL NERVOUS SYSTEM
Cerebral tumour (neurological signs)
Migraine (nausea, photophobia, vertigo)
Cerebrovascular accident (neurological signs)
Cerebral haemorrhage (subdural or subarachnoid)
Trigeminal neuralgia (face, frontal, unilateral)
Cluster headaches (sudden, unilateral, lacrimation)
Neuralgia (sharp localised pain)
Prolactinoma (visual defect, cranial nerve palsy)
Psychiatric disorders (eg. phobia, anxiety)

ENDOCRINE
Adrenal insufficiency (fatigue, nausea, diarrhoea)
Acromegaly (gigantism, vision loss, amenorrhoea)
Diabetes insipidus (polyuria, polydipsia)
Hypothyroidism (dry skin, fatigue, cold intolerance)
Phaeochromocytoma (hypertension, sweating, abdominal pain)
Menopause (flushes, lightheaded, amenorrhoea)

SYNDROMES (see SYNDROMES SECTION 6)
Chinese restaurant syn. (nausea, facial pressure)
Chronic fatigue syn. (fever, poor exercise tolerance)
Cushing's syn. (hirsute, obese, ecchymoses, plethora)
Gradenigo's syn. (diplopia, facial pain)
Post-traumatic cerebral syn. (vertigo, mental changes)
Premenstrual tension syn. (mastalgia, nausea)
Scapulocostal syn. (neck and arm pain)
Sick building syn. (fatigue, malaise)
Sticky platelet syn. (strokes, migraines)
SUNCT syn. (very brief, unilateral)
Toxic shock syn. (vomiting, diarrhoea, fever)
Vogt-Koyanagi-Harada syn. (blind, fever)

OTHER
Hypertension (fatigue, tinnitus)
Anaemia (fatigue, palpitations)
Polycythaemia vera (malaise, pruritus)
Uraemia (fatigue, pruritus, thirst)
Glomerulonephritis (oliguria, malaise, oedema)
Temporomandibular joint dysfunction
Vascular anomalies
Cervical osteoarthritis
Temporal arteritis (unilateral, visual disturbances)
Glaucoma (visual disturbance)
Pre-eclampsia (pregnancy, hypertension)
SLE (rash, arthralgia)
Carotodynia (neck pain, unilateral, tender carotid artery)
Paget's disease (bone pain)
Anaphylaxis

Head, Large
Acromegaly (large jaw, large hands)
Hydrocephalus
Dandy-Walker syn. (vomiting, nystagmus, cleft palate)
Proteus syn. (gross disfigurement)
Stewart-Morgagni-Morel syn. (hyperostosis frontalis)

See also Growth and Height, Excessive

Hearing Loss
See Deafness

Heart
See Cardiac Associated Syndromes

Heartburn (Pyrosis)
Reflux oesophagitis (worse recumbent, waterbrash, cough)
Hiatus hernia (waterbrash, burping)
Peptic ulcer (tender, nausea, epigastric pain)
Stomach carcinoma (nausea, fullness, burping)
Over eating (flatulence, fullness)
Pregnancy
Excess alcohol use

See also Chest Pain; Dyspepsia

Height, Excessive
See Growth and Height, Excessive

Hemianopia
Loss of half visual field in eye
Cerebral abscess (preceding infection, headache)
Migraine (transient, headache)
Cerebral tumour (neurological signs)
Temporal arteritis (pain, unilateral)
Cerebrovascular accident (neurological signs)
Acromegaly (headache, gigantism, amenorrhoea)
Pituitary tumour (headache)

See also Blindness, Partial or Total

Hemiplegia
See Paralysis and Muscular Weakness; Paraplegia and Quadriplegia

Hepatomegaly
See SIGNS SECTION 2: Hepatomegaly

Hiccup (Hiccough)
Repeated spasm of diaphragm
Phrenic nerve irritation from any cause
Peptic oesophagitis and hiatus hernia
Cardiorespiratory disorders (eg. pneumonia, infarct)
Gastrointestinal disorders (eg. indigestion)
Emotional stress

Aerophagia
Encephalitis
Meningitis (neck stiff, headache, fever)
CNS infarct, tumour or abscess
Uraemia (fatigue, headache, thirst)
Diaphragmatic irritation (eg. subphrenic abscess)
Oesophageal obstruction (dysphagia)
Small bowel obstruction
Aortic aneurysm
Mediastinal mass
Foreign body in ear canal
Hyponatraemia
Hypocalcaemia
Addison's disease (skin pigmentation)
Sudden temperature change
Excess alcohol intake
Smoking
Psychogenic

Hip
See Leg Pain

Hirsutism and Hypertrichosis
Excess body hair
Racial, familial and genetic causes
Pregnancy or hormone therapy (eg. oral contraceptives)
Puberty or menopause
Acromegaly (coarse facies, backache)
Pituitary tumour
Various neoplastic diseases
Hypothyroidism (fatigue, cold intolerance, dry skin)
Porphyria (urine turns red when left standing)
Ovarian tumours and polycystic ovaries
Head injury
Starvation
Amenorrhoea (see separate entry)
Severe psychological stress
Hyperprolactinaemia
Drugs (eg. cortisone, diazoxide, streptomycin, minoxidil, penicillamine, danazol, cyclosporin A, hormones, anabolic steroids, metoclopramide, phenytoin)

SYNDROMES (see SYNDROMES SECTION 6)
Adrenogenital syn. (amenorrhoea, acne, rough skin)
Coffin-Siris syn. (mental retardation, hypoplastic toe nails)
Cushing syn. (moon face, bruising, obese)
De Lange syn. (microcephaly, dwarf)
Fetal alcohol syn. (face abnormal, mental retardation)
Sanfilippo syn. (mental retardation, gross facies)
Stein-Leventhal syn. (polycystic ovaries)

See also Puberty, Early; Virilism Associated Syndromes

Hoarseness
Laryngeal strain or trauma (eg. shouting)
Upper respiratory tract viral, bacterial or fungal infections
Intubation
Gastro-oesophageal reflux (retrosternal pain, waterbrash)

Laryngeal web (child)
Recurrent laryngeal nerve palsy
Diphtheria (throat pain and membrane, myocarditis)
Syphilis (various symptoms)
Laryngeal foreign body (cough, stridor, gagging)
Laryngeal or vocal cord tumour or polyp
Hypothyroidism (fatigue, dry skin, cold intolerance)
Acromegaly (gigantism, headache, amenorrhoea)
Angioneurotic oedema (allergic reaction)
Goitre (Pemberton's sign, see SIGNS SECTION 2)
Amyloidosis
Tuberculosis (cough, haemoptysis, malaise)
Neurological causes
Cerebrovascular accident
Aortic aneurysm (pain, dysphagia, dyspnoea)
Adrenogenital syn. (hirsute, amenorrhoea)
Smith-Magenis syn. (brachycephaly)
Inhalation of refluxed acid
Hot gas burns (eg. in fire)
Glottic web

Homosexuality Associated Syndromes
AIDS (splenomegaly, fever, skin lesions)
Gay bowel syn. (diarrhoea, tenesmus)
Idiopathic lymphadenopathy syn. (adenitis)

See also SYNDROMES SECTION 6

Hot Flush
See Flush; Facial Erythema

Hunger, Excess
(Bulimia, Polyphagia)
Excess appetite
Pregnancy
Thyrotoxicosis (sweating, heat intolerance)
Diabetes mellitus (polyuria, polydipsia)
Islet cell adenoma
Hypothalamic lesion (somnolence, hypogonadism)
Acromegaly
Peptic ulcer (epigastric pain)
Compulsive personality trait
Other psychiatric disorders
Drugs (eg. thioridazine)

Hydrophobia
Fear of drinking
Psychiatric disorders
Rabies (animal bite, paraesthesiae)

Hyperactivity
See Overactive

Hyperhidrosis
See Sweating, Excessive and Abnormal

Hypertension
See SIGNS SECTION 2: Hypertension

Hypertonicity
See SIGNS SECTION 2: Hypertonicity

Hypertrichosis
See Hirsutism and Hypertrichosis

Hyperventilation
See SIGNS SECTION 2: Hyperventilation

Hypocalcaemia
See Tetany

Hypochondria Associated Syndromes
Briquet syn.
Münchausen syn. (excess surgery)
SHAFT syn
See also SYNDROMES SECTION 6

Hypogastric Pain
See Pelvic Pain

Hypospadias
See Penis, Abnormal

Hypotension
See SIGNS SECTION 2: Hypotension

Hypotonia
See Paralysis and Muscular Weakness
See also symptoms listed under Neurological Symptoms

Ichthyosis
Generalised dryness and scaling of skin
Congenital
Ichthyosis vulgaris (widespread, inherited)
Acquired ichthyosis (precipitated by disease)
Hypothyrodisim (cold intolerance, lethargy)
Lymphomas (eg. Hodgkin's disease)
Sarcoidosis
Leprosy
Vitamin A deficiency
Harlequin syn. (see SYNDROMES SECTION 6)
Refsum's syn. (deaf, ataxia, polyneuritis)
Sjögren-Larsson syn. (spastic diplegia)
Drugs (eg. cimetidine, nicotinic acid, retinoids)

Icterus
See Jaundice

Impotence
Lack of male potency and libido
Psychogenic
Pituitary adenoma
Addison's disease (fatigue, anaemia, irritable)
Testicular disease or tumours
Diabetes mellitus (polyuria, polydipsia, blurred vision)
Thyrotoxicosis (sweating, fatigue, weight loss)
Alcohol and poisons (eg. lead, mercury)
Panhypopituitarism (fatigue, hypothermia)
Hypothyroidism
Hyperprolactinaemia
Multiple sclerosis (weakness, abnormal sensation)
Hypogonadism (tall, shrill voice, hairless)
Atherosclerosis
Hypercholesterolaemia
Pelvic or penile arterial obstruction
Hypertension
Prostatic carcinoma
Peyronie's disease
Paraplegia
Fractured penis (haematoma)
Depression (insomnia, loss of interest)
Fractured pelvis
Drugs (eg. antihypertensives, sedatives, tricyclics, clofibrate, cimetidine, thiazides, spironolactone, beta-blockers, digoxin, nicotine, marijuana)

SYNDROMES (see SYNDROMES SECTION 6)
Cushing syn. (obese, hirsute, ecchymoses)
Fröhlich syn. (thin skin, scanty hair, obese)
Klinefelter syn. (delayed puberty, hypoplastic genitalia)
Lariche syn. (claudication, poor pulses)

See also Ejaculation, Retarded; Ejaculation, Retrograde;
Infertility; Libido, Reduced

Incontinence of Faeces
Normal Sphincter
Diarrhoea (see separate entry)
Rectal carcinoma (irregular bowel habits, blood)
Ulcerative colitis (abdo. pain, diarrhoea)
Haemorrhoids (pain on defaecation, bright blood)
Mucosal prolapse
Diabetes mellitus (thirst, polyuria, malaise)

Abnormal Sphincter
Fissure-in-ano (pain on defaecation)
Recent childbirth
Neurogenic (demented)
Neurological conditions
Rectal prolapse
Anal or reianal infection
Sphincter trauma
Anal sexual intercourse

Incontinence of Urine

Urinary tract infections (dysuria, frequency, fever)
Urethral sphincter incompetence
Cerebrovascular accidents (neurological signs)
Senility (confusion of old age)
Diabetes mellitus (polydipsia, polyuria)
Diabetes insipidus (polydipsia, polyuria)
Oestrogen deficiency
Renal failure
Hypercalcaemia
Parkinson's disease (tremor, shuffling gait)
Spinal cord injuries, disease and tumours
Neurogenic bladder
Bladder tumour or stone (haematuria)
Enuresis
Anaphylaxis
Bladder distension due to partial obstruction
Vesico-vaginal fistulae
Urethrotrigonitis
Multiple sclerosis (diffuse neurological anomalies)
Reactive depression (anxiety, agitation, anger)
Urge syn. (nocturia, frequency, micturitional urgency)
Congenital malformations
Trauma to perineum (eg. parturition)
Surgery and radiation injury to perineum
Shock (eg. anaphylaxis)
Loss of consciousness (eg. convulsions)
Alcohol excess
Drugs (eg. alpha-blockers, caffeine, hypnotics, lithium, tranquillizers, diuretics, tricyclic antidepressants)

Incoordination

See Clumsiness

Indigestion

See Abdominal Pain; Burping, Excessive; Chest Pain; Dyspepsia; Heartburn

Infection (Recurrent) Associated Syndromes

AIDS (rash, fever, adenitis)
DiGeorge syn. (neonate, tetany, hypertelorism)
Myelodysplastic syn. (anaemia, abnormal white cells)
Nezelof syn. (diarrhoea, failure to thrive)
Schiei syn. (recurrent respiratory infections, kyphosis)
Sly syn. (recurrent respiratory infections, kyphosis)

See also Fever
See also SYNDROMES SECTION 6

Infertility

MALE

Poor coital technique
Psychosexual impotence
Premature ejaculation
Prostatectomy
Retrograde or retarded ejaculation (see separate entry)
Anatomical abnormalities of penis (eg. absent vas, hypospadias)

Genetic disease (eg. Klinefelter's syndrome)
Undescended testes
Hypogonadism
Diabetes mellitus
Overheating of testes (eg. tight clothing)
Testicular trauma or irradiation
Testicular torsion
Mumps orchitis
Syphilis
Testicular tumours
Pituitary disorders
Hypothyroidism
Zinc deficiency (reduced growth, dermatitis)
Vasectomy
Drugs (eg. guanethidine, cyclophosphamide, marijuana, steroids, heroin)

FEMALE

Vaginismus
Sperm antibodies
Cervical surgery or trauma
Endometriosis (abdominal pain)
Uterine maldevelopment
Uterine fibroids or polyps
Fallopian tube adhesions from peritonitis etc.
Salpingitis (pain, fever)
Pelvic inflammatory disease
Hydrosalpinx
Tuberculosis
Ovarian cysts or tumours
Pituitary disease
Asherman's syn. (amenorrhoea, post curette)
Sheehan's syn. (postpartum haemorrhage)
Stein-Leventhal syn. (polycystic ovaries)
Turner's syn. (genital hypoplasia, breast agenesis)

See also Impotence; Investigation: Infertility, Female; Infertility, Male

Inflamed Eye

See Eye, Inflamed or Red

Inguinal Pain

See Groin Pain

Insomnia

Inability to sleep

Anxiety and pain
Behaviour (eg. day time naps)
Evening exercise
Elderly (depression, irritable)
Psychiatric disorders (eg. schizophrenia, affective disorders)
Menopause (flush, sweating, mood changes)
Depression (anxiety, phobia)
Postpartum depression
Obstructive sleep apnoea (snoring)
Chorea (involuntary jerks, aphasia, weakness)
Sleep apnoea (snoring)

Alcohol withdrawal
Drugs (eg. anorectics, caffeine, pseudoephedrine)

SYNDROMES (see SYNDROMES SECTION 6)

Cushing syn. (obese, striae, weakness)
Post-traumatic stress syn. (after catastrophe, psychiatric problems)
Premenstrual syn. (headache, irritable)
Restless legs syn. (hyperkinesia)

See also Psychiatric Disturbance Associated Syndromes

Intellectual Disability

See Mental Retardation

Intercourse, Painful

See Dyspareunia

Intestine

See Abdominal Pain; Constipation; Diarrhoea; Dyspepsia; Dysphagia; Exomphalos; Malabsorption; Melaena and Rectal Bleeding; Nausea and Vomiting; Obesity; Oesophageal Associated Syndromes; Weight Loss

Iris Abnormality Associated Syndromes

Pseudoexfoliation syn. (glaucoma)
Rieger syn. (iris dysgenesis, small teeth)
WAGR syn. (Wilms' tumour, mental retardation)
Williams' syn. (blue iris, prominent lips)

See also SYNDROMES SECTION 6

Irritable

See Psychiatric Disturbance Associated Syndromes

Itch

See Pruritus; Pruritus Ani and Proctitis; Pruritus Vulvae

Jaundice (Icterus)
Yellow skin

HEPATOBILIARY

Biliary tract obstruction (pain, pruritus, fever)
Cholecystitis (pain, nausea, fever)
Cirrhosis (pruritus, RUQ pain fever)
Carcinoma of head of pancreas (pain, pruritus, cachexia)
Cholelithiasis (colic)
Primary or secondary hepatic malignancy
Alcoholic liver disease
Hepatic vein stenosis
Gaucher's disease (hepatosplenomegaly, anaemia)
Primary sclerosing cholangiitis

INFECTIONS

Hepatitis, infectious and serum (anorexia, nausea, fever)
Malaria (paroxysmal fevers, nausea, headache)
Clostridial gangrene (pain, foul smell, tissue crepitations)
Yellow fever (purpura, muscle pain, oliguria)
Pancreatitis (severe pain, shock)
Cytomegalovirus (neonate, purpura, haematuria)
Syphilis (variable symptoms)
Echinococcus (wheeze, urticaria)

SYNDROMES (see SYNDROMES SECTION 6)

Bard-Pic syn. (carcinoma of pancreas)
Crigler-Najjar syn. (kernicterus, neonate)
Dubin-Johnson syn. (neonate, asymptomatic)
Gilbert syn. (benign asymptomatic jaundice)
Lissencephaly syn. (fits, hypotonia)
Patau syn. (neonate, asymptomatic)

OTHER

Neonatal icterus
Familial causes
Hodgkin's disease (adenitis, fever, weight loss)
Sickle cell anaemia (fever, abdominal pain, negroid)
Post upper abdominal surgery
Haemolytic anaemia (fatigue, malaise, pallor)
Thalassaemia major (hepatosplenomegaly, lethargy)
Drugs (eg. chlorinates, chromates, sulphonamides, halothane)
Carotenaemia (excess ingestion of orange coloured food, headache, white conjunctivae)

Jaw Anomaly Associated Syndromes

Gardner's syn. (mandibular osteomas, melaena)
Gorlin-Goltz syn. (multiple BCC, jaw keratocysts)
Neu-Lexova syn. (oedema, facial anomalies)
Siccard syn. (paralysis of cranial nerves 9, 10, 11, 12)
Smith-Magenis syn. (prognathism)

See also Micrognathia
See also SYNDROMES SECTION 6

Jellyfish Sting

Irukandji syn. (severe pain, sweating, tachycardia)

Jerks

See Tremor; Chorea

Jewish Race Associated Syndromes

Bloom's syn. (photosensitive skin, small at birth)
Riley-Day syn. (no lacrimation, excess sweating)

See also SYNDROMES SECTION 6

Joint Disease and Pain

See Arthritis and Arthralgia; Shoulder Pain; Knee Pain; Joint, Swollen; Joint, Abnormal Movement; Erythema, Joint

Joint, Abnormal Movement

Ehlers-Danlos syn. (pseudotumours, hyperextensible joints)
Hypermobility syn. (excess joint mobility)

See also Arthritis and Arthralgia; Joint, Swollen

Joint, Swollen

Rheumatoid arthritis (red, painful)
Septic arthritis (hot, tender, inflamed)
Trauma (pain, history)
Gout (red, painful, acutely tender)
Mechanical derangement
Avascular necrosis
Tumours
Sarcoidosis (dyspnoea, malaise, fever)
Charcot joint (painless joint swelling)
Bursitis (fluid filled cyst)
Baker's cyst (posterior to knee)
Tendinitis (pain on movement)
Synovitis
Metabolic disorders

See also Arthritis and Arthralgia; Joint, Abnormal Movement
See also SIGNS SECTION 2: Joint Erythema

Kidney; Kidney Pain

See Loin Pain; Renal Disease Associated Syndromes

Knee

See Knee, Locked; Knee Pain; Knee, Swollen; Knee, Unstable; Leg Pain; Patella, Abnormal

Knee Pain

Trauma causing periarticular fracture, bruising, ligamentous tear or meniscal tear
Haemarthrosis
Meniscal strain (joint line pain, limited movement)
Ligamentous instability (abnormal joint laxity)
Osteoarthritis (night pain, elderly)
Osteochondritis dessicans (adolescent, effusion)
Chondromalacia (pain after rest, adolescent girls)
Osgood-Schlatter's disease (tibial tubercle tender, adolescent)
Popliteal cyst (child, mass in popliteal fossa)
Discoid meniscus (lateral joint line tender)
Genu valgum and varus (child)
Varus deformity of foot
Referred pain (eg. sciatica)
Plica syn. (see SYNDROMES SECTION 6)
Iliotibial band friction syn. (see SYNDROMES SECTION 6)
Johansson-Sinding-Larsen syn. (patella tender)
Tendinitis
Still's disease (child) (juvenile rheumatoid arthritis)
Bursitis
Paget's disease (leg bowing, acromegaly)
Septic arthritis (fever, swelling, erythema)

See also Arthritis and Arthralgia; Joint, Swollen; Leg Pain; Leg, Swollen; Patella, Abnormal

Knee, Locked

Difficult or impossible to move knee
Bucket handle tear of medial meniscus
Loose body in joint
Anterior cruciate ligament tear

Knee, Swollen

Meniscal tear
Osteoarthritis
Inflammatory or infective arthritis
Pigmented villonodular synovitis
Synovial osteochondomatosis
Cruciate ligament rupture
Fracture

Knee, Unstable

Patella dislocation or subluxation
Ligamentous tear
Cruciate ligament rupture
Patellofemoral arthritis
Osteochondritis
Meniscal pain (quadriceps inhibition)
Loose body in joint
Proprioceptive loss

Labour, Premature

Multiple pregnancy
Polyhydramnios (overlarge uterus)
Uterine malformations
Premature rupture of membranes
Cervical incompetence (post-trauma or surgery)
Alcohol dependence
Grand multiparity
Previous abortion
Heavy smoker
Previous premature births

Lacrimation, Abnormal

Facial nerve palsy
Crocodile tears syn. (lacrimation with eating after Bell's palsy)
Mikulicz syn. (parotitis, enlarged lacrimal glands)
Riley-Day syn. (Jewish, excess sweating, fever)
Sicca syn. (dry eyes, adenitis)
Sjögren's syn. (dry eyes and mucous membranes)
SUNCT syn. (severe brief headache)

Lactation, Failure of

Sheehan's syn. (failure of lactation after postpartum haemorrhage)
Anxiety and stress
Malnutrition

Laryngitis

See Hoarseness

Leg Pain

Arterial claudication (intermittent, hair loss, wasting)
Venous claudication (eased by leg elevation, oedema)
Embolism (numb, cold, weak)
Osteoarthritis, fibrositis and tenosynovitis
Buerger's disease (smoker, inflamed arteries, cold leg)
Causalgia (trauma, skin and temperature changes)
Shin splints (tibial tenderness)
Osteomyelitis (tender, hot)
Fibromyositis (fatigue, stiffness)
Varicose veins (oedema)
Thrombophlebitis (oedema, tender)
Baker's cyst rupture (posterior to knee)
Polymyalgia rheumatica (muscle pain, weakness, recurrent)
Sickle cell anaemia (jaundice, fever, negroid)
Multiple myeloma (bone pain, malaise, anaemia)
Osgood-Schlatter's disease (tibial tuberosity tender)
Bursitis
Referred pain (eg. sciatica)
Tendon strain or rupture
Haemarthrosis
Tendinitis
Osteochondrosis
Septic arthritis
Perthe's disease
Bone tumours
Paget's disease (bone deformity)
Calcium or phosphorus deficiency
Rickets
Osteomalacia
Scurvy (bleeding gums)
Rheological claudication (hyperviscosity, whole leg pain)
Neurological claudication (dermatome distribution)
Polyneuritis (paralysis, anaesthesia, wasting)
Beriberi (anorexia, paraesthesia)
Gas gangrene (wound, oedema, tachycardia)
Deep fasciitis (fever)
Other musculoskeletal disorders
Trauma (eg. fracture, sprain, bruise)

SYNDROMES (see SYNDROMES SECTION 6)

Anterior compartment syn. (tibial pain)
Anterior impingement syn. (ankle, anterior)
Posterior impingement syn. (ankle, posterior)
Eosinophilia-myalgia syn. (dyspnoea, arthralgia)
Fibrositis syn. (tender, stiff muscles)
Iliotibial band friction syn. (runner, pain on lateral side of knee)
Leriche syn. (calf claudication, impotence)
Limb pain syn. (child, nocturnal)
Patello-femoral pain syn. (anterior knee pain)
Piriformis syn. (sciatica)
Posterior facet syn. (back pain)
Restless legs syn. (leg movement)
Seckel syn. (hip and elbow dislocation)
Synovial plica syn. (knee pain and effusion)
Tibial stress syn. ('Shin splints')

See also Arm Pain; Arthritis and Arthralgia; Bone Mass or Tumour; Foot Anomaly Associated Syndromes; Knee Pain

Leg, Swollen

Congestive cardiac failure
Deep venous thrombosis (tender calf, Homan's sign)
Superficial venous insufficiency
Lymphoedema
Renal failure
Nutritional insufficiency
Lipoedema
Constrictive clothing or bandages
Prolonged sitting or standing

Lethargy

See Fatigue, Abnormal

Leucoplakia of Mouth

White lesions in mouth

Trauma to oral mucosa
Chemicals (eg. aspirin held in mouth)
Thermal trauma
Candidiasis/thrush (bright white plaques, inflamed surrounds)
Leucoderma (more common in negro population)
Gingivostomatitis
Herpes simplex
Lichen planus
SLE (face rash, arthritis, weight loss)
Pemphigus (skin blisters, crusts, ulcers)
Erythema multiforme (papules, wheals, blisters)
Aphthous ulcers (pain)
Carcinoma (firm, fixed)
Keratosis (due to tooth friction on mucosa)
Dental amalgam tattoo
Smoker's keratosis
Drugs (eg. ACE inhibitors, allopurinol, diuretics, methyldopa, NSAIDs)

Leucorrhoea

See Vagina, Discharge, Excessive

Libido, Reduced

Reduced desire for sexual activity

BOTH SEXES

Psychological stress
Pituitary disease (eg. adenoma)
Hyperprolactinaemia
Hypothyroidism (constipation, hoarse, dry skin)
Addison's disease (pigmentation, fatigue, nausea)
Diabetes mellitus (polyuria, polydipsia)
Cerebrovascular accident
Parkinson's disease (tremor, rigidity)
Cerebral space occupying lesions
Psychiatric disease (eg. depression)
Chronic renal failure
Chronic hepatic failure
Carcinoid syn. (flushing)
Cushing's syn. (obese, striae)
Malignancies
Drugs (eg. alcohol, steroids, antihistamines, benzodiazepines, antihypertensives, diuretics)

MALE

Testicular atrophy or disease
Prostate infection or enlargement

FEMALE

Climacteric syn. (menopausal symptoms)
Stage of menstrual cycle
Pregnancy

See also Frigidity; Impotence; Infertility; Orgasm, Lack of

Light Reactions

See Photophobia; Photosensitive Skin

Lightheadedness

Vertigo (see separate entry)
Postural hypotension
Lack of sleep
Stress and anxiety
Malnutrition/starvation
Excess alcohol intake
Migraine (headache, visual disturbances, nausea)
Hyperventilation (tetany, vertigo, paraesthesiae)
Cervical spondylosis
Transient ischaemic attacks (various CNS symptoms)
Visual deterioration (eg. cataracts)
Viral or bacterial infection
Fever of any cause
Impaired vestibular function
Deafness
Peripheral neuropathy
Psychiatric conditions
Drugs (eg. antihistamines, tranquillizers,
antihypertensives)

Limb Pain

See Arm Pain; Arthritis and Arthralgia; Groin Pain; Hand Pain; Knee Pain; Leg Pain

Lip

See Cleft Lip and/or Palate; Facial Anomaly Associated Syndromes

Loin Pain

Renal or ureteric stone (severe pain radiates to groin)
Pancreatitis (nausea, acute pain)
Pyelonephritis (fever, polyuria)
Renal tumour
Hepatobiliary disease (eg. cholecystitis)
Nerve root pain
Lumbar hernia
Colonic disease (eg. diverticulitis, ulcerative colitis)
Splenic disease

See also Abdominal Pain; Groin Pain

Love, Unrequited

de Clerambault's syn. (monomania, erotomania, female)

Lumps

*See Breast Lump; Bone Mass or Tumour; Adenitis and Lymphadenopathy; Nodules; Goitre; Neck Lump; Testicular or Scrotal Mass or Tumour; Throat Lump
See also symptoms listed under Tumours*

Lung

See Chest Pain; Cough; Dyspnoea; Haemoptysis; Wheeze

Lymph Nodes (Lymphadenitis)

See Adenitis and Lymphadenopathy

Macroglossia

See Tongue Abnormality Associated Syndromes

Macular Rash

See Rash, Macular

Malabsorption

Thyrotoxicosis (heat intolerance, proptosis, tachycardia)
Cystic fibrosis (pulmonary disease, steatorrhoea)
Gastric or intestinal surgery
Gastric or intestinal tumour
Lactase deficiency
Lipase deficiency
Crohn's disease (colic, pain, diarrhoea)
Chronic pancreatitis or carcinoma of pancreas
Irradiation to abdomen
Hepatic diseases (eg. cholestasis, cirrhosis)
Cholelithiasis (intermittent RUQ pain)
Scleroderma (skin thickening, arthritis)
Diverticulitis (varied bowel habits, pain)
Amyloidosis (pulmonary symptoms)
Diabetes mellitus (polydipsia, polyuria)
Coeliac disease (foul faeces, weight loss, anaemia)
Tropical sprue (travel history, diarrhoea)
Giardiasis (diarrhoea, flatus, often asymptomatic)
Mesenteric vascular disease (postprandial pain)
Lymphomas
Hypogammaglobulinaemia
Whipple's disease (pain, diarrhoea, melaena)
Postgastrectomy syn.
Pernicious anaemia (fatigue, sore tongue)
Zollinger-Ellison syn. (peptic ulcer)
Hartnup disease
Afferent loop syn. (abdominal pain relieved by food)
Bassen-Kornzweig syn. (low weight, ataxia)
Alcohol dependence
Drugs (eg. neomycin, cholestyramine, metformin)

*See also Weight Loss; Failure to Thrive
See also SIGNS SECTION 2: Cachexia*

Malaise

See Fatigue, Abnormal

Malnutrition
See Failure to Thrive; Weight Loss
See also SIGNS SECTION 2: Cachexia

Mastalgia
See Breast Pain

Melaena and Rectal Bleeding

MELAENA (DARK, ALTERED BLOOD)
Peptic ulcer (epigastric pain and tenderness, nausea)
Carcinoma of stomach or oesophagus (fullness, pain, anorexia)
Small intestine tumours and disease (pain, nausea)
Portal hypertension (hepatomegaly)
Lymphoma
Leiomyoma
Gardner's syn. (sebaceous cysts, colonic adenomas)

FRESH BLOOD LOSS
Ulcerative colitis (colic, diarrhoea, fever)
Colonic polyps (often painless)
Diverticulitis (diarrhoea, abdominal pain)
Colonic carcinoma (alt. diarrhoea and constipation)
Haemorrhoids (pain, discharge, pruritus)
Fissure-in-ano (pain, constipation)
Salmonellosis
Dieulafoy's disease (massive haemorrhage)
Amoebiasis (diarrhoea, colic)
Peutz-Jegher syn. (pigmented mouth and fingers)

VARIABLE BLOOD FORM
Endometriosis (dysmenorrhoea, dyspareunia)
Crohn's disease (abdominal mass and pain, diarrhoea)
Infective colitis (fever, malaise, diarrhoea)
Defibrination syn. (generalised excessive bleeding)
Henoch-Schoenlein syn. (purpura, abdominal pain)
Vascular malformations
Haemophilia and other coagulation disorders
Intestinal foreign body
Drugs (eg. warfarin, salicylates)

See also Bleeding, Excessive

Melanoma
See Pigmentation of Skin, Excess

Memory Disturbance
Cerebral trauma or tumour
Alzheimer's disease
Acute brain syn. (elderly, psychotic, disorientation)
Amnestic syn. (alcohol dependence, thiamine deficiency)
Organic brain syn. (multiple psychiatric changes)

See also Amnesia; Psychiatric Disturbance Associated Syndromes

Memory Loss
See Amnesia; Memory Disturbance

Menarche
See Puberty, Delayed; Puberty, Early

Menorrhagia
Excessive blood loss during menstruation
Menopause (flushes, mood changes)
Uterine myomata or fibroids
Intrauterine contraceptive device
Endometrial polyps
Hypothyroidism (dry skin, psychoses, myalgia)
Psychological disturbances
Follicular or corpus luteal ovarian cysts
Ovarian or uterine tumours and neoplasms
Menopause (flushes, mood changes)
Cervical ectropion (leucorrhoea)
Stein-Leventhal syn. (polycystic ovarian syn.)
Pelvic arteriovenous malformations
Thrombocytopenia (see Pathology)
Abortion or miscarriage
Ectopic pregnancy (hypogastric pain)
Endometriosis (cyclical pelvic pain)
Pelvic inflammatory disease
Endometrial hyperplasia
Leukaemia
SLE
Congestive cardiac failure (dyspnoea, oedema)
Liver diseases
Blood dyscrasias and coagulopathies
Pituitary diseases
Oestrogen therapy

See also symptoms listed under Gynaecology

Menstrual Disturbances
See Amenorrhoea and Oligomenorrhoea; Dysmenorrhoea; Menorrhagia; Vaginal and Uterine Bleeding, Abnormal

Menstruation
See Dysmenorrhoea; Menorrhagia; Vaginal and Uterine Bleeding, Abnormal

Menstruation, Lack of
See Amenorrhoea and Oligomenorrhoea; Puberty, Delayed

Mental Disorders
See Amnesia; Anorexia; Anxiety; Déjà Vu; Depression; Insomnia; Phobia; Psychiatric Disturbance Associated Syndromes; Mental Retardation

Mental Retardation

GENETIC OR CHROMOSOMAL
Cretinism
Lysosomal storage disease
Niemann-Pick disease

Duchenne muscular dystrophy
Gaucher's disease
Galactosaemia
Phenylketonuria
Tuberous sclerosis
Microcephaly

ENVIRONMENTAL

Lead and other toxins
Drugs
Toxoplasmosis
Rubella
Cytomegalovirus
Other viral and bacterial diseases
Congenital syphilis
Sclerosing panencephalitis
Wilson's disease

PSYCHOLOGICAL

Psychoses
Autism
Stimulus deprivation etc.

OTHER

Cerebral space occupying lesion (eg. tumours, abscess, haematoma)
Diabetes mellitus (polydipsia, polyuria)
Chronic epilepsy
Birth trauma
Brain trauma
Cerebral palsy
Multiple sclerosis (slow onset)
Hydrocephalus
Deafness may mimic subnormality

SYNDROMES (see SYNDROMES SECTION 6)

Angelman syn. (mute, laughter, ataxic)
Blue diaper syn. (nephrocalcinosis, hypercalcaemia)
Coffin-Lowry syn. (prominent lips, coarse facies)
Coffin-Siris syn. (hypoplastic toe nails)
Conrad's syn. (deaf, cataracts)
Cri-du-chat syn. (cat cry, ocular hypertelorism)
De Lange syn. (microcephaly, 'Amsterdam dwarf')
Down syn. (typical facies, reduced growth)
Dubowitz syn. (micrognathia, ptosis)
Fetal alcohol syn. (hirsute, reduced growth)
Fragile X syn. (hyperactive, autistic, epilepsy, large)
Hunter syn. (gross facies, arthralgia, hepatomegaly)
Hurler syn. (dwarf, gross facies, arthralgia)
Johanson-Blizzard syn. (deaf, anal atresia)
Klinefelter syn. (XXY, male, hypoplastic genitals)
Laurence-Moon-Biedl syn. (retinitis pigmentosa)
Lennox-Gastaut syn. (convulsions)
Lesch-Nyhan syn. (gout, athetosis, mutilation)
Louis-Bar syn. (telangiectasia of face and eye)
Lowe syn. (cataracts, epicanthal folds)
Miller-Dieker syn. (abnormal facies)
Neu-Lexova syn. (face anomalies, oedema)
Patau syn. (cleft lip, polydactyly)
Pompe syn. (hypotonia, cardiac anomalies)
Prader-Willi syn. (hypotonia, male, obese)
Rett's syn. (female, hyperventilation, seizures)
Richner-Hanhart syn. (uveitis, keratoderma)

Sanfilippo syn. (gross facies, hepatosplenomegaly)
Savant syn. (specific talent)
Seckel syn. (hip and elbow dislocation)
Smith-Lemli-Opitz syn. (ptosis, hypospadias)
Sturge-Weber syn. (port wine stain, convulsions)
WAGR syn. (Wilms' tumour, iris abnormality)
Wolf-Hirschhorn syn. (cleft lip)

Microcephaly
Small head
Angelman syn. (mental retardation, ataxic, laughter)
De Lange syn. (mental retardation, low hair line)
Langer-Giedion syn. (sparse hair, exostoses)

Micrognathia
Small jaw
Dubowitz syn. (ptosis, growth reduced)
Edward syn. (rocker-bottom feet, cardiac anomalies)
Fetal alcohol syn. (slow growth, retarded)
Neu-Lexova syn. (facial abnormalities)
Pierre-Robin syn. (cleft palate)
Potter syn. (renal agenesis, hypoplastic lungs)
Treacher-Collins syn. (deaf, hairy cheeks)

See also Jaw Anomaly Associated Syndromes

Microphthalmia
Small eyes
Patau's syn. (polydactyly, cardiac anomalies)

Micturition, Abnormal
See Dysuria; Oliguria and Anuria; Pneumaturia; Polyuria and Pollakiuria; Strangury; Urinary Retention

Miscarriage
See Abortion, Recurrent

Mood Changes
See Psychiatric Disturbance Associated Syndromes

Mouth
See Leucoplakia of Mouth; Mouth, Dry; Mouth Swellings; Mouth Ulcer; Mucous Membranes, Dry; Pigmentation of Mouth; Stomatitis and Gingivitis; Tongue Abnormality Associated Syndromes; Tongue Pain; Trismus; Facial Anomaly Associated Syndromes

Mouth Rash
See Leucoplakia of Mouth

Mouth Swellings
Buccal malignancy (hard, painful)
Antral polyp
Hyperplasia of gums secondary to dentures
Salivary gland calculus (pain with salivation)

Epulis (gingival)
Fibroepithelial polyp
Osteoma (hard, midline palate)
Dental cyst (painless, alveolus)
Mucous cyst (lip, bluish, fluctuant)
Oro-antral fistula
Drugs (eg. phenytoin, cyclosporin A)

Mouth Ulcer

Trauma (eg. biting bone, dentures)
Burn (eg. hot food)
Aphthous ulceration (transient, recurrent)
Malignancy (chronic, squamous cell)
Herpetic stomatitis (scattered, irregular)
Chickenpox
Infectious mononucleosis (adenitis, fever)
Trigeminal herpes (painful, facial rash)
Syphilis (form depends on stage)
Hand, foot, mouth disease (vesicles on hands and feet)
TB (tongue, irregular, undermined edges)
Pernicious anaemia (glossitis, asthenia)
Iron or folic acid deficiency
Acute leukaemia
Coeliac disease (foul faeces, weight loss)
Crohn's disease (diarrhoea, abdominal pain)
Lichen planus (persistent, irregular, white)
Pemphigoid (persistent, blister initially)
SLE (butterfly rash, arthralgia)
Erythema multiforme (recurrent, haemorrhagic)
Pemphigus vulgaris (blisters initially, persistent)
Behcet syn. (uveitis, arthritis, convulsions)
Food sensitivity
Anaphylaxis
Drugs (eg. cytotoxics)

See also Stomatitis and Gingivitis

Mouth, Dry (Xerostomia)

Fever
Anxiety (palpitations, sweating)
Dehydration
Diabetes mellitus (polydipsia, polyuria)
Diabetes insipidus
Primary biliary cirrhosis (dry eyes, pruritus, cholestasis)
Cystic fibrosis (lung and bowel symptoms)
Sialadenitis (swelling, pain)
Ductal stones (pain with eating, swelling)
Postradiation therapy
Botulism (diplopia, dysphagia, paralysis)
Salivary gland agenesis or atrophy
Autoimmune diseases
AIDS
Graft versus host reaction
Hypolipoproteinaemia
Sarcoidosis
Anaemia
Elderly
Drugs (eg. atropine, antidepressants, antihistamines)

See also Glossitis; Mucous Membranes, Dry

Mouth, Sore

See Glossitis

Movement, Abnormal

See Tremor; Chorea; Bradykinesia
See also SIGNS SECTION 2: Movement, Abnormal

Mucocutaneous Disorders

See Leucoplakia of Mouth

Mucopolysaccharide Associated Syndromes

Hunter syn.
Hurler syn.
Maroteaux-Lamy syn.
Morquio's syn.
Sanfilippo syn.
Schiei syn.
Sly syn.

Mucous Membranes, Dry

Sicca syn. (dry eyes, adenitis)
Sjögren syn. (dry eyes, mouth, nose, dysphagia, etc.)

See also Mouth, Dry

Multilation, Self

See Violence
See also symptoms listed under Neurological Symptoms

Muscle Pain

See Myalgia

Muscle Spasm

See Chorea; Cramps, Muscular; Myoclonus; Tremor
See also SIGNS SECTION 2: Hypertonicity

Muscular Weakness

See Paralysis and Muscular Weakness; Fatigue, Abnormal

Myalgia
Muscular pain

Viral infections (eg. influenza, arbovirus)
Hepatitis (jaundice, hepatomegaly, malaise)
Encephalitis (fever, neck stiff, nausea)
Malaria (intermittent fevers, jaundice, hepatomegaly)
Poliomyelitis (headache, stiff neck, weakness)
Rheumatic fever (carditis, chorea, nodules, arthritis)
Menopause (flushes, depression, amenorrhoea)
Trichinosis (fever, splinter haemorrhages)
Brucellosis (fatigue, fever, headache)
Dengue fever (chills, headache, prostration)
Measles (fever, coryza, rash)
Glanders (suppuration, lymphangitis, fever)
Infectious mononucleosis (adenitis, fever)

Polymyalgia rheumatica (stiffness, malaise, weakness)
Motor neurone disease (weakness, variable course)
Lyme disease (erythema, adenitis, fever)
Toxoplasmosis (encephalitis or pneumonitis or myocarditis)
Weil's disease (fever, abdominal pain, vomiting)
Leptospirosis (fever, conjunctival infection)
Tularaemia (papule, fever, nausea, adenitis)
Bornholm's disease (pleurodynia) (localised pain)
Herpes zoster [shingles] (segmental vesicular rash)
Fibrositis (painful muscle group with firmness)
Hypoglycaemia (blurred vision, headache, weak)
Hyperparathyroidism (joint pain, polyuria)
Renal tubular acidosis
Fibrositis syn. (see SYNDROMES SECTION 6)
Chronic fatigue syn. (poor exercise tolerance, fever)
Guillain-Barré syn. (weakness, postviral)
Scurvy (bleeding gums)
Thiamine deficiency (? alcoholism)
Psychiatric causes
Drugs (eg. methyldopa)

See also Arm Pain; Arthritis and Arthralgia; Knee Pain; Leg Pain

Myoclonus
Brief sudden muscle jerks
Hypnic jerks (occur while falling asleep)
Startle reflex (sudden loud noise)
Drug or alcohol intoxication
Focal epilepsy
Spinocerebellar degenerations
Lesions of cortex or brainstem
Spinal lesions (segmental, localised)
Post-anoxic
Demyelinating diseases
Metabolic encepalopathy
Baltic myoclonus
Hereditary
Lafora body disease (child to teens, dementia)

Nail Pain
Trauma
Subungual haematoma
Ingrowing nail edge
Paronychia
Whitlow (herpetic)
Acropustulosis
Nail bed tumour
Subungual fibroma

Nail, Abnormal
See SIGNS SECTION 2: Nail Changes

Nasal Discharge
See Rhinitis and Rhinorrhoea

Nasal Obstruction
Sinusitis
Viral or allergic rhinitis

Deviated nasal septum
Nasal tumours (eg. carcinoma, angiofibroma)
Turbinate hypertrophy
Atrophic rhinitis (yellow crusts)
Nasal polyps
Nasal trauma (eg. fracture)
Adenoid hypertrophy
Fungal infections (candidiasis or aspergillosis)
Diphtheria (membrane, mucopurulent discharge)
Tuberculosis
Drugs (eg. methyldopa, decongestant spray overuse)

Nausea and Vomiting

INFECTIONS
Bacterial and viral gastrointestinal and systemic infections (eg. cholera, salmonelloses, actinomycoses)
Metazoal and protozoal infestations (eg. malaria, trichinosis, leptospirosis)
Meningitis (headache, fever, neck stiffness)
Sinusitis and catarrh

GASTROINTESTINAL
Gastritis (anorexia, pain, haematemesis)
Peptic ulcer (epigastric pain and tenderness, melaena)
Stomach carcinoma (fullness, heartburn, melaena)
Intussusception (bloody diarrhoea, infant)
Small intestinal tumours (melaena, pain)
Mesenteric artery occlusion (pain, diarrhoea)
Gut obstruction and ileus (colic, distension)
Appendicitis (RIF pain, anorexia, fever)
Mesenteric adenitis (pain, anorexia, fever)

HEPATOBILIARY
Cholecystitis (RUQ pain, jaundice, fever)
Hepatitis (anorexia, jaundice, fever)
Cirrhosis (RUQ pain, anorexia, fatigue)
Biliary colic (RUQ pain, shock)
Pancreatitis (severe pain, shock, fever)

CEREBRAL
Migraine (headache, photophobia, vertigo)
Cerebrovascular accident (neurological signs)
Intracranial tumours (headache, neurological signs)
Increased intracranial pressure (various signs)
Cerebral hypoxia (anoxia or circulatory causes)
Epilepsy (convulsion, amnesia, micturition)
Ménière's disease (tinnitus, vertigo)
Motion sickness
Labyrinthine disease (vertigo, pain)

ENDOCRINE
Hyperparathyroidism (polyuria, polydipsia, bone pain)
Hyperthyroidism (sweating, cold intolerance)
Adrenal insufficiency [Addison's disease] (headache, fatigue, diarrhoea)
Phaeochromocytoma (hypertension, headache, sweating)
Diabetes mellitus (polyuria, paraesthesiae, blurred vision)
Hypercalcaemia (anorexia, constipated)

URINARY

Acute renal failure (oliguria or diuresis, haematuria)
Urinary tract infections (fever, dysuria, pain)
Renal colic (severe pain, haematuria)

SYNDROMES (see SYNDROMES SECTION 6)

AIDS (fever, arthralgia, rash)
Chinese restaurant syn. (face pressure, chest pain)
Dandy-Walker syn. (craniomegaly, cleft palate)
Diencephalic syn. (cachexia, pallor, sweating)
Dumping syn. (postgastrectomy, postprandial)
Haemolytic-uraemic syn. (haematuria,
thrombocytopenia)
Leigh's syn. (encephalitis)
Lightwood's syn. (weight loss, child, constipation)
Mallory-Weiss syn. (haematemesis, forceful vomiting)
Premenstrual syn. (mastalgia, headache)
Serotonin syn. (tremor, antidepressant drugs)
Toxic shock syn. (fever, diarrhoea, hypotension)
Xiphoid syn. (sternal pain)

OTHER

Bulimia
Morning sickness of pregnancy
Myocarditis (asthenia, vertigo, dyspnoea)
Haemolytic anaemia (fever, abdominal pain, jaundice)
Altitude sickness (vertigo, headache, fatigue)
Polyarteritis nodosa (arthritis, nodules, rash)
Porphyria (abdominal colic, sweating, tachycardia)
Severe hypertension (headache)
Alcohol dependence (liver disease)
Acidosis or alkalosis
Myocardial infarct (chest pain, shock, dyspnoea)
Glaucoma (eye pain, visual disturbance)
Congestive cardiac failure (oedema, dyspnoea)
Electrolyte disturbances
Severe pain, fright or shock
Anaphylaxis
Psychogenic
Ciguatera poisoning (paraesthesia)
Radiotherapy
Effects of hormones and toxins
Drugs (eg. digoxin, theophylline, narcotics, cytotoxics)

See also Haematemesis

Neck Abnormality Associated Syndromes

Klippel-Feil syn. (short neck with limited movement)
Noonan syn. (short, shield chest)
Scapulocostal syn. (neck pain radiating to arm)
Sicard syn. (paralysis of cranial nerves 9, 10, 11, 12)
Superior vena cava syn. (neck oedema)
Turner's syn. (webbed neck, amenorrhoea, female)

See also Neck Lump; Neck Pain; Shoulder Pain
See also SYNDROMES SECTION 6

Neck Lump

Lymph node (infection)
Thyroid enlargement (eg. goitre)
Lipoma (subcutaneous)
Sebaceous cyst (punctum, fluctuant)

Thyroglossal cyst (midline, child)
Dermoid cyst
Salivary gland tumour, infection or obstruction
Carotid body tumour
Lymphoma
Pharyngeal pouch (varies in size)
Branchial cyst (lateral)
Thyroid tumour
Haemangioma or other vascular malformation
Oropharyngeal carcinoma
Metastatic carcinoma
Neuroma
Abscess

See also Neck Abnormality Associated Syndromes

Neck Pain

Lymph node disease (eg. mumps, other infections,
tumours)
Cervical vertebral fractures or dislocation
Clavicle fracture or dislocation
Oesophageal foreign bodies and tumours
Intervertebral disc lesions (muscle spasms, hyporeflexia)
Vertebral joint osteoarthritis (limited movement)
Torticollis (eg. sternomastoid tumour, positional,
neurological)
Cervical rib (muscle wasting, sensory loss)
Respiratory tract infections (fever)
Thyroid diseases, infections or tumours
Primary and secondary tumours
Rheumatoid arthritis
Osteomyelitis (fever, tenderness)
Pott's disease
Myocardial infarct
Pancoast's tumour
Aortic dissection
Thymic tumours
Branchial cyst (lump, tender)
Thyroglossal cyst (midline)
Carotodynia (tender, unilateral, headache)
Rabies (hydrophobia, animal bite)
Thoracic outlet syn. (see SYNDROMES SECTION 6)

*See also Neck Abnormality Associated Syndromes;
Shoulder Pain*

Neurological Symptoms

*See Athetosis; Chorea; Convulsions; Headache;
Memory Disturbance;Paraesthesia; Paralysis and
Muscular Weakness; Psychiatric Disturbance
Associated Syndromes; Ptosis; Rigidity, Muscular;
Anaesthesia; Syncope; Thirst, Excessive: Tremor;
Vertigo; Violence*

Night Sweats

See Sweating, Nocturnal

Nipple Discharge

Pregnancy and lactation
Hormonal therapy and other drugs (eg. methyldopa,
reserpine, tricyclic antidepressants)

Breast carcinoma (lump, pain, bloody discharge)
Intraductal papilloma (painless lump)
Mammary dysplasia (pain, cyclical, lumps)
Pituitary tumour (headache, neurological signs)
Thyroid disease (eg. hypothyroidism, thyroid cancer)
Mastitis (red tender breast)
Oral contraceptives
Renal failure
Breast stimulation
Acromegaly (large hands, feet and jaw, amenorrhoea)
Adrenal tumours (Cushing syn.)
Newborn infant ('witch's milk')

Nocturia
See Polyuria and Pollakiuria

Nodules

DERMATOLOGICAL
Warts (irregular surface, varied shape, crops)
Haemangioma (blood vessel malformation)
Basal cell carcinoma (rounded, pearly, telangiectatic vessels)
Lipoma (soft, diffuse)
Prurigo nodularis (itchy, red, hard, scaly)
Neurofibromatosis (café-au-lait spots)
Molluscum sebaceum and contagiosum
Chilblains (red, itching, extremities)
Granuloma inguinale (ulcerates, painless, sexually transmitted)
Melanoma (pigmented, metastases)
Hyperlipidaemia (xanthomata) (see SIGNS SECTION 2)
Stewart-Treves syn. (see SYNDROMES SECTION 6)

SYSTEMIC
Erythema nodosum (tender, fever, legs)
Rheumatic fever (heart murmur, polyarthralgia, rash)
Rheumatic arthritis (arthralgia, malaise, paraesthesiae)
Heberden's nodes (see SIGNS SECTION 2)
Polyarteritis nodosa (arthritis, pruritus, rash)
Gout (severe pain in acute stage)
SLE
Sarcoidosis (lung symptoms)
Syphilis (second stage symptom with rash)

Noise, Abdominal
See Borborygmi

Noises in Ears
See Tinnitus

Nose
See Nasal Obstruction; Facial Anomaly Associated Syndromes; Epistaxis; Rhinitis and Rhinorrhoea

Nose Bleed
See Epistaxis

Nose Discharge
See Rhinitis and Rhinorrhoea

Numbness
See Anaesthesia; Paraesthesia; Formication

Nystagmus
See SIGNS SECTION 2: Nystagmus
See also symptoms listed under Eye

Obesity
Diet, exercise and lifestyle
Familial or genetic
Hypothalamic lesions
Hypothyroidism (fatigue, cold intolerance, dry skin)

SYNDROMES (see SYNDROMES SECTION 6)
Cushing syn. (amenorrhoea, hirsute, central obesity, moon face)
Fröhlich syn. (obese genitals and buttocks)
Laurence-Moon-Biedl syn. (retinitis pigmentosa)
Mauriac syn. (dwarf, diabetes, hepatomegaly)
Menopausal syn. (weight gain, menstrual changes)
Pickwickian syn. (cyanosis, cardiac failure)
Prader-Willi syn. (hypotonia, mental retardation)
Reaven syn. (hypertension)
Stein-Leventhal syn. (amenorrhoea, hirsute)

See also Growth and Height, Excessive; Weight Gain

Odynophagia
Pain on swallowing
Reflux oesophagitis (burping, waterbrash)
Infective oesophagitis (fever)
Oesophageal stenosis (dysphagia)
Corrosive oesophagitis
Drugs (eg. NSAIDs, iron, tetracyclines)

See also Dysphagia

Oedema
Tissue swelling

DERMATOLOGICAL
Contact dermatitis (erythema, vesiculation, crusts)
Stasis dermatitis (pruritus, erythema, ulceration)
Photodermatitis [sunburn] (erythema, vesiculation, pain)
Urticaria (wheals, erythema, pruritus)
Erysipelas (hot, erythema, pain, malaise)
Cellulitis (hot, diffuse)

CARDIOVASCULAR
Cardiac failure (dyspnoea, cough, dependent, pitting)
Aortic aneurysm (neck and arms involved, pain, dyspnoea)
Varicose veins (leg pain)
Beriberi (leg cramps, paraesthesiae)
Thrombophlebitis (pain, tenderness)
Lymphoedema (painless, pitting to brawny)

SYNDROMES (see SYNDROMES SECTION 6)

Carcinoid syn. (head and neck oedema, flush)
Cushing syn. (obese, striae, moon face)
Eosinophilia-myalgia syn. (dyspnoea, arthralgia)
Nephrotic syn. (ascites, anorexia, dyspnoea, hypertension, striae)
Neu-Lexova syn. (facial abnormalities)
Postphlebitic syn. (leg oedema and ulcers)
Premenstrual syn. (mastalgia, nausea, irritable)
Raynaud's phenomenon (finger oedema and pain)
Superior vena cava syn. (head and neck oedema)

OTHER

Trauma
Anaphylaxis
Glomerulonephritis (oliguria, headache, malaise)
Myxoedema (fatigue, dry skin, cold intolerance)
Hepatic failure (jaundice)
Renal failure
Trypanosomiasis (anaemia, myocarditis)
Filariasis (adenitis, fever, orchitis)
Protein deficiency
Thiamine deficiency (?alcohol dependence)
Drugs (eg. indomethacin, steroids, clonidine, prazosin)

See also Oedema, Eyelid
See also SIGNS SECTION 2: Ankle Oedema; Pitting Oedema

Oedema, Eyelid

Angioneurotic oedema (pruritus, diffuse)
Insect bites and trauma
Thyrotoxicosis (fatigue, sweating, weight loss)
Superior vena cava obstruction (cyanosis, venomegaly)
Hypothyroidism (dry skin, myalgia, deaf)
Trichinosis (myalgia, nausea, diarrhoea)

See also Oedema

Oesophageal Associated Syndromes

Barrett's syn. (reflux, ulcers)
CREST syn. (Raynaud's phenomenon, calcinosis, sclerodactyly)
Denervation syn. (bloated, diarrhoea, oesophageal surgery)

See also Dysphagia

Oligomenorrhoea

See Amenorrhoea and Oligomenorrhoea

Oliguria and Anuria

Low or absent urinary output
Glomerulonephritis (headache, oedema, malaise)
Acute renal failure (haematuria, nausea)
Gram-negative septicaemia (fever, shock)
Shock (hypotension) (various causes)
Yellow fever (jaundice, muscle pain, purpura)
Dehydration (poor skin turgor, dry mucous membranes)

Cholera (odourless liquid stools, vomiting)
Drugs (eg. mercurials, sulfonamides, CCl_4)

See also Renal Disease Associated Syndromes

Optic

See symptoms listed under Eye

Optic Paralysis

Cogan syn. (no horizontal eye movement)
Duane syn. (deficient horizontal eye movement)
Moebius syn. (ptosis, fixed facies)
Parinaud syn. (loss of upward gaze)
Steele-Richardson-Olszewski syn. (rigidity, dementia)
Tolosa-Hunt syn. (unilateral, ptosis, mydriasis)
Wernicke-Korsakoff syn. (dementia)

See also symptoms listed under Eye

Orgasm, Lack of

Alcohol
Fatigue
Psychological stress
Inadequate stimulation
Dyspareunia (see separate entry)
Lumbar vertebral disc herniation
Vaginal infection
Vulval or vaginal pain (eg. ulcers)
Diabetes mellitus (neuropathy)
Pelvic or spinal surgery
Paraplegia
Hypothyroidism (fatigue, cold intolerance)
Hypopituitarism
Hypoadrenalism
Sex hormone deficiencies
Drugs (eg. MAOIs, sedatives, narcotics, alpha-adrenergic blockers)

Orthopnoea

Shortness of breath while supine
Mitral stenosis (fatigue)
Left ventricular failure (dyspnoea, cough, fatigue)

See also Dyspnoea

Otalgia

See Earache

Otic

See Tinnitus
See also symptoms listed under Ear

Otorrhoea

See Ear Discharge

Ovary

See symptoms listed under Gynaecology

Overactivity

Autism
Attention deficit hyperactivity disorder
Behavioural problem
Minimal brain dysfunction
Fragile X syn. (male, subnormal intelligence, epilepsy)
Hyperkinetic syn. (poor coordination)

Pain

See Abdominal Pain; Arm Pain; Arthritis and Arthralgia;
Back and Vertebral Pain; Breast Pain; Chest Pain;
Dyspareunia; Dysuria; Earache; Facial Pain; Fractures,
Pathological; Groin Pain; Hand Pain; Headache; Knee
Pain; Leg Pain; Loin Pain; Myalgia; Neck Pain; Shoulder
Pain; Throat Pain; Odynophagia

Pallor

Pale skin

Anaemia (lassitude, dyspnoea, palpitations)
Leukaemia (fever, arthralgia, malaise)
Haemolytic anaemia (fever, nausea, abdominal pain)
Pernicious anaemia (anorexia, sore tongue,
paraesthesiae)
Chronic renal failure (nausea, pruritus)
Aplastic anaemia (lethargy, purpura)
Shock (eg. myocardial infarct and other causes of
hypotension)
Ischaemic limb (pain, pulseless)
Racial or genetic characteristic

SYNDROMES (see SYNDROMES SECTION 6)

Diencephalic syn. (cachexia, vomiting, sweating)
Dumping syn. (postgastrectomy, postprandial)
Raynaud's phenomenon (cyanosis and oedema of
fingers)
Vasovagal syn. (hypotension, syncope, bradycardia)
Waterhouse-Friderichsen syn. (petechiae, prostration)

Palpitations

Rapid, forceful or irregular heartbeat

Normal heart (anxiety, asthenia)
Pyrexia of any cause
Viral infections
Anaemia (pallor, fatigue, dyspnoea)
Thyrotoxicosis (fatigue, weight loss, sweating)
Paroxysmal atrial tachycardia (healthy, sudden, vertigo)
Myocardial infarct (pain, shock)
Atrial fibrillation (irregular, rapid)
Ventricular ectopics (intermittent, irregularly irregular)
Myocarditis
Hypokalaemia (weakness, convulsions)
Mitral valve disease (murmur)
Menopause (flush, sweating, mood changes)
Phaeochromocytoma (hypertension)
Gastro-oesophageal reflux (burping, chest pain)
da Costa's syn. (chronic, stress induced)
Serotonin syn. (tremor, antidepressant drugs)
Pregnancy
Heavy smoking

Alcohol excess
Foods (eg. chocolate, cheese, preservatives, cola, coffee)
Drugs (eg. salbutamol, caffeine, glyceryl trinitrate,
imipramine, terbutaline, aminophylline)

Palsy

See Paralysis and Muscular Weakness

Papules

See Rash, Papular

Paraesthesia (Pins and Needles)

Psychiatric and emotional causes
Nerve compression (eg. bruising, inflammation, joint
overuse)
Transient ischaemic attack (temporary, clumsiness,
confusion)
Pernicious anaemia (pallor, anorexia, dyspepsia)
Diabetes mellitus (polyuria, blurred vision, fatigue)
Ischaemic limb (pallor, pain, pulseless)
Chronic renal failure (nausea, pruritus)
Multiple sclerosis (muscle weakness)
Posterolateral sclerosis (weakness, sensory loss)
Beriberi (leg cramps, oedema, anorexia)
Tetanus (muscle spasm, dysarthria, wound)
Rabies (hydrophobia, animal bite)
Leprosy (macular rash, anaesthesia)
Acromegaly (psychic changes, coarse facies)
Ciguatera poisoning (tropical fish ingestion)
Other poisons

SYNDROMES (see SYNDROMES SECTION 6)

Carpal tunnel syn. (arm pain, burning)
Cervical rib syn. (arm pain and weakness)
Conn syn. (weak, hypertension)
Painful bruising syn. (female, spontaneous bruises)
Raynaud's phenomenon (finger pain, pallor and cyanosis)
Refsum's syn. (distal polyneuropathy)
Restless legs syn. (leg movement)

See also Hand Pain
See also symptoms listed under Neurological Symptoms

Paralysis and Muscular Weakness

Loss of motor power

CEREBRAL

Cerebrovascular accident (confusion, aphasia, anaesthesia)
Head trauma (headache, ocular signs)
Bell's palsy (face involved, spontaneous onset and
recovery)
Myasthenia gravis (ptosis, diplopia, dysarthria)
Transient ischaemic attack (clumsiness, temporary,
confusion)

NERVOUS SYSTEM

Zoster paresis (follows shingles)
Multiple sclerosis (diffuse neurological symptoms)
Polyneuritis (pain, anaesthesia, limbs)

Motor neurone disease (progressive, several forms)
Familial periodic paralysis (intermittent)
Poliomyelitis (stiff neck, sore throat, flaccid)

MUSCULOSKELETAL

Vertebral disc herniation (back pain, hyporeflexia)
Muscular dystrophy (child, proximal weakness)
Rheumatoid arthritis (joint pain, nodules)
Ischaemic limb (pain, pallor)
Dermatomyositis (proximal weakness, rash)
Osteomalacia and rickets (bone bowing, fatigue)
Duchenne muscular dystrophy
Inclusion body myositis (elderly, white, male, peripheral)

SYNDROMES (see SYNDROMES SECTION 6)

Bartter syn. (polyuria, weakness, polydipsia, short)
Behcet syn. (uveitis, arthritis, ulcer)
Bell's palsy (facial, unilateral)
Brown-Sequard syn. (hemisection of cord)
Carpal tunnel syn. (hand pain and weakness)
Cervical rib syn. (arm involved, pain)
Conn syn. (weak, hypertension)
Cori syn. (glycogen storage disease)
Creutzfeldt-Jakob syn. (jerks, seizures)
Cushing syn. (obese, ecchymoses, hirsute)
Eaton-Lambert syn. (myasthenic symptoms)
Erb-Duchenne palsy (shoulder girdle paralysis)
Floppy baby syn. (partial widespread muscular paralysis)
Guillain-Barré syn. (progressive, dysphagia, polyneuritis)
Klumpke's palsy (neonate, limp wrist)
Kugelberg-Welander syn. (shoulder girdle weakness)
Locked-in syn. (total paralysis of body)
McArdle syn. (cramps, myopathy)
Parkinsonism (tremor, rigidity, reduced strength)
Pompe syn. (hypotonia, mental retardation)
Potassium wastage syn. (polyuria, weak, dilute urine)
Prader-Willi syn. (hypotonia, obese, mental retardation)
Refsum syn. (distal sensorimotor polyneuropathy)
Roussy-Levy syn. (hypotonia, ataxia, kyphoscoliosis)
Shy-Drager syn. (hypotension, vertigo, tremor)
Sicard syn. (paralysis of cranial nerves 9, 10, 11, 12)
Sturge-Weber syn. (hemiplegia, port wine stain)
Uveoparotid syn. (facial paralysis, uveitis)
Werdnig-Hoffman syn. (progressive dystrophy, neonate)

OTHER

Psychological stress
Hyperparathyroidism (polyuria, polydipsia, bone pain)
Tick bite (child more common)
Hyperaldosteronism (tetany, headache, polyuria)
Hyperthyroidism (sweaty, proximal myopathy)
Porphyria (nausea, abdominal colic, sweating)
Botulism (dry mouth, diplopia, dysphagia)
Syphilis (rash, sexually transmitted, various symptoms)

See also Facial Weakness; Floppy Baby; Optic Paralysis; Paraplegia and Quadriplegia
See also symptoms listed under Neurological Symptoms

Paralysis, Optic
See Optic Paralysis

Paraplegia and Quadriplegia
Paralysis of the lower or all four limbs
Trauma to vertebral column and spinal cord
Vertebral disc herniation (pain, hyporeflexia)
Cord tumour or vascular malformation
Multiple sclerosis (intermittent, variable)
Infections of spinal cord (fever, backache)
Meningitis (neck stiffness, headache, fever)

See also Paralysis and Muscular Weakness

Paresis
See Paralysis and Muscular Weakness

Patella, Abnormal
Patella dislocation
Chondromalacia
Nail-patella syn. (small or absent patella, gross nail defects)
Synovial plica syn. (knee pain and effusion)

See also Knee Pain

Pelvic Pain

GYNAECOLOGY
Dysmenorrhoea (primary or secondary)
Ectopic pregnancy (abnormal vaginal bleeding)
Abortion
Intrauterine contraceptive device
Hydrosalpinx
Salpingitis (fever, discharge)
Endometriosis (infertile, intermittent)
Ovarian cyst or neoplasm
Pelvic congestion syndrome
Ovarian torsion (acute onset)
Pelvic inflammatory disease (fever)
Gynaecological carcinoma
Uterine fibroids
Retrograde menstruation

OTHER
Peritonitis (acutely tender, fever, malaise)
Appendicitis (anorexia, nausea, rebound)
Cystitis (dysuria, frequency)
Ureteric calculus (haematuria, nausea)
Ulcerative colitis (diarrhoea, fever, rectal blood)
Diverticulitis (variable bowel habits)
Irritable bowel syn. (intermittent pain, variable bowel habits)
Constipation (tenesmus)
Adhesions
Bowel obstruction
Prostatitis (difficult micturition)
Testicular torsion
Inguinal or femoral hernia

See also Abdominal Pain; Back and Vertebral Pain; Groin Pain; Loin Pain

Penile Ulcers
See Genital Ulcer

Penis Discharge
See Urethral Discharge

Penis, Abnormal
Idiopathic
Lichen sclerosis (white area around urethral meatus)
Smith-Lemli-Opitz syn. (ptosis, mental retardation, hypospadias)

See also Priapism; Urethral Discharge

Personality Change

PSYCHIATRIC
Paranoid personality disorder (eccentric)
Schizophrenia (antisocial, unemotional)
Histrionics (demands attention)
Narcissistic personality disorder (reacts badly to criticism)
Obsessive compulsive disorder
Antisocial personality (conduct disorder)
Borderline personality disorder (unstable)
Phobic disorders (avoidance behaviour)
Manic depressive psychosis (mood swings)
Stress reaction

OTHER
Frontal lobe tumours
Cerebral space occupying lesions
Alzheimer's disease
Arteriosclerosis

Pes Cavus
See SIGNS SECTION 2: Pes Cavus

Petechiae
See Purpura and Petechiae

Pharyngitis
See Throat Pain

Phobia
Abnormal fear
Neuroses (anxiety, headache, hyperventilation)
Depression (insomnia, anxiety)
Obsessional (compulsions)
Schizophrenia

Photophobia
Eye pain with bright light
Migraine (headache, nausea, vertigo)

Iritis (pain, blurred vision, small pupil)
Corneal inflammation (eg. herpetic ulcer) (discharge, blurred vision)
Hypoparathyroidism (tetany, wheeze, convulsions)
Corneal foreign body (red, pain)
Acute glaucoma (severe pain, poor vision)
Episcleritis (pain, discharge)
Rickettsial and viral infections (eg. measles)
Trichinosis (myalgia, nausea, diarrhoea)
Richner-Hanhart syn. (tyrosinaemia, mental retardation)

Photosensitive Skin
Rashes that develop in response to sunlight
Polymorphic light eruption
Photocontact dermatitis
SLE
Porphyria cutanea tarda
Pellagra
Phenylketonuria
Hartnup disease
Xeroderma pigmentosum
Congenital photosensitivity
Bloom's syn. (Jewish, reduced growth, leukaemia)
Drugs (very wide range incl. tetracycline, phenothiazines, sulfonamides, thiazides, frusemide, antimalarials, griseofulvin, nalidixic acid)

Pigmentation of Mouth
Addison's disease (weak, anaemia, nausea)
Melanoma (variable colouration)
Haemochromatosis (arthropathy, hepatomegaly)
Peutz-Jegher syn. (hereditary intestinal polyposis)
Kaposi's sarcoma (purple, raised, AIDS)
Racial

See also Leucoplakia of Mouth; Pigmentation of Skin, Excess
See also SIGNS SECTION 2: Tongue, Discoloured

Pigmentation of Skin, Excess

DERMATOLOGICAL
Freckles
Chloasma (pregnancy or oral contraceptives)
Malignant melanoma (irregular border, varying colour)
Naevi (benign, demarcated, hairy)
Haemangiomas (red, benign)
Mongoloid spot (lower back, hereditary)
Lentigo (normal in most people)
Xeroderma pigmentosa
Café-au-lait spots (see Signs)
Kaposi's sarcoma (purple, raised, AIDS)
Sunburn and skin trauma (eg. keloids)

SYNDROMES (SEE SYNDROMES SECTION 6)
Albright syn. (precocious puberty, polyostotic fibrous dysplasia)
Bloch-Sulzberger syn. (neonate, pigmented streaks, incontentia pigmenti)
Blue rubber bleb syn. (multiple blue tinged rubbery blebs, small bowel haemangiomas)

Cushing syn. (central obesity, plethora, headache)
Cronkhite syn. (pigmented hands and feet)
Dysplastic naevus syn. (multiple large moles)
Felty syn. (polyarthritis, splenomegaly)
Leopard syn. (multiple spots, cardiac changes)
Leschke syn. (spots, asthenia, hyperglycaemia)
Nelson syn. (postadrenalectomy)
Peutz-Jegher's syn. (pigmented mouth, lips and fingers)
Rothmund-Thomson syn. (erythema, telangiectasia)
Russell-Silver syn. (café-au-lait spots, dwarf)

OTHER

Varicose veins (oedema, leg ache)
Addisonism (fatigue, anorexia, nausea)
Neurofibromatosis (eg. von Recklinghausen's disease,
phaeochromocytoma)
Haemochromatosis (hepatomegaly, hepatic and cardiac
failure)
Scleroderma (arthritis, Raynaud's phenomenon)
Sprue (bulky foul stools, weight loss, anaemia)
Pregnancy (face, nipples and flexure lines)
Thyrotoxicosis (sweating, fatigue, weight loss)
Pituitary tumours (eg. acromegaly)
Carotenaemia (yellow palms and soles)
Familial and racial factors
Acanthosis nigricans
Drugs (eg. chloroquine, tetracyclines, amantadine,
phenothiazines, chlorpromazine, arsenic, busulphan,
bleomycin, amiodarone, gold, psoralens, oral
contraceptives)

Pigmentation of Skin, Lack of
See Skin, Depigmented

Piles
See Haemorrhoids

Pimples
See Acne; Rash, Papular

Pins and Needles
See Paraesthesia

Plethora
See Flush

Pneumaturia
Passing gas with urine
Recto-vesical fistula (eg. Crohn's disease, colonic
carcinoma, diverticulitis, bladder carcinoma, appendix
abscess)
Urinary infection with gas forming organisms
Fractured pelvis

Polyarthritis
Arthritis in more than one joint
Ross River fever (epidemic polyarthralgia)

Parvovirus infection
Other viraemias
Rheumatoid arthritis
Osteoarthritis
Polymyalgia rheumatica (elderly)
Psoriatic arthritis
Chondrocalcinosis
Gout (severe pain, red swollen joint)

Polydactyly
Extra fingers or toes
Laurence-Moon-Biedl syn. (retinitis pigmentosa)
Meckel syn. (renal cysts, cleft lip and palate)
Patau's syn. (cardiac anomalies, cleft lip)

Polydipsia
See Thirst, Excessive

Polyphagia
See Hunger, Excess

Polyuria and Pollakiuria
Excessive urinary output or frequency
Cystitis (dysuria, hypogastric pain)
Acute renal failure (in end stage only)
Prostatitis (discharge, pain, dysuria)
Diabetes insipidus (polydipsia, low urine SG)
Diabetes mellitus (fatigue, blurred vision, paraesthesiae)
Pregnancy (amenorrhoea, breast fullness)
Cystocele (pelvic pain, urgency)
Hypoparathyroidism (tetany, wheeze, convulsions)
Hyperparathyroidism (polydipsia, bone pain, nausea)
Addison's disease (nocturia, pigmentation, weakness)
SLE (macular rash, polyarthritis)
Hypercalcaemia (constipation, nausea)
Menopause (flushes, depression, amenorrhoea)
Obstructive sleep apnoea (snoring)
Anxiety neurosis
Hand-Schuller-Christian disease (eczema, adenitis)
Acromegaly (coarse features, back pain, psychoses)
Hyperaldosteronism (polydipsia, weakness, tetany)
Bilharzia (urticaria, fever, haematuria)
Drugs (eg. lead, diuretics)

SYNDROMES (see SYNDROMES SECTION 6)
Bartter syn. (child, short, polydipsia)
Cushing syn. (obese, moon face, striae)
Diencephalic syn. (cachexia, vomiting, pallor)
Potassium wastage syn. (weak, hypokalaemia)
Urethral syn. (dysuria, sterile urine)
Urge syn. (nocturia, urge incontinence)

Port Wine Stain
Idiopathic
Klippel-Trenaunay syn. (tissue overgrowth)
Sturge-Weber syn. (convulsions, mental retardation)
Spinal cord abnormalities (eg. spina bifida)

Postviral Infection Associated Syndromes

Guillain-Barré syn. (paralysis, polyneuritis)
Reye syn. (encephalopathy, hepatic failure)
Chronic fatigue syn. (lethargy, depression)

See also SYNDROMES SECTION 6

Pregnancy Associated Syndromes

HELLP syn. (haemolysis, liver abnormal, thrombocytopenia)
Painless thyroiditis syn. (postpartum, variable thyroid function)
Sheehan's syn. (postpartum haemorrhage, pituitary necrosis)

See also Abortion, Recurrent; Labour, Premature
See also SYNDROMES SECTION 6

Priapism

Painful, persistent penile erection
Bladder calculus
Spinal cord lesions
Leukaemia
Polycythaemia rubra vera
Multiple myeloma
Cerebrovascular accident (CNS signs)
Diabetes mellitus (polyuria, polydipsia)
Urethritis (dysuria)
Sickle cell anaemia
Leukaemia (child)
Metastatic carcinoma
Psychiatric disorders
Excess sexual stimulation
Penile trauma
Drugs (eg. prazosin, psychotropics, heparin, vasodilators, alcohol, cocaine, marijuana)

Proctitis

See Pruritus Ani and Proctitis

Pruritus

Itching of the skin with a skin abnormality

Rash Usually present

DERMATOLOGICAL

Overcleaning of skin
Ichthyosis (dry, rough, scaly skin)
Pressure areas
Atopic eczema (exudate, skin folds, allergic history)
Seborrhoeic dermatitis (fine scale)
Contact dermatitis
Stasis dermatitis (erythema, ulceration, oedema)
Lichen simplex (pigmented lichenified lesions)
Exfoliative dermatitis (scaling, erythema, malaise)
Lichen planus (flat papules along scratches, anxiety)
Psoriasis (red plaques, scales, nail changes)
Pityriasis rosea (herald patch, fawn scaly eruption)
Urticaria (wheals, malaise, oedema)
Intertrigo (body folds, erythema, stinging)
Miliaria [heat rash] (burning, vesicles, hot climate)
Dermatitis herpetiformis

Prurigo nodularis (nodules, red, hard, scaly)
Mastocytosis (red/brown skin spots)
Pemphigoid

INFECTIONS AND INFESTATIONS

Impetigo (pustules, crusts)
Tinea (ring, scaling, erythema)
Scabies (vesicles, 'runs', finger webs involved)
Bilharzia (rash, haematuria, diarrhoea)

SYNDROMES (see SYNDROMES SECTION 6)

AIDS
Red man syn. (vancomycin infusion)
Sézary syn. (erythroderma)
Sjögren syn.

OTHER

Allergy (oedema, erythema)
Insect bites (eg. fleas)
Hepatitis (anorexia, nausea, jaundice)
Cholecystitis (RUQ pain, nausea, jaundice)
Fibreglass and other irritants

No Rash Usually present

HEPATOBILIARY

Hepatomas (fever, polycythaemia, hypoglycaemia)
Cirrhosis (anorexia, jaundice, RUQ pain, alcoholic)
Obstructive hepatobiliary disease
Haemochromatosis

INFECTIONS AND INFESTATIONS

Pediculosis (excoriation, lice on skin and clothes)
Echinococcus (wheeze, allergies)
Other metazoal infestations (eg. hookworm, hydatids)
Other intestinal parasites

OTHER

Diabetes mellitus (polyuria, blurred vision, fatigue)
Thyrotoxicosis (weak, weight loss, diarrhoea)
Hypothyroidism (dry skin, fatigue, cold intolerance)
Hypoparathyroidism (tetany, wheeze, abdominal pain)
Nephritis (reaction to disease or toxins)
Uraemia (fatigue, thirst, headache)
Lymphomas and Hodgkin's disease (fever, adenitis, fatigue)
Leukaemia (malaise, arthralgia, pallor)
Neoplastic diseases
Multiple myeloma
Polycythaemia vera (fatigue, headache)
Iron deficiency anaemia
Itchy upper arm syn. (sun damage, no rash)
Fibreglass and other irritants
Pregnancy
Ciguatera poisoning (paraesthesiae)
Emotional and psychogenic causes
Drugs of addiction (abrupt onset, malaise, fever, headache)
Medications (eg. aspirin, dextran, narcotics, scopolamine)

See also Pruritus Ani and Proctitis; Pruritus Vulvae

Pruritus Ani and Proctitis
Perianal itch
Haemorrhoids (bleeding, pain, lump)
Fissure-in-ano (discharge, bleeding, pain)
Perianal fistula (pain, oedema, erythema)
Leucorrhoea (physiological, any vaginal infection)
Candidiasis and other superficial fungal infections
Diarrhoea of any cause
Enterobiasis and other metazoal infections
Diabetes mellitus (polyuria, fatigue, blurred vision)
Crohn's disease (abdominal pain and mass, diarrhoea)
Intertrigo (erythema, stinging, body folds)
Lichen simplex (pigmented lichenified lesions)
Seborrhoeic dermatitis (erythematous vesicles)
Contact dermatitis (erythema, vesicles, oedema)
Psoriasis (red plaques, nail changes, scaling)
Papillomata and skin tags
Molluscum contagiosum (umbilicated blisters)
Rectal prolapse
Condylomata accuminata
Sexually transmitted disease (eg. syphilis, gonorrhoea)
Bowen's disease
Poor hygiene

See also Pruritus; Pruritus Vulvae

Pruritus Vulvae
Itchy vulva
Candidiasis (rash, white vaginal discharge)
Bacterial vaginitis (pain, foul discharge)
Excessive sweating
Tight clothing (particularly nylon)
Over washing of area
Allergic reaction to soaps, material, toiletries, etc.
Atopic dermatitis
Seborrhoeic dermatitis
Psoriasis (plaques, scaling)
Urinary tract infection (frequency, dysuria)
Pediculosis (lice seen in pubic hair)
Scabies (burrows, inflamed skin)
Human papilloma virus infection (warts)
Oestrogen deficiency (postmenopause, postoophorectomy)
Diabetes mellitus (polyuria, polydipsia)
Depression (poor sleep pattern, loss of interest)
Lichen sclerosis (burning, fissures)
Autoimmune diseases
Lichen simplex chronicus (hyperkeratosis)
Vulval carcinoma (induration, erythema)
Trichomoniasis (yellow vaginal discharge, smell)
Genital herpes (vesicles or ulcers, pain)
Burning vulva syn. (see SYNDROMES SECTION 6)
Contraceptive foam or cream sensitivity

See also Pruritus Ani and Proctitis; Pruritus

Psychiatric Disturbance Associated Syndromes
Acute brain syn. (confusion, elderly, disoriented)
Asperger syn. (violent, no emotion)
Behcet syn. (uveitis, arthritis, mouth ulcers)
Capgras' syn. (delusion of doubles)
Charles Bonnet syn. (hallucinations)

Chronic fatigue syn. (depressed, postviral)
Cushing syn. (moon face, bruising, hirsute)
Episodic dyscontrol syn. (alcohol dependent, abusive)
Lesch-Nyhan syn. (mental retardation, gout, self-mutilation)
Kleine-Levin syn. (excess sleep, sexually overactive)
Menopausal syn. (menstrual changes, flushes)
Münchausen syn. (demands surgery)
Organic brain syn. (multiple changes)
Organic personality syn. (labile emotions)
Polle syn. (child abuse, Münchausen's syn. by proxy)
Post-traumatic cerebral syn. (vertigo, headache, personality change)
Post-traumatic stress syn. (after catastrophe, insomnia, fear)
Premenstrual syn. (mastalgia, headache)
Rett syn. (female, hyperventilation, seizures)
Reye syn. (confusion, hepatic failure, encephalopathy)
SHAFT syn. (neurosis)
Steele-Richardson-Olszewski syn. (dementia, rigidity)
Wernicke-Korsakoff syn. (ataxia, dementia)

See also Insomnia; Violence
See also symptoms listed under Neurological Symptoms
See also SYNDROMES SECTION 6

Ptosis
Drooping eyelid(s)
Bell's palsy (unilateral, spontaneous, painless)
Myasthenia gravis (generalised weakness)
Third cranial nerve palsy from any cause

SYNDROMES (see SYNDROMES SECTION 6)
Dubowitz syn. (reduced growth, mental retardation)
Eaton-Lambert syn. (myasthenic symptoms)
Guillain-Barré syn. (progressive palsy)
Horner syn. (myosis, exophthalmos, anhydrosis)
Moebius's syn. (ophthalmoplegia, dysphagia, drool)
Pancoast syn. (arm and chest pain, lung cancer)
Parinaud syn. (loss of upward gaze)
Smith-Lemli-Opitz syn. (mental retardation, hypospadias)
Tolosa-Hunt syn. (pain, mydriasis)
Uveoparotid syn. (facial paralysis, uveitis)
Wernicke-Korsakoff syn. (ataxia, dementia)

See also Eyelid Disease; Eyelids, Abnormal

Puberty, Delayed
Anorchia and gonadal dysgenesis
Gonadal infection or trauma (eg. tortion of testes)
Undescended testes
Adrenal hypoplasia or trauma
Pituitary neoplasms or hypophysectomy
Chronic systemic illness
Chronic emotional stress
Hormonal deficiencies
Constitutional and hereditary factors
Malnutrition and other causes of growth retardation (see Growth, Reduced)
Hypothyroidism (dry skin, lethargy)
Anorexia nervosa
Sarcoidosis
Haemochromatosis
Histiocytosis X

Cystic fibrosis
Exercise stress
Cranial irradiation
Cytotoxic therapy

SYNDROMES (see SYNDROMES SECTION 6)

Kallmann's syn. (anosmia, familial hypogonadism)
Klinefelter's syn. (XXY, hypoplastic genitals)
Noonan's syn. (female morphology)
Laurence-Moon-Biedl syn.
Prader-Willi syn. (male, hyptonia, obese)
Rothmund-Thomson syn. (erythema, pigmentation)
Soto's syn. (facial anomalies, accelerated growth)
Turner's syn. (short, neck webbing)

See also symptoms listed under Gynaecology
See also INVESTIGATIONS SECTION 3: Puberty,
Delayed

Puberty, Early

Ovarian or testicular tumours
Ingestion of hormones (eg. androgens, oestrogens,
chorionic gonadotrophin)
Hypothyroidism (dry skin, fatigue, cold intolerance)
Congenital adrenal hyperplasia
Hormone producing tumours
Hydroxylase deficiency
Hydrocephalus and other developmental defects
Encephalitis
Craniopharyngiomas and other cerebral tumours
Tuberous sclerosis (convulsions, mental retardation)
Idiopathic

SYNDROMES (SEE SYNDROMES SECTION 6)

Albright syn. (hypocorticalism, child)
Cushing syn. (central obesity, moon face)
Russell-Silver syn. (dwarf, café-au-lait spots)

See also Hirsutism and Hypertrichosis; Virilism
Associated Syndromes
See also SIGNS SECTION 2: Precocious Puberty
See also symptoms listed under Gynaecology

Puberty, Precocious

See Puberty, Early
See also SIGNS SECTION 2: Precocious Puberty

Pulse

See Cardiac Associated Syndromes; Palpitations
See also SIGNS SECTION 2: Pulse

Pupil Changes

See SIGNS SECTION 2: Miosis; Mydriasis

Purpura and Petechiae
Cutaneous haemorrhages

HAEMATOLOGICAL
Idiopathic thrombocytopenia (epistaxis, ecchymoses)

Vasculitis
Platelet or coagulation factor disorders
Aplastic anaemia (lassitude, pallor, bleeding)
Acute leukaemias (malaise, arthralgia, fever)
Disseminated intravascular coagulation (secondary to
severe disease)

OTHER

Viral exanthema (eg. measles)
Senile purpura (ecchymoses on arms, elderly)
Allergic conditions
Cytomegalovirus (neonate, haematuria, jaundice)
Severe generalised bacterial infections
Polyarteritis nodosa (arthritis, skin disorders, nodules)
Uraemia (fatigue, headaches, pruritus)
Yellow fever (jaundice, muscle pain, oliguria)
Scurvy (gingivitis, arthralgia, anaemia)
Amyloidosis (symptoms vary with involved organ)
Meningococcal septicaemia
Vitamin K deficit
Miliary tuberculosis
Bacterial endocarditis (murmur, fever)
Meningococcal meningitis (fever, headache, vomiting)
Trauma
Drugs (eg. quinine, thiazides, heparin, aspirin,
trimethoprim/sulfamethoxazole)

SYNDROMES (see SYNDROMES SECTION 6)

Bernard-Soulier syn. (excess bleeding)
Cushing syn. (central obesity, plethora, fatigue)
Defibrination syn. (excess bleeding)
Glanzmann syn. (mucocutaneous bleeding)
Henoch-Schoenlein syn. (abdominal pain, excess
bleeding)
Waterhouse-Friderichsen syn. (petechiae, pallor)

See also Bleeding, Excessive; Ecchymosis

Pustules

See Rash, Pustular

Pyrexia

See Fever

Pyrosis

See Heartburn

Quadriplegia

See Paraplegia and Quadriplegia

Rash

See Rash, Bullous; Rash, Linear; Rash, Macular; Rash,
Papular; Rash, Pustular; Rash, Vesicular; Ecchymosis;
Purpura and Petechiae; Skin Lesion Associated
Syndromes
See also symptoms listed under Skin Disorders
See also SIGNS SECTION 2: Spider Naevi

Rash, Bullous

Large fluid filled blisters
Impetigo (crusts, vesicles, pruritic)
Herpes zoster (severe pain, dermatome distribution)
Herpes simplex (pain)
Cellulitis (red, hot, fever)
Toxic epidermal necrolysis
Contact dermatitis (erythema, itch)
Drug eruptions
Insect and arachnid bites
Erythema multiforme (target lesions, erythema, extensor surfaces)
Pemphigus (normal skin surrounds, relapsing crops)
Pemphigoid (large, tense, elderly)
Dermatitis herpetiformis (vesicles, papules, erythema)
Pompholyx (soles and palms, tense blisters)
Porphyria cutanea tarda
Epidermolysis bullosa
Lichen planus
Burns (heat or irradiation)

Rash, Erythematous

See Erythema; Facial Erythema

Rash, Face

See Facial Erythema

Rash, Linear

Longitudinal skin rash
Lichen planus
Flat warts
Psoriasis
Epidermal naevi
Contact dermatitis (eg. perfumes)
Scabies (vesicles, 'runs', finger webs involved)
Dermographia
Lichen striatus
Koebner phenomenon
Jellyfish stings
Stinging and irritating plants

Rash, Macular

Flat, circumscribed, discoloured lesions

DERMATOLOGICAL

Psoriasis (red, scaling)
Dermatomyositis (weakness, oedema, myalgia)
Vitiligo (white patches)
Tinea corporis (white centred erythematous patches)
Pityriasis rosea (scales, erythematous, trunk)
Tinea versicolor (red patches, do not tan in sun)
Seborrhoeic dermatitis (red/brown, scaly)
Mycosis fungoides
Lichen planus (glossitis)
Leprosy (anaesthetic, erythematous, peripheral)

INFECTIONS

Measles (cough, rhinitis, conjunctivitis)
Roseola infantum (high fever, adenitis, infant)
Rubella (fever, coryza, adenitis)

Rheumatic fever (erythematous margin, nodules, arthritis)
Infectious mononucleosis (often after penicillin therapy)
Epidemic polyarthralgia (lethargy, arthritis)
Meningococcal infection (meningism, vomiting)
Leprosy (raised edge, anaesthetic)
Pinta (itch, lymphadenopathy)

OTHER

SLE (arthritis, malaise, anorexia)
Addison's disease (dark patches, fatigue, nausea)
Neurofibromatosis (eg. phaeochromocytoma, von Recklinghausen's disease)
Sweet syn. (see SYNDROMES SECTION 6)
Kawasaki syn. (adenitis, fever)
Drug eruptions

Rash, Nodular

See Nodules

Rash, Papular

Firm, raised, circumscribed lesions
Acne (comedones, cysts, erythema) (see separate entry)
Naevi (pigmented)
Melanoma (black, irregular)
Basal cell carcinoma (pearly, telangiectasia)
Folliculitis
Xanthoma (yellow, cholesterol containing)
Molluscum contagiosum (smooth, rounded, apical depression)
Granuloma (singular, soft)
Psoriasis (scales, erythema, nail changes)
Contact and atopic dermatitis
Lichen planus (flat topped, itchy scales)
Neurodermatitis (itch, thickened skin)
Miliaria (flexures)
Scabies
Pinta (itch, lymphadenopathy)
Cutaneous anthrax (oedema, surrounding vesicles)
Tularaemia (one papule that ulcerates, adenitis)
Drug eruption (itchy, red)

Rash, Plaque and Patch Formation

RED

Psoriasis vulgaris
Tinea corporis, capitis and cruris
Discoid lupus erythematosus
Parapsoriasis
Mycosis fungoides

WHITE

Pityriasis alba
Pityriasis versicolor
Vitiligo
Postinflammatory hypopigmentation

BROWN

Café-au-lait patches
Postinflammatory hyperpigmentation
Congenital naevi

Rash, Pustular
Elevated lesions filled with purulent fluid
Acne (comedones, erythema)
Rosacea (face, telangiectasia, chronic)
Folliculitis (hairy areas, chronic)
Chickenpox (itch, varying stages, central distribution)
Herpes zoster and *Herpes simplex*
Smallpox (historic only)
Impetigo (crusts, erythema, itch)
Melioidosis (cough, chest pain)
Chancroid (sexually transmitted, ulcerates, painful)

Rash, Scaly
See Icthyosis; Scalp, Scaly

Rash, Vesicular
Well defined small collections of fluid
Herpes zoster and *Herpes simplex*
Insect and arachnid bites
Burns
Chickenpox (fever, malaise, different stages)
Contact and atopic dermatitis
Scabies (burrows, itch)
Molluscum contagiosum (central umbilication)
Dermatitis herpetiformis (erythema, bullae, crops)
Vaccinia (secondary to vaccination, umbilicated vesicles)
Ramsay Hunt syn. (shingles)
Anthrax (oedema, sloughs)
Hand-foot-mouth disease (fever, irritable, child)
Dracunculiasis (west Africa)

Red Eye
See Eye, Inflamed or Red

Red Skin
See Erythema

Red Urine
See Haematuria and Red Urine

Renal Disease Associated Syndromes
Alport syn. (deaf, cataract, otitis media)
DeToni-Fanconi-Debre syn. (osteomalacia)
Goodpasture syn. (haemoptysis, cough, dyspnoea)
Haemolytic-uraemic syn. (haematuria,
thrombocytopenia)
Meckel syn. (polydactyly, cleft lip)
Potter syn. (renal agenesis, hypoplastic lungs)
Shock syn. (oliguria, hypotension, tachycardia)
Toxic shock syn. (renal failure, vomiting, diarrhoea)
Weil syn. (leptospirosis)

*See also Dysuria; Haematuria and Red Urine; Polyuria
and Pollakiuria*
See also SYNDROMES SECTION 6

Renal Pain
See Loin Pain

Retarded Mentality
See Mental Retardation

Retention of Urine
See Urinary Retention and Difficult Micturition

Retrograde Ejaculation
See Ejaculation, Retrograde

Rheumatism
See Arthritis and Arthralgia; Back and Vertebral Pain

Rhinitis and Rhinorrhoea (Cattarh)
Nasal discharge
Coryza (malaise, fever, sore throat, cough)
Allergy (sneezing, eye itch)
Anaphylaxis
Sinusitis (purulent discharge, face ache, fever)
Nasal tumour (blockage, unilateral, epistaxis)
Nasal foreign body
Vasomotor rhinitis (response to ambient temperature
change)
Nasal polyp
Adenoid hypertrophy or infection
Senile atrophy of nasal mucosa
Cleft palate
Hypothyroidism (constipation, dry skin)
Ozaena (foul smell, atrophic mucosa)
Other upper respiratory tract infections
Post-traumatic CSF loss
Hormonal (eg. pregnancy, oral contraceptives)
France's triad (aspirin sensitivity, asthma)
Smoking and other inhaled irritants
Drugs (eg. reserpine, guanethidine)

Rigidity, Muscular
Wilson's disease (cirrhosis, tremor, green-brown cornea)
Frontal lobe disease
Upper motor neurone lesions (hyperreflexia)
Extrapyramidal lesions (cogwheel rigidity)
Parkinson's disease (tremor, weakness, fixed facies)
Multiple sclerosis
Severe hypothyroidism (bradycardia, weak)
Machado-Joseph syn. (dysarthria, limb weakness)

SYNDROMES (see SYNDROMES SECTION 6)
Neuroleptic malignant syn. (fever, tranquillizer use)
Shy-Drager syn. (tremor, vertigo, hypotension)
Steele-Richardson-Olszewski syn. (dementia, gaze
paralysis)
Stiff man syn. (idiopathic toxic muscular rigidity)

See also Tetany
See also symptoms listed under Neurological Symptoms

Rigor
See Convulsions; Shivering and Rigors

Salivary Gland Pain and/or Swelling

Duct obstruction (intermittent pain)
Malignancy (pain, swelling)
Parotitis (pain, swelling, tender)
Sialadenitis (unilateral swelling)
Mumps (fever)
Infectious mononucleosis (fever, pharyngitis)
Other viral or bacterial infection (pain, fever, erythema)
Tuberculosis
Sarcoidosis (pulmonary symptoms)
Sjögren syndrome

Scalp, Scaly

Dandruff (loose, grey scales)
Seborrhoeic dermatitis (fungal cause, inflamed scalp)
Eczema (widespread, marked erythema, fine white scale)
Neurodermatitis (thick crusts, erythema)
Psoriasis (erythema, firmly adherent scale, nail changes)
Pityriasis amiantacea (very thick plaque, localised)
Tinea capitis (slightly pruritic, fractured hairs)
SLE (plaques, scarring)
Kerion (pustules, crusts)

Scoliosis

Lateral curvature of spinal column
Structural abnormality
Developmental abnormality
Disc prolapse
Coffin-Lowry syn. (coarse face, prominent lips)
Marfan syn. (arachnodactyly, kyphoscoliosis)
Roussy-Levy syn. (ataxia, hypotonia)

See also Arthritis and Arthralgia; Back and Vertebral Pain

Scrotal Mass

See Testicular or Scrotal Mass or Tumour

Scrotal Pain

See Testicular or Scrotal Pain

Seizure

See Convulsions

Sensation, Loss of

See Anaesthesia

Sensory Suppression

See Agnosia

Sex, Painful

See Dyspareunia

Sexual Dysfunction

See Ejaculation, Retarded; Ejaculation, Retrograde; Genital Ulcer; Impotence; Infertility; Libido, Reduced; Orgasm, Lack of; Puberty, Delayed; Puberty, Early; Virilism Associated Syndromes
See also symptoms listed under Gynaecology

Shingles Associated Syndromes

Ramsay Hunt syn. (face involved)

Shivering and Rigors

Fever from any cause (eg. infection, malignancy)
Hypothermia (environmental cold)
Fear
Malaria (jaundice, cyclical, hepatomegaly)
Addictive drug withdrawal

See also Convulsions

Shock

See SIGNS SECTION 2: Hypotension

Short Stature

See Growth, Reduced

Shortness of Breath

See Dyspnoea

Shoulder Pain

Supraspinatus tendinitis (mid-range abduction pain)
Osteoarthritis (pain with movement)
Subacromial bursitis
Cervical dysfunction
Polymyalgia rheumatica
Acromioclavicular joint dysfunction
Partial or complete tendon rupture
Tendon calcification
Capsulitis (generalised stiffness)
Biceps tendon subluxation
Fracture or dislocation
Septic arthritis (inflamed, tender)
Rheumatoid arthritis
Ankylosing spondylitis (back pain)
Bone tumour
Avascular necrosis
Cardiac pain (eg. myocardial infarct, angina)
Neuropathies

SYNDROMES (SEE SYNDROMES SECTION 6)

Painful arc syn. (mid-range movement pain)
Pancoast's syn. (lung cancer, Horner's syn.)
Rotator cuff syn. (limited abduction)
Scapulo-costal syn. (neck and arm pain)
Shoulder-hand syn. (arthritis, hand atrophy)

See also Arm Pain; Arthritis and Arthralgia; Chest Pain; Joint, Swollen; Neck Pain

Shoulder Tip Pain

Peptic ulceration (epigastric pain, tender, nausea)
Ruptured viscus (shock, abdominal pain)
Intraperitoneal bleeding from any cause
Diaphragmatic irritation from any cause
Local musculoskeletal trauma or disease

Singultus

See Hiccup

Sinusitis Associated Syndromes

Kartagener syn. (dextrocardia, bronchiectasis)

Skeletal Anomalies

*See Arthritis and Arthralgia; Back and Vertebral Pain;
Fractures, Pathological; Scoliosis; Spinal Abnormality
Associated Syndromes*

Skin Disorders

*See Ecchymosis; Erythema; Ichthyosis; Nodules;
Photosensitive Skin; Pigmentation of Skin, Excess;
Pruritus; Purpura and Petechiae; Rash, Bullous; Rash,
Linear; Rash, Macular; Rash, Papular; Rash, Pustular;
Rash, Vesicular; Skin, Depigmented; Skin, Dry; Skin
Lesion Associated Syndromes; Skin Pain; Skin
Thickening; Skin Thinning; Striae*

Skin Lesion Associated Syndromes

AIDS (fever, high risk group, splenomegaly)
Bloch-Sulzberger syn. (vesicles fade to pigmented
streaks)
Bloom syn. (photosensitive skin, Jewish)
Carney's complex (spotty pigmentation, atrial myxoma)
Chediak-Higashi syn. (skin infections, albinism)
Cogan syn. (interstitial keratitis, tinnitus)
Conradi-Hunermann syn. (large skin pores, cardiac lesions)
Dubowitz syn. (ptosis, micrognathia)
Ehlers-Danlos syn. (fragile skin, joint pseudotumours)
Felty syn. (leg ulcers, polyarthritis)
Fröhlich syn. (thin skin, scanty hair, obese)
Gardner syn. (sebaceous cysts, melaena)
Goltz syn. (scar-like skin atrophy)
Gorlin-Goltz syn. (multiple BCC, jaw keratocysts)
Hand-Schuller-Christian syn. (diabetes insipidus)
Harlequin syn. (severe ichthyosis)
Johanson-Blizzard syn. (aplasia cutis, anal atresia)
Kawasaki syn. (polymorphous rash, fever, red hands and
feet)
Koebner phenomenon (linear psoriasis)
Leschke syn. (brown spots, hyperglycaemia, asthenia)
Letterer-Siwe syn. (pruritic, papular rash)
Nephrotic syn. (striae, ascites, oedema)
Neu-Lexova syn. (collodion skin, face abnormal)
Nezelof syn. (infant, diarrhoea, rashes, infections)
Postphlebitic syn. (stasis dermatitis, leg ulcers)
Proteus syn. (gross disfigurement)
Ramsay Hunt syn. (herpetic vesicles, earache)
Red man syn. (vancomycin infusion)
Reiter syn. (arthritis, conjunctivitis, urethritis)

Richner-Hanhart syn. (keratoderma, uveitis)
Rothmund-Thomson syn. (skin pigmentation and atrophy)
Scalded skin syn. (infant, Staphylococcal infection)
Sjögren-Larsson syn. (ichthyosis, spastic)
Stevens-Johnson syn. (mucous membrane vesicles)
Sweet syn. (tender plaques, myalgia)
Toxic shock syn. (fever, vomiting, diarrhoea)
Vogt-Koyanagi-Harada syn. (vitiligo, blind)
Wiskott-Aldrich syn. (eczema, thrombocytopenia)

*See also Acne; Albinism; Erythema; Pigmentation of Skin,
Excess; Photosensitive Skin; Port Wine Stain; Purpura
and Petechiae; Skin Ulcer*
See also SYNDROMES SECTION 6

Skin Pain

Photodermatitis [sunburn] (erythema, oedema,
vesiculation)
Herpes zoster [shingles] (dermatome distribution,
vesicular lesions, unilateral)
Cellulitis (erythema, oedema, fever)
Trauma

Skin Thickening

Sun exposure
Scleroderma (arthritis, Raynaud's phenomenon)
Neurodermatitis (itch, papules)
Leprosy
Icthyosis (scales, dry)
Lichen sclerosis
Porphyria cutanea tarda
Eosinophilia-myalgia syn. (muscle pain, cough)
Neu-Lexova syn. (nose and eyelid abnormalities)
Ichthyosiform erythroderma (infant, bullae)

Skin Thinning

Aging
Cushing syn. (obese, striae, moon face)
Ehlers-Danlos syn. (joint pseudotumours)
Fröhlich syn. (late puberty, fine hair)
Goltz syn. (scalp, thighs, iliac crests)
Topical or systemic steroids
Scars

Skin Ulcer

Stasis dermatitis (erythema, pruritus, oedema)
Decubitus ulcer (pressure area, elderly or debilitated)
Squamous cell carcinoma (red, hard, scales)
Varicose veins (pain and oedema of legs)
Polyarteritis nodosa (nodules, arthritis, fever)
Trauma and pressure
Basal cell carcinoma (telangiectasia, pearly edge)
Venous thrombosis (leg, tender vein)
Venous or arterial insufficiency
Buerger's disease (smoker)
Peripheral neuropathy
Chilblains
Diabetes mellitus (poor circulation)
Malignant melanoma (not always black)
Other malignancies

TB (symptoms vary with organs involved)
Rheumatoid arthritis
Syphilitic gummata (sexually transmitted, painless, adenitis)
Chancroid (sexually transmitted, painful)
Tularaemia (fever, adenitis, headache)
Granuloma inguinale (large, painless, sexually transmitted)
Lymphogranuloma venereum (adenitis, prostatitis)
Coagulation disorders
Behcet's syn. (uveitis, arthritis, convulsions)
Postphlebitic syn. (stasis dermatitis, leg oedema)
Leprosy
Cutaneous leishmaniasis
Tabes dorsalis
Yaws (adenitis, painless, poor hygiene)

See also Skin Lesion Associated Syndromes

Skin, Depigmented

Pityriasis versicolor (reddish, scaling)
Pityriasis alba (eczematous, asymptomatic)
Vitiligo (dead white, well demarcated patches)
Halo naevus
Leprosy
Postinflammatory
Albinism
Tuberous sclerosis (subnormal)
Hypopituitarism
Kwashiorkor (malnutrition)
Vogt-Koyanagi-Harada syn. (see Syndromes)
Scars and burns
Chemicals (eg. phenols)

Skin, Dry (Xeroderma)

Fever
Seborrhoeic dermatitis (scales, erythema)
Hypothyroidism (mental retardation, reduced growth)
Constitutional reasons (eg. genetic, familial)
Psoriasis (red, scaling, patchy)
Hypovitaminosis A (night blindness, hyperkeratoses)
Ichthyosis (rough, scabs)
Typhoid fever (abdominal pain)
Other dermatoses

See also Ichthyosis

Skull Anomalies

See Facial Anomaly Associate Syndromes; Head, Large; Microcephaly

Sleep Disturbance

See Insomnia; Sleep, Excess; Snoring

Sleep, Excess

Cerebral space occupying lesion
Head injury
Narcolepsy
Other forms of epilepsy

Kleine-Levin syn. (hungry, sexually overactive)
Psychiatric conditions
Drugs (eg. sedatives, antihistamines, antidepressants)

Slow Movement

See Bradykinesia; Rigidity, Muscular

Small Stature

See Growth, Reduced

Smell, Loss of

See Anosmia

Sneezing

See Rhinitis and Rhinorrhoea

Snoring

Adenoid or tonsillar hypertrophy
Congenital malformations of the posterior nasal space
Deflected nasal septum
Allergic rhinitis (rhinorrhoea, swollen mucous membranes)
Nasal polyps
Nasal trauma
Collapsed alae nasi
Obstructive sleep apnoea (drowsy, nocturnal apnoea)
Narcolepsy (frequent periods of sleep)
Sedative or alcohol abuse
Smoking

Sore Throat

See Throat Pain

Spasm, Muscular

See Chorea; Convulsions; Cramps, Muscular; Rigidity, Muscular; Tetany; Tremor

Speech Defects

See Aphasia and Dysarthria; Hoarseness

Spider Naevi

See SIGNS SECTION 2: Spider Naevi

Spinal Abnormality Associated Syndromes

Brown-Sequard syn. (hemisection of cord)
Kugelberg-Welander syn. (lordosis, shoulder girdle weak)
Maroteaux-Lamy syn. (bone dysplasia)
Morquio'syn. (bone dysplasia, cataracts)
Schiei syn. (recurrent respiratory infections, kyphosis)
Sly syn. (recurrent respiratory infections, kyphosis)

See also Back and Vertebral Pain; Scoliosis
See also SYNDROMES SECTION 6

Splenomegaly
See SIGNS SECTION 2: Splenomegaly

Spots in Vision
See Vision, Black Spots in Field of

Squint (Strabismus)
Deviation of eye axes
Paralytic (limited movement of affected eye caused by trauma, vascular disease, cerebrovascular accident, tumour, multiple sclerosis, hyperthyroidism, etc.)
Concomitant (deviation constant at all angles of gaze due to congenital cataract, infantile lazy eye, etc.)
Crouzon's syn. (facial distortion, exophthalmos)

See also Diplopia

Stomatitis and Gingivitis
Inflammation of the mouth
 Dental disease
Aphthous ulcer (pain, erythema, tender)
Trauma (eg. false teeth, heat, irradiation)
Vincent's angina and other infections (pain, bleeding)
Thrush [candidiasis] (white plaques, pain, fever)
Geographic tongue (see SIGNS SECTION 2)
Agranulocytosis (fever, fatigue)
Erythema multiforme (skin lesions, extensor surfaces)
Tuberculosis (cough, malaise, fever, haemoptysis)
Leukaemia (malaise, fever, anorexia, pallor)
Herpetic stomatitis (ulcers, pain, erythema)
Uraemia (nausea, anorexia, malaise, halitosis)
Pernicious anaemia (anorexia, dyspepsia, pallor)
Ulcerative colitis (ulcer, diarrhoea, rectal blood)
Pemphigus vulgaris
Lichen planus (red skin, spots)
Pemphigoid
Crohn's disease (abdominal pain, diarrhoea)
Oral cancer (leucoplakia, ulcer or plaque)
Scurvy (arthritis, bleeding tendency)
Iron deficiency
Vitamin B deficiency
Drugs (eg. phenytoin, captopril)

SYNDROMES (see SYNDROMES SECTION 6)
Behcet syn. (uveitis, arthritis)
Hand-Schuller-Christian syn. (diabetes insipidus)
Kawasaki syn. (infant, fever, red hands and feet)
Plummer-Vinson syn. (dysphagia, splenomegaly)
Reiter syn. (urethritis, conjunctivitis, arthritis)
Stevens-Johnson syn. (adenitis, fever, coryza, erythema, conjunctivitis)

See also Mouth Ulcer; Tongue Pain

Strabismus
See Squint

Strangury
Very slow, painful micturition
Bladder infection (frequency, hypogastric pain)
Prostatitis
Bladder tumours (haematuria)
Urethritis (dysuria, proteinuria, discharge)
Gonorrhoea (urethral discharge)
Nonspecific urethritis (discharge)
Urethral tumour, trauma, stone or foreign body

See also Dysuria

Stress Incontinence
See Incontinence of Urine

Stretch Marks
See Striae

Striae (Stretch Marks)
Band, streak or strip in skin
Obesity
Pregnancy (striae gravidarum on abdomen)
Cushing syn. (obese, ecchymoses)
Nephrotic syn. (ascites, oedema)
Pituitary malfunction

Stridor
Harsh whistling with inspiration
Laryngotracheobronchitis (child, catarrh, fever)
Epiglottitis (acute, fever, dyspnoea)
Laryngitis (nocturnal, fever)
Croup (cough, hoarse)
Infectious mononucleosis (adenitis, fever)
Diphtheria (dyspnoea, membrane, fever)
Foreign body in larynx or trachea
Laryngeal papillomata
Congenital cysts, tumours and membranes
Laryngomalacia (congenital, worse on exertion)
Retropharyngeal abscess (rare)
Subglottic haemangioma

See also Cough; Wheeze

Subnormal Mentality
See Mental Retardation

Sudden Death
See Death, Sudden, Unexpected

Sun Exposure Related Syndromes
Bloom's syn. (photosensitive skin, Jewish)
Itchy upper arm syn. (no rash, intense pruritus)

See also SYNDROMES SECTION 6

Surgery, Excess

Münchausen's syn. (false symptoms and signs, many old surgery scars)
SHAFT syn.

Swallowing Difficulty

See Dysphagia; Odynophagia

Swearing, Uncontrolled

Attention deficit hyperactivity disorder
Gilles de la Tourette syn. (convulsions, spasms)

Sweating, Excessive and Abnormal (Hyperhidrosis, Diaphoresis)

Any infective state (eg. bacterial [TB], viral, parasitic [malaria])
Exercise
Obesity
Smoking
Anxiety and neuroses
Pregnancy
Menopause (flush, palpitations, mood changes)
Many forms of carcinoma
Thyrotoxicosis (weak, weight loss, diarrhoea)
Myocardial infarct (pain, shock)
Pulmonary embolus (chest pain)
Diabetes mellitus (polyuria, polydipsia, blurred vision)
Gustatory reflex (stimulated by spicy food, chocolate, cheese, etc.)
Gout (joint pain, tophi)
Rheumatoid arthritis (small joint involvement)
Hyperpituitarism
Acromegaly (coarse facies, backache)
Organic cerebral disease
Parkinson's disease (tremor, stiff gait)
Spinal cord lesions
Peripheral nerve lesions
Pulmonary oedema (cold)
Shock (hypotension)
Phaeochromocytoma (hypertension, headache)
Porphyria (tachycardia, muscular pain, nausea)
Drugs (eg. alcohol, aspirin, tricyclic antidepressants, heroin abuse)

SYNDROMES (see SYNDROMES SECTION 6)

AIDS (rash, adenitis, weight loss)
Chorda tympani syn. (associated with eating)
Diencephalic syn. (cachexia, vomiting, pallor)
Dumping syn. (postgastrectomy, postprandial)
Frey syn. (face sweating when eating)
Irukandji syn. (jellyfish sting, severe pain, tachycardia, respiratory failure)
Riley-Day syn. (Jewish, no lacrimation, fever)

See also Sweating, Nocturnal

Sweating, Lack of (Anhidrosis)

Multiple sclerosis
Erythroderma (red skin)

Severe dehydration
Miliaria
Leprosy
Peripheral nerve lesions
Multiple myeloma
Hypothyroidism (tired, dry skin)
Polyarteritis nodosa
Rheumatoid arthritis
Diabetes mellitus (polydipsia, polyuria)
Carcinoma of bronchus
Quadriplegia
Horner syn. (exophthalmos, ptosis, miosis)
Congenital absence of sweat glands
Premature infant
Postirradiation
Hodgkin's disease
Drugs (eg. arsenic, mepacrine)

Sweating, Nocturnal

Warm climate, clothing, ambient termperature
Anxiety and fear
Menopause (menstrual irregularities)
Viral or bacterial infection of any type
Thyrotoxicosis (heat intolerance, tachycardia)
Hypoglycaemia (light headedness, cold)
Lymphomas
Other neoplasms
Hypothalamic lesions (eg. tumour, abscess)
Use of drugs with cholinergic effects
Withdrawal from narcotics
Idiopathic

Swelling

See Adenitis and Lymphadenopathy; Ascites; Joint, Swollen; Knee, Swollen; Leg, Swollen; Mouth Swellings; Oedema
See also symptoms listed under Tumours

Syncope (Faint)

CARDIOVASCULAR

Stokes-Adams attack (heart block, bradycardia)
Myocardial infarct (chest pain, hypotension)
Hypotension from any cause (eg. blood loss, shock, postural)
Aortic stenosis (bruit, poor pulses)
Paroxysmal tachycardia (rapid irregular pulse, shock)
Pulmonary hypertension
Pulmonary artery stenosis
Atrioventricular block
Bradycardia (eg. heart block, infarct)
Vasovagal syncope (emotional, trauma)
Atrial fibrillation (irregularly irregular pulse)
Ventricular tachycardia
Carotid sinus syn. (after head turning)
Mitral stenosis (murmur)
Anaemia (fatigue, pallor, dyspnoea)
Arteriosclerosis (mental deterioration)
Atrial myxoma
Cardiac tamponade
Hypertrophic cardiomyopathy

PULMONARY

Pulmonary embolism (shock, chest pain, cough)
Hypoxia from any cause (cyanosis, bradycardia)
Pulmonary hypertension (hepatomegaly)
Severe coughing fit
Hyperventilation due to tetany or fright

CEREBRAL

Emotional states, fear or pain
Cerebrovascular accident (headache, confusion, convulsion)
Transient ischaemic attack (brief, headache, confusion)
Migraine (headache, nausea, photophobia)
Cerebral tumours (neurological anomalies)
Cerebral abscess or cyst
Narcolepsy (excessive sleep)
Epilepsy (convulsions, amnesia, paroxysmal)
Vertebrobasilar disease (vertigo)
Parkinson's disease (tremor, rigidity)
Meningitis (headache, fever)
Carotid ischaemia

SYNDROMES (see SYNDROMES SECTION 6)

Dumping syn. (postgastrectomy, postprandial)
Jervell-Lange-Nielsen syn. (deaf)
Sick sinus syn. (variable heart rate)
Subclavian steal syn. (arm claudication)
Wolf-Parkinson-White syn. (loud first heart sound)

OTHER

Severe infections (eg. myocarditis)
Hypoglycaemia (blurred vision, weakness, convulsions)
Micturition syncope
Addison's disease (weak, nausea, diarrhoea)
Pregnancy (causes postural hypotension)
Acidosis (hyperventilation, confusion)
Autonomic peripheral neuropathy
Anaphylaxis
Dehydration (primary, or secondary to excess diuretics)
Psychogenic (attention seeking)
Alcohol dependence
Drugs (eg. hypotensives, tricyclics, phenothiazines, narcotics, hypnotics)

See also Coma; Drop Attack
See also symptoms listed under Neurological Symptoms

Syndactyly

Fingers or toes partially or completely fused
Russell-Silver syn. (dwarf, precocious puberty)
Smith-Lemli-Opitz syn. (ptosis, mental retardation)
Idiopathic

Tachycardia

See SIGNS SECTION 2: Tachycardia

Tall Stature

See Growth and Height, Excessive (Gigantism)

Taste, Abnormal (Dysgeusia)

Reduced or altered taste sensation
Xerostomia
Heavy metal poisoning
Smoking
Dentures
Radiation therapy
Bacterial or viral infections of mouth, tongue or pharynx
Neoplasms of mouth, tongue or pharynx
Inflammation of mouth, tongue or pharynx
Trauma to gustatory nerve pathways
Migraine
Hypothyroidism
Cerebrovascular accident
Cerebral neoplasm, trauma or abscess
Sjögren syn. (see SYNDROMES SECTION 6)
Elderly
Drugs (eg. antithyroid, antineoplastic, ACE inhibitors)

Tears

See Lacrimation, Abnormal

Teeth

See Tooth, Discoloured; Tooth, Loose

Telangiectasia

See SIGNS SECTION 2: Spider Naevi

Tenesmus

Abnormal desire to defaecate
Diarrhoea from any cause (see separate entry)
Haemorrhoids (blood on faeces, pain)
Rectal carcinoma
Ulcerative colitis (bloody diarrhoea)
Rectal polyps
Pelvic inflammatory disease (abdominal pain, vaginal discharge)
Carcinoid syn. (flushes, asthma, oedema)

Testes, Small

Pituitary adenoma
Hyperprolactinaemia
Craniopharyngioma
Kallman syn. (see SYNDROMES SECTION 6)
Cryptorchidism
Mumps orchitis
Testicular torsion or trauma
Irradiation
Klinefelter syn. (see SYNDROMES SECTION 6)
Severe diabetes mellitus
Hepatic cirrhosis
Thyrotoxicosis
Spinal cord disease or injury
Anorexia nervosa
Haemochromatosis
Tuberculosis
Drugs (eg. cytotoxics, digitalis, spironolactone, ketaconazole, opiates, marijuana, alcohol)

Testicular or Scrotal Mass or Tumour

Testicular carcinoma or teratoma (often painless)
Hydrocele (transilluminates)
Spermatocele (above and behind testes, transilluminates)
Inguinal hernia (continuous with abdomen)
Torted testes (severe pain, nausea)
Epididymo-orchitis (pain, fever)
Epididymal cyst
Syphilitic gumma (solid)
Haematoma
Varicocele (above testes, soft)
Idiopathic scrotal oedema (erythema, slight pain)
Filariasis (elephantiasis) (adenitis, fever)
Fragile X syn. (subnormal intelligence, epilepsy, testis enlarged)

Testicular or Scrotal Pain

Epididymo-orchitis (pain, fever, bacterial or viral)
Torted testicular appendage [torted hydatid of Morgagni] (prepubertal, testes palpable)
Testicular tumour (firm, gynaecomastia)
Torted testes (severe pain, nausea, oedema)
Mumps orchitis (parotid pain and swelling, fever)
Gonorrhoea (discharge, dysuria)
Filariasis (oedema, fever, adenitis)
Brucellosis (fever, myalgia, confusion)
Referred pain from back or ureter

Tetany

Neuromuscular hyperactivity causing spasm
Hyperventilation from any cause
Hypoparathyroidism (stridor, wheeze, polyuria)
Osteomalacia and rickets (weakness, bone ache)
Acute pancreatitis (severe abdominal pain, shock)
Epilepsy (convulsions, amnesia, faints)
Hyperaldosteronism (hypertension, polyuria, weakness)
Tetanus (rigid jaw, wounded, rigors)
Hypovitaminosis D (osteomalacia or rickets)
DiGeorge syn. (neonate, severe infections)

See also Rigidity, Muscular; Tremor
See also symptoms listed under Neurological Symptoms

Thirst, Excessive (Polydipsia)

Diabetes insipidus (polyuria, low urine SG)
Diabetes mellitus (fatigue, blurred vision, paraesthesiae)
Dehydration (oliguria, dry mouth, poor skin turgor)
Uraemia (fatigue, anaemia, nausea)
Psychogenic (concentrated urine with fluid restriction)
Acromegaly (coarse facies, back pain, psychoses)
Hyperparathyroidism (polyuria, bone pain)
Hyperaldosteronism (weakness, tetany, polyuria)
Hypercalcaemia (constipation, nausea)

SYNDROMES (see SYNDROMES SECTION 6)

Bartter syn. (child, short, polyuria)
Cushing syn. (obese, moon face, striae)
Shock syn. (hypotension, pallor, oliguria)

Thoracic Pain
See Chest Pain

Throat Lump

Trauma from swallowing sharp or hard object or food
Foreign body (eg. fish bone)
Tonsillitis (pain, fever)
Smoke irritation (passive or active smoking)
Pharyngitis (pain, fever)
Chemical irritation
Laryngitis (hoarse)
Epiglottitis
Cancer of larynx or pharynx
Benign tumours
Pharyngeal pouch
Globus hystericus (psychological)
Hiatus hernia (burping)
Reflux oesophagitis (pain, waterbrash)
Sjögren's syn.
Diabetes mellitus (polyuria, polydipsia)
Dry mouth (eg. mouth breathing)
Lymphadenopathy
Cervical osteoarthritis
Thyroglossal cyst
Brachial cyst
Long styloid process
Irritation from chronic cough
Motor neurone disease
Bulbar palsy
Myocardial ischaemia (worse with exercise)

Throat Pain

Coryza (malaise, rhinitis, cough)
Pharyngitis (fever, malaise)
Tonsillitis (fever, headache, anorexia)
Quinsy (dysphagia, fever, trismus)
Pharyngeal abscess (dysphagia, dyspnoea, fever)
Infectious mononucleosis (adenitis, anorexia, fever)
Measles (rash, adenitis, conjunctivitis)
Diphtheria (membrane, hoarse, myocarditis)
Vincent's angina
Oesophageal reflux (burping, waterbrash)
Gonococcal pharyngitis
Syphilis
Leukaemia
Other viral and bacterial respiratory tract infections
Pharyngeal carcinoma
Cervical arthritis (neck stiff)
Chronic fatigue syn. (fever, poor exercise tolerance)
Foreign body (eg. fish bone)
Agranulocytosis (fever, fatigue, ulcers)
Rabies (hydrophobia, animal bite, convulsions)
Lassa fever (malaise, cough, abdominal pain)

See also Neck Pain

Thymus Associated Syndromes

Good syn. (thymic hypoplasia, hypothyroidism)

See also SYNDROMES SECTION 6

Thyroid Disease

See Goitre; Neck Pain

Tics

Repetitive muscular movement
Emotional (habit, stress induced)
Degenerative nervous disease
Epilepsy (amnesia, variation in mental state)
Basal ganglia disease
Chorea (see separate entry)
Psychoses (other psychiatric symptoms)

Tingling

See Paraesthesia

Tinnitus

Noise in ears
Menière's disease (deaf, vertigo, nausea)
Vascular disease (eg. atherosclerosis)
Labyrinthitis (nystagmus, stagger, vertigo)
Hypertension (headache, fatigue)
Neuroses
Temporomandibular joint dysfunction
Chronic otitis media
Chronic noise exposure
Aneurysms and vascular tumours
Patulous tympanic membrane
Otosclerosis
Cochlear degeneration
Otic trauma (eg. barotrauma, surgery)
Cogan syn. (vertigo, deaf)
Costen syn. (ear pain, deaf)
Altitude sickness (vertigo, dyspnoea, headache)
Caffeine (eg. coffee, tea, cola)
Drugs (eg. salicylates, quinine)

See also Earache; Vertigo

Tiredness

See Fatigue, Abnormal

Toe

See Foot Pain; Leg Pain; Polydactyly; Syndactyly

Tone, Increased

See SIGNS SECTION 2: Hypertonicity

Tongue Abnormality Associated Syndromes

Beckwith syn. (exomphalos, neonate, macroglossia)
Down syn. (mental retardation, typical facies, macroglossia)
Sicard syn. (paralysis of cranial nerves 9, 10, 11, 12)

See also SYNDROMES SECTION 6
See also SIGNS SECTION 2: Tongue, abnormal

Tongue Pain

Thrush (white adherent plaque)
Aphthous ulcers
Hand, foot, mouth disease (palm and sole blisters)
Pernicious anaemia (anorexia, dyspepsia, pallor)
Tongue carcinoma (stiffness, mass)
Iron deficiency (smooth, red tongue)
Folic acid deficiency

See also Stomatitis and Gingivitis

Tooth, Discoloured

Extrinsic Causes
Smoking
Coloured food and drinks
Poor dental hygiene
Fungal infections
Drugs (eg. iron, chorhexidine, tetracycline)

Intrinsic Causes
Dental caries
Dental amalgam
Trauma (dead tooth)
Internal resorption (pink spots)
Fluorosis (fluoride supplements)
Kernicterus
Amelogenesis imperfecta
Dentinogenesis imperfecta
Porphyria (port wine urine)

Tooth, Loose

Local Causes
Trauma to tooth, mandible, maxilla or gums
Periodontitis
Neoplasms of gum
Papillon-LeFevre syn. (wide tooth spaces)

Systemic Causes
Down syn. (see SYNDROMES SECTION 6)
Diabetes mellitus
Leucopenia
Scurvy (nutritional deficit)
AIDS

Genetic Causes
Hypophosphatasia
Ehlers-Danlos syn. (joint hypermobility, cutaneous fragility)
Chediak-Higashi syn. (oculocutaneous albinism, immunodeficiency)
Eosinophilic granulomas

Tremor

Senile tremor
Muscular fatigue
Essential [benign familial] tremor
Anxiety and stress
Physiological tremor (minimal, arms, postural)
Essential [benign familial] tremor (postural, arms, legs, head)
Orthostatic tremor (14-6 Hz., axial, unsteady)

Anxiety and stress
Muscular fatigue
Cerebrovascular accident (intention tremor)
Cerebral dysfunction (intention tremor)
Cerebral trauma (tremor at rest)
Cerebellar lesions (intention tremor)
Cerebral tumour
Multiple sclerosis (neurological signs, young adult)
Wilson's disease (cirrhosis, rigidity, brown cornea)
Chorea (involuntary jerks, speech impaired, weakness)
Delirium tremens (alcohol, anxiety)
Thyrotoxicosis (weak, sweating, weight loss)
Peripheral neuropathy
Neurosyphilis
Hypoglycaemia
Trypanosomiasis (apathy, neurological signs)
Phaeochromocytoma (hypertension)
Mercury or arsenic poisoning
Addictive drug withdrawal
Drugs (eg. alcohol, caffeine, salbutamol, lithium, phenytoin)

SYNDROMES (see SYNDROMES SECTION 6)

Diencephalic syn. (cachexia, pallor, vomiting)
Neuroleptic malignant syn. (tranquillizer use, fever)
Parkinsonism (rigidity, worse at rest, limbs, head, jaw)
Punch drunk syn. (gait abnormal, boxer)
Serotonin syn. (tremor, antidepressant drugs)
Shy-Drager syn. (hypotension, dysarthria, vertigo)

See also Chorea; Tetany
See also SIGNS SECTION 2: Flapping Tremor
See also symptoms listed under Neurological Symptoms

Trismus

Inability to open the mouth fully
Masticatory muscle spasm
Temporomandibular joint trauma or arthritis
Acute pericoronitis (pain)
Scleroderma (thick skin, pulmonary lesions)
Submucous fibrosis or scarring
Fracture/dislocation of mandibular condyle
Myofascial syn. (face pain, bruxism)
Freeman-Sheldon syn. (see SYNDROMES SECTION 6)

Tumours

See Breast Lump; Bone Mass or Tumour; Goitre; Mouth Swellings; Nodules; Testicular or Scrotal Mass or Tumour

Twitch

See Tremor

Ulcer, Genital

See Genital Ulcer

Ulcer, Mouth

See Mouth Ulcer

Ulcer, Skin

See Skin Ulcer

Unconscious

See Coma; Drop Attack; Syncope (Faint)

Underweight

See Failure to Thrive; Weight Loss

Urethral Discharge

Prostatitis (dysuria, frequency, pain)
Gonorrhoea (dysuria, milky discharge)
Nonspecific urethritis [Chlamydia]
Mycoplasma / Ureoplasma infection

Urethritis

See Dysuria; Urethral Discharge

Urinary Retention and Difficult Micturition

Prostatic hyperplasia (poor stream, infection)
Prostatic carcinoma (back pain, renal failure)
Bladder tumours (haematuria, pain)
Bladder calculus or blood clot
Foreign body in urethra or bladder
Urethral stricture or tumour
Neurogenic bladder
Typhoid fever (abdominal tenderness, cough)
Stress and anxiety

Urine

See Dysuria; Haematuria and Red Urine; Polyuria and Pollakiuria; Renal Disease Associated Syndromes

Urine, Abnormal Colour

See Haematuria and Red Urine
See also SIGNS SECTION 2: Urine, Abnormal Colour

Urine, Bloody

See Haematuria and Red Urine

Urine, Excessive

See Polyuria and Pollakiuria

Urine, Gaseous

See Pneumaturia

Urine, Reduced Volume

See Oliguria and Anuria

Urticaria

See Oedema; Pruritus

Uterine Bleeding

See Vaginal and Uterine Bleeding, Abnormal

Uveitis

See Eye, Inflamed or Red

Vaginal and Uterine Bleeding, Abnormal

UTERINE

Fibroma (bulky uterus, leucorrhoea, dysmenorrhoea)
Endometrial polyps
Adenomyosis
Endometritis (foul discharge, pain, fever)
Salpingitis (pain, leucorrhoea, fever)
Threatened, inevitable or missed abortion
Endometrial hyperplasia or cancer
Hydatidiform mole (nausea, large uterus)

VAGINAL

Vaginitis (leucorrhoea)
Ulcers of cervix (leucorrhoea, back pain, dyspareunia)
Erosion or eversion of cervix
Carcinoma of cervix
Vaginal tumours or polyps

OVARIAN

Ovulation [mittelschmerz] (mid-cycle, pain)
Anovulatory haemorrhage
Ovarian tumours (eg. follicular cysts, corpus luteum cyst)

GENERAL GYNAECOLOGY

Hormonal imbalance (eg. pituitary disease, hormone therapy)
Menopause (flush, depression)
Gynaecological carcinoma (noncyclical pain and bleeding)
Endometriosis (dysmenorrhoea, dyspareunia, rectal blood)
Ectopic pregnancy (abdominal pain, pregnancy symptoms)
Oral contraceptives and other hormones
Uterine or vaginal wall prolapses

OTHER

Blood dyscrasias (bruising, epistaxis)
Coagulopathies
Systemic malignancy
Liver diseases
Hypothyroidism (weak, cold intolerance, dry skin)
Psychological or physical trauma

See also Menorrhagia; Gynaecology; Vagina, Discharge, Excessive

Vagina, Discharge, Excessive

Leucorrhoea [excessive normal discharge]
Hormonal imbalance or therapy (eg. oral contraceptives)
Gynaecological infections (eg. thrush, Trichomonas, bacteria)
Sexual stimulation
Gynaecological tumours (bleeding, pain)
Cervicitis and vaginitis
Eversion of cervix
Sexually transmitted disease (eg. gonorrhoea)
Uterine fibroids (pelvic mass)
Polyps of vagina or endometrium
Pregnancy
Pelvic inflammatory disease (abdominal pain, dysuria)
Nonspecific urethritis (Chlamydia)
Vaginal worms
Sexual abuse in child
Septic abortion
Intrauterine contraceptive device
Trauma (eg. dildo)
Retained vaginal tampon or other foreign body
Chemical irritants (eg. douche)

Vagina, Dry

Senile atrophy
Hypothyroidism (cold intolerance, tired)
Lack of sexual stimulation
Menopause
Vaginismus
Pituitary or adrenal diseases
Vaginal prolapse
Vaginal malignancy

Vertebral Pain

See Back and Vertebral Pain

Vertigo
Dizziness/giddiness

OTIC

Menière's disease (deaf, tinnitus, nausea)
Labyrinthitis (nystagmus, stagger, tinnitus)
Eighth cranial nerve damage (eg. neuroma)
Otitis media (pain, fever)
Eustachian tube blockage (ear discomfort, deaf)
Vestibular neuronitis (nystagmus, resting vertigo)
Mastoiditis (pain, mastoid tender, fever)
Perilymphatic fistula

CARDIOVASCULAR AND CIRCULATORY

Myocardial infarct (shock, chest pain)
Postural hypotension
Vertebrobasilar insufficiency (diplopia, dysarthria, faint)
Myocarditis (asthenia, dyspnoea, nausea)
Arteriosclerosis (mental deterioration and confusion)
Anaemia (pallor, fatigue, palpitations)
Hypertension (headache)
Cardiac arrhythmias

CENTRAL NERVOUS SYSTEM

Motion sickness
Temporal lobe epilepsy (aura, faint)
Cerebellar lesions (incoordination, headache, nausea)

Psychiatric disorders
Cerebrovascular accident (confusion, headache, aphasia)
Transient ischaemic attack (brief, confusion, headache)
Migraine (headache, nausea, photophobia)
Multiple sclerosis (weakness, abnormal sensation)
Parkinson's disease (tremor, stiffness)
Subdural haematoma
Cerebral tumours

SYNDROMES (see SYNDROMES SECTION 6)

Cogan syn. (tinnitus, deaf)
Dandy syn. (bilateral loss of vestibular function, loss of foveation)
Post-traumatic cerebral syn. (headache, mental changes)
Ramsay Hunt syn. (earache, *Herpes zoster*)
Shy-Drager syn. (hypotension, tremor, ataxia)

OTHER

Hyperventilation from any cause
Cervical spine osteophytes (neck pain and stiffness)
Thyrotoxicosis (sweating, heat intolerance, warm skin)
Hypothyroidism (cold intolerance, dry skin)
Diabetes mellitus (paraesthesiae, blurred vision, polyuria)
Hypoglycaemia (insulin overdosage)
Benign paroxysmal positional vertigo (worse lying)
Addison's disease (weak, pigmentation)
Acromegaly (coarse facies, psychoses, back pain)
Pre-eclampsia (pregnancy, hypertension, proteinuria)
Syphilis (various neurological symptoms)
Trauma (eg. fractured temporal bone)
Altitude sickness (headache, drowsiness, nausea)
Drugs (eg. phenytoin, benzodiazepines, phenobarbitone, salicylates, gentamicin, streptomycin)

See also Balance, Disturbed

Vesicles

See Rash, Vesicular

Violence

Alcohol intoxication
Drug abuse (eg. barbiturates, LSD)
Attention deficit hyperactivity disorder
Hypoglycaemia (slurred speech, mental changes)
Head injury (disorientation, pupil changes)
Epilepsy (amnesia, collapse, spasmodic)
Hypomania
Schizophrenia (hallucination, delusions)

SYNDROMES (see SYNDROMES SECTION 6)

Acute brain syn.
Asperger's syn. (no emotion, poor communication)
Episodic dyscontrol syn. (alcohol dependence, sex crimes)
Hyperkinetic syn. (overactive, poor coordination)
Klinefelter's syn. (hypoplastic genitals, XXY)
Lesch-Nyhan syn. (mental retardation, self-mutilation, gout)
Organic personality syn. (labile emotions)
XXY syn. (male, tall)

See also symptoms listed under Neurological Symptoms

Viral

See Postviral Infection Associated Syndromes

Virilism Associated Syndromes

Adrenogenital syn. (child, hypocorticalism)
Albright syn. (polyostotic fibrous dysplasia)

See also Hirsutism and Hypertrichosis; Puberty, Early
See also SYNDROMES SECTION 6

Vision, Black Spots in Field of

Migraine (headache, nausea, photophobia)
Vitreous floater
Epilepsy (convulsions, absences)
Detached retina (fixed spot)
Cataract (small central opacity)
Optic nerve tumour
Poor cerebral blood flow (eg. before faint)
Noticing blind spot in visual field

Vision, Blurred

OPHTHALMIC

Refractive error
Corneal opacities
Cataract (progressive, lens opacity, painless)
Retinal detachment (no pain or redness)
Iritis (pain, red eye)
Glaucoma (pain, red eye, small pupil)
Conjunctivitis (discharge, red eye, no pain)
Corneal ulcer (discharge, pain)
Optic vascular disease
Arc or UV eye (pain, red)
Herpetic keratitis (pain, photophobia)
Optic neuritis (pain)

OTHER

Diabetes mellitus (fatigue, polyuria, polydipsia)
Cerebrovascular accident (unilateral, sudden)
Anaphylaxis
Migraine (headache)
Uraemia (fatigue, headache, pruritus)
Hypoparathyroidism (tetany, wheeze, convulsions)
Phaeochromocytoma (sweating, hypertension, headache)
Drugs (eg. atropine, cocaine, nicotine)

See also Blindness, Partial or Total

Vision, Double

See Diplopia

Vision, Loss

See Blindness, Partial or Total; Hemianopia; Vision, Black Spots in Field of; Vision, Blurred

Visual Halos

See Halos, Visual

Vitiligo

See Skin, Depigmented

Voice, Abnormal

See Aphasia and Dysarthria; Hoarseness

Vomiting

See Nausea and Vomiting; Haematemesis

Vulval Itch

See Pruritus Vulvae

Waterbrash

Bitter tasting fluid in mouth

Reflux oesophagitis (heartburn, cough, nausea when recumbant)
Hiatus hernia (burping, heartburn)
Peptic ulcer (epigastric pain and tenderness, food related)

Weakness, Muscular

See Paralysis and Muscular Weakness; Fatigue, Abnormal; Floppy Baby; Facial Weakness

Weight Gain

Excess caloric intake
Lack of exercise
Hypothyroidism (cold intolerance, depression, dry skin)
Congestive cardiac failure (dyspnoea, oedema)
Cushing's syn. (see SYNDROMES SECTION 6)
Prader-Willi syn. (see SYNDROMES SECTION 6)
Hypogonadism (lack of secondary sexual characteristics)
Insulinoma (hypoglycaemia)
Craniopharyngioma (headache, visual changes, vomiting)
Drugs (eg. steroids, tricyclics, thioridazine)

See also Obesity

Weight Loss

GASTROINTESTINAL

Oesophageal stricture or neoplasm (dysphagia)
Peptic ulcer (epigastric pain, burping, melaena)
Cirrhosis (jaundice, pruritus, hepatomegaly)
Hepatitis of any cause or type
Intestinal parasites (altered bowel habits)
Cholestasis and cholelithiasis (RUQ pain)
Chronic pancreatitis (cachexia, back pain)
Ulcerative colitis (fever, altered bowel habits)
Crohn's disease (abdominal pain, diarrhoea)
Chronic vomiting or diarrhoea
Intestinal obstruction (eg. colonic carcinoma)

SYNDROMES (see SYNDROMES SECTION 6)

AIDS (adenitis, rash, fever, splenomegaly)
Diencephalic syn. (pallor, vomiting, tremor)
Leschke syn. (brown spots, hyperglycaemia)

Letterer-Siwe syn. (rash, infant, fever)
Lightwood syn. (vomiting, constipatation, child)
Malabsorption syn. (eg. sprue)
Trousseau syn. (carcinoma, thrombophlebitis)

OTHER

Neoplasms of any sort
Deliberate dieting or malnutrition
Anorexia nervosa (amenorrhoea, female)
Schizophrenia (no insight)
Other psychiatric problems (eg. depression)
Chronic infection (eg. TB, hepatitis, AIDS, brucellosis)
Autoimmune disorders (eg. SLE, scleroderma, dermatomyositis)
Depression (insomnia, loss of interest)
Cerebrovascular accident
Parkinson's disease (tremor, rigidity)
Systemic fungal infections
Reticuloses
Hyperthyroidism (rapid pulse, exophthalmos)
Rheumatoid arthritis (joint swelling and pain)
Renal failure
Chronic congestive cardiac failure (dyspnoea)
Phaeochromocytoma (hypertension)
Addison's disease (pigmentation)
Endocarditis
Asthma (wheeze, cough)
Emphysema (dyspnoea, cough, oedema)
Diabetes mellitus (polyuria, weak, neuropathy)
Diabetes insipidus (polydipsia, polyuria)
Hypercalcaemia (nausea, constipation, weak)
Alcohol and drug dependence

See also Anorexia; Failure to Thrive

Weight, Low

See Failure to Thrive; Growth, Reduced; Weight Loss

Wheals

See Pruritus; Rash, Bullous; Erythema

Wheeze

Bronchial or tracheal foreign body (cough)
Asthma (dyspnoea, cough, prolonged expiration)
Anaphylaxis
Acute left ventricular failure (cough, oedema)
Bronchitis (cough, fever, chest pain)
Bronchial carcinoma (cough, haemoptysis, malaise)
Bronchiectasis (foul sputum, chest pain)
Emphysema (dyspnoea, cough, barrel chest)
Hypoparathyroidism (tetany, stridor, polyuria)
Bronchiolitis (fever, tachypnoea, overinflation, child)
Echinococcosis (urticaria, jaundice)
Cystic fibrosis (recurrent lung infections)
Aspergillosis
Alpha$_1$-antitrypsin deficiency (child)
Gastro-oesophageal reflux
Pneumonitis

SYNDROMES (see SYNDROMES SECTION 6)

Carcinoid syn. (flush, abdominal cramps, diarrhoea)

Churg-Strauss syn. (vasculitis)
France's triad (aspirin sensitivity, rhinitis)
Loeffler syn. (cough, fever, pulmonary eosinophilia)
Mendelson's syn. (pneumonitis, bronchospasm)

See also Cough; Dyspnoea; Stridor

White Mouth Lesions
See Leucoplakia

Worm Associated Diseases

CESTODES (tapeworms)
Diphyllobothriasis [fish] (rare)
Echinococcus [Hydatid disease] (jaundice, chest pain, epilepsy)
Taeniasis [beef and pork] (intestinal symptoms)

NEMATODES (roundworms)
Ancylostoma [hookworm, cutaneous larva migrans]
Ascariasis (asymptomatic or intestinal symptoms)
Dracunculiais [guinea worm]
Enterobiasis [threadworm] (pruritis ani)
Filariasis [loiasis, onchocerciasis etc.] (fever, lymph blockage)
Necator americanus [hookworm anaemia]
Strongyloidiasis (rash, lung and gut symptoms)
Trichinosis (asymptomatic, gut or muscle symptoms)
Trichuriasis [whipworm] (colitis)
Toxocariasis [visceral larva migrans] (intestinal and lung symptoms, epilepsy)

TREMATODES (flukes)
Clonorchiasis [oriental liver fluke] (asymptomatic, jaundice)
Fascioliasis [liver fluke] (urticaria, liver pain, jaundice)
Fasciolopiasis [intestinal fluke] (intestinal symptoms)
Schistosomiasis [bilharzia] (fever, gut symptoms, haematuria)

Wrist Pain
Carpal tunnel syn. (radiates to hand)
Osteoarthritis (inflammation)
Synovitis
Sprain or strain to wrist ligaments
Ganglion (lump)
Tendinitis (eg. de Quervain's) (movement pain)
Tendon avulsion
Ulnar nerve entrapment
Wrist joint instability
Ulnar or radius fracture
Scaphoid or other wrist bone fracture
Carpal bone or wrist dislocation
Carpal bone chondromalacia
Avascular necrosis of carpal bone
Bone cyst or tumour
Cartilaginous tears
Ulnar artery thrombosis
Forearm compartment strain
Madelung deformity

See also Arm Pain; Hand Pain

Writhing Movements
See Athetosis

Writing Disability
See Agraphia

Xanthomata
See SIGNS SECTION 2: Xanthomatosis

Xeroderma
See Skin, Dry

Xerophthalmia
See Eye, Dry

Xerostomia
See Mouth, Dry

Yellow Skin
See Jaundice

SECTION TWO
SIGNS

CLINICAL SIGNS AND THEIR INTERPRETATION

SIGN: Objective evidence of disease or deformity.

Butterworths Medical Dictionary

FORMAT

Sign (Alternate Name) [Abbreviation]
EXP: An explanation of the sign, with its methodology described in sufficient detail to enable the practitioner to perform the test
INT: The interpretation of the sign.
+) The disease, syndromes etc., that should be considered if the test is positive.
++) The interpretation of an exaggerated or grossly positive result.
−) Ditto for a negative test.
AB) Ditto for an abnormal test result
PHYS: The pathophysiology of the sign to enable its significance to be better understood.
See also Other Signs of Significance

Alternate Name
See Sign Name

Abdominal Mass

EXP: Palpation of an abnormal structure in the abdominal cavity

INT: (+ Superficial) – Lipoma, sebaceous cyst, umbilical hernia, inguinal hernia, incisional hernia, post-traumatic scarring, rectus sheath haematoma, divarication of the recti
(+ Deep) – Carcinoma of bowel or stomach, Crohn's disease, Hodgkin's disease, other lymphomas, metastatic carcinoma, appendiceal abscess, pancreatic tumour, aortic aneurysm, pregnancy, uterine fibroid or tumour, ovarian tumour or cyst, hydatid cyst, distended gall bladder, enlarged liver (see Hepatomegaly), enlarged spleen (see Splenomegaly), enlarged kidney (see Kidney, Large), pyloric stenosis, bladder carcinoma, vertebral tumours, neuroblastoma

PHYS: Any organ in the abdominal cavity may become diseased and distended

Abdominal Rigidity

EXP: Unrelaxable firmness of the abdominal wall on palpation

INT: (+) Appendicitis, pancreatitis, perforated viscus (eg. peptic ulcer), acute Crohn's disease, intraperitoneal haemorrhage, ectopic pregnancy, ruptured ovarian cyst, peritonitis, pelvic inflammatory disease

PHYS: Involuntary muscular spasm due to irritation of the peritoneum by blood, pus, acid, enzymes or inflamed tissue

See also Carnett's Test

Adie's pupil

See also Holmes-Aide Syndrome in SYNDROMES SECTION 6

Adson's Test

EXP: Patient is seated with hands on thighs, and takes and holds a very deep breath. The neck is then hyperextended, and the head turned from side to side. Positive if radial pulse on one side is obliterated

INT: (+) Cervical rib syn., thoracic outlet syn., scalenus anticus syn.

PHYS: Compression of subclavian artery against abnormal cervical rib or scalenus anticus

Adventitious Sounds

See Crepitations, Pulmonary; Crepitations, Tissue; Rhonchi
See also SYMPTOMS SECTION 1: Stridor

Amphoric Breathing

EXP: High pitched, metallic toned, bronchial breathing heard on auscultation

INT: (+) Open pneumothorax, tuberculous cavities

PHYS: Named after Greek amphora (pottery vessel), as breath sounds similar to blowing over the top of a bottle

Anaesthesia

See SYMPTOMS SECTION 1: Anaesthesia

Anal Examination

See Rectal Mass

Aniscoria

EXP: Pupils are different sizes

INT: (+) Physiological (20% of population), raised intracranial pressure, abnormal migraine, third nerve palsy, Adie's pupil (ciliary muscle paresis), Horner syndrome, Pancoast tumour, penetrating trauma, medications (eg. atropine)

PHYS: causes may be physiological, structural, pharmacological or neurological

Ankle Clonus

EXP: Sharp dorsiflexion of foot causes repeated spasm of calf muscles and plantar flexion of foot

INT: (+) Upper motor neurone lesions and disease, functional nervous disorders, epilepsy, tuberous sclerosis, Wilson's disease, uraemia, encephalitis, multiple sclerosis, CVA, cirrhosis, Creutzfeldt-Jakob disease, encephalitis lethargica, alcohol withdrawal, drugs, benign idiopathic

PHYS: With an upper motor neurone lesion there is no inhibition of the tendon stretch reflex

See also Ankle Jerk

Ankle Jerk

EXP: With patient kneeling on a chair, or supine, the Achilles tendon is struck firmly, causing spasm of the calf musculature

INT: (–) Peripheral neuropathies, polio, tabes dorsalis, posterior root tumour, spinal tumours, subacute combined degeneration of the cord, syringomyelia, multiple sclerosis, hypothyroidism, diabetes mellitus, beriberi, often absent in elderly
(++) Upper motor neurone lesions, encephalitis, anxiety, tetanus, hyperthyroidism, cord transection

PHYS: Reflex absence due to interruption of the reflex arc or muscular disease. Exaggeration due to lack of suppression of reflex by cortical centres. Acts at L2, L3, L4

See also other signs listed under Reflexes

Ankle Oedema

EXP: Swelling of the ankle due to excess fluid accumulation

INT: (+) Congestive cardiac failure, venous valve

incompetence, venous thrombosis, hypoproteinaemia, malnutrition,cirrhosis, glomerulonephritis, nephrotic syn., secondary hyperaldosteronism, intra-abdominal tumour, filariasis, cellulitis, gout,SLE, pregnancy, pre-eclampsia, prolonged sitting or rest, heat, drugs (eg. felodipine, nifedipine)

PHYS: Reduced venous return from the legs, excess body fluid load or localised inflammation

See also Pitting Oedema
See also SYMPTOMS SECTION 1: Oedema

Apex Beat

EXP: Palpation of the cardiac apex beat and assessing its duration, force, site (see Apex Beat Displacement below) and area covered. Felt with patient supine, or erect and leaning forwards

INT: Forceful, displaced laterally, slightly prolonged – Hypertension
Displaced laterally, rapid rise and fall, brief duration – Aortic or mitral regurgitation
Powerful, prolonged, not displaced – Aortic stenosis

Apex Beat Displacement

EXP: Palpation of chest wall with flat of finger tips to detect point of maximal cardiac pulsation. Normally 7 to10 cm to left of midline in 5th intercostal space

INT: Displaced to left – Cardiomegaly (eg. valvular disease,hypertension, pulmonary disease, cardiomyopathies, congenital heart disease, aneurysm,rheumatic fever), pulmonary fibrosis, scoliosis, pectus excavatum, elevated diaphragm, bronchiectasis
Displaced to right – Pneumothorax, pleural effusion, dextrocardia

PHYS: Commonly due to cardiac or pulmonary disease

Apley's Grind Test

EXP: With the patient prone, flex the knee to be tested to 90°. Apply pressure to the bottom of the heel in order to force the tibia into femoral articulation, then twist the tibia. If pain is felt at the knee, the test is positive

INT: (+) Cartilage damage in knee joint, septic arthritis

Arcus Senilis

EXP: An opaque ring in the peripheral cornea with a clear zone separating it from the limbus

INT: (+) Occurs invariably with advancing age, hypercholesterolaemia

Phys: Deposition of lipids in periphery of cornea

See also Xanthomatosis

Areolar Pigmentation

EXP: Darkening of areola and nipple

INT: (+) Present or past pregnancy, hormone therapy, familial, racial

PHYS: Enlargement of Montgomery's follicles in areola should also be noted in current pregnancy or hormone therapy

Argyll Robertson Pupil

EXP: Small, irregular, unequal pupils that do not react to light, but do react to convergence

INT: (+) Neurosyphilis, tabes dorsalis, diabetes

PHYS: Damage to the midbrain section of the optic tract

Arlt's Line

EXP: Cicatricial scarring of upper eyelid causing entropion

INT: (+) Chronic trachoma

PHYS: Chronic inflammation of subepithelial tissue of the tarsus

See also Entropion

Arrhythmias, Cardiac

See Bradycardia; Dicrotic Pulse; Extrasystolic Beats; Gallop Rhythm; Tachycardia; INVESTIGATIONS SECTION 3: Arrhythmias, Cardiac
See also signs listed under Heart; Pulse

Arteriovenous Nipping, Retinal

EXP: Ophthalmoscopic or slit lamp examination of the retina reveals narrowing of venules where they are crossed by arterioles

INT: (+)Hypertension, arteriosclerosis

PHYS: Increased pressure on the venule in the shared adventitial sheath where vessels cross

Ascites

See Shifting Dullness; Thrill, Fluid;
See also SYMPTOMS SECTION 1: Ascites

Asterixis

See Tremor, Flapping

Ataxia

EXP: Lack of proper coordination. An unsteady, uncontrolled gait and/or a clumsy nose-finger test

INT: (+) Subacute combined degeneration of cord, multiple sclerosis, Friedreich's ataxia, tabes dorsalis, cerebellar lesions, posterior column lesions, poliomyelitis, hydrocephalus, postviral transient ischaemic attack, foramen magnum lesions, Creutzfeldt-Jakob disease, metabolic disorders, alcohol abuse, Angelman syn., Bassen-Kornzweig syn.,Louis-Bar syn., Machado-Joseph syn., Marinesco-Sjögren syn., Roussy-Levy syn., Shy-Drager syn., Strachan syn., Wernicke-Korsakoff syn.

PHYS: Sensory (posterior column) and motor

(cerebellar) forms. Former may be compensated for by ocular impressions (poorer coordination with eyes shut)

See also Heel-Knee Test; Nose-Finger Test; Romberg's Sign
See also INVESTIGATIONS SECTION 3: Achilles Tendon Rupture

Athetosis (Torsion Dystonia)

EXP: Involuntary, slow, writhing movements; particularly of hands and arms
INT: (+) Infantile hemiplegia, extrapyramidal lesions, basal ganglia lesions, cerebral palsy, encephalitis lethargica, Wilson's disease, juvenile Huntington's chorea, Lesch-Nyhan disease, kernicterus, Hallervorden-Spatz disease, idiopathic and paroxysmal dystonias, drugs (eg. phenothiazines, diazoxide)
PHYS: Release mechanism associated with various forms of damage to basal ganglia and related motor pathways, particularly in children with birth trauma or anoxia

See also Choreiform Movements

Atrial Fibrillation

EXP: On an ECG, numerous disorganised waves (f waves) can be seen circulating rapidly and randomly through the atria at a rate between 300 and 600 per minute
INT: (+) Ischaemic heart disease, myocardial infarct, mitral valve disease, rheumatic valve disease, congestive cardiac failure, cardiomyopathies, myocarditis, pericarditis, thyrotoxicosis, Wolff-Parkinson-White syn., cardiac trauma, cardiac tumours
PHYS: AV node receives f waves at a rate higher than it can conduct. A random minority of these pulses are transmitted to the ventricles, giving the irregular pattern of beats

See also Irregularly Irregular Pulse

Atrophy, Muscular

EXP: Wasting of musculature in one or more limbs. Careful comparative measurements of limbs advisable
INT: (+) Lower motor neurone lesions, muscular dystrophies, rheumatoid arthritis, dystrophia myotonica, peroneal muscular atrophy, polio, motor neurone disease, prolonged immobilisation
PHYS: Interruption to muscular nerve supply or disuse due to pain causes wasting

Auspitz's Sign

EXP: When white scale is removed from a plaque of scale covered dermatitis on the shins, a bleeding area results
INT: (+) Psoriasis
PHYS: In psoriasis, the plaque has a microcapillary circulation that is disrupted by its removal

Austin-Flint Murmur

EXP: When listening to the cardiac apex, a murmur is heard that has its onset associated with a 3rd heart sound, is loudest at mid-diastole and may have some presystolic accentuation
INT: (+) Aortic regurgitation
PHYS: The full opening of the mitral valve is prevented by the regurgitant jet from the aortic valve defect and the more rapid rise in the left ventricular than the left atrial diastolic pressure. Inadequate function of the mitral valve subsequent to the aortic regurgitation produces the characteristic murmur

Babinski's Sign (Plantar Reflex)

EXP: Normally, slow dorsiflexion of the great toe and fanning of the other toes occurs when the lateral side of the sole is stroked firmly with a pointed object, from the heel towards the toes. Positive with extension of great toe
INT: (+) Corticospinal tract lesions, coma, post epileptic seizure, upper motor neurone lesions, multiple sclerosis, CVA, subacute combined degeneration of cord, paraplegia, normal infants
PHYS: Acts at S1, S2 level

Barford Test

EXP: Place both legs of patient in mirror-image positions. A stethoscope is placed over the symphysis pubis, and a comparison is made between the sound heard from a vibrating 128Hz tuning fork placed on each medial femoral condyle or patella in turn. Positive if reduced conduction of sound occurs on the injured side
INT: (+) Fracture of neck of femur
PHYS: Fracture disrupts conduction of sound from distal femur to pelvis

Barlow Test

EXP: With the infant supine, the hips are adducted with the examiner's thumb over the medial aspect of the femoral head. Pressure is applied forwards and laterally by the thumb in an attempt to dislocate the hip. The hip is then abducted, and a clunk will be felt if the hip joint has been displaced. Test should be done without any significant force being applied
INT: (+) Unstable hip that has the potential for dislocation

See also Ortolani Test

Barrel Chest

EXP: Chest fixed in inspiration. Increased anteroposterior diameter to give impression of a cylindrical chest

INT: (+) Emphysema, asthma
PHYS: Permanent overinflation of distal air spaces due
       to chronic infections or expiratory airway
       obstruction

See also Pink Puffer

Battle's Sign

EXP: Retromastoid bruising behind the ear
INT: (+) Fracture of the petrous bone
PHYS: Blood tracks to this subcutaneous point from
       fracture site

See also Racoon Sign

Beau's Line

See Nail Ridging

Beighton Score

See Joint Hypermobility

Biceps Jerk

EXP: With elbow flexed and forearm slightly
       pronated, a finger placed on the biceps tendon
       is struck firmly. Normal reaction is flexion of the
       elbow
INT: (–) Polio, peripheral neuropathy (eg. diabetes,
       alcoholism), tabes dorsalis, posterior root and
       cord tumours, syringomyelia, subacute
       combined degeneration of cord, cord trauma,
       muscular dystrophy, coma, peripheral nerve
       lesions, elderly
       (++) Upper motor neurone lesions, tetanus,
       encephalitis
PHYS: Acts at C5, C6 level

See also other signs listed under Reflexes

Black Eyes, Bilateral

EXP: Both eyelids spontaneously blackened after
       trauma excluded. May be precipitated by
       sigmoidoscopy
INT: (+) Amyloidosis
PHYS: The Valsalva manoeuvre of sigmoidoscopy
       may be a precipitant

Black Urine

See Urine, Abnormal Colour

Blood Pressure

See Hypertension; Hypotension

Blue Bloater

EXP: Oedematous patient with cyanosis at rest, warm
       extremities, generalised plethora, shortness of
       breath, productive cough, polycythaemia and a
       large heart

INT: (+) Bronchitic chronic obstructive airways
       disease
PHYS: Greatly increased airways resistance and
       cardiac failure

See also Pink Puffer

Blue Cervix and Vagina

EXP: Vagina and cervix are a dark blue to purple
       colour on speculum examination
INT: (+) Pregnancy
PHYS: Increased progesterone levels cause venous
       dilatation

See also Hegar's Sign; Areolar Pigmentation

Blue Line on Gums

See Gums, Blue Line on

Blue Sclera

See Sclera, Blue

Blue Skin

*See SYMPTOMS SECTION 1: Cyanosis, Central;
Cyanosis, Peripheral*

Borborygmus

EXP: Greatly exaggerated, high pitched, tinkling
       abdominal sounds
INT: (+) Intestinal obstruction or infection, food
       poisoning, toxic enteritis
PHYS: Sound due to compression of air-fluid mixture
       by excessive peristaltic movements of gut
       attempting to overcome obstruction or being
       irritated by infection

Bossing

See Frontal Bossing

Bouchard's Nodes

EXP: Bony prominences at the dorsal margins of
       proximal interphalangeal joints
INT: (+) Severe osteoarthritis

See also Heberden's Nodes

Bounding Pulse

EXP: Full, exaggerated arterial pulsation
INT: (+) Thyrotoxicosis, fever, pregnancy, anaemia,
       other hyperkinetic circulatory states, drugs (eg.
       adrenaline)
PHYS: Vasodilatation and increased cardiac output
       exaggerates peripheral pulsations

Boutonnière (Button Hole) Deformity

EXP: Painful, fixed flexion of proximal interphalangeal
       finger joint with marked prominence of distal

end of proximal phalanx and swelling of joint

INT: (+) Disruption of central slip of extensor digitorum tendon allows joint to protrude between medial and lateral slips of extensor tendon, rheumatoid arthritis

PHYS: May be associated with a fracture avulsion of central slip which will require surgical repair if displaced

Bradycardia

EXP: Slow heart (pulse) rate, generally below 60 per minute

INT: (+) Healthy athlete, elderly, fright, hypothermia, postinfective states, increased intracranial pressure, serious liver disease, cerebral tumours, hypothyroidism, electrolyte imbalances, syncope, anaphylaxis, myocardial infarct, heart block, sick sinus syn., congestive cardiac failure, Stokes-Adams syn., Romano-Ward syn., vasovagal syn., septicaemia, drugs (eg. digitalis, beta-blockers, narcotics, verapamil, diltiazem, amiodarone)

PHYS: Normal heart rate maintained by cardiac sinus and appropriate conduction by bundle of His to ventricles. Vagal centres in medulla slow heart rate with increased cerebral pressure

Breathing

See Barrel Chest; Blue Bloater; Bronchial Breathing; Cavernous Breathing; Cheyne-Stokes Respiration; Crepitations, Pulmonary; Hyperventilation; Hypoventilation; Kussmaul's Breathing or Sign; Rhonchi; Pink Puffer; Pleural Effusion

Bronchial Breathing

EXP: Harsh, clear, breath sound that is equal in inspiration and expiration

INT: (+) Pneumonia, pulmonary tumours, TB, pulmonary consolidation

PHYS: Suppression of vesicular component of breath sound when alveoli not working results in bronchial breathing

Brudzinski's Sign

EXP: The head is flexed on the chest, causing the lower limbs to be drawn up

INT: (+) Meningeal irritation, meningitis, cerebral abscess, subdural empyema, subarachnoid haemorrhage, other cerebral haemorrhages, typhus, leptospirosis

PHYS: Traction of the inflamed meninges on spinal nerves causes a protective flexor reflex

See also Neck Stiffness; Kernig's Sign

Bruit

See Thrill, Cardiac
See also signs listed under Murmur, Cardiac

Buffalo Hump

EXP: Excess deposition of fatty tissue over upper thoracic vertebrae

INT: (+) Cushing's disease, steroid medication

Buphthalmos

See Exophthalmos

Burn's Test

EXP: A patient with sciatica is asked to kneel sideways on a chair, bend forwards and touch the floor with the finger tips

INT: (+) Patients with sciatica can usually achieve this task

(–) Patients who are malingering are unable to reach the floor or overbalance

Butterfly Rash

EXP: Erythematous, scaly rash spreading across both cheeks and meeting on the nasal bridge

INT: (+) SLE, photodermatitis, discoid lupus, atopic dermatitis, serum sickness

PHYS: Occurs in 45% of patients with SLE

Button Hole Deformity

See Boutonnière (Button Hole) Deformity

Cachexia

EXP: Widespread muscular wasting, grey pallor, dry and wrinkled skin

INT: (+) Malignant diseases (eg. carcinoma of lung, stomach, ovary), Hodgkin's disease, leukaemia, anorexia nervosa, chronic renal or hepatic disease, advanced diabetes, chronic TB, malnutrition, chronic cardiac failure, chronic malaria, ancylostomiasis, sprue, scurvy, Addison's disease, fluorosis, thyrotoxicosis, Simmonds' disease, lead or mercury poisoning

PHYS: Many serious diseases, particularly when chronic, cause the loss of protein and ketones through the urine. A loss of muscle tissue and anaemia results

See also SYMPTOMS SECTION 1: Weight Loss

Café-au-Lait Spots

EXP: Light brown spots on skin

INT: (+) Von Recklinghausen's disease of multiple neurofibromata, pityriasis versicolor, tuberous sclerosis

See also SYMPTOMS SECTION 1: Pigmentation of Skin, Excess

Calf Squeeze Test (Simmond's Test)

EXP: Lie patient prone with both feet extending beyond the end of the couch by 10 cm. With one hand, grip the sides of the gastrocnemius/

soleus and squeeze. Foot should plantar flex. Compare with other side

INT: (+) Normal Achilles tendon
(–) Ruptured Achilles tendon

PHYS: A complete rupture of the Achilles tendon may be missed because the foot may be plantar flexed using the deep long flexors. This test specifically demonstrates the integrity of the Achilles tendon

Caloric Stimulation

EXP: Irrigation of the external auditory canal with ice-cold water while the head is at 30° to the horizontal and the eyes looking at a fixed object, causes the gaze to turn laterally towards the side of the irrigated ear

INT: (+) Brain stem intact
(+ nystagmus and vertigo) Vestibular disease
(–) Brain stem damage

PHYS: Used for assessing comatose patients. Check that there is no excess wax in ear canal and that tympanic membrane is intact before proceeding.

Cardiac Displacement

See Apex Beat Displacement

Cardiomegaly

See Apex Beat Displacement; Cor Pulmonale

Carnett's Test

EXP: In cases of abdominal tenderness, locate point of maximal tenderness, ask patient to cross arms and sit half way forward, and palpate area again. Positive if tenderness increases

INT: (+) Abdominal wall tenderness, not visceral pain

PHYS: Differentiates intra-abdominal source of pain from abdominal wall pain in cases of acute abdomen

See also Abdominal Rigidity

Carpal Spasm

See Obstetric Hand

Cat Cry

See Cri-du-Chat

Cataract

See Lens Opacity

Cavernous Breathing

EXP: Hollow quality, low toned breath sound that is equal in inspiration and expiration

INT: (+) Open pneumothorax, lung cavities (eg. TB, bronchiectasis, pulmonary abscess)

PHYS: Due to lung cavity surrounded by partially consolidated lung tissue

Central Venous Pressure

See Jugular Venous Pressure

Cervical Fleche

EXP: With heels and back placed against wall, patient tries to touch wall with back of head without raising chin above horizontal. Positive if unable to do so

INT: (+) Ankylosing spondylitis, cervical vertebral trauma

PHYS: Indicates involvement of cervical vertebrae in disease

Cervix, Tender

EXP: Pain on movement of cervix by examining doctor's fingers

INT: (+) Pelvic inflammatory disease, ectopic pregnancy, ovarian cysts, advanced carcinoma of cervix, endometriosis, salpingitis, pelvic abscess

Charcot's Joints

EXP: A totally disorganised and apparently severely arthritic major joint which remains completely pain free

INT: (+) Tabes dorsalis, syringomyelia, diabetic neuropathy, myelomeningocele, leprosy

PHYS: Impairment of pain and proprioceptive sensation deprives the joint of the normal protective reflexes when exposed to stress

Chaussier's Sign

EXP: Epigastric pain in a pregnant woman with pre-eclampsia

INT: (+) Imminent eclampsia

Cheyne-Stokes Respiration

EXP: Respirations that gradually decrease in frequency until a temporary cessation occurs. Respiration then restarts and the frequency builds to a maximum before the cycle repeats itself

INT: (+) CVA, meningitis, uraemia, narcotic or barbiturate overdose, advanced cardiac disease (eg. left ventricular failure), terminal stage of many chronic diseases, cerebral tumours, raised intracranial pressure

PHYS: Damage to cerebral respiratory centre. One full cycle equates to twice the circulation time

See also Papilloedema

Chip Sign

EXP: Skin blotches covered with fine, nonadherent scabs that are easily removed by a fingernail or blunt edge

INT: (+) Pityriasis versicolor

PHYS: Superficial fungal infection

Chloasma
EXP: Yellow-brown spotty skin pigmentation, often on upper cheeks and forehead
INT: (+) Pregnancy, oral contraceptives, sun exposure, syphilis, malaria, TB,cirrhosis, chronic trauma, some drugs
PHYS: Melanocyte stimulation

Choreiform Movements
EXP: Irregular, spontaneous, rapid, random, purposeless movements of the larger joints. Increased by voluntary effort and emotion
INT: (+) Sydenham's chorea, Huntington's chorea (slower movements), encephalitis, rheumatic fever, hyperthyroidism,SLE, cerebral tumours, CO poisoning, basal ganglia disease, senility, chorea gravidarum, oral contraceptive sensitivity, polycythaemia rubra vera, neuroleptic or phenytoin overdose, kernicterus, hemiballismus
PHYS: Damage in the area of the caudate nucleus and putamen

Chvostek's Sign
EXP: A light tap on the facial nerve as it emerges from the stylomastoid foramen causes contraction of the facial muscles on that side
INT: (+) Hypoparathyroidism, hypocalcaemia, rickets, alkalosis, magnesium deficit, some normal people
PHYS: Low serum calcium or magnesium causes muscular hyperexcitability and may lead to tetany

See also Trousseau's Sign

Circumoral Pallor
EXP: Relatively white area around mouth
INT: (+) Fever of any cause (eg. scarlet fever)
PHYS: Dilatation of superficial blood vessels in looser skin further away from mouth causes darkening and reddening of that area (rather than blanching of circumoral tissue)

Clasp-Knife Rigidity
EXP: When a limb joint is flexed by an examiner, there is considerable initial resistance which, once overcome, results in relative ease of movement
INT: (+) Upper motor neurone lesion, spasticity
PHYS: A lengthening reaction due to hyperactivity or sensitivity of alpha or gamma motor neurones

See also Cogwheel Rigidity

Claw Hand (Main–en–Griffe)
EXP: Chronic spasmodic hand position characterised by flexion of wrist and interphalangeal joints and extension of metacarpophalangeal joints
INT: (+) Lower motor neurone lesions, progressive muscular dystrophy, ulnar and median nerve paralysis, gargoylism, carpal tunnel syn.

PHYS: Due to wasting of small hand muscles and overactivity of long muscles with interruption to peripheral motor nerve supply

Clay Stool
See Faeces, Abnormal Colour

Clonus
See Ankle Clonus

Clubbing of Fingers
EXP: Soft terminal part of fingers and/or toes immediately proximal to nail is bulbous, and nail is excessively curved in lateral and longitudinal planes
INT: (+) Chronic diseases of heart, lungs or alimentary system (eg. lung carcinoma, pneumoconioses, bacterial endocarditis, TB, bronchiectasis, sarcoidosis,cirrhosis, lung abscess, regional enteritis, tetralogy of Fallot), congenital, in association with hypertrophic pulmonary osteoarthropathy, subphrenic abscess, cystic fibrosis, fibrosing alveolitis, asbestosis, arteriovenous fistula, atrial myxoma, Crohn's disease, benign intrathoracic tumours, thoracic empyema, mesothelioma, familial
PHYS: Due to overgrowth of soft tissues and subjacent periosteum. Exact cause unknown but may be due to increase in peripheral blood flow and reduced pO_2

See also Schamroth's Sign

Coffee-Grounds Vomitus
EXP: Dark brown granular vomitus
INT: (+) Peptic ulcer, stomach carcinoma, oesophageal varices, portal cirrhosis, yellow fever
PHYS: Alteration of blood due to action of gastric acid

Cogwheel Rigidity
EXP: Resistance to passive movement diminishes in jerky steps
INT: (+) Extrapyramidal lesions, athetosis, paralysis agitans (parkinsonism), cerebral palsy
PHYS: Static tremor masked by rigidity

See also Lead-Pipe Rigidity; Clasp-Knife Rigidity
See also Festination under Gait, Abnormal

Coilonychia
See Koilonychia

Coin Test
EXP: When a coin on the chest wall is struck by another coin, a metallic noise is heard through a stethoscope placed on the chest wall at a distance from the coin. Two sides of chest should be compared

INT: (+) Pneumothorax
PHYS: Conduction of sound is altered by the partial collapse of a lung

Collapsing Pulse
See Water-Hammer Pulse

Consensual Reflex
EXP: Light shone into one eye causes the pupils of both eyes to contract
INT: (–) (only opposite eye contracts) Retrobulbar neuritis, multiple sclerosis
PHYS: Afferent path of reflex arc is interrupted, but efferent path remains intact

Consolidation of Lung
See Dull Percussion Note, Thoracic

Convulsions
See SYMPTOMS SECTION 1: Convulsions

Cor Pulmonale
EXP: Pulmonary arterial hypertension and right ventricular enlargement. Confirmed by ECG and chest X-ray
INT: (+) Chronic obstructive airways disease, pulmonary vascular disease, multiple pulmonary emboli, diffuse interstitial pulmonary disease, sleep apnoea, kyphoscoliosis, neuromuscular diseases of chest wall, Pickwickian syn., high altitude sickness
PHYS: Primarily a sign of obstructed circulation of blood through the lungs, and not cardiac disease. Congenital heart disease and left heart disease must be excluded

Corneal Anaesthesia
EXP: Loss of corneal sensation to light touch
INT: (+) Riley-Day syn.

Corneal Reflex
EXP: Lightly touching one cornea with a piece of cotton wool produces blinking in both eyes
INT: (– bilateral) Coma, general anaesthesia, death
        (– unilateral) Lesion of 7th or ophthalmic division of 5th nerve
PHYS: Tests for anaesthesia of cornea, or interruption of reflex arc

Corrigan's Sign
EXP: Vigorous, jerky pulsation of major arteries causing ears to move or head to nod
INT: (+) Aortic regurgitation, patent ductus arteriosus, ventricular septal defect

See also Water-Hammer Pulse

Cough
See SYMPTOMS SECTION 1: Cough

Courvoisier's Law
EXP: A distended gall bladder (found by palpation) in the presence of jaundice is due to some cause other than gallstones
INT: (+) Carcinoma of head of pancreas, cholelithiasis not absolutely excluded
PHYS: Chronic gallstones cause fibrosis of the gall bladder, thus preventing its later expansion

See also Hepatomegaly

Cremasteric Reflex
EXP: Retraction of the testicle by the cremaster muscle when the inner side of the thigh is gently stroked, or pressure is applied to the subsartorial canal
INT: (– bilateral) Old age
        (– unilateral) Corticospinal lesions
PHYS: Acts at L1 level. Do not confuse with Dartos reflex where scrotum contracts with cold

Crepitations, Pulmonary (Moist Rales)
EXP: Moist sounds on chest auscultation that vary from bubbling (coarse) to crackling (medium) and inspiratory tinkling (fine)
INT: (Coarse +) bronchiectasis, bronchitis
        (Fine +) Pneumonia, TB, pulmonary collapse, pulmonary oedema, pulmonary embolism, elderly
PHYS: Due to passage of air through fluid (mucus, pus, oedema fluid, exudate, etc.)

Crepitations, Tissue
EXP: Spongy crackling sensation and/or sound when affected tissue is palpated
INT: (+) Subcutaneous emphysema (eg. lung trauma, surgery, fractured rib), gas gangrene, crepitant cellulitis, gross tissue trauma, laryngeal or tracheal trauma
PHYS: Due to gas (air) in subcutaneous tissues

Cri-du-Chat
EXP: Cat-like cry in newborn infant
INT: (+) Cri-du-chat syn. (see SYNDROMES SECTION 6)
PHYS: Temporary maldevelopment of larynx that corrects with age. Due to deletion of short arm of 5th chromosome

Cullen's Sign
EXP: Spontaneous umbilical bruising
INT: (+) Ruptured ectopic pregnancy, carcinoma of pancreas, haemorrhagic pancreatitis, other causes of haemoperitoneum
PHYS: Tracking of free intraperitoneal blood to umbilicus

Cyanosis
See SYMPTOMS SECTION 1: Cyanosis, Central; Cyanosis, Peripheral

Dance's Sign
EXP: Palpable right iliac fossa depression in a distressed infant
INT: (+) Intussusception
PHYS: Intussusception causes large bowel (normally present in right iliac fossa) to be drawn into centre of abdomen

Darier's Sign
EXP: Rubbing a finger or blunt object firmly over a skin lesion causes oedema and erythema around the lesion
INT: (+) Mastocytosis
PHYS: Pressure releases histamine from increased number of mast cells in lesion

Dartos Reflex
See Cremasteric Reflex

Dehydration
EXP: <5% – Thirst, dry mucous membranes, normal pulse, depressed fontanelle in infant
5-10% – Loss of skin turgor, sunken eyes, tachycardia, oliguria, markedly depressed fontanelle in infant
> 10% – Altered mood or consciousness (irritable or drowsy), weak pulse, poor peripheral circulation, marked loss of skin turgor
INT: (+) Dehydrated because of excess fluid loss (eg. diarrhoea, excess sweating, diabetes insipidus, diuretic abuse), or reduced fluid intake (eg. fluid deprivation)

See also SYMPTOMS SECTION 1: Diarrhoea; Sweating, Excessive and Abnormal

Diarrhoea
See SYMPTOMS SECTION 1: Diarrhoea

Diastolic Murmur
EXP: Auscultation reveals a murmur between the 2nd and 1st heart sounds
INT: (+) Mitral stenosis, aortic incompetence, ventricular septal defects, hyperdynamic conditions (eg. anaemias, thyrotoxicosis), pulmonary incompetence, patent ductus arteriosus, tricuspid stenosis, carcinoid syn.
PHYS: Damaged valve or increase in flow rate causes turbulence

Dicrotic Pulse
EXP: Arterial palpation reveals a double pulsation, the latter being lesser in strength, for each heart beat
INT: (+) Acute infections (eg. typhoid fever)
PHYS: Small stroke volume causes brief pulsation, and subsequent closure of aortic valve causes further pulsation. Normally the two are merged

Displacement of Heart
See Apex Beat Displacement

Doll's Head Manoeuvre
EXP: In a comatose patient, rolling the head to one side causes counter-rolling of the eyes to the other side
INT: (+) Brain stem intact
(−) Brain stem damage
PHYS: Used in assessment of comatose patient. Should not be used if there is any possibility of neck injury

Dowager's Hump
EXP: Hump caused by crush fractures of the upper thoracic vertebrae
INT: (+) Osteoporosis

Dull Percussion Note, Thoracic
EXP: One index finger is laid flat on the chest wall and is struck firmly with the other index finger. Lower than normal pitch of percussion is dullness
INT: (+) Pneumonia, fibrosis, consolidation, TB, pleural effusion, extensive carcinoma
PHYS: Solid lung tissue does not reflect sound as readily as aerated lung

See also Tympany, Thoracic; Pectoriloquy, Whispering; Pleural Effusion

Dysdiadochokinesia
EXP: With the arms extended in front, patient pronates and supinates the forearms rapidly. Positive if action is uncoordinated
INT: (+) Cerebellar lesions (eg. tumours, abscess, CVA), other extrapyramidal motor lesions
PHYS: Agonist and antagonist muscle bundles cannot be coordinated due to hypotonia secondary to the central lesion

See also Tremor, Intention; Ataxia

Dyskinesia, Tardive
EXP: Impairment of voluntary movement causing incomplete or partial actions
INT: (+) Side effects of drugs used for psychoses (eg. phenothiazines, tricyclics, droperidol, haloperidol, pimozide, thioxanthines) and Parkinson's disease (eg. biperiden, benzhexol) and other drugs (eg. phenytoin, antihistamines)
PHYS: Iatrogenic

See also INVESTIGATIONS SECTION 3: Dyskinesia, Tardive

Dysmetria
See Tremor, Intention

Dystonia, Torsion
See Athetosis

Ear Lobe Crease
EXP: Diagonal crease across ear lobe
INT: (+) Increased risk of aortic and coronary atherosclerosis
PHYS: Statistically significant correlation. Reason unknown

Ectopic Beats
See Extrasystolic Beats

Edema
See Pulmonary Oedema; Pitting Oedema; SYMPTOMS SECTION 1: Oedema

Ely's Sign
EXP: With patient prone, flexion of knee causes pelvic elevation and hip abduction
INT: (+) Sacroiliac disease, contracture of lateral fascia of thigh

Emphysema, Subcutaneous
See Crepitations, Tissue

Engorgement, Venous
See Jugular Venous Pressure

Enophthalmos (Enophthalmia)
EXP: Recession of eyeballs within sockets
INT: (+) Dehydration, cachexia, malnutrition, advanced carcinoma, other wasting diseases, lacrimal gland tumour, Horner's syn.
PHYS: Take care to avoid confusion with ptosis. Due to loss of turgor of tissue supporting eyeball

Entropion
EXP: Inversion of eyelid edge that may result in eyelashes rubbing on eye surface to cause irritation
INT: (+) Chronic conjunctivitis, chronic trachoma, blepharitis, iritis, eyelid trauma, congenital, obesity, elderly

See also Arlt's Line; Trichiasis

Erythema, Joint
See Joint Erythema

Exophthalmos (Proptosis)
EXP: Protrusion of eyeballs within sockets. Marked amount of sclera visible above iris in normal forward vision
INT: (+) Hyperthyroidism, cerebral tumour, optic or orbital tumour, Cushing's disease, cavernous sinus thrombosis, Hand-Schueller-Christian disease, pituitary tumours, osteomas, neurofibromatosis, Wegener's granulomatosis, metastatic carcinoma, xanthomas, malignant hypertension, uraemia, cellulitis, vascular malformation, lacrimal tumours, mucocele, rhabdomyosarcoma, Apert syn., Crouzon syn., Sturge-Weber syn.
PHYS: Increase in the volume of orbital contents

Extrasystolic Beats
EXP: Occasional irregularities noted when feeling pulse or listening to heart. May disappear when heart rate increases
INT: (+) Idiopathic, stress, anoxia, drugs (eg. tobacco, caffeine, alcohol, sympathomimetics, digoxin), exercise, myocardial infarct, hypertension, cardiomyopathy, anaphylaxis, rheumatic heart disease, valve prostheses, hypokalaemia, hyperthyroidism, may be associated with all forms of heart disease
PHYS: Premature beating of heart or missed beat due to failure of normal pacemaker and/or conduction mechanisms

Exudates, Retinal
See Retinal Exudates

Eye Signs
See Arcus Senilis; Arlt's Line; Consensual Reflex; Corneal Reflex; Enophthalmos; Entropion; Exophthalmos; Foster Kennedy Sign; Kayser-Fleischer Ring; Lens Opacity; Miosis; Mydriasis; Nystagmus; Optic Atrophy; Papilloedema; Paralysis of Upward Gaze; Pupil, Irregular; Pupil, White; Retinal Exudates; Retinal Haemorrhages; Retinal Pigmentation; Roth's Spots; Sclera, Blue; Third Eyelid of Morgan-Denny; Trichiasis; Xanthelasma
See also SYMPTOMS SECTION 1: Amaurosis Fugax; Blindness, Partial or Total; Cataract; Diplopia; Eye Discharge; Eye, Dry; Eye, Inflamed or Red; Eye Pain; Eye, Watery; Eyelids, Abnormal; Eyelid Disease; Flashes, Visual; Hemianopia; Iris Abnormality Associated Syndromes; Lacrimation, Abnormal; Microphthalmia; Optic Paralysis; Photophobia; Ptosis; Squint; Vision, Black Spots in Field of; Vision, Blurred; Xerophthalmia

Facies
See Parkinsonian Facies; Moon Face; Risus Sardonicus

Faeces, Abnormal Colour
INT: Dark – Red wine, certain fruits, iron or bismuth medications

Green/yellow (excess bile) – Intestinal hurry,
bowel infections, starvation
Canary yellow – Diet primarily of dairy products
Clay – Lack of bile from biliary obstruction
Pale yellow – Steatorrhoea (excess fat)
Red – Blood from lower intestine (eg.
haemorrhoids, cancer, polyps)
Black – Melaena, excess iron

See also SYMPTOMS SECTION 1: Melaena and Rectal
Bleeding

Fasciculation, Muscular (Twitching)

EXP: Fibrillary twitching of voluntary muscles visible
        through the skin. Exacerbated by tapping
        muscle bundles
INT: (+) Depolarising drugs, muscular dystrophies,
        amyotrophic lateral sclerosis, lower motor
        neurone lesions, motor neurone disease,
        poliomyelitis, Guillain-Barré syn.,
        syringomyelia, hypocalcaemia, severe viral
        diseases, thyrotoxicosis, polymyositis
PHYS: May occur without neurological cause. Due to
        uncoordinated depolarisation of muscle fibres

See also Tremor, Intention; Tremor, Postural; Tremor,
Resting; Myotonia

Feces
See Faeces

Festination
See Gait, Abnormal; Cogwheel Rigidity

Fetal Growth, Reduced
See Intrauterine Growth Retardation

Fever
See SYMPTOMS SECTION 1: Fever

Finger Clubbing
See Clubbing of Fingers

Finkelstein's Test

EXP: The patient folds the thumb into the palm, with
        the fingers folded over the thumb. The doctor
        rotates the wrist medially (towards the ulnar) to
        stretch the involved tendons. Positive if pain
        worsened or reproduced
INT: (+) De Quervain's disease of stenosing
        tenosynovitis
PHYS: Abductor pollicus longus and/or extensor
        pollicus brevis are tendons involved. Caused by
        repetitive wrist action

Flaccid Paralysis
See Paralysis, Flaccid

Flapping Tremor (Asterixis)
See Tremor, Flapping

Flint-Austin Murmur
See Austin-Flint Murmur

Fluid Thrills
See Thrill, Fluid

Flush
See SYMPTOMS SECTION 1: Flush

Foot Lesions
See Pes Cavus

Foster Kennedy Sign

EXP: Unilateral papilloedema with contralateral optic
        atrophy
INT: (+) Cerebral tumour adjacent to optic nerve of
        atrophied eye
PHYS: Pressure on one optic nerve causes optic
        atrophy while increasing intracranial pressure to
        cause papilloedema of the other eye

Fremitus
See Vocal Fremitus

Friction Rub, Pericardial

EXP: Cardiac auscultation reveals a localised or
        generalised grating sound associated with each
        contraction
INT: (+) Pericarditis, pleurisy, rheumatic fever,
        pneumonia, TB, myocardial infarct, uraemia,
        dissecting aortic aneurysm
PHYS: Friction between the two pericardial layers in the
        presence of an exudate

Friction Rub, Pleural

EXP: Chest auscultation reveals a grating sound
        associated with each breath
INT: (+) Pleurisy, pulmonary thrombosis, lung
        cancer, empyema
PHYS: Friction between the two inflamed layers of
        pleura

Froment's Sign

EXP: Patient holds a piece of thin cardboard with both
        hands with thumbs on top of cardboard and
        closed hands under cardboard so that each
        thumb presses down through the cardboard
        onto the side of index finger proximal
        interphalangeal joint. Doctor holds opposite
        side of cardboard in same way. Doctor and
        patient both try to pull cardboard towards

themselves. Sign positive if the interphalangeal joint of the patient's thumb flexes to hump upwards
INT: (+) Ulnar nerve paralysis
PHYS: Ulnar nerve may be compressed at the olecranon or Guyton's canal. Alternatively, the nerve roots in the neck may be compressed

Frontal Bossing
EXP: Protruberant enlargement of the frontal bones
INT: (+) Rickets, congenital syphilis, bruising

Gaenslen's Sign
EXP: Patient lies on side on firm couch. Bottom leg is hyperflexed onto abdomen. Upper leg is hyperextended. Positive if sacroiliac pain
INT: (+) Sacroiliac joint involved in disease (eg. ankylosing spondylitis, ligamentous tear)

Gag Reflex
See Pharyngeal Reflex

Gait, Abnormal
EXP: Ataxic gait – Unsteady, unbalanced, lack of confidence
          Extrapyramidal gait – Slow, rigid gait, no arm swinging
          Festination – Quick, shuffling, trunk bent
          'Marche-a-petit-pas' – 'Gait of little steps', jerky, unbalanced, muscle spasm, feet 'stick' to floor on turning or starting, asymmetrical brisk reflexes
          Scissors gait – Legs cross left to right and vice versa when walking
          Spastic ataxic gait – Muscle spasm, jerky, unsteady, unbalanced
          Waddling gait – Exaggerated elevation of the hip on the stepping side and abnormal yielding of the hip on the grounded side, giving excessive lateral movement to the trunk
INT: Ataxic gait – (+) Drug induced cerebellar ataxia, alcoholic cerebellar degeneration, hypothyroidism, transient ischaemic attack, Gerstmann-Straussler-Scheinker syn., other cerebellar disease
          Extrapyramidal gait – (+) Parkinson's disease, drug induced parkinsonism (eg. prochlorperazine, metoclopramide)
          Festination – (+) Parkinson's disease, extrapyramidal lesions
          'Marche-a-petit-pas' – (+) Multiple lacunar strokes
          Scissors gait – (+) Cerebral diplegia, diseases of hip joint, spastic paraplegia
          Spastic ataxic gait – (+) Multiple strokes, transient ischaemic attacks, cerebral palsy, vitamin B_{12} deficiency, cervical myelopathy, spinocerebellar degeneration
          Waddling gait – (+) Progressive muscular dystrophy, congenital dislocation of hips, Huntington's chorea, pseudohypertrophic muscular paralysis, inclusion body myositis
PHYS: Ataxic gait – Midline or vermian cerebellar degeneration
          Festination – Muscular rigidity
          'Marche-a-petit-pas' – Pseudobulbar lesion. Commonly confused with parkinsonian gaits
          Scissors gait – Acute adduction of both hips from hip joint disease or adductor muscle contracture
          Spastic ataxic gait – May be associated with incontinence and cognitive disturbances in elderly
          Waddling gait – Weakness of gluteal muscles

See also Cogwheel Rigidity; Parkinsonism

Gallop Rhythm (Triple Rhythm)
EXP: Cardiac auscultation reveals a triple rhythm with a 3rd or 4th heart sound
INT: Protodiastolic 3rd sound – Distended heart, mitral incompetence or stenosis, left ventricular failure, alveolitis, constrictive pericarditis, physiological
          Presystolic 4th sound – Left ventricular failure, aortic stenosis, atrial hypertrophy, prolonged PR interval
PHYS: Various flow and valve movement abnormalities

Geographic Tongue
EXP: Smooth red patches with greyish margin scattered on tongue
INT: (+) Filiform papillae desquamation (benign condition), TB, allergies

See also Strawberry Tongue

Glaucoma
See Horizontal Light Test; Swinging Torch Sign

Goitre
See SYMPTOMS SECTION 1: Goitre

Golden's Sign
EXP: Pallor of cervix
INT: (+) Ectopic pregnancy, cervical infections or infiltrations

Gottron's Sign
EXP: Scaly patches over dorsum of proximal interphalangeal and metacarpophalangeal joints, subungual erythema and cuticular telangiectasiae
INT: (+) Polymyositis, dermatomyositis

Gower's Manoeuvre
EXP: Child attempts to rise by walking hands up legs
INT: (+) Duchenne muscular dystrophy
PHYS: Muscular weakness prevents rising to standing position in normal manner

Graham Steell Murmur

EXP: Soft, high pitched murmur heard in the 2nd left
intercostal space on early diastole
INT: (+) Pulmonary hypertension or pulmonary
artery dilatation in association with severe mitral
stenosis or septal defects
PHYS: Pulmonary vascular regurgitation

Grasp Reflex

EXP: Automatic grasping of objects placed against
palm of hand
INT: (+) Normal neonate, upper prefrontal lobe
lesions and tumours
PHYS: Prefrontal lobes concerned with intellect and the
origination of motor movements. Patient is
unable to prevent a primitive reflex with lesions
to this area

Green Urine

See Urine, Abnormal Colour

Gums, Blue Line on

EXP: Blue line that cannot be cleaned away noted at
gum margins
INT: (+) Lead poisoning
PHYS: Deposit of lead sulphide in gums

Haematuria

*See SYMPTOMS SECTION 1: Haematuria and Red
Urine*
See PATHOLOGY SECTION 4: Haematuria

Haemorrhages

*See Retinal Haemorrhages; Splinter Haemorrhages;
Hess Test*
*See also SYMPTOMS SECTION 1: Purpura and
Petechiae; Bleeding, Excessive*

Hair, Transverse Depigmentation

EXP: Band across hair of different (usually lighter)
colour from rest of hair
INT: (+) Protein deficiency, copper deficiency

Halitosis

See SYMPTOMS SECTION 1: Halitosis

Hall Pike Test

EXP: The patient is carefully seated on an
examination couch with legs on the couch.
There should be no pillow and no wall or other
obstruction for 50 cm beyond the head of the
couch. The patient's head is turned at 45° to one
side. The patient is then quickly lowered, with
the support of the examiner, so that the head is
hanging over the edge of the table and extended

to 30° still in a 45° orientation. The test is then
repeated with the head turned 45° in the
opposite direction, and with the head in the
direct anteroposterior position. Immediately
after each test, any vertigo is recorded and the
patient's eyes are checked for nystagmus, its
character and duration being noted
INT: (+ marked vertigo, delayed nystagmus with
rapid movement away from lower ear that
fatigues easily) – Benign positional vertigo,
common in elderly
(+ mild vertigo, immediate nystagmus with
variable direction, and prolonged) – Central
positional nystagmus, cerebellopontine or brain
stem lesions

See also Nystagmus

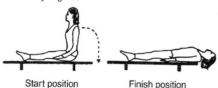

Start position   Finish position

Halo

See Rainbow Halo

Hand

See Obstetric Hand; Waiter's Hand; Claw Hand

Harrison's Sulcus

EXP: Diagonal groove on anterior and lateral side of
chest along line of attachment of diaphragm
INT: (+) Asthma, rickets
PHYS: Chest deformity from over exertion of
diaphragmatic muscle

Heaf Test

See PATHOLOGY SECTION 4: Tuberculin Skin Test

Heart

*See Apex Beat Displacement; Atrial Fibrillation;
Bradycardia; Extrasystolic Beats; Gallop Rhythm; Heart
Sounds; Jugular Venous Pressure; Split Heart Sounds;
Tachycardia; Thrill, Cardiac*
See also signs listed under Murmur, Cardiac; Pulse

Heart Sounds

PHYS: First sound – Closure of mitral and tricuspid
valves at beginning of systole
Second sound – Closure of aortic and
pulmonary valves at end of systole
Third sound – Rapid ventricular filling in early
diastole
Fourth sound – Atrial contraction in late diastole

Heberden's Nodes

EXP: Bony prominence at the dorsal margins of distal interphalangeal joints
INT: (+) Osteoarthritis, osteoarthrosis
PHYS: More common in women. May be due to a single autosomal gene

See also Bouchard's Nodes

Heel-Knee Test

EXP: While supine, the patient is told to touch one knee with the opposite heel, and then to run the heel down the shin
INT: (+) Ataxia (eg. tabes dorsalis, posterior column lesions, cerebellar lesions, Friedreich's ataxia), poliomyelitis
PHYS: Loss of integrity of sensory pathway along posterior columns to cerebellum

See also Ataxia; Romberg's Sign; Nose-Finger Test

Hegar's Sign

EXP: On bimanual examination of vagina an empty softened area can be palpated between the firmer cervix and globular uterus
INT: (+) Pregnancy between 6th and 10th weeks
PHYS: Hormones of pregnancy cause softening of uterus, but fetus occupies only upper pole in early stages

See also Areolar Pigmentation; Blue Cervix

Henoch-Schönlein Purpura

EXP: Extensive elevated purpuric or ecchymotic lesions on extensor surfaces of arms and legs. May be recurrent and can occur on the face, in the gut (causing haemorrhage and colic), and in the kidney (causing haematuria)
INT: (+) Idiopathic, after sensitising foods, poststreptococcal infection, drugs
PHYS: Immunological reaction, more common in children

See also SYNDROMES SECTION 6: Henoch-Schoenlein Syndrome

Hepatomegaly

EXP: Palpation of abdominal RUQ reveals a mass that may extend below the umbilicus, may be hard or soft, and may be tender
INT: (+) Congestive cardiac failure, hepatitis, infectious mononucleosis, malaria, other infectious agents, primary or metastatic tumour, cirrhosis, fatty liver, lymphoma, leukaemia, bile duct obstruction, amoebiasis, hepatic abscess, actinomycosis, polycystic disease, hepatic fibrosis, TB, sarcoid, haemosiderosis, amyloidosis, diabetes mellitus, myelofibrosis, glycogen storage diseases, galactosaemia, lipidoses, anaemias, pericarditis, polyarteritis nodosa, schistosomiasis, Gaucher's disease, Hand-Schueller-Christian disease, histiocytosis X, hydatid, thalassaemia, hepatic vein thrombosis, protein deficiency, starvation, syphilis, rheumatoid arthritis, Andersen syn., Budd-Chiari syn., carcinoid syn., Cori syn., Felty syn., Hers syn., Hunter syn., Hurler syn., Letterer-Siwe syn., Mauriac syn., Pompe syn., Sanfilippo syn., Scheie syn., Sly syn., von Gierke syn., drugs and innumerable other causes
(false +) Depressed right diaphragm, subdiaphragmatic abscess, Riedel's lobe, asthma
PHYS: Liver enlargement may be due to vascular, biliary tract, infiltrative, inflammatory or tumorous causes

See also Courvoisier's Law

Herald Patch

EXP: Oval, discoid or annular, solitary, reddish, slightly raised and scaly patch on the trunk. Followed by multiple smaller lesions
INT: (+) Pityriasis rosea, drug eruptions
PHYS: Pityriasis rosea is a self-limiting inflammatory condition

Hering-Breuer Reflexes

EXP: The desire to inspire when the breath is held in expiration, and vice versa
INT: No clinical significance
PHYS: Activated through receptors sensitive to stretch and deflation

Hess Test

EXP: A sphygmomanometer cuff inflated to 80 mmHg (10.6 kPa) around the upper arm for five minutes causes purpuric spots to appear below the cuff
INT: (+) Diseases associated with purpura (eg. thrombocytopenia, diseases of vascular endothelium, thromboasthenia, uraemia)
PHYS: Tests the resistance of capillaries to increased venous pressure. Obsolete test that should not be performed if more sophisticated tests for vascular disease available.

See also SYMPTOMS SECTION 1: Purpura and Petechiae; INVESTIGATIONS SECTION 3: Bleeding, Excessive

Hirsutism

See Precocious Puberty
See also SYMPTOMS SECTION 1: Puberty, Early

Hoffmann's Sign or Reflex

EXP: Dorsiflexion of the foot produces calf muscle spasm and/or pain
INT: (+) Thrombophlebitis of deep vein of calf, cellulitis of calf, musculoskeletal trauma

PHYS: Tensing of muscle bundle puts pressure on
        thrombosed and inflamed vein

Hoover's Sign

EXP: With the patient lying, the doctor cups both
        heels in his or her hands, and asks the patient to
        push down with the heel on the affected side.
        Normally, the heel on the unaffected side
        becomes lighter in the examiner's hand as
        counterpressure is exerted. Positive if this does
        not occur
INT: (+) Muscular power in affected leg is limited by
        pain, malingering, or hysterical reaction

Horizontal Light Test

EXP: Shine a bright narrow beam of light horizontally
        onto the eye from its temporal aspect. Observe
        the iris shadow pattern
INT: Iris evenly illuminated or shadow on temporal side
        – Deep anterior chamber (glaucoma unlikely)
        Shadow on nasal side – Shallow anterior
        chamber (potential for acute angle closure
        glaucoma)
PHYS: The iris is normally concave, but when convex it
        narrows the anterior chamber and casts a
        shadow on the nasal side

See also Swinging Torch Sign

Hydrocephalus

EXP: Accumulation of excess CSF under presssure
        to cause skull enlargement in children and
        cerebral damage in adults
INT: (+) Congenital malformations, ventricular
        colloid cyst, pineal tumours, intraventricular
        haemorrhage, aqueduct stenosis, pituitary
        tumours, craniopharyngioma, ependymoma,
        choroid plexus disease or tumour, astrocytoma
        of cerebellum, medulloblastoma, Arnold-Chiari
        malformation
PHYS: Any obstruction of the CSF circulation will lead
        to hydrocephalus

Hydrophobia

EXP: Patient asks for water, but when offered, there is
        spasm of inspiratory muscles and inexplicable
        terror
INT: (+) Rabies

Hydrothorax

EXP: Fluid transudate in pleural cavity proven by
        pleural tap
INT: (+) Nephrotic syn., Meigs syn., congestive
        cardiac failure, obstruction of thoracic veins and
        lymphatics, other renal diseases

Hypermobility, Joint

See Joint Hypermobility

Hypertension

EXP: Blood pressure above 160 mmHg (21.3 kPa)
        systolic and/or 95 mmHg (12.6 kPa) diastolic.
        Significant variations for age, sex and
        circumstances
INT: (+) Anxiety, exertion, essential hypertension,
        renal artery stenosis, acute and chronic
        glomerulonephritis, polycystic kidneys,
        nephrotic syn., other renal diseases,
        phaeochromocytoma, aortic coarctation, pre-
        eclampsia of pregnancy, hyperthyroidism,
        raised intracranial pressure (tumour or trauma),
        overdistended neurogenic bladder, polyarteritis
        nodosa, SLE, scleroderma, Conn syn.,
        malignant hypertension, Cushing syn.,
        porphyria, ovarian tumours, lead poisoning,
        diabetes mellitus, pseudohermaphroditism,
        polycystic kidneys, Liddle syn., Irukandji syn.,
        Riley-Day syn., alcoholism, drug and food
        interactions (eg. MAOIs and cheese), drugs (eg.
        analgesics, anorectics, antidepressants,
        cyclosporin, carbenoxolone, liquorice, MAOIs,
        NSAIDs, oral contraceptives, steroids)
PHYS: 85% essential form. Generally due to increased
        peripheral resistance, abnormalities of the
        renin-angiotensin-aldosterone system,
        increased levels of adrenaline or noradrenaline,
        or increased cardiac output (eg. thyrotoxicosis)

Hyperthermia

See SYMPTOMS SECTION 1: Fever (Pyrexia)

Hypertonicity

EXP: Involuntary resistance is encountered when
        limb is passively moved. Muscles are firm to
        touch
INT: (+) Upper motor neurone lesions,
        extrapyramidal system lesions, CVA,
        parkinsonism, cord transection, postasphyxia,
        kernicterus, premature infant, encephalitis,
        cerebral oedema, trauma, meningitis,
        hydrocephalus, cerebral space occupying
        lesion, cerebral palsy
PHYS: Disinhibition of the stretch reflex

See also Myotonia

Hypertrophy, Cardiac

See Apex Beat Displacement

Hyperventilation

EXP: Rapid respiratory rate (generally above 35
        breaths per minute in adult)
INT: (+) Anxiety, pain, fever, hysteria, pulmonary
        embolism, metabolic acidosis (diabetic
        ketoacidosis, renal disease), most infections,
        cerebral haemorrhage, pneumothorax, anoxia,
        congenital heart lesions, drugs (eg. adrenaline),
        Rett syn.

PHYS: Due to low pO_2, high pCO_2, or direct cerebral
        action

See also Kussmaul's Breathing or Sign

Hypotension

EXP: Blood pressure below 100mmHg (13.3kPa)
        systolic and/or 50mmHg (6.6kPa) diastolic
INT: (+) Cardiac failure, cardiogenic shock, acute
        blood loss, orthostatic hypotension, fright,
        familial, myocardial infarct, anaphylaxis, acute
        major pulmonary embolus, coma,
        haemorrhagic nephrosonephritis, carcinoid
        syn., dehydration, sympathectomy, Addison's
        disease, diabetes mellitus, autonomic
        degeneration, amyloidosis, alcoholism,
        prolonged rest or standing, excess heat or
        humidity, fever, septicaemia, micturition
        syncope, postprandial, electrolyte imbalance,
        pregnancy, anaemia, gastrectomy,
        malnutrition, constrictive pericarditis, heart
        block, carcinomatosis, bradycardia,
        hypothyroidism, hypopituitarism, porphyria,
        Conn syn., Riley-Day syn., Sheehan syn., Shy-
        Drager syn., toxic shock syn.,vasovagal syn.,
        neurological trauma, autonomic disease or
        trauma, drugs (eg. diuretics, antianginal
        nitrates, hypnotics, tranquillizers, tricyclic
        antidepressants, levodopa, antipsychotics,
        insulin excess)
PHYS: Overdilatation of peripheral blood vessels, loss
        of blood volume or low cardiac output

Hypothermia

EXP: Core body temperature below 35°C
INT: (+) Exposure, immersion, newborn infant, very
        elderly, severe sepsis, severe trauma,
        cerebrovascular accident, congestive cardiac
        failure, diabetic ketoacidosis, hypoglycaemia,
        uraemia, hypothyroidism, major transfusion,
        alcohol abuse, drug overdose (eg. barbiturates)
PHYS: Medical emergency requiring slow and steady
        warming. Ventricular fibrillation a risk

See also TREATMENT SECTION 5

Hypotonia

EXP: Passive limb movement freely accomplished
        with greater range than usual. Muscles are soft
        and flabby
INT: (+) Lower motor neurone lesion, cerebellar
        lesions, grossly debilitating diseases,
        poliomyelitis, tabes dorsalis, spinal shock,
        myopathies, Sydenham's chorea, premature
        infant
PHYS: Loss, or blocking, of motor innervation of muscles

Hypoventilation

EXP: Low respiratory rate (generally below 10
        breaths per minute)

INT: (+) Raised intracranial pressure (eg. tumour,
        abscess, haemorrhage), drugs (eg. sedatives),
        pleural effusion, pulmonary collapse, asthma,
        pneumonia, pneumothorax, bronchiectasis,
        neuromuscular disease, kyphoscoliosis
PHYS: Direct action on respiratory centre, or physical
        limitation of lung expansion

Incoordination

See Dysdiadochokinesia

Intention Tremor

See Tremor, Intention

Intrauterine Growth Retardation

EXP: Failure of fetus to achieve its full growth
        potential antenatally. Assessed clinically and by
        ultrasound
INT: (+) Maternal hypertension, congenital
        abnormalities, genetic and chromosomal
        abnormalities, cerebral palsy, rubella,
        toxoplasmosis, Herpes infection,
        cytomegalovirus, other fetal infections,
        cytotoxics, irradiation, twins, alcoholism, heavy
        smoker, high altitude, abruptio placentae,
        diabetes, chronic renal disease, malnutrition,
        anaemia, family history, drug abuse
PHYS: Due to fetal, maternal or placental factors

*See also INVESTIGATIONS SECTION 3: Failure to
Thrive*

Irregularly Irregular Pulse

EXP: Pulse that is totally random in its rate and
        volume
INT: (+) Atrial fibrillation, multiple extrasystoles,
        thyrotoxicosis
PHYS: Atrial rate of 400–600 per minute (due to
        ischaemia, pressure or metabolic influences) is
        transmitted randomly via the AV node to the
        ventricles. Pulse deficit notable

See also Atrial Fibrillation

Itard-Cholewa's Sign

EXP: Anaesthesia of tympanic membrane,
        anaesthesia of external auditory meatus, deafness
INT: (+) Otosclerosis

Jacobsen-Holdsnedt Phenomenon

EXP: Expiratory and inspiratory chest X-rays taken.
        Positive if mediastinum displaced away from
        affected side on expiration
INT: (+) Unilateral obstructive emphysema
PHYS: Valve-like mechanism allows air to enter lung
        but not escape. May be due to foreign body or
        tumour

Janeway Lesion

EXP: Small purplish/red nodule on palms or soles
INT: (+) Infective endocarditis
PHYS: Infected embolic lesion

See also Osler's Nodes; Splinter Haemorrhages

Jaundice

See SYMPTOMS SECTION 1: Jaundice

Jaw Jerk

EXP: With the jaw relaxed and the mouth hanging
open, a finger is placed across the front of the
jaw and struck with a rubber hammer.
Contraction of masseters may result
INT: (+) Lesion of both corticospinal tracts
PHYS: Acts at the level of the pons

Jerk

*See Ankle Jerk; Biceps Jerk; Jaw Jerk; Knee Jerk;
Triceps Jerk*
See also signs listed under Reflexes

Joint Erythema

EXP: Redness and inflammation of tissue overlying a
joint
INT: (+) Septic arthritis, cellulitis, gout, pseudogout,
rheumatoid arthritis, reactive arthropathy,
Reiter syn. (see SYNDROMES SECTION 6),
Heberden's node, Bouchard's node, erythema
nodosum, inflammatory osteoarthritis,
rheumatic fever

Joint Hypermobility

EXP: Beighton Score:
Little finger extension > 90° (1 point each finger)
Extend thumb parallel to forearm (1 point each
thumb)
Extend elbow > 10° (1 point each elbow)
Extend knee > 10° (1 point each knee)
Touch floor with palms while keeping knees
straight (1 point)
Score of 6 or more positive for joint hypermobility
INT: (+) Increased incidence of dislocation,
enthesopathy, Marfan syn., Ehlers-Danlos syn.,
acromegaly
PHYS: Often familial

Jugular Venous Pressure [JVP]

EXP: With patient reclining at 30°, the distance that a
distended jugular vein rises vertically above the
horizontal level of the sternal angle is noted.
Normally veins are collapsed above this level
INT: High – Congestive cardiac failure, constrictive
pericarditis, tricuspid stenosis, pulmonary
stenosis, cardiomyopathies, superior
mediastinal tumour, enlarged thymus,
obstructed superior vena cava, increased

intrathoracic or intra-abdominal pressure
Low – Shock, dehydration, severe infections
PHYS: Increased back pressure due to obstructed flow
through the right side of the heart causes an
increase in systemic venous pressure. Blood
loss or vasodilatation causes it to drop

Kayser-Fleischer Ring

EXP: Greenish-brown ring at the outer edge of the
cornea
INT: (+) Wilson's disease
PHYS: Deposition of copper compounds in cornea
(diagnostic sign)

Kehr's Sign

EXP: Left shoulder tip pain, acute abdomen
INT: (+) Ruptured spleen
PHYS: Referred pain via phrenic nerve, caused by
irritation of diaphragm

See also Shoulder Tip Pain

Kerley B Lines

EXP: A plain AP X-ray of the chest shows fine
horizontal lines in the lower zones of the lungs,
lateral to the down curve of the diaphragm
INT: (+) Interstitial pulmonary oedema
PHYS: Perilymphatic oedema

Kernig's Sign

EXP: One hip of supine patient is fully flexed. Any
subsequent attempt to straighten the knee
results in painful spasm of the hamstrings when
positive
INT: (+) Meningeal irritation, bacterial and aseptic
meningitis, cerebral or spinal cord abscess,
subdural empyema, subarachnoid
haemorrhage, encephalitis, typhus,
leptospirosis, other cerebral haemorrhages
PHYS: Activation of protective flexor reflexes which
shorten and immobilise the spine

See also Neck Stiffness; Brudzinski's Sign

Kidney, Large

EXP: Large kidney(s) noted on abdominal palpation
or X-ray
INT: (+) Unilateral – Acute or chronic obstruction,
ureteric or renal stone, acute pyelonephritis,
duplicate pelvicalyceal system, subcapsular
renal haematoma, renal cyst, renal vein
thrombosis, renal neoplasm, compensatory
hypertrophy, hydronephrosis
(+) Bilateral – SLE, polyarteritis nodosa, allergic
angiitis, diabetes, Wegener's granulomatosis,
acute glomerulonephritis, multiple myeloma,
leukaemia, lymphoma, amyloidosis, acromegaly,
polycystic kidneys, acute tubular necrosis
PHYS: Depends on individual disease process

Kidney, Small

EXP: Abnormally small kidney(s) noted on abdominal X-ray or ultrasound
INT: (+) Unilateral – Infarction or ischaemia, renal artery stenosis, reflux pyelitis, postobstructive atrophy, postinflammatory atrophy, partial nephrectomy, irradiation atrophy, congenital (+) Bilateral – Amyloidosis, chronic glomerulonephritis, papillary necrosis, bilateral ischaemia, medullary cystic disease, urate nephropathy

Knee Jerk

EXP: With the patient seated and one knee crossed over the other, the patellar tendon is tapped firmly. Quadriceps contraction and knee extension occurs
INT: Sustained – Chorea
Pendular – Acute cerebellar disease
(++) Hyperthyroidism, encephalitis, upper motor neurone lesion, anxiety, tetanus, cord transection
(–) Peripheral neuropathies, polio, tabes dorsalis, posterior root tumours, cord tumours, subacute combined degeneration of cord, syringomyelia, cord shock, coma, muscular dystrophies, hypothyroidism, beriberi
PHYS: Acts at L2, L3, L4 level

See also signs listed under Reflexes

Koilonychia

EXP: Spooning of nails
INT: (+) Iron deficiency anaemias, Plummer-Vinson syn.

Kussmaul's Breathing or Sign

EXP: An increased depth and frequency of respirations associated with increased respiratory effort. Often described as hissing respiration
INT: (+) Diabetic acidosis, uraemia, other causes of acidosis, neurogenic hyperpnoea, midbrain and upper pontine brain lesions

Labyrinth Tests

EXP: Each ear is irrigated with hot or cold water to produce vertigo and/or nystagmus. The response from both ears should be equal
INT: Unequal – Inner ear dysfunction (nonspecific)

Lachman's Test

EXP: With the knee in nearly full extension, the femur is held firmly in one hand and the tibia is moved forward on the femoral condyle. Positive test if significant forward movement elicited
INT: (+) Anterior cruciate ligament laxity
PHYS: Rupture or stretching of the anterior cruciate ligament allows excess tibial movement

Lasegue's Sign

EXP: With patient supine, the extended leg is lifted from the bed. The presence of pain and amount of passive elevation possible is noted and compared to other leg and normal person
INT: (+) Radiculopathy (eg. disc herniation), other musculoskeletal disorders of the back
PHYS: Elevating extended leg stretches nerve roots and causes pain if they are inflamed

Lead-Pipe Rigidity

EXP: Heavy passive stiffness of limb throughout range
INT: (+) Extrapyramidal lesions, parkinsonism, basal ganglia disease
PHYS: Chronic overactive lengthening reaction

See also Cogwheel Rigidity; Clasp-Knife Rigidity

Lens Opacity

EXP: White opacity within pupil
INT: (+) Cataract, diabetes, interstitial keratitis, galactosaemia, congenital syphilis, hypoparathyroidism, hypocalcaemia, drugs (eg. chlorpromazine, steroids)
PHYS: Inflammation, senile degeneration, radiation or disordered metabolism

See also SYMPTOMS SECTION 1: Blindness, Partial or Total; Cataract

Leser-Trelat Sign

EXP: Abrupt appearance, and rapid increase in size, of many seborrhoeic keratoses
INT: (+) Underlying carcinoma (eg. adenocarcinoma)
PHYS: May also occur during lysis of tumour with cytotoxics

Leucocoria

See Pupil, White

Leuconychia

See Nail Discolouration

Liver, Enlarged

See Hepatomegaly

Lung Consolidation

See Dull Percussion Note, Thoracic; Tracheal Displacement

Machinery Murmur

EXP: Continuous cardiac murmur that waxes and wanes
INT: (+) Patent ductus arteriosus (maximal in aortic and pulmonary areas), arteriovenous fistula, aortic coarctation, aortopulmonary septal defect

Macroglossia
See Tongue, Enlarged

Main d'Accoucheur
See Obstetric Hand

Main-en-Griffe
See Claw Hand

Malnutrition
See SYMPTOMS SECTION 1: Weight Loss; Failure to Thrive

Mass Reflex
EXP: Various stimulations to a point below the level of the neurological lesion causes sudden drawing up of the legs, evacuation of the bladder and sweating below lesion level
INT: (+) Severe spinal cord lesions, paraplegia

McMurray Sign
EXP: One hand grasps ankle firmly, other hand rests on patient's knee. The knee is fully flexed and the tibia is fully laterally rotated. The knee is then extended while rotation is maintained. A 'click' or 'clunk' felt by the hand on the knee is a positive sign. The test is repeated from varying angles of knee flexion
INT: (+) Torn knee meniscus
PHYS: Manoeuvre attempts to catch torn tag of meniscus between bone ends to cause a 'click'

Mediastinal Mass
EXP: Mass detected in mediastinum by X-ray or CT scan
INT: (+) Superior mediastinum – Bronchogenic cyst, retrosternal goitre, ectopic thyroid tissue, oesophageal enterogenous cyst
        (+) Inferior mediastinum – Hiatus hernia, abscess, pericardial cyst
        (+) Posterior mediastinum – Neurogenic tumours, neurofibroma, neuroblastoma, paravertebral abscess, aortic aneurysm
        (+) Anterior mediastinum – Thymic tissue, thymoma, ectopic thyroid tissue, germ cell tumour, teratoma, dermoid cyst, aortic aneurysm
        (+) Varied position in mediastinum – Sarcoidosis, TB, lymphoma, Hodgkin's disease, metastatic carcinoma
PHYS: Any of the structures of the mediastinum may become enlarged, infected or neoplastic. CT scans and MRI can accurately position mass and sometimes determine its structure

Melaena
See SYMPTOMS SECTION 1: Melaena and Rectal Bleeding

Meningism
See Neck Stiffness; Kernig's Sign; Brudzinski's Sign; Opisthotonos

Miosis
EXP: Abnormally contracted pupils (diameter <2mm)
INT: (+) Bright light, convergence, syphilis (tabes dorsalis), narcotics, sympathetic nerve paralysis, pontine lesions, congenital, hysteria, Horner syn., Holmes-Adie syn., insecticide poisoning, drugs (eg. pilocarpine, physostigmine, narcotics, beta-blockers)

Moon Face
EXP: Fat, rounded face with loss of skin wrinkles
INT: (+) Cushing syn. and disease
PHYS: Excess intrinsic or extrinsic cortisol causes deposition of fat in face and trunk, but loss from limbs

See also Buffalo Hump

Morgan-Denny Eyelid
See Third Eyelid of Morgan-Denny

Moro Reflex (Startle Reflex)
EXP: While supporting an infant prone, allow the head to fall back sharply for a short distance. Results in extension of trunk and extension and abduction of limbs, followed by flexion and adduction of limbs
INT: (+) Normal infant up to 4 months
        (–) Over 4 months age, severe brain damage, premature infant
        (–) Unilateral – Limb fracture, peripheral neuropathy, Erb's palsy

Movement, Abnormal
See Athetosis; Choreiform Movements; Dyskinesia, Tardive; Gait, Abnormal;Tremor, Flapping ; Tremor, Intention; Tremor, Postural; Tremor, Resting
See also SYMPTOMS SECTION 1: Chorea; Tremor

Murmur, Cardiac
See Diastolic Murmur; Graham Steell Murmur; Gallop Rhythm; Machinery Murmur; Split Heart Sounds; Still's Murmur; Systolic Murmur; Thrill, Cardiac

Murphy's Law
EXP: Jaundice due to cholelithiasis is preceded by colic. Jaundice due to neoplasm or external obstruction of the biliary tract has no history of colic

Murphy's Sign
EXP: With the examiner's fingers pressed firmly over

the patient's abdominal RUQ, the patient inhales slowly and deeply. A momentary interruption of inhalation occurs due to pain

INT: (+) Cholecystitis
PHYS: The inflamed gall bladder is pressed against the examiner's fingers by the descending diaphragm

Muscular Spasm

See Myotonia

Muscular Weakness

See Hypotonia; Paralysis, Flaccid

Mydriasis

EXP: Abnormal dilatation of pupils
INT: (+) Dark room, hyperthyroidism, anxiety, iritis, traumatic or inflammatory adhesions, iris sphincter paralysis, iris dilator muscle spasm, syphilis, lead or carbon monoxide poisoning, post-seizure; botulism, diphtheria, syringomyelia, midbrain lesions, third nerve, palsy, Parinaud's syn., Tolosa-Hunt syn., Holmes-Adie syn., coma, drugs (eg. atropine, cocaine, amphetamines, cannabis)
PHYS: Damage to or inhibition of the iris and its musculature or innervation

Myoclonus

See Ankle Clonus

Myosis

See Miosis

Myotonia

EXP: Delayed muscular relaxation following forceful muscular contraction (eg. repeated muscular fasciculation after tap with rubber hammer)
INT: (+) Myotonic dystrophy, myotonia congenita, hyperkalaemia, Talma's disease
PHYS: Usually reduced by repeated activity. Often worse in cold

See also Hypertonicity; Fasciculation, Muscular

Naevi

See Spider Naevi

Nail Banding

EXP: Transverse white bands across nails
INT: (+) Hypoalbuminaemia (see Albumin, Serum in PATHOLOGY SECTION 4), steroid therapy, cytotoxics, arsenic
PHYS: Return to normal after serum albumin corrected

See also Beau's line in Nail Ridging

Nail Changes

See Clubbing of Fingers; Koilonychia; Nail banding; Nail Discolouration; Nail Pitting; Nail Ridging; Nail, Brittle; Nail, Hypoplastic; Nail, Thickened; Onychogryphosis; Onycholysis; Splinter Haemorrhages; Subungal Hyperkeratosis

Nail Discolouration

EXP: Nail or subungual tissue colour change
INT: Black – Haematoma, melanoma, naevi, pseudomonas infection, fungal infection, chronic paronychia
  Brown – Uraemia, psoriasis, nicotine, Addison's disease, mercury poisoning, silver poisoning, chemical stains
  Yellow – Tinea, jaundice, yellow nail syn., slow growth, lymphoedema, tetracyclines
  Blue – Cyanosis, mepacrine, chloroquine, Wilson's disease, argyria, amodiaquine
  White – Trauma, cardiac disease, renal disease, psoriasis, dermatophyte infection, hypoalbuminaemia, cytotoxics, arsenic, liver disease
  Red – Haemorrhage, congestive cardiac failure (half moons red), cold exposure
  Green – Pseudomonas, aspergillus or candida infections

Nail Pain

See SYMPTOMS SECTION 1: Nail Pain

Nail Pitting

EXP: Small isolated or confluent pits on the nail plate
INT: (+) Psoriasis, chronic paronychia, digital eczema, alopecia areata, familial
PHYS: Inflammatory damage to nail matrix

Nail Ridging

EXP: Longitudinal or transverse ridging of nail plate
INT: (+) Longitudinal – Elderly, nail matrix tumours, lichen planus, alopecia areata, rheumatoid arthritis, Darier's disease, mucous cyst of matrix, peripheral vascular disease, nail dystrophy
  (+) Multiple transverse – Eczema, chronic paronychia, habit tics, chronic inflammation of digit, chronically wet nails (eg. housework), severe dysmenorrhoea, Raynaud's disease, severe carpal tunnel syn., protein deficiency
  (+) Single transverse 'Beau's line' – Occurs after severe physical or emotional illness of any cause
PHYS: Transverse ridging due to temporary cessation of nail formation. When cause removed, nail growth resumes, and the ridge moves forward with the nail plate growth

See also Splinter Haemorrhages

Nail, Brittle
EXP: Nails that break and split very easily
INT: Trauma, excessive dampness, chemicals (eg. detergents), lichen planus, psoriasis, iron deficiency, circulatory deficiency (eg. diabetes), vitamin deficiency (eg. vitamin A, B_6 or C), arsenic poisoning, oral retinoids, excessive use of nail polish remover
Phys: Caused by damage to keratin filaments

Nail, Hypoplastic
EXP: Underdeveloped nails
INT: (+) Coffin–Siris syn., fetal alcohol syn., Goltz syn., nail-patella syn.

Nail, Separation from Bed
See Onycholysis; Subungal Hyperkeratosis

Nail, Thickened
EXP: Thicker than usual nail plate
INT: (+) Onychogryphosis, psoriasis, lichen planus, chronic fungal infection, chronic paronychia, congenital

Neck Stiffness
EXP: Passive flexion of the neck causes undue tautness of neck muscles
INT: (+) Meningeal irritation (eg. aseptic or bacterial meningitis, encephalitis, cerebral abscess, subdural empyema, typhus, leptospirosis, subarachnoid or other cerebral haemorrhage, migraine), cervical arthritis, torticollis and other neck muscular spasms and strains, adenitis
PHYS: Traction of inflamed meninges on spinal nerves activates a protective reflex which shortens and immobilises spine

See also Brudzinski's Sign; Kernig's Sign; Opisthotonos

Neck Webbing
See Webbing of Neck

Nikolsky Sign
EXP: Gentle lateral pressure with a finger to apparently normal skin causes epidermis to immediately slough off leaving a raw area
INT: (+) Pemphigus, toxic epidermal naevus

Nipping, Arteriovenous, Retinal
See Arteriovenous Nipping, Retinal

Nipple Pigmentation
See Areolar Pigmentation

Nose-Finger Test
EXP: Using the index finger, patient touches own nose then examiner's finger, back and forth as rapidly as possible. Examiner changes position of finger between touches. Positive if clumsy
INT: See Ataxia
PHYS: See Ataxia

See also Heel-Knee Test

Nuchal Rigidity
See Neck Stiffness

Nystagmus
EXP: Involuntary rhythmic movement of eyeball. Two types:
Pendular (oscillating) – with regular movements
Jerk (rhythmic) – with movement faster in one direction than the other
INT: (+) Normal with acute lateral vision and watching a moving object, barbiturates, labyrinthine and vestibular disease, brain stem lesions (often vertical nystagmus), demyelinating diseases (eg. multiple sclerosis), during epileptic fit (eg. petit mal), brain tumours, syringobulbia, Dandy-Walker syn., Parinaud syn., diencephalic syn., pinealoma, central vision loss (eg. albinism, retinal disease), other visual disturbances, cerebral abscess, coma, Friedreich's ataxia, congenital, alcohol, some normal infants
PHYS: Jerk form more common and is neurological in aetiology. Pendular is due to a visual defect. Direction of nystagmus can give further clue to localise lesion

See also Hall Pike Test

Obstetric Hand (Main d'Accoucheur , Carpal Spasm, Tetany)
EXP: The fingers and wrist are in painful spasm. The fingers are tightly apposed, the thumb is opposed across the palm, the terminal phalanges hyperextended and the wrist flexed
INT: (+) Tetany from hypocalcaemia or alkalosis (eg. renal insufficiency, hypoparathyroidism, hyperventilation, gastrointestinal diseases, calcium or magnesium deficiency)
PHYS: Low levels of blood calcium cause neuromuscular hyperexcitability

See also Chvostek's Sign; Trousseau's Sign

Oculogyric Crisis
EXP: Varies from mild cases with abnormal uncontrolled random eye movements, to severe cases with fixed elevated gaze associated with painful extension of the neck which may be so severe that the occiput nearly touches the thoracic vertebrae and the airway may be compromised

INT: (+) Rare side effect of prochlorperazine, encephalitis or Parkinson's disease
PHYS: Effect rapidly reversed by IV benztropine

Oedema, Pitting
See Pitting Oedema
See also SYMPTOMS SECTION 1: Oedema

Oedema, Pulmonary
See Pulmonary Oedema

Oliguria
See SYMPTOMS SECTION 1: Oliguria and Anuria

Onychogryphosis
EXP: Gross thickening of the nail plate
INT: (+) Chronic trauma from poorly fitting shoes, subungual tinea, psoriasis, subungual hyperkeratosis, old age
PHYS: Chronic inflammation of nail bed

Onycholysis
EXP: Distal separation of nail plate from nail bed
INT: (+) Trauma, chemicals, fungal infections, psoriasis, eczema, lichen planus, pemphigus, Raynaud's phenomenon, diabetes mellitus, other causes of impaired peripheral circulation, hypothyroidism, hyperthyroidism, SLE, iron deficiency, yellow nail syn., drugs (eg. tetracycline)
PHYS: Impaired viability of distal nail bed

See also Subungal Hyperkeratosis

Opacity of Lens
See Lens Opacity

Opisthotonos
EXP: Acute rigid arching of the body due to spasm of the back muscles
INT: (+) Tetanus, spinal meningitis, infantile meningitis, cerebellar lesions, other causes of meningeal irritation
PHYS: Overactivation of protective flexor reflexes designed to shorten and immobilise spine

See also Neck Stiffness; Kernig's Sign

Optic Atrophy
EXP: On ophthalmoscopic examination of retina, a pale optic disc with blurred margins is noted. Disc cupping may also occur, and patient complains of reduced visual acuity. Field defects may be found
INT: (+) Glaucoma, arteriosclerosis, retinal ischaemia, optic neuritis, Paget's disease, tumour pressing on optic nerve, retinitis pigmentosa, vitamin B deficiency, methanol poisoning
PHYS: Ischaemia or chronic inflammation of optic disc

Optic Cup/Disc Ratio
EXP: Ratio of the vertical diameter of the optic cup to that of the optic disc, measured on ophthalmoscopic or slit lamp examination of the retina
INT: Normal Optic Cup/Disc Ratio = 0.2
<0.5 – Probably normal
>0.5 – Suspicious of glaucoma
>0.8 – Usually diagnostic of glaucoma
PHYS: The optic cup is a depression within the pale optic disc on the inferomedial part of the retina caused by the optic nerve. Rising pressure of intraocular contents flattens and enlarges the optic cup

Measurement of Optic Cup/Disc Ratio

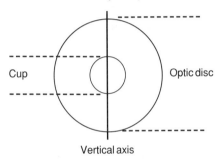

Cup

Optic disc

Vertical axis

Optic Disc, Abnormal
EXP: Characteristics noted during ophthalmoscopic examination of retina
INT: (+) Extra vascularity – Optic neuritis
(+) Papilloedema (bulging of disc) – Increased intracranial pressure
(+) Atrophy (reduced vascularity) – Optic nerve disease (see Optic Atrophy)
(+) Pale disc – Central retinal artery occlusion
(+) Haemorrhages – Central retinal vein occlusion

See also Optic Cup/Disc Ratio

Orange Urine
See Urine, Abnormal Colour

Ortolani Test
EXP: Child is placed on a firm surface with the knees and hips flexed at 90°. The legs are grasped by the examiner so that the knee is in the palm, the finger tips are behind the greater trochanters and the thumb rests on the anteromedial surface of the thigh. The hips are then abducted to 90°. When resistance is felt, forward pressure

is applied by the fingertips to the back of the greater trochanters. Test is positive if a distinct clunk is felt as the head of the femur slips forward into the acetabulum

INT:　(+) Congenital dislocation of the hip

Osler's Manoeuvre

EXP:　Inflate sphygmomanometer to level that obliterates radial pulse. Positive if a sclerotic radial artery can be palpated against the underlying radius
INT:　(+) Arteriosclerosis
PHYS:　May result in significant overestimation of systolic blood pressure

See also Ear Lobe Crease; Arteriovenous Nipping, Retinal

Osler's Nodes

EXP:　Small, tender, raised, red, transient patch on tips of fingers or toes
INT:　(+) Bacterial endocarditis
PHYS:　Caused by infected cutaneous embolus

See also Janeway Lesion; Splinter Haemorrhages

Ovarian Mass

EXP:　Enlarged ovary found on bimanual examination or ultrasound scan
INT:　(+) Simple cyst, follicular cyst, cystadenoma, polycystic ovarian syn., adenocarcinoma, teratoma, tubal abscess, stromal tumour

See also Pelvic Mass

Pallor

See SYMPTOMS SECTION 1: Pallor

Pallor, Circumoral

See Circumoral Pallor

Papanicolaou Smear (Smear Test)

EXP:　Using a vaginal speculum, the cervix is exposed, and a wooden or plastic spatula is used to scrape cells from the cervical os and body. The scraping is then smeared onto a glass slide which is immediately fixed in alcohol. The slide is later stained and examined for abnormal cells, bacteria, fungi, trichomonads, etc.
INT:　Reported as showing no malignant cells, dysplasia, atypical cells or carcinoma. Inflammatory or infected elements are also reported
PHYS:　Screening test that should be performed at regular intervals to exclude pre-cancerous changes of the cervix

Papilloedema

EXP:　On ophthalmoscopic or slit lamp examination, the optic disc is noted to be flattened, swollen or protruberant bilaterally with blurred edges. Absent venous pulsation, dilated retinal veins, and flame shaped haemorrhages may also be noted
INT:　(+) Increased intracranial pressure (eg. haemorrhage, tumour, meningitis, cerebral abscess, emphysema, hypoparathyroidism), optic neuritis, hypertension, multiple sclerosis, Guillain-Barré syn.
PHYS:　Increased CSF pressure, due to an increase in CSF volume (caused by haemorrhage or increased protein content) or blocked CSF circulation, is transmitted along the sheath of the optic nerve to the optic disc. Vision remains unimpaired in early stages

See also Cheyne-Stokes Respiration

Paralysis of Upward Gaze

EXP:　Unable to look upwards
INT:　(+) Pinealoma

Paralysis, Flaccid

EXP:　Relaxed and flabby muscles that cannot be moved voluntarily
INT:　(+) Poliomyelitis, infantile muscular atrophy, cerebral atonic diplegia, amyotonia congenita, glycogen storage diseases (weak rather than paralysed muscles), plexus palsies, multiple sclerosis, hyperkalaemia, Conn syn., spinal cord shock, botulism, poisons (eg. organo-phosphates), neuropathies, motor neurone disease, encephalitis, other lower motor neurone lesions, Guillain-Barré syn., myasthenia gravis, hysteria, drugs (eg. curare derivatives)
PHYS:　Inflammation, interruption or disease of motor nerve supplying a muscle prevents the voluntary contraction of that muscle. Reflexes usually absent

Paralysis, Spastic

EXP:　Involuntary spasm of muscles
INT:　(+) Spinal cord transection, cerebral or cord tumours, vascular accidents of cerebrum or cord, cerebral or cord infections, upper motor neurone lesions, multiple sclerosis
PHYS:　Loss of inhibition of reflex arc by pyramidal centres causes hyperreflexia and recurrent muscular spasm

Paraplegia

See Paralysis, Flaccid; Paralysis, Spastic
See also SYMPTOMS SECTION 1: Paraplegia and Quadriplegia

Parkinsonian Facies

EXP: Rigidity of facial muscles that gives a characteristic loss of facial expressiveness

INT: (+) Parkinson's disease (paralysis agitans), encephalitis lethargica, cerebral arteriosclerosis, Wilson's disease, phenothiazines, manganese poisoning

PHYS: Degeneration of or damage to the basal ganglia results in muscular hypertonicity

Parkinsonism

EXP: Hypokinesia, tremor and rigidity

INT: (+) Parkinson's disease, familial, encephalitis lethargica, syphilitic mesencephalitis, tuberculoma, brain stem tumours, drugs (eg. phenothiazines, butyrophenones, tetrabenazine, rauwolfia alkaloids)

PHYS: Parkinson's disease and iatrogenic causes most common. Caused by degeneration of the substantia nigra and locus ceruleus

See also Cogwheel Rigidity; Festination; Lead-Pipe Rigidity; Parkinsonian Facies; Tremor, Resting
See also Festination under Gait, Abnormal

Patellar Tap

EXP: One hand is used to apply pressure to the suprapatellar pouch forcing fluid out of this and under the patella. The middle and index fingers of the other hand are used to push down sharply on the patella. A tap is felt when the patella hits the femoral condyles

INT: (+) Knee effusion from trauma, arthritis or other cause of inflammation

PHYS: Any inflammatory process causes the production of an exudate (excess synovial fluid) within the knee joint

Patrick's Sign

EXP: In supine patient, heel of leg being tested is placed on opposite knee. Knee of leg being tested is then pushed down to the couch by the examiner. Positive if pain and involuntary muscular spasm occur

INT: (+) Hip joint disease, musculoskeletal trauma
(–) Sciatic cause of hip pain

Pectoriloquy, Whispering

EXP: Auscultation of the chest while the patient whispers (often the phrase 'ninety-nine' is repeated). If intense broncophony is present, individual syllables can be identified

INT: (+) Lung consolidation or cavitation, TB, pneumonia

PHYS: Solid lung tissue conducts sound better than normally aerated tissue

Pel-Ebstein Phenomenon

EXP: Temperature chart over several weeks shows a remittent fever that occurs daily, reaches a peak level after about a week, then gradually subsides, to recycle again

INT: (+) Hodgkin's disease, other lymphadenomas, undulant fever (*Brucella abortus, B. melitensis*)

PHYS: Malaria, relapsing fever, etc. cause a more rapid alternation

Pelvic Mass

EXP: Abnormal mass felt in pelvis on vaginal and/or abdominal palpation

INT: (+) Pregnancy, faecal impaction, uterine fibroids, congenital uterine abnormality, lymphoma, endometriosis, pelvic malignancy, pelvic inflammatory disease, ovarian cyst or malignancy, teratoma, ectopic pregnancy, hydrosalpinx, pelvic abscess, rectal carcinoma, bladder carcinoma, pelvic kidney

See also Ovarian Mass

Pemberton's Sign

EXP: When patient raises both hands above head, dyspnoea, vertigo, facial flushing, dysphagia and syncope occur

INT: (+) Large intrathoracic goitre

PHYS: Superior mediastinal pressure on the trachea, oesophagus and surrounding veins and arteries

Percussion

See Dull Percussion Note, Thoracic; Tympany, Thoracic

Pericardial Friction Rub

See Friction Rub, Pericardial

Peristalsis, Visible

EXP: Observation of abdomen in relaxed patient reveals peristaltic waves moving vaguely across an often distended abdomen

INT: (+) Pyloric stenosis, acute gastrointestinal obstruction at any level, congenital adrenal insufficiency, thin children

PHYS: Blockage of the intestine causes dilatation of the gut above the blockage and increased peristaltic activity by the gut in an attempt to overcome the obstruction. Ileus results from prolonged blockage

Pes Cavus

EXP: Excessive concave curvature of sole (foot)

INT: (+) Friedreich's ataxia, peroneal muscular atrophy, familial, spina bifida, sacral dermoid, cerebral palsy, poliomyelitis

PHYS: Progressive wasting of extensor muscles of foot and/or spasm of flexor muscles of foot; idiopathic

Phalen's Sign

EXP: Tingling or sudden pain in hand within one minute of acute wrist flexion
INT: (+) Carpal tunnel syn.
PHYS: Median nerve compression. The faster the test is positive, the more likely surgery will be required

See also Tinel's Sign

Pharyngeal Reflex

EXP: A spatula lightly touched against pharynx causes contraction of pharyngeal muscles and gagging
INT: (–) 9th cranial nerve lesions, hysteria, anaesthesia
PHYS: Innervation of the pharynx is via a reflex arc involving the glossopharyngeal (9th) nerve

Phlebitis

EXP: Inflammation of a vein
INT: (+) Venous thrombosis, trauma (eg. IV cannula), infection, syphilis, TB, typhoid, pulmonary embolism, antiphospholipid syn., gout, puerperal phlebitis

Pigmentation

See Areolar Pigmentation; Nail Discolouration
See also SYMPTOMS SECTION 1: Pigmentation of Mouth; Pigmentation of Skin, Excess

Pink Puffer

EXP: Underweight patient who is very breathless on exertion, has markedly pink mucous membranes and an overinflated chest. Narrow heart on X-ray
INT: (+) Emphysematous chronic obstructive airways disease
PHYS: Overinflation and underperfusion of lungs

See also Blue Bloater; Barrel Chest

Pitting Oedema

EXP: Persistent indentation of skin following pressure
INT: (+) Congestive cardiac failure, nephrotic syn., acute glomerulonephritis, cirrhosis, cellulitis, hypoproteinaemia (anorexia nervosa, marasmus, kwashiorkor), beriberi, thrombophlebitis, lymphangitis, filariasis, operative disruption of lymphatic or venous drainage, pregnancy and eclampsia, premenstrual
PHYS: Movement of fluid from vascular to extravascular tissue occurs with increases in interstitial colloid osmotic pressure or intravascular hydrostatic pressure

See also Ankle Oedema
See also SYMPTOMS SECTION 1: Oedema

Plantar Reflex

See Babinski's Sign

Plateau Pulse

EXP: Prolonged duration of pulse summit on palpation
INT: (+) Aortic stenosis, aortic coarctation
PHYS: Systole sustained due to slowing of blood flow

Pleural Effusion

EXP: Restricted chest wall movement, reduced vocal fremitus, dullness on percussion, and decreased breath sounds may be noted. May be found by chest X-ray
INT: (+) Transudate – Cardiac failure, hepatic cirrhosis, nephrotic syn., Meigs syn., constrictive pericarditis
(+) Exudate – Primary or metastatic pleural malignancy, lymphoma, TB, pulmonary infarct, infection, subphrenic abscess, pancreatitis,SLE, rheumatoid disease, trauma, hypothyroidism, postmyocardial infarct, drugs (eg. methysergide)
PHYS: Exudate and transudate distinguished biochemically after thoracocentesis

See also Vocal Fremitus; Dull Percussion Note, Thoracic

Pleural Friction Rub

See Friction Rub, Pleural

Pneumothorax

EXP: Presence of gas in pleural space, detected clinically or radiologically
INT: (+) Spontaneous, traumatic, asthma, bacterial pneumonia, whooping cough, cystic fibrosis, emphysema, chronic bronchitis, congenital bullae, positive pressure assisted ventilation, TB, oesophageal rupture, pleural malignancy, subphrenic abscess, tuberous sclerosis, histiocytosis X, sarcoidosis, iatrogenic (eg. biopsy of lung, aspiration cannula, external cardiac massage)

See also INVESTIGATIONS SECTION 3: Pneumothorax, Spontaneous

Precocious Puberty

(Sexual Precocity)

EXP: Premature genital, axillary and facial hair; breast, clitoris or penis enlargement; voice changes; or menstruation
INT: (+) Adrenal cortical hyperplasia, cerebral or pineal tumours, Albright's syn., hypothalamic cysts or tumours, gonadal tumours, postencephalitic or postmeningitic lesions, hypothyroidism, constitutional
PHYS: Premature release of gonadotrophic hormones from the hypothalamus occurs with various forms of stimulation of that part of the cerebrum

Proprioceptive Sense, Loss of

EXP: Inability to detect vibration or joint movement
INT: (+) Posterior column lesions, tabes dorsalis, subacute combined degeneration of cord, medullary lesions, spinal tumours
PHYS: Proprioceptive fibres run independent of pain, temperature and some touch fibres, not decussating until the medial lemniscus

See also Ataxia; Heel-Knee Test; Romberg's Sign

Proptosis

See Exophthalmos

Prostatomegaly

EXP: Rectal digital examination reveals an enlarged prostate gland
INT: (+) Benign hyperplasia, adenocarcinoma, prostatitis
PHYS: Benign hyperplasia very common over 50 years due to hyperplasia of fibromuscular stroma. Cause unknown. Carcinomas often involve posterior lobe and present late due to minimal urethral obstruction

Ptosis

See SYMPTOMS SECTION 1: Ptosis

Puberty

See Precocious Puberty

Puff Reflex

See Santmyer Swallow

Pulmonary Nodule

EXP: Pulmonary nodule seen on chest X-ray
INT: (+) Lung cancer, metastatic carcinoma, lymphoma, mesothelioma, tuberculosis, abscess, localised pneumonia, benign tumour (eg. haemangioma, chondroma, carcinoid), bronchogenic cyst, hydatid cyst, Wegner's granulomatosis, arteriovenous malformation, pulmonary infarct, rheumatoid nodule

Pulmonary Oedema

EXP: Fluid detected in the lungs by auscultation (see Crepitations, Pulmonary) or characteristic X-ray appearance
INT: (+) Left ventricular failure, atrial fibrillation, mitral stenosis, hypertensive heart disease, fluid overload, severe asthma, smoke inhalation, lymphatic blockage, diffuse pulmonary infections, aspiration pneumonia, shock, adult respiratory distress syn., various neurogenic causes, organophosphate poisoning, snake bite, heroin toxicity, high altitude
PHYS: Physiology dependent upon cause. Primarily due to an imbalance in Starling's forces as related to capillary pressure gradients

Pulse

See Bounding Pulse; Bradycardia; Corrigan's Sign; Dicrotic Pulse; Extrasystolic Beats; Irregularly Irregular Pulse; Plateau Pulse; Pulse, Absent; Pulsus Alternans; Pulsus Paradoxus; Tachycardia; Water-Hammer Pulse
See also signs listed under Heart

Pulse, Absent

EXP: Distal pulse absent or diminished
INT: (+) Arteriosclerosis, diabetes mellitus, thrombosus, Leriche syn., embolism

Pulsus Alternans

EXP: Alternate variation in size of pulse wave, often detected by sphygmomanometry
INT: (+) Paroxysmal tachycardia, left ventricular failure, cardiomyopathy, hypertension, ischaemic heart disease
PHYS: Not all fibres of myocardium able to contract with each beat due to disease

Pulsus Paradoxus

EXP: Pulse volume decreases with inspiration, the reverse of normal
INT: (+) Thoracic respiration, certain postures, pericardial effusion, constrictive pericarditis, pericardial tamponade
PHYS: Due to distension of right atrium and ventricle with venous return in inspiration, compressing the left side of the heart and reducing its output; or due to reduction in pressure gradient between pulmonary veins and left atrium

Pupil Changes

See Aniscoria; Miosis; Mydriasis; Lens Opacity; Pupil, Irregular; Pupil, White

Pupil, Dilated

See Aniscoria

Pupil Irregular

EXP: Pupil of eye is irregular in outline
INT: (+) Iritis, surgery, trauma, pupillary membrne, congenital

Pupil, White (Leucocoria)

EXP: Pupil of eye is white and reflects light
INT: (+) Cataract, retinoblastoma, retinal fibroplasia, corneal scarring, persistent tunica vasculosa lentis

See also Lens Opacity

Purpura

See Hess Test
See also SYMPTOMS SECTION 1: Purpura and Petechiae

Queckenstedt's Test

EXP: Pressure on either or both jugular veins during lumbar puncture normally produces a rise in the CSF manometric pressure, and then a drop when pressure on veins released
INT: (−) Block of spinal subarachnoid space or blocking of CSF escape from cerebral cavity (eg. vertebral fracture, TB, tumours of cord or vertebrae, haematomas)
PHYS: Physical block of fluid connection via jugular veins, cerebral CSF and spinal CSF causes test to be negative

Racoon Sign

EXP: Periorbital ecchymosis (dark bruise rings around eyes)
INT: (+) Fracture at base of skull
PHYS: X-rays may be negative despite positive sign. Caused by tracking of blood through tissue planes from fracture site

See also Battle's Sign

Radial Jerk

EXP: With the elbow flexed at 90° and the forearm in neutral position, the styloid process of the radius is tapped with a rubber hammer. Normal result is flexion of elbow and supination of forearm
INT: (−) Lower motor neurone lesion, peripheral neuropathy, polio, tabes dorsalis, posterior root tumours, syringomyelia, muscular dystrophies, subacute combined degeneration of cord, coma (++) Upper motor neurone lesion, tetanus, CVA
PHYS: Due to contraction of brachioradialis. Acts at C7, C8 level

See also other signs listed under Reflexes

Rainbow Halo

EXP: Rainbow coloured halo seen around lights, particularly at night
INT: (+) Acute angle closure glaucoma, corneal oedema, incipient cataract, allergic conjunctivitis
PHYS: Distortion of light, as in a prism, by unequal alignment of inner and outer surfaces of cornea

Rales

See Crepitations, Pulmonary; Rhonchi

Rash

See Butterfly Rash; Café-au-Lait Spots; Chloasma; Spider Naevi
See also SYMPTOMS SECTION 1: Rash

Rash, Butterfly

See Butterfly Rash

Rebound Tenderness, Abdominal

EXP: Gentle pressure on the abdomen followed by rapid removal of pressure causes sudden, acute pain
INT: (+) Peritonitis, peritonism due to any inflamed intra-abdominal viscus (eg. appendicitis, pancreatitis, perforated ulcer, cholecystitis, Crohn's disease, diverticulitis, cystitis, adenitis), intraperitoneal haemorrhage (eg. ectopic pregnancy, leaking aneurysm, endometriosis)
PHYS: The sudden release of pressure causes movement of the viscus within an inflamed peritoneum, and thus pain

See also SYMPTOMS SECTION 1: Abdominal Pain

Rectal Mass

EXP: Palpable mass on digital examination of the rectum
INT: (+) Thrombosed internal pile, rectal polyp, rectal carcinoma, metastatic carcinoma, prostatomegaly, prostate carcinoma, ovarian cyst or carcinoma, uterine fibroids, pelvic malignancy, mesorectal lymph nodes, endometriosis, enlarged or cancerous uterine cervix, bone cyst of sacrum, tampon or othr object in vagina, foreign body in rectum, impacted faeces

Red Urine

See Urine, Abnormal Colour
See also PATHOLOGY SECTION 4: Haematuria

Reflexes

See Ankle Jerk; Babinski's Sign; Biceps Jerk; Consensual Reflex; Corneal Reflex; Cremasteric Reflex; Grasp Reflex; Hering-Breuer Reflexes; Hoffmann's Sign or Reflex; Knee Jerk; Mass Reflex; Moro Reflex; Pharyngeal Reflex; Radial Jerk; Santmyer Swallow; Triceps Jerk

Renal

See Kidney, Large; Kidney, Small

Retinal Arteriovenous Nipping

See Arteriovenous Nipping, Retinal

Retinal Exudates

EXP: Ophthalmoscopic examination of retina reveals white fluffy patches
INT: (+) Diabetes mellitus, hypertension, increased intracranial pressure, massive blood loss
PHYS: Occlusion of retinal capillaries

Retinal Haemorrhages

EXP: Red spots and patches adjacent to blood vessels are noted on ophthalmoscopic examination of the retina. Various types described as punctate, splinter and flame

INT: (+) Pernicious anaemia, leukaemia, aplastic anaemia, hypertension, diabetes mellitus, bacterial endocarditis, anticoagulants, haemorrhagic disease

PHYS: Damaged retinal capillaries

Retinal Pigmentation
(Retinitis Pigmentosa)

EXP: Cells filled with epithelial pigment congregate beside retinal blood vessels

INT: (+) Bassen-Kornzweig syn., Laurence-Moon-Biedl syn., other genetic conditions

PHYS: Night blindness and tunnel vision early symptoms

Rhonchi (Dry Rales)

EXP: Musical wheezing sounds caused by air flow through narrowed or congested bronchi, heard on chest auscultation. Deeper pitched sonorous rhonchi originate in large bronchi. Higher pitched sibilant rhonchi originate in smaller bronchi

INT: (+) Bronchitis, tracheobronchitis, asthma, pulmonary tumours, bronchial oedema or spasm

PHYS: Air passing through the narrowed part of a tube becomes turbulent and produces a sound

See also Crepitations, Pulmonary

Rib Notching

EXP: A plain AP X-ray of the chest shows notching on the lower surface of the 4th to 8th ribs posteriorly. Usually bilateral

INT: Congenital coarctation of aorta

Rigidity

See Lead-Pipe Rigidity; Cogwheel Rigidity; Abdominal Rigidity; Clasp-Knife Rigidity; Neck Stiffness; Opisthotonos

Rinne's Test

EXP: A vibrating tuning fork (512 cps) is placed on the mastoid process. When it becomes inaudible to the patient, the vibrating end is placed near the external auditory meatus. If heard at the external auditory meatus, air conduction is greater than bone conduction (i.e. Rinne positive). In reverse situation, if heard on mastoid process after air conduction lost, the test is Rinne negative

INT: (+) Air conduction < bone conduction – Conductive deafness (eg. wax, perforated tympanum, otosclerosis, glue ear, otitis media, foreign body, dislocated ossicles, tumours, meatal stenosis, exostoses, barotrauma)

(+) Air conduction > bone conduction – Normal hearing

(+) Reduced time – Perceptive deafness (eg. presbycousis, vascular causes, measles, mumps, influenza, meningitis, labyrinthitis, congenital causes [maternal rubella], trauma [blast], prolonged noise exposure, drugs (eg. streptomycin, aspirin, quinine), Menière's disease, late otosclerosis, CNS tumours, haemorrhage, leukaemia, multiple sclerosis, vitamin B deficit), psychogenic

See also Weber's Test

Risus Sardonicus

EXP: Fixed, immobile grin

INT: (+) Tetanus

PHYS: Excess tension of facial musculature

Rogoff's Sign

EXP: Costovertebral angle pain and tenderness

INT: (+) Adrenal crisis

PHYS: Adrenal inflammation due to steroid withdrawal; or adrenal infection or destruction

Romana's Sign

EXP: Unilateral persistent oedema of upper and lower eyelids

INT: (+) Chagas' disease

PHYS: Occurs when conjunctiva is portal of trypanasome entry

Romberg's Sign

EXP: Patient stands at attention with heels close together and then shuts eyes. Positive when severe swaying or falling occurs

INT: (+) Tabes dorsalis, posterior column lesion, subacute combined degeneration of cord, intoxication

PHYS: Due to loss of proprioceptive sensation. Negative in cerebellar disease

See also Ataxia; Proprioceptive Sense, Loss of; Heel-Knee Test; Tandem Romberg Test

Rosary, Thoracic

EXP: Nodular swelling of costochondral junctions of the ribs bilateral to the sternum in a child

INT: (+) Rickets

PHYS: Calcium deficient diet

Roth's Spots

EXP: Superficial retinal haemorrhages with pale or white centres

INT: (+) Retinal infarct, leukaemia, retinal haemorrhage with central resolution

PHYS: In leukaemia, due to extravasation of excess white corpuscles from a retinal haemorrhage

Rubin Test

EXP: A cannula of sufficient diameter to make the os cervix airtight is introduced through the cervix into the uterus. Carbon dioxide is passed through the tube into the uterus, while a side arm to a manometer measures the pressure, which should not exceed 200mmHg. A stethoscope is used to listen to gas bubbling through tubular ostia. Any abdominal or shoulder tip pain is also noted

INT: (– no gas heard) Nonpatent fallopian tubes

PHYS: Test of tubal patency in infertility. May help clear mildly blocked tubes. Should be performed immediately after menstruation, before ovulation

Saddle Nose

EXP: Characteristic 'saddle' or dip at junction of bony and cartilaginous parts of dorsum of nose

INT: (+) Wegener's granulomatosis, congenital syphilis

Santmyer Swallow (Puff Reflex)

EXP: Blowing gently on the face of an infant induces a reflex swallow

INT: Useful procedure for easing the passage of a nasogastric tube or medication. Developmental assessment test – should have disappeared by 24 months of age

Scanning Speech (Staccato Speech)

EXP: A speech form in which there are marked, and sometimes rhythmic, pauses between syllables and/or words

INT: (+) Cerebellar ataxia, multiple sclerosis

See also Slurred Speech

Schamroth's Sign

EXP: Same fingers of both hands are held with nails touching. In normal nails, there is a gap between the nails at their bases. If fingers are clubbed, gap between nails occurs at tips of nails

INT: (+) Clubbing present

PHYS: Used to note presence of clubbing

See also Clubbing of Fingers

Schiller Test

EXP: The cervix is painted with aqueous iodine solution. Normal areas stain dark brown

INT: (+) Nonstained areas – Cervical carcinoma, erosion, eversion, scars, leucoplakia, cystic mucous glands

PHYS: Normal cells take up stain because they contain glycogen. Test shows abnormal areas, but is not specific for any cause

Schober's Test

EXP: With patient erect, mark skin over L5 level and a point 10cm above. Patient bends forward maximally and distance between marks is measured

INT: (+) Increase <5 cm – Lumbar ankylosing spondylitis, other degenerative lumbar vertebral disease

Scissors Gait

See Gait, Abnormal

Sclera, Blue

EXP: Markedly blue sclera (not iris) noted

INT: (+) Fragilitas ossium (osteogenesis imperfecta)

PHYS: Congenital disease transmitted by a dominant mutant gene

Sexual Precocity

See Precocious Puberty

Shifting Dullness

EXP: Percussion of an abdomen with patient lying on one side reveals a dullness on the side nearest the bed, and a tympanic note on the high side, regardless of which side the patient is lying

INT: (+) Free intraperitoneal fluid (ascites) (eg. cirrhosis, intraperitoneal neoplasms, TB, peritonitis, congestive cardiac failure, nephrosis, hepatoma, constrictive pericarditis, hepatic vein obstruction, myxoedema, Meigs syn.).

PHYS: Fluid flows from one side of abdomen to other as patient turns

See also Thrill, Fluid
See also SYMPTOMS SECTION 1: Ascites

Shirmer's Test

EXP: A strip of filter paper 5mm x 35mm is folded 5mm from one end. The short flap is inserted under the lower lid of each eye and the eye is closed lightly. After 5 minutes, length of strip from ciliary margin that has been dampened by tears is measured. Normal > 5mm

INT: (<5 mm) Xerophthalmia

See also SYMPTOMS SECTION 1: Xerophthalmia

Shock

EXP: Hypotension, oliguria, tachycardia, reduced mental acuity, peripheral hypoperfusion, peripheral vasoconstriction, (metabolic acidosis)

INT: (+) Severe diarrhoea and/or vomiting, dehydration, excessive sweating, severe injury, haemorrhage (internal or external), cardiac arrhythmia, cardiac failure (eg. infarct, myopathy), cardiac valve failure or stenosis, tension

pneumothorax, pericardial tamponade, pulmonary embolus, severe burns, diabetic ketoacidosis, pancreatitis, ascites, bowel obstruction, septicaemia, toxic shock syndrome, anaphylaxis, acute adrenal insufficiency, drugs (eg. vasodilators, narcotics, phenothiazines)
PHYS: Caused by inadequate circulation of arterial blood

See also Hypotension

Shoulder Tip Pain

EXP: Pain at tip of shoulder
INT: (+) Blood, pus or air under diaphragm, inflammation of subphrenic organs (eg. liver, spleen), after abdominal operations in which air may have been introduced (eg. laparoscopy)
PHYS: Referred pain via phrenic nerve, caused by irritation of diaphragm. Exclude local causes

See also Kehr's Sign

Simmond's Test

See Calf Squeeze Test

Sister Mary Joseph's Nodule

EXP: Raised umbilical nodule, often erythematous and painless
INT: (+) Disseminated intra-abdominal malignancy (eg. ovarian or gastric carcinoma)
PHYS: Retrograde lymphatic spread of carcinoma to form an umbilical deposit

Skin, Abnormal

See Areolar Pigmentation; Butterfly Rash; Café-au-Lait Spots; Chip Sign; Chloasma; Dermographia; Gottron's Sign; Leser-Trelat Sign; Nikolsky Sign; Spider Naevi; Xanthomatosis
See also SYMPTOMS SECTION 1: Skin Disorders

Slurred Speech

EXP: Marked difficulty or trembling in attempts to pronounce words of several syllables
INT: (+) Drugs (eg. alcohol, sedatives), general paralysis of insane, Friedreich's ataxia, bulbar palsy

See also Scanning Speech

Small for Dates

See Intrauterine Growth Retardation

Smear Test

See Papanicolaou Smear

Sounds, Heart

See Murmur, Cardiac

Spalding's Sign

EXP: Overlapping of cranial bones seen on X-ray examination of intrauterine fetus
INT: (+) Intrauterine fetal death, labour
PHYS: Loss of tissue turgor in death

Spasm, Muscular

See Myotonia; Hypertonicity

Spastic Paralysis

See Paralysis, Spastic

Speech

See Scanning Speech; Slurred Speech

Spider Naevi (Telangiectasia)

EXP: Skin area where several capillaries can be seen radiating from a central point
INT: (+) Cirrhosis of liver, thyrotoxicosis, rheumatoid arthritis, pregnancy, sun damaged skin, irradiation, carcinoid syn., CREST syn., Louis-Bar syn., Rendu-Osler-Weber syn., Rothmund-Thomson syn., systemic sclerosis, acute alcoholic and viral hepatitis, hereditary tendency

Spleen, Enlarged

See Splenomegaly

Splenomegaly

EXP: Enlarged spleen found on bimanual palpation of abdominal LUQ
INT: (+) Systemic infection, (eg. infectious mononucleosis, hepatitis, AIDS, septicaemia, subacute bacterial endocarditis, malaria, TB, brucellosis, typhoid fever), portal hypertension (due to cirrhosis, portal or splenic vein thrombosis or obstruction), Gaucher's disease, Niemann-Pick disease, congestive cardiac failure, Letterer-Siwe disease, sarcoidosis, leukaemias, lymphoma, various haemoglobino-pathies, thalassaemia major, myelofibrosis, kala-azar, SLE,polyarteritis nodosa, poly-cythaemia vera, spherocytosis, thrombocyto-penia, haemolytic anaemias, splenic cysts or neoplasms, Hand-Schueller-Christian disease, amyloidosis, Budd-Chiari syn., Felty syn., Hunter syn., Hurler syn., Plummer-Vinson syn., Pompe syn., Sanfilippo syn., Schiei syn., Sly syn., protein deficiency, starvation
PHYS: Deposition of matter in the spleen, venous outlet obstruction or increased red blood cell production

Splinter Haemorrhages

EXP: Linear haemorrhages of the nail bed
INT: (+) Subacute bacterial endocarditis, blood dyscrasias, psoriasis, eczema, rheumatoid arthritis, tinea, trauma

PHYS: Due to microemboli in subacute bacterial endocarditis

See also Janeway Lesion; Osler's Nodes

Split Heart Sounds

EXP: Double heart sound in which the two elements are very close together
INT: (+) 1st sound – Not pathological
          (+) 2nd sound – Normal in inspiration, left bundle branch block, atrial septal defect, aortic valve stenosis, patent ductus arteriosus, left ventricular failure due to hypertension or ischaemia
PHYS: Asynchronous closure of mitral and tricuspid valves (1st sound) or pulmonary and aortic valves (2nd sound)

Spooning Nails

See Koilonychia

Squint

See SYMPTOMS SECTION 1: Squint

Staccato Speech

See Scanning Speech

Startle Reflex

See Moro Reflex

Steatorrhoea

See PATHOLOGY SECTION 4: Fat, Faecal

Steell Murmur

See Graham Steell Murmur

Still's Murmur

EXP: Musical or vibrating soft early to mid-systolic murmur in a child heard maximally over third left intercostal space, that becomes more noticeable with a fever
INT: (+) Innocent murmur of no clinical significance
Phys: Left ventricular outflow murmur

See also Systolic Murmur

Stool, Abnormal Colour

See Faeces, Abnormal Colour

Strawberry Tongue

EXP: Red glazed tongue with prominent papillae
INT: (+) Scarlet fever (may have thick white fur between papillae for first 2 days)

See also Geographic Tongue

Striae

See SYMPTOMS SECTION 1: Striae

Subcutaneous Emphysema

See Crepitations, Tissue

Subungal Hyperkeratosis

EXP: Deposition of keratin under nail
INT: (+) Psoriasis, fungal infection (onychomychosis), recurrent trauma, chronic eczema, chronic paronychia, lichen planus, pityriaisis rubra pilaris, Norwegian scabies
Phys: Chronic inflammation of the nail bed results in keratin deposition

See also Onycholysis

Swinging Torch Sign

EXP: In a darkened room, shine a torch in normal eye and there is immediate bilateral constriction of pupils. Swinging torch to affected eye causes initial bilateral dilatation with subsequent constriction. Swinging torch back to normal eye results in immediate pupil constriction again
INT: (+) Glaucoma (more advanced in affected eye), optic nerve demyelination, tumour or disease
PHYS: As the light shifts from the less to the more diseased eye, the direct afferent stimulus passes along the more damaged optic nerve; it is now no longer sufficient in intensity to keep the pupils as small as they had been when the better eye was illuminated, both pupils thus dilate

Systolic Murmur

EXP: Cardiac auscultation reveals a murmur between 1st and 2nd heart sounds
INT: (+) Physiological, exercise, mitral valve incompetence, atrial and ventricular septal defect, patent ductus arteriosus, gross anaemia, aortic stenosis, dilatation of base of aorta, high fever, hyperthyroidism, pulmonary stenosis, aortic coarctation, tricuspid incompetence, carcinoid syn., cardiomyopathies
PHYS: Due to flow disturbances within the heart. Mitral incompetence and associated states tend to be heard at the apex; aortic valve disease is heard maximally at right sternal margin in 2nd intercostal space

See also Still's Murmur

Tachycardia

EXP: Heart (pulse) rate significantly higher than average (generally > 100 per minute)
INT: (+) Exercise, emotion, pain, shock, infections, sarcoidosis, thyrotoxicosis and other hypermetabolic diseases, endocarditis,

hypotension, cardiac failure, atrial flutter and fibrillation, paroxysmal tachycardia, pacemaker and conductive anomalies, nodal tachycardia, sick sinus syn., anaphylaxis, pulmonary oedema, phaeochromocytoma, venous hypertension, mitral valve disease, coronary artery disease, pulmonary thromboembolism, polyarteritis nodosa, other connective tissue diseases, dumping syn., Irukandji syn., serotonin syn., drugs (eg. alcohol, adrenaline, atropine, amphetamines, cocaine)

PHYS: Due to metabolic or mechanical influences on the cardiac pacemaker, or the occurrence of a more rapidly depolarising ectopic pacemaker

See also Torsades de Pointes

Tachypnoea
See Hyperventilation

Tandem Romberg Test
EXP: Patient stands with one foot in front of the other (toe to heel in tandem), then closes eyes. Positive if patient sways or is unsteady within 60 seconds
INT: (+) Labyrinth, posterior column lesions, tabes dorsalis, subacute combined degeneration of cord, intoxication
PHYS: More sensitive than standard Romberg's sign

See also Romberg's Sign

Tardive Dyskinesia
See Dyskinesia, Tardive

Target Lesions
EXP: Round, erythematous macule that becomes papular, enlarges and develops concentric rings of colour to resemble a target. Centre of lesion may blister, erode and crust. May become pigmented during resolution
INT: (+) Erythema multiforme
PHYS: Precursor target lesion often not identified as erythema multiforme until widespread lesions erupt

Telangiectasia
See Spider Naevi

Temperature, Reduced
See Hypothermia

Tetany
See Obstetric Hand

Third Eyelid of Morgan-Denny
EXP: Extra fold of skin above upper eyelid

INT: (+) Atopic eczema of eyelid, allergic conjunctivitis, other chronic irritating conditions of eye
PHYS: Caused by chronic rubbing of eye. More common in children

Thorn's Sign
EXP: Stiffness of cartilage in ear
INT: (+) Addison's disease

Thrill, Cardiac
EXP: Vibration that emanates from the heart or great vessels felt by the palpating hand. Analogous to murmur
INT: (+ systolic) Aortic stenosis, aortic aneurysm, pulmonary stenosis, infundibular stenosis, ventricular septal defect, mitral regurgitation, patent ductus arteriosus, other arteriovenous aneurysms
(+ diastolic) Mitral stenosis, patent ductus arteriosus, pulmonary incompetence
PHYS: Rapid movement of blood through abnormally narrowed or dilated passage

See also Diastolic Murmur; Systolic Murmur

Thrill, Fluid
EXP: The patient or a third person places his or her hand vertically on edge along the linea alba. Examiner places flat of hand on one side of abdomen and sharply taps opposite flank. A sudden change in abdominal pressure is noted by the palpating hand
INT: (+) Intraperitoneal fluid (ascites) (due to cirrhosis, cardiac failure, hepatitis, carcinoma of liver, pericarditis, nephrotic syn., etc.)
PHYS: Fluid thrill may be felt due to subcutaneous fat transmission of impulse unless this is obstructed by hand on linea alba

See also Shifting Dullness
See also SYMPTOMS SECTION 1: Ascites

Thrombophlebitis
See Phlebitis

Thyroid Glitter
EXP: 'Glitter' of light in the eyes
INT: (+) Thyrotoxicosis
PHYS: Conjunctival oedema

Tinel's Sign
EXP: Tingling or sudden pain on volar wrist percussion
INT: (+) Carpal tunnel syn.
PHYS: Median nerve compression

See also Phalen's Sign

Tone, Decreased Muscular

See Hypotonia

Tone, Increased Muscular

See Hypertonicity

Tongue, Abnormal

See Fasciculation, Muscular; Geographic Tongue;
Strawberry Tongue; Tongue, Discoloured; Tongue,
Enlarged; Tongue, Fissured
See also SYMPTOMS SECTION 1

Tongue, Discoloured

EXP: Abnormal tongue colour
INT: White – Thrush (fungal infection), leucoplakia, lichen planus, erythema multiforme, pemphigus vulgaris, squamous cell carcinoma, Reiter's syn., milk curds, burns
Black – Filiform papillae hypertrophy, tobacco, penicillin, chromogenic bacteria, antiarthritic drugs, melanoma
Red – Scarlet fever, poststreptococcal infection, pernicious anaemia, erythema multiforme, ariboflavinosis, pellagra, sprue, vitamin B deficit, Reiter's syn. vascular hamartoma
Blue – Central cyanosis from heart or lung disease
Patchy – Geographic tongue

Tongue, Enlarged (Macroglossia)

EXP: Oversize tongue for mouth
INT: (+) Down syn. (see SYNDROMES SECTION 6), haemangioma, lymphangioma, primary amyloidosis, acromegaly, cretinism

Tongue, Fissured

EXP: Deep fissures on tongue surface
INT: (+) Niacin deficiency, congenital

Torsades de Pointes

(Twisting of the Points)

EXP: Variant of ventricular tachycardia characterised by bursts of ventricular tachycardia complicating a junctional bradycardia. On an ECG, the bradycardia element shows a long QT interval, and the ventricular tachycardia shows a swinging axis ('twisting of the points') in a series of ectopic QRS complexes that vary in their form. Abnormal T waves may be present in bradycardia phase
INT: (+) Complete heart block, acute myocardial infarction, myocarditis, hypokalaemia, congenital, drugs (eg. phenothiazines, tricyclics, some antiarrhythmics)
PHYS: Abnormality in ventricular repolarisation. Normally self-terminating condition, but may terminate in syncope or sudden death

Torsion Dystonia

See Athetosis

Torticollis

EXP: Spasm of the muscles in one side of the neck which causes the head to twist to that side. Straightening of the head usually causes pain
INT: (+) Muscle trauma, hysteria, rheumatoid arthritis, corpus striatum disease, adenitis of neck glands, neck abscess, ocular diseases, 11th cranial nerve disease, fibrositis, thermal trauma to neck, habitual tic, labyrinthine disease, tissue scarring, congenital
PHYS: Sternomastoid muscle most commonly involved

Tracheal Displacement

EXP: Deviation of the trachea from the midline to the suprasternal notch
INT: (+ towards lesion) Pulmonary fibrosis, TB, pulmonary collapse
(+ away from lesion) Pleural effusion, pneumothorax
PHYS: Base of trachea moved laterally by variations in the normal volume of the chest contents

See also Dull Percussion Note, Thoracic

Tremor, Flapping (Asterixis)

EXP: With arms, hands and fingers outstretched, the patient dorsiflexes the wrists and spreads the fingers. An irregular but synchronous tremor of a flapping nature is seen, with maximum activity at the wrist and metacarpophalangeal joints. May also involve feet and tongue
INT: (+) Encephalopathy, liver failure, metabolic diseases, subdural haematomas, cerebral infarcts in diencephalon region
PHYS: Distortion of proprioceptive cerebral pathways and inappropriate motor stimulation

Tremor, Intention (Dysmetria)

EXP: Attempt to touch nose with finger or perform any other definite movement causes increasing shaking of hand until movement is completed. Precision movement lost
INT: (+) Cerebellar lesions (eg. tumours, CVA, abscess), multiple sclerosis, brain stem disease, Friedreich's ataxia, spinocerebellar degenerations, mercury poisoning
PHYS: Loss of appreciation of the force and rate of muscular contraction necessary for a movement

See also Dysdiadochokinesia

Tremor, Postural

EXP: Tremor obvious in certain postures such as outstretched hands
INT: (+) Anxiety, thyrotoxicosis, alcohol, drugs (eg. bronchodilators, tricyclics), heavy metal

poisoning, Wilson's disease, neurosyphilis, cerebellar lesions, familial

PHYS: Loss of fine control of flexor/extensor reflex

Tremor, Resting

EXP: Rhythmic sinusoidal movement of limbs and/or head at rest

INT: (+) Parkinson's disease (paralysis agitans), postencephalitic, cerebral tumours, drugs (eg. reserpine, phenothiazines)

PHYS: Degeneration of substantia nigra and associated pathways

See also Festination under Gait, Abnormal
See also Cogwheel Rigidity

Trendelenburg Test

EXP: Observe patient from behind while each leg in turn is lifted from the ground and the hip flexed forward. Positive if pelvis tilts towards side on which leg is lifted

INT: (−) Normal
(+) Lesion of contralateral gluteal nerve supply at radicular level, congenital dislocation of hip, muscular dystrophy

PHYS: Superior gluteal nerve separates from the sciatic distribution of the L4–5 nerve roots at lumbar plexus level

Triceps Jerk

EXP: With the elbows at 90° and relaxed, the triceps tendon is tapped just above the point of the elbow. This results in extension of the elbow

INT: (−) Poliomyelitis, peripheral neuropathies, posterior root disease, tabes dorsalis, spinal cord tumours or degenerations, spinal shock, syringomyelia, muscle dystrophies, coma
(++) Upper motor neurone lesion, tetanus, hyperthyroidism, anxiety, cord transection

PHYS: Acts at C6, C7, C8 level. Due to contraction of triceps brachii muscle

See also other signs listed under Reflexes

Trichiasis

EXP: Ingrown eyelash causes irritation of conjunctiva
INT: (+) Trachoma, eyelid trauma

See also Entropion

Triple Rhythm

See Gallop Rhythm

Trousseau's Sign

EXP: Circumferential pressure (eg. by sphygmonanometer cuff) on a limb causes carpopedal spasm

INT: (+) Hypoparathyroidism, hypocalcaemia, rickets, alkalosis, Bartter syn. (see SYNDROMES SECTION 6)

PHYS: Low serum calcium causes hyperexcitability of muscles that may lead to tetany

See also Chvostek's Sign

Twitching

See Fasciculation, Muscular

Tympany, Thoracic

EXP: One index finger is laid flat on the chest and is struck firmly with the other index finger. Higher than normal pitch of percussion note is tympany

INT: (+) Pneumothorax, overinflation of lungs (eg. asthma, emphysema), cavitation of lungs

PHYS: Large air masses reflect sound more readily

Umbilical Bruising

See Cullen's Sign

Unterberger's Test

EXP: Patient is asked to walk on the spot with eyes closed for one minute while holding arms out horizontally in front and counting aloud with each step. The knees must be raised as high as possible while stepping. A positive test occurs if the patient turns about his axis in a particular direction by more than 45°.

INT: (+) Unilateral vestibular disorder

Urine, Abnormal Colour

INT: White – Gross excess protein, gross excess white cells, chyle
Red – Blood (see Haematuria), porphyria, myoglobin, beetroot and other red foods, drugs (eg.phenytoin, phenindione, rifampicin, desferrioxamine, phenothiazines)
Brown/black – Porphyria, alkaptonuria, old blood, melanin, drugs (eg. nitrofurantoin, methyldopa, cascara), foods (eg. rhubarb, fava beans)
Orange – Dehydration, jaundice, drugs (eg. primaquine, riboflavine, sulfasalazine)
Blue/green – Biliverdin, drugs (eg. amitriptyline, triamterene, phenol, indigo)

Urine, Smelly

EXP: Fishy smell – E. coli infection, tyrosinaemia
Ammonia – Common in infants, occurs in urine that has been left standing
Mousy – Phenylketonuria
Maple syrup – Maple syrup urine disease
Cabbage – Methionine malabsorption

Uterus, Enlarged

See Pelvic Mass

Venous Engorgement and Pressure
See Jugular Venous Pressure

Vocal Fremitus
EXP: Ulnar border of hand is used to detect variations in the vibrations transmitted from the larynx through the airways and lungs to the chest wall when a patient repeats a phrase (eg. 'ninety-nine')

INT: (–) Feeble voice, blocked bronchus from foreign body, bronchial tumour, pleural effusion, pneumothorax, collapsed lung
(++) Pneumonia, consolidation around major bronchus, TB

PHYS: Variations depend on the degree of interference of vibration conduction through lung tissue

See also Pleural Effusion

Vomit
See SYMPTOMS SECTION 1: Nausea and Vomiting

Waddling Gait
See Gait, Abnormal

Waiter's Hand
EXP: The arm is adducted and extended at the elbow and the forearm is pronated, with the palm facing backwards as though accepting a surreptitious tip

INT: (+) Erb-Duchenne paralysis
PHYS: Damage (usually at birth) to the 5th cervical anterior nerve root and subsequent paralysis of deltoid, brachioradialis and biceps

Walk, Abnormal
See Gait, Abnormal

Wasting, Muscular
EXP: Reduction in muscle bulk
INT: Localised – Paralysis of muscle bundle (eg. paraplegia, motor neurone disease, plexus palsy), congenital
Generalised – Diabetes mellitus, thyrotoxicosis, Addison's disease, phaeochromocytoma, occult carcinoma, hypopituitarism, anorexia nervosa, fad diets

Water-Hammer Pulse
(Collapsing Pulse)
EXP: With patient's hand raised as high as possible above head, a pulse is felt that appears to hammer at the examiner's fingers and then suddenly collapse
INT: (+) Aortic incompetence, arteriovenous fistula (eg. patent ductus arteriosus), severe anaemia, ventricular septal defect, complete heart block,

fever, thyrotoxicosis, vasodilatory drugs
PHYS: Low diastolic pressure and subsequent flaccidity of arterial walls

See also Corrigan's Sign

Weakness, Muscular
See Paralysis, Flaccid; Hypotonia

Webbing of Neck
EXP: Anterior aspect of neck is broadened due to an exaggerated skin fold from the mastoid process to the shoulder
INT: (+) Noonan syn., Turner syn.

Weber's Test
EXP: Vibrating tuning fork placed on midline of forehead or a central incisor, is normally heard at midline
INT: In conductive deafness sound is referred to deafer ear. In perceptive deafness sound is referred to the better ear
PHYS: Often unreliable. In conductive deafness the cochlear is undisturbed by extraneous noises encountered by the better ear

See also Rinne's Test

Wheeze
See SYMPTOMS SECTION 1: Wheeze

Whispering Pectoriloquy
See Pectoriloquy, Whispering

White Pupil (Leucocoria)
See Pupil, White

Windlass Test
EXP: Passive hyperextension of the hallux (great toe) causes the plantar medial longitudinal arch of the foot to reform in a flat-footed patient
INT: (+) Physiological flat foot
(–) Pathological flat foot
PHYS: Physiological flat foot due to ligamentous laxity is asymptomatic, common and requires no treatment

Wodak Sign
EXP: The patient is seated with back and elbows unsupported. With the arms slightly extended, the patient points the index fingers while keeping the other fingers in a fist. The examiner sits opposite the patient and points his or her index fingers close to those of the patient, but has his or her elbows supported on the arms of a chair. The patient closes his or her eyes. Positive test if patient's fingers drift away from

those of the examiner

INT: (+) Labyrinth disease

PHYS: If nystagmus of labyrinthine origin is present,
the fingers will drift in the direction of the slow
phase when the patient's eyes are closed

Wrist Drop

EXP: Inability to extend wrist

INT: (+) Radial nerve lesion, peripheral neuropathy,
muscular dystrophy, lead poisoning

PHYS: Lower motor neurone lesion of wrist extensors

Xanthelasma

(Xantheloma Palpebrarum)

EXP: Yellow-brown nodules in soft tissues around
eye

INT: (+) Primary biliary cirrhosis, elderly,
hyperlipidaemia, cholestasis

See also Xanthomatosis

Xanthomatosis

EXP: Cluster of pale yellow papules on a red patch of
skin, often on buttocks

INT: (+) Hypertriglyceridaemia, other
hyperlipidaemias, diabetes mellitus, biliary
cirrhosis, cholestasis

PHYS: Deposition of excess circulating lipids in skin

See also Arcus senilis

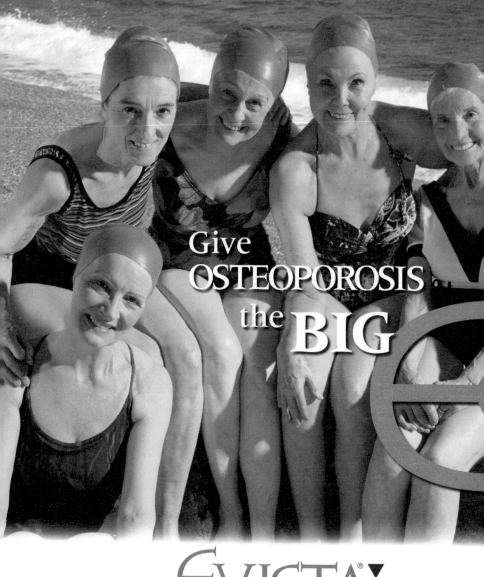

Give
OSTEOPOROSIS
the **BIG**

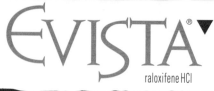

EVISTA®▼

raloxifene HCl

Proven prevention and treatment of osteoporo

Further information is available on request from Eli Lilly and Company Limited,
Dextra Court, Chapel Hill, Basingstoke, Hants RG21 5SY.

EV 766 December 2001 [POM]

Lil

SECTION THREE
INVESTIGATION

THE PATHOLOGY TESTS AND CLINICAL SIGNS
THAT WILL CONFIRM A DIAGNOSIS
AND THE DIFFERENTIAL DIAGNOSES OF DISEASES

FORMAT

Suspect Diagnosis [Abbreviation] (Alternate Name)

TEST: The pathology tests (biochemistry, haematology, cytology and bacteriology) that should be considered when a history and examination indicate that this is a probable diagnosis. The result that may be expected with this diagnosis is shown in (brackets) after each test. Physiological, electrophysiological (eg: ECG) and radiological tests are not always included. See PATHOLOGY SECTION 4 for the explanation and interpretation of these tests

SIGN: Signs (not symptoms), methods of examination and clinical findings that may be useful in the diagnosis of, or may be found in association with this disease or syndrome. See SYMPTOMS SECTION 2 for the explanation and interpretation of these signs.

DD: Differential diagnoses. Other diseases with which this diagnosis may be confused.

PHYS: The basic physiology of the disease, to enable the reason for abnormal pathology tests to be better understood.

See also Other Entries or Sections of Significance

Abbreviation
See Suspect Diagnosis

Alternative Name
See Suspect Diagnosis

Please note:
See SECTION 2 for explanation and interpretation of SIGNS.
See SECTION 4 for explanation and interpretation of TESTS.

Abortion, Recurrent (Miscarriage, Recurrent)

TEST: Any abnormal result in the following tests may
        indicate a possible cause: S.ANA, S.anti-DNA
        antibodies, B.LE cells, S.LH, parental
        karyotype, TFT, GTT, vaginal swab M/C/S,
        hysterosalpingogram.

See also SYMPTOMS SECTION 1: Abortion, Recurrent

Abscess

TEST: Choose antibiotic or antifungal on result of pus
        M/C/S or abscess wall biopsy and culture. Other
        tests to be considered include FBC, ESR, CRP,
        amoebic antibodies
SIGN: Fluctuant mass
DD: Bacterial, fungal, helminthic or amoebic causes;
        cyst, hernia

Achilles Tendon Rupture

SIGN: Calf squeeze test.
DD: Tendon avulsion, sprain.

Acquired Immune Deficiency Syndrome [AIDS]

TEST: **GROUP I (Acute infection):**
        S.HIV-3 (HTLV-3) antibodies (+), S.p24 antigen
        (+), S.p24 antibody (–), Hb (N), ESR (H or N),
        B.lymphocytes (H), B.neutrophils (N), platelets
        (N), S.immunoglobulins (N), S.complement (N
        or H).
        GROUP II (Asymptomatic):
        S.HIV-3 (HTLV-3) antibodies (+), S.p24 antigen
        (–), S.p24 antibody (+), Hb (N), ESR (N),
        B.lymphocytes (N), B.neutrophils (N), platelets
        (N), S.immunoglobulins (H), S.complement (H).
        **GROUP III (Persistent generalised
        lymphadenopathy):**
        S.HIV-3 (HTLV-3) antibodies (+), S.p24 antigen
        (–), S.p24 antibody (+), Hb (N), ESR (N),
        B.lymphocytes (N), B.neutrophils (N), platelets
        (N), S.immunoglobulins (H), S.complement (H).
        GROUP IV (AIDS related complex):
        S.HIV-3 (HTLV-3) antibodies (+), S.p24 antigen
        (+), S.p24 antibody (+), lymphocyte CD4 (L), Hb
        (L), ESR (H), B.lymphocytes (L), B.neutrophils
        (L), platelets (L), S.immunoglobulins (H),
        S.complement (H).
        GROUP V (AIDS):
        S.HIV-3 (HTLV-3) antibodies (+), S.p24 antigen
        (+), S.p24 antibody (–), lymphocyte CD4 (L), Hb
        (VL), ESR (VH), B.lymphocytes (VL),
        B.neutrophils (VL), platelets (VL),
        S.immunoglobulins (H), S.complement (VH).
SIGN: Fever, skin nodules, adenitis, splenomegaly,
        oral candidiasis, hairy leukoplakia, sarcomas,
        absent reflexes.
DD: Idiopathic lymphadenopathy syn., viraemia,
        fungaemia, metastatic carcinoma, other causes
        of reduced immunity (see separate entry).
PHYS: Caused by human immunodeficiency virus
        (HIV). Transmitted by blood and semen. Occurs

mainly in homosexuals, IV drug users and blood
product recipients. Eventual mortality close to
100% but may be kept in early stages for
prolonged period by appropriate medication

Acromegaly

TEST: S. growth hormone (H, remains H with GTT),
        S.IGF-1 (H), thyrotrophin releasing hormone
        test (AB), GTT (H), S.phosphorus (H or N).
DD: Gigantism, hypothyroidism, phenytoin therapy.
PHYS: Due to excessive secretion of growth hormone
        by an adenoma of the pituitary.

Actinomycosis (Lumpy Jaw)

TEST: Pus culture (+ for *A.israeli*), lesion biopsy (+),
        sputum culture (+ or N), pus microscopy ('sulphur
        granules' seen), ESR (H), WCC (H), Hb (L).
SIGN: Hepatomegaly, cachexia (abdominal).
DD: Cellulitis, bacterial abscess, TB, malignancies.
PHYS: Due to infection of jaw (often via decayed teeth)
        or other areas by *Actinomycetes israeli*, which is
        an anaerobic bacterium.

Acute Leukaemia

See Leukaemia, Acute

Addiction

See Alcoholism; Narcotic Addiction

Addison's Disease
(Chronic Hypoadrenocorticism)

TEST: P.cortisol (fails to increase after IM or IV ACTH –
        synacthen test), S.ACTH (H), S.sodium (L),
        S.potassium (H), S.adrenal cell antibodies (+),
        S.HLA-DR3 (+), BUN(H), B.neutrophils (H),
        B.lymphocytes (H), haematocrit (H), B.glucose
        (L).
SIGN: Cachexia, hypotension, nail discoloration,
        pigmentation, Rogoff's sign, alopecia (groin and
        axilla), Thorn's sign.
DD: Haemochromatosis, porphyria, thyrotoxicosis,
        anorexia nervosa, malnutrition, malignancy,
        renal disease, malabsorption, anaemia,
        postural hypotension, anxiety, stress, hepatic
        cirrhosis, myasthenia gravis, polyglandular
        autoimmune syn.
PHYS: A deficiency in cortisol and/or aldosterone
        production by the adrenal cortex.

Adenitis (Swollen and Inflamed Lymph Nodes)

TEST: WCC (AB), ESR (H), specific viral serology (N or
        AB), chest X-ray (N or AB), lymph node biopsy
        (AB).
DD: Viral, bacterial or fungal disease of affected
        region, infectious mononucleosis, carcinoma,
        leukaemia, brucellosis, toxoplasmosis,
        encephalitis, otitis, conjunctivitis, pharyngitis,

measles, mumps, rubella, hepatitis, sarcoidosis, STDs, TB, Hodgkin's disease, reaction to foreign body, cytomegalovirus infection, allergic reaction, mesenteric adenitis, sialadenitis.

PHYS: Lymph nodes in many areas of the body may become enlarged and inflamed from a vast range of illnesses that may affect anatomical areas significantly removed from the swollen glands.

Adrenal Hyperplasia
See Cushing's Syndrome

Adrenal Insufficiency
See Addison's Disease

AIDS
See Acquired Immune Deficiency Syndrome

Alcoholism
TEST: S.ethanol (H or N), B. carbohydrate-deficient transferrin, S.glucose (L), U.glucose (+), LFT (AB), S.GGT (H), MCV (H), S.platelets (N or L), prothrombin time (N or H), S.AST (H), S.urate (H), S.triglycerides (H).
SIGN: Nystagmus, postural tremor, biceps jerk and other reflexes.
DD: Drug intoxication or overdose, cerebral injury, CVA, diabetic coma, psychiatric disorders.
PHYS: Habitual excessive alcohol intake causes liver damage and inability to mobilise glucose from storage.

Aldosteronism
See Conn Syndrome

Alkaptonuria
TEST: U. Homogentisic acid (+)
SIGN: Urine that darkens on standing
DD: Rheumatoid arthritis, ankylosing spondylitis, other causes of pigmented skin (see SYMPTOMS SECTION 1: Pigmentation of Skin, Excess
PHYS: Rare inherited disorder of tyrosine metabolism causing arthritis and pigmentation

Allergic Rhinitis (Hay Fever)
TEST: RAST test for specific allergen Igs (+), nasal mucus microscopy (eosinophils present), skin tests for common allergens (+), B.eosinophils (H), S.IgE (H).
DD: Polycythaemia rubra vera, coryza, vasomotor rhinitis, noxious fumes, viral and bacterial infections.

PHYS: Wind borne pollens contacting the nasal mucosa release proteins that act as allergens, causing the release of histamine and hypersecretion by the nasal mucosa of thin watery mucus.

Allergy
TEST: RAST (+), S.IgE (H), intradermal skin test (+), S.tryptase (H in anaphylaxis), S.Complement (H in anaphylaxis).
SIGN: Dermographia, geographic tongue.
PHYS: Allergy reactions may present in any major system depending on allergen and site of entry. Clinical diagnosis is more important than tests. Diseases with an allergy component include asthma, bronchitis, coryza, colitis, dermatitis, eczema, hay fever, cluster headaches, migraine, diarrhoea, etc.

Alveolitis
See Cryptogenic Fibrosing Alveolitis

Alzheimer's Disease
TEST: No specific diagnostic test. Tests to exclude other causes of dementia (eg. hypothyroidism) should be performed
DD: Cerebrovascular insufficiency, depression, Parkinson's disease, alcoholism, mental retardation, encephalopathy, Creutzfeldt-Jakob disease, hydrocephalus, social isolation, medications (eg. sedatives).
PHYS: Clinical diagnostic criteria are:
• Multiple cognitive deficits manifested by both
  − memory impairment
  − one or more of aphasia, apraxia, agnosia, or failure of planning or organising
• Other causes of dementia excluded
• Gradual onset and continuing decline
• Decline from previous level of social function

Amenorrhoea, Secondary
TEST: S.FSH, S.prolactin, S.progesterone, P.oestradiol, S.LH, TFT, x-ray of sella turcica. For interpretation, see PATHOLOGY SECTION 4.
DD: Pregnancy, present or recent past use of the oral contraceptive pill, ectopic pregnancy, choriocarcinoma, obesity, rapid weight loss, anorexia nervosa, strenuous exercise, prolactin secreting tumour, pituitary tumour, polycystic ovary syn., premature menopause, virilising tumours, Asherman syn., adrenal tumours, hypothroidism, thyrotoxicosis, debilitating disease.
PHYS: It is essential to determine cause of amenorrhoea in all cases as some tumours may be difficult to detect, but relatively easy to treat.

Hormonal Changes in Menstruating Women

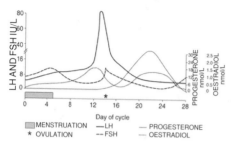

MENSTRUATION   —LH   — PROGESTERONE
* OVULATION   --FSH   — OESTRADIOL

Amoebiasis

TEST: Faeces M/C/S (+ *Entamoeba histolytica*), colonic biopsy (+), specific antimicrobial antibodies (+).

SIGN: Diarrhoea, fever, abdominal tenderness, abdominal rebound.

DD: Ulcerative colitis, diverticulitis, bacterial dysentery, gastroenteritis, Crohn's disease, carcinoma.

PHYS: Infection of bowel by *E. histolytica*.

Amyloidosis

TEST: S.amyloid protein scintigraphy (+), organ biopsy (+), Congo red test (60%+ loss of dye from serum in 1 hour), ESR (H), CRP (H), abnormal tests of involved organ function.

SIGN: Hepatomegaly, splenomegaly, bilateral black eyes.

DD: Multiple myeloma, familial Mediterranean fever, chronic infection, specific diseases of involved organs

PHYS: An abnormal glycoprotein (with an affinity for Congo red dye) accumulates in one or more major organs.

Anaemia

TEST: Hb (L), RBC (L or hypochromic or AB), MCV (L-microcytic anaemias, H-macrocytic anaemias), MCHC (L or N), MCH (L-hypochromic, H-macrocytic), WCC (N or AB), platelets (N or AB), Heinz bodies (+ or –)

SIGN: Bounding pulse, diastolic murmur, hepatomegaly, koilonychia (iron deficiency), retinal haemorrhages (pernicious and aplastic), splenomegaly (haemolytic), systolic murmur (severe), water-hammer pulse (severe).

DD: Symptoms of various anaemias differ, but include lethargy, vertigo, headache, malaise, fever, CCF and jaundice. DD includes any disease that may cause these symptoms.

PHYS: Anaemia may be due to excess blood loss, deficient RBC production, iron deficit, vit.B$_{12}$ deficiency, bone marrow failure, haemolysis of RBC, chronic disease, neoplasia, hepatic and renal disease. It is vital to determine the cause of any anaemia.

See also specific anaemia types below.

Anaemia, Acute Haemolytic

TEST: Hb (L), RBC (normocytic, normochromic), RCC (L), WCC (VH), platelets (H), B.reticulocytes (H), marrow biopsy (hyperplastic), U.Hb (+), U.urobilinogen (+), S.G6PD (L), HbS (+ or –).

DD: Acute infection, all causes of acute abdomen, blood loss.

PHYS: Induced by drugs, infection, cancer, malaria or unknown causes.

Anaemia, Aplastic

TEST: Hb (L), RCC (L), B.reticulocytes (L), WCC (L), platelets (L), S.bilirubin (L), bone marrow biopsy (fatty).

DD: Hypersplenism, myelofibrosis, leukaemia, Hodgkin's disease, lymphomas, other anaemias.

PHYS: Aetiology often unknown, but may be due to drugs, toxins or radiation. Depression of blood cell production occurs.

Anaemia, Iron Deficiency

TEST: Hb (L), RCC (L or N, microcytic, hypochromic), B.reticulocytes (H), platelets (H or N), WCC (N), S.iron (L), iron binding capacity (H), marrow stain for haemosiderin (–), S.ferritin (L).

Sign: Brittle nails, onycholysis

DD: Thalassaemia minor, anaemia of infection, haemoglobinopathies, other anaemias.

PHYS: Due to blood loss, pregnancy, haemosiderosis or malnutrition.

Anaemia, Pernicious (Megaloblastic Anaemia)

TEST: Schilling test (AB), S.vit.B$_{12}$ (L), B.intrinsic factor autoantibodies (+), Hb (L), WCC (L), platelets (L), bone marrow biopsy (megaloblastic), S.folic acid (L or N), S.bilirubin (N or H), S.LDH (H), LFT (AB), gastric pH (H), S.parietal cell antibodies (+).

DD: Folic acid deficit, other anaemias, hepatic disease

PHYS: There are causes of megaloblastic anaemia other than pernicious anaemia. Due to lack of intrinsic factor in the stomach and subsequent failure of vit. B$_{12}$ absorption

Anaphylaxis

See Allergy

Aneurysm, Aortic

TEST: Chest or abdominal x-ray, chest or abdominal CT, abdominal ultrasound.

SIGN: Aortic regurgitation, pericardial friction rub, pleural effusion, loss of peripheral pulse.

DD: Myocardial infarct, pulmonary embolism,

pericarditis, oesophageal pain, musculoskeletal pain, any cause of abdominal pain (see SYMPTOMS SECTION 1).

ngina Pectoris (Coronary Artery Disease)

EST: ECG (N or AB), exercise ECG (AB), coronary angiography (AB), coronary artery calcification on CT scan (+), pO_2 (L), S.cholesterol (N or H), S.triglycerides (N or H), Hb (L or N), S.glucose (N or L), Holter monitor (AB), coronary angiography (AB).

D: Myocardial infarct, hiatus hernia, gastritis, peptic ulcer, oesophagitis, biliary disease, pleurisy, myositis, pericarditis, Tietze syn., vertebral disease.

HYS: Narrowed or diseased coronary arteries prevent sufficient blood, and thus oxygen, reaching the heart muscles.

ee also Myocardial Infarct

ngina, Vincent's

ee Vincent's Angina

nkylosing Spondylitis

EST: HLA-B27 (+), ESR (H), rheumatoid factor (–, occ. +) Hb (L), WCC (AB), S.IgA (H), S.CK (H), vertebral x-ray (AB).

GN: Cervical fleche, Gaenslen's sign, Schober's test.

D: Osteoarthritis, rheumatoid arthritis, Pott's disease, degenerative disc disease, spinal tumours, osteoporosis, psoriatic arthritis, brucellosis, fluoride poisoning.

HYS: Chronic inflammatory condition of the axial skeletal joints that causes progressive stiffening of the spine and pain.

norexia Nervosa and Bulimia Nervosa

EST: None diagnostic. Screening tests to exclude other pathology or complicaitons may include FBC, LFT, S.electrolytes, S.creatinine and ECG

GN: Amenorrhoea, cachexia, muscular wasting, pitting oedema

D: Other psychiatric disturbances, malnutrition, AIDS, Addison's disease, malignancy, hypopituitarism

HYS: Bulimia nervosa is a milder form. Affects up to 2% of caucasian females. Diagnostic criteria for anorexia nervosa are:
– Refusal to maintain minimal bodyweight
– intense fear of gaining weight
– Body image distortion
– Amenorrhoea

ntenatal Care

e Pregnancy, Antenatal Care

Anthrax

TEST: Lesion and sputum gram stain (+), lesion and sputum culture (+), S.antibodies (+), B.cultures (+), WCC (AB).

DD: Pneumonias, CCF, carcinoma of lung, meningitis, influenza, furunculosis, erysipelas, orf, glanders, tularaemia.

PHYS: Highly infectious disease of sheep, goats, cattle and horses caused by *Bacillus anthracis* that is transmissible to man.

Aortic Valve Disease

TEST: Echocardiography (AB).

SIGN: INCOMPETENCE - Apex beat displacement, Corrigan's sign, diastolic murmur, water-hammer pulse, Austin-Flint murmur.
STENOSIS - Apex beat displacement, gallop rhythm, plateau pulse, split heart sounds, systolic murmur, systolic cardiac thrill.

Aplastic Anaemia

See Anaemia, Aplastic

Appendicitis

TEST: WCC (H), urine M/C/S (–), B.neutrophils (H).

SIGN: Abdominal rigidity, abdominal mass, abdominal rebound tenderness.

DD: Gastroenteritis, mesenteric adenitis, peritonitis, pneumonia, ectopic pregnancy, salpingitis, torsion of ovarian cyst, cholecystitis, diverticulitis, Meckel's diverticulitis, pyelonephritis, ureteric colic, ovarian follicle rupture, carcinoma of colon.

PHYS: Inflammation of the vermiform appendix, often due to obstruction by a faecalith.

Arrythmias, Cardiac

TEST: ECG (AB). To exclude cardiac pathology, the following tests may be ordered: AST, LDH, CPK, aldolase. For interpretation see PATHOLOGY SECTION 4 .

SIGN: Atrial fibrillation, apex beat, extrasystolic beats, tachycardia, bradycardia, gallop rhythm, dicrotic pulse.

PHYS: Cause of arrythmia must be determined, and may include myocardial infarct, cardiomyopathy, valvular disease, hyperthyroidism, exercise, alcohol, drugs.

See also SIGNS SECTION 2: Arrhythmias, Cardiac

Arteriosclerosis

See Atherosclerosis

Arthritis

See Arthritis, Septic; Epidemic Polyarthritis; Gout; Osteoarthritis; Pseudogout; Reactive Arthritis; Rheumatoid Arthritis; Rheumatic Fever

Arthritis, Septic

TEST: Synovial fluid culture (+), B.culture (+ or –), WCC (H), synovial WCC (H), synovial sugar (L), rheumatoid factor (+ or –), antinuclear antibodies (–), ultrasound or x-ray.
DD: Rheumatoid arthritis, gout, pseudogout, trauma, osteoarthritis.
PHYS: Often due to *Staphylococcus aureus* or haemolytic streptococci.

Asbestosis

TEST: Chest x-ray (AB), sputum cytology (asbestos bodies +)
DD: Lung cancer, mesothelioma, interstitial lung disease
PHYS: Exposure to asbestos may have been remote in time and minimal

Ascaris

See Roundworms, Intestinal

Ascites

TEST: Paracentesis fluid (AB), serum-ascites albumin gradient (AB)
Sign: Shifting dullness, fluid thrill
DD: See SYMPTOMS SECTIONS 1: Ascites

Aspergillosis

TEST: S.IgE (H), sputum or swab M/C/S (+), biopsy fungal culture (+), specific serological antigen test (+).
DD: Bronchitis, pneumonia, TB, sarcoidosis, empyema, histoplasmosis.
PHYS: Fungal disease that may occur in any aerobic body cavity.

Asthma, Pulmonary

TEST: Respiratory function tests (AB), chest x-ray (AB), sputum microscopy (eosinophils, Curschmann spirals), WCC (eosinophilia), allergen sensitivity testing (AB), B.pO$_2$ (L or N), B.pCO$_2$ (H or N), B.pH (AB), S.IgE (H).
SIGN: Barrel chest, Harrison's sulcus, rhonchi, hypoventilation.
DD: CCF, obstructive emphysema, lung carcinoma, pulmonary embolism, TB, bronchitis, Mycoplasma pneumonia.
PHYS: Obstruction of air outflow in smaller bronchi due to tenacious mucus and bronchial wall thickening. May be allergic, infective, emotional or exertional in origin.

See also Allergy

Atherosclerosis (Arteriosclerosis)

TEST: S.cholesterol (H or N), S.homocysteine (H), arteriography (AB).
SIGN: Retinal arteriovenous nipping, parkinsonian facies, ear lobe crease, Osler's manoeuvre premature arcus senilis.
DD: May be cause of stenosis, thrombosis or aneurysm in any limb or organ (eg. angina pectoris, myocardial infarct, stroke).
PHYS: Thickening of the arterial intima due to localised accumulations of lipids in the form of atheromatous plaques.

Atopic Dermatitis

See Eczema

Bacillary Dysentery

See Shigellosis

Back Pain

TEST: X-ray (N or AB), myelogram (N or AB), CT (N or AB) MRI (N or AB).
SIGN: Lasegue's sign, Patrick's sign, Trendelenburg test, Ely's sign, Burn's test.
DD: See SYMPTOMS SECTION 1: Back Pain.

Bacterial Endocarditis

See Endocarditis, Bacterial, Subacute

Barmah Forest Virus

TEST: S. specific IgM serology (+).
DD: Ross River fever (epidemic polymyalgia), dengue fever.
PHYS: Arbovirus infection spread by mosquito bite.

Bell's Palsy

TEST: None significant.
DD: Carotid body tumour, cholesteatoma, Ramsay Hunt syn., acoustic neuroma, CVA.
PHYS: Due to spontaneous inflammation of the facial nerve at the level of the stylomastoid foramen.

Beriberi

TEST: S. and U.thiamine (L), S.pyruvic acid (H after exercise glucose stress).
SIGN: Pitting oedema, knee jerk, ankle jerk.
DD: Wernicke syndrome, CCF, deep vein thrombosis of calf, diabetic polyneuropathy.
PHYS: A deficiency in thiamine and consequently of coenzyme cocarboxylase results in degeneration of the medullary sheath around distal nerves. Other lesions may appear in the brain and heart.

Bilharzia (Schistosomiasis)

TEST: Faeces and urine microscopy (eggs seen), rectal or bladder biopsy (+), skin sensitivity testing (+), WCC (eosinophilia), specific serology (+).
SIGN: Hepatomegaly, splenomegaly, ascites, rash.

D: Urticaria, cystitis, gastroenteritis, cirrhosis, amoebiasis.
HYS: Infection of the bladder, intestine and other ogans by the parasitic fluke, Schistosoma.

Black Death
See Plague, Bubonic

Blackwater Fever
TEST: U.Hb (+), Hb (L), B.smear (+), WCC (lymphocytes and monocytes H), BUN (H).
DD: Bilharzia, bladder carcinoma, cystitis, pyelonephritis.
PHYS: Form of malaria in which there is intravascular haemolysis and haemoglobinuria due to chronic infection with Plasmodium falciparum.

Blastomycosis
TEST: Sputum microscopy (+), skin biopsy (+), pus M/C/S (+), specific complement fixation test (+), WCC (H), Hb (L), ESR (H).
DD: TB, lung carcinoma, actinomycosis, aspiration pneumonia, histoplasmosis.
PHYS: Fungal infection of skin, lung and viscera caused by Blastomyces dermatitidis.

Bleeding Disorders
See Bruising, Excessive

Bone Cancer
TEST: S.ALP(H), ESR (H or N), U.cross-linked N-telopeptides (H). X-ray (AB), bone scan (AB).
SIGN: Fracture with minimal trauma, bone pain, bone swelling.
DD: Osteosarcoma, metastatic cancer, bone cyst, osteomyelitis.
PHYS: Many different types of bone cancer known. Metastatic most common. Others include osteosarcoma, Ewing's sarcoma, fibrosarcomas, osteoclastomas, etc.

Bornholm Disease
See Pleurodynia

Botulism
TEST: S. or faecal botulinum toxin assay (+), faeces culture (+ C. botulinum)
DD: Other forms of food poisoning
PHYS: Caused by Clostridium botulinum from preserved food

Brain
See Cerebellar Lesions; Cerebral Lesions; Infarct, Cerebral; Transient Ischaemic Attack

Breast Cancer
TEST: Biopsy or excision cytology (+), S.CA 15–3 (H), S.CA 549 (H), S.CEA (AB), nipple exudate cytology (+ or –), mamography (+ or –), ESR (H), S.calcium (H with bone metastases), S.ALP (H with liver metastases).
DD: Fibroadenoma, cysts, mastitis, Paget's disease of nipple.
PHYS: Commonest female cancer. Metastasises early. Diagnosis is surgical.

Bronchial Carcinoma
See Lung Cancer

Bronchiectasis
TEST: Sputum culture (+ or –), sputum blood (+), sputum microscopy (pus and plugs), Hb (L), WCC (H).
SIGN: Cavernous breathing, clubbing of fingers, crepitations, hypoventilation, yellow nail syn.
DD: Bronchitis, pneumonia, lung cancer, amyloidosis, TB.
PHYS: Irreversible dilation of the bronchial tree which may be patchy, or throughout the lung. Secondary infection and mucopurulent sputum almost invariably occur.

Bronchiolitis
TEST: Nasal or pharyngeal swab viral M/C/S (+), chest x-ray (N)
DD: Asthma, bronchitis, pneumonia
PHYS: Infection of infants caused by respiratory syncitial virus. Primarily a clinical diagnosis

Bronchitis, Acute
TEST: Sputum M/C/S (+ or –), FBC (AB), chest x-ray (AB).
DD: Pneumonia, TB, bronchiectasis, bronchiolitis.
PHYS: Often viral.

Bronchitis, Chronic (Chronic Obstructive Airways Disease)
TEST: Sputum M/C/S (+ with exacerbations), WCC (H), spirometry (AB), chest x-ray (AB).
SIGN: Blue bloater, clubbing of fingers, cor pulmonale, whispering pectoriloquy, pink puffer, Schamroth's sign.
DD: Pneumonia, TB, bronchiectasis, bronchial carcinoma, emphysema, asthma, cystic fibrosis, airway obstruction, aspergillosis.
PHYS: Cigarette smoking most common cause.

See also Emphysema

Brucellosis (Undulant Fever)
TEST: Specific agglutination test (RT), CSF or B.culture (+), WCC (L or N), B. lymphocytes (H), ESR (H), LFT (AB), S.complement fixation test

DD: (RT), antihuman globulin test (RT), Hb (L).
Influenza, URTI, coryza, typhoid fever, infectious mononucleosis, other viral infections, TB, Q fever, SLE, tularemia, malaria, histoplasmosis, blastomycosis, protozoal infections.

PHYS: Infection of humans by animals (usually cattle), with Brucella organisms. Causes bacteremia with fever, malaise and nasopharyngeal symptoms. May become chronic. Incubation period 1-3 weeks.

Bruising, Excessive

TEST: Screening tests include: Bleeding time, fibrinogen, APTT, prothrombin time, thrombin clotting time, platelet count, FBC. Further detailed investigations may include full blood count, vit. K assay,LFT, individual factor assays (eg. factors I, II, VII, IX, X), fibrin degradation products [D-dimer].

DD: Physiological, vascular defects, psychogenic, hormonal, haemophilia, Christmas disease, other rare hereditary disorders, thrombocytopenia, cirrhosis, vit. K deficiency, malnutrition, renal failure, disseminated intravascular coagulation, multiple myeloma, renal failure, SLE, aspirin, anticoagulants.

PHYS: Any interference with the complex clotting factors and the involved factors and cells may lead to excessive bruising.

Bubonic Plague
See Plague, Bubonic

Buerger's Disease (Thromboangiitis Obliterans)

TEST: None diagnostic. S.IgA (H).
DD: Arterial insufficiency, diabetes, superficial phlebitis, atherosclerosis, frostbite, Raynaud's disease.
PHYS: Segmental phlebitis of peripheral blood vessels leading to their occlusion. Aggravated by smoking.

Bulimia Nervosa
See Anorexia Nervosa and Bulimia Nervosa

Calculi, Renal
See Nephrolithiasis

Cancer (Carcinoma)

TEST: No test to diagnose or exclude all cancer available, but the following may be used in appropriate circumstances: biopsy or swab microscopy, FBC, Hb, S.Ca, CEA, ESR,CRP, ferritin, iron saturation, carbohydrate antigen, lymphocyte CD16.
SIGN: Abdominal mass, cachexia, clubbing fingers, coffee grounds vomitus, Courvoisier's law, Foster-Kennedy sign, hepatomegaly, Leser-

Trelat sign, Pel-Ebstein phenomenon, pelvic mass, prostatomegaly, Schiller Test, Sister MaryJoseph's nodule, splenomegaly.
Phys: Carbohydrate antigens (CA) cannot be used for diagnosis, only monitoring progress of cancer

See also Bone Cancer, Breast Cancer, Colorectal Carcinoma; Hepatic Metastases; Lung Cancer, Stomach Carcinoma; Testicular Cancer; Thyroid Carcinoma

Candidiasis (Thrush) (Moniliasis)

TEST: Skin scraping, vaginal or mouth swab M/C/S (+), blood culture (+ in fungaemia), B.glucose (H or N, candidiasis common with diabetes).
DD: Mouth – milk plaques, stomatitis.
Skin – eczema, psoriasis.
Vagina – leukorrhoea, trichomoniasis, gonorrhoea, mixed bacterial infections.
PHYS: *Candida albicans* is a normal resident of mucous membranes, but may overgrow with antibiotic or steroid therapy, malaise, pregnancy, or hypoparathyroidism. May infect vagina, mouth, skin or nails.

Carcinoid Syndrome

TEST: U.5HIAA (H), platelet serotonin (H), provocative IV adrenalin test (+).
SIGN: Hypotension, oedema of head and neck, diastolic murmur, systolic murmur, spider naevi
DD: Asthma, thyrotoxicosis, other causes of acute abdomen (see Abdominal Pain in SYMPTOMS SECTION 1), cardiac failure, septicaemia.
PHYS: Argentaffine cell tumours secrete vasoactive agents that can cause a wide variety of vascular symptoms

See also SYNDROMES SECTION 6: Carcinoid Syndrome

Carcinoma
See Cancer

Cardiac Failure

TEST: Chest x-ray (AB), ECG (N or AB)
SIGN: Bradycardia (congestive), atrial fibrillation, cachexia, Cheyne-Stokes respiration, clubbing of fingers (chronic), extrasystolic beats, gallop rhythm (left ventricle failure), hepatomegaly (congestive), hypotension, jugular venous pressure raised (congestive), pitting oedema (congestive), pleural effusion, pulsus alterans (left ventricle failure), shifting dullness (ascites), splenomegaly (congestive), split heart sounds (left ventricle failure), tachycardia, fluid thrills (ascites).
DD: Pericardial effusion, constrictive pericarditis, pulmonary disease, asthma, chronic bronchitis, emphysema, cirrhosis, carcinoma of lung, nephritis, nephrotic syn., pulmonary emboli, severe anaemia, vena caval obstruction, mediastinal tumour.

PHYS: Due to failure of pump action of heart from coronary artery disease, myocarditis, cardiomyopathies, hypertension, valvular disease, anaemia, thyrotoxicosis or arteriovenous shunts.

Cardiac Ischaemia
TEST: Hb (– or N), ECG (N or AB).
SIGN: Hypertension, signs of peripheral vascular disease, cardiac failure.
DD: Cardiac failure, myocardial infarct, aortic aneurysm, pericarditis, pulmonary embolism, oesophageal pain, musculoskeletal pain.

Carotenaemia (Hypervitaminosis A)
TEST: S.vit.A (H), S.bilirubin (N).
DD: Jaundice due to hepatitis or other liver disease.
PHYS: Caused by excessive ingestion of carotene containing foods (eg. carrots, paw paw, pumpkin, etc). Conjunctivae are not yellow; in jaundice, they are.

Carpal Tunnel Syndrome
SIGN: Claw hand, Tinel's sign, Phalen's sign, flaccid paralysis of hand.
DD: Compression of median nerve in arm, other cervical and brachial plexus nerve lesions, fractured scaphoid.
PHYS: Due to compression of median nerve in the carpal tunnel of the wrist.

Cat-Scratch Disease
TEST: Lymph node histology (AB, acid fast bacilli), specific serum antibody test (+), specific intradermal skin test (+), WCC (N or H), ESR (H).
DD: TB, bacterial adenitis, Hodgkin's disease, tularaemia, toxoplasmosis.
PHYS: May occur without association with cats. Often due to Bartonella henselae.

Cellulitis
TEST: Lesion swab M/C/S (+), S.ASOT (+ if caused by Streptococcus), blood culture (+ or N)
DD: Erysipelas, abscess, dermatitis, eczema, venous thrombus

Cerebellar Lesions
SIGN: Ataxia, dysdiadochokinesia, heel-knee test, hypotonia, knee jerk and other reflexes, nose-finger test, opisthotonus, scanning speech, intention tremor, postural tremor.
PHYS: Cerebellum responsible for muscular coordination.

Cerebral Lesions
SIGN: Athetosis, Brudzinski's sign, choreiform movements, cogwheel rigidity, grasp reflex, jaw jerk, Kernig's sign, Kussmaul's breathing, Moro reflex, mydriasis (midbrain), miosis (pontine), neck stiffness, nystagmus (brain stem), papilloedema, pharyngeal reflex (9th cranial nerve), retinal exudates, scissor gait, slurred speech (bulbar).

Cerebral Thrombosis
See Infarct, Cerebral

Cerebral Trauma
See Head Injury

Cerebrovascular Accident [CVA]
See Infarct, Cerebral; Transient Ischaemic Attack

Cestodes
See Tapeworms

Chagas' Disease
TEST: B.microscopy (fresh, stained and centrifuged) (+), lymph node biopsy (+), specific serological test (+).
SIGN: Romana's sign.
DD: Cretinism hypothyroidism, myositis, trichinosis, meningitis, CCF.
PHYS: Due to systemic infection by Trypanosoma cruzi.

Chancroid
TEST: Lesion smear and culture for Haemophilus ducreyi (+), specific skin test (+ for life).
DD: Syphilis, gonorrhoea, impetigo, lympho-granuloma venereum, other pyogenic lesions.
PHYS: Genital lesions degenerate to ragged, undermined, painful ulcers 2-14 days after contact. Adenitis common.

Chickenpox (Varicella, Herpes Zoster)
TEST: Virus isolation from lesions (+), sputum or vesicular lesion microscopy (multinucleated giant cells), WCC (N or L).
DD: Smallpox, vaccinia, Herpes simplex, rickettsioses, shingles.
PHYS: Herpes zoster infection.

Chlamydial Infection
TEST: Specific urine or swab PCR test (+), specific urine or swab LCR test (+)
PHYS: Chlamydia trachomatis responsible. false negative test results common.

See also Lymphogranuloma Venereum

Cholecystitis
TEST: WCC (H), S.bilirubin (N or H), ALP (H), BSP (H),

AST (N or H), ALT (N OR H), S.amylase (H), B.culture (N or +), ultrasound (AB), cholangiogram (AB).

SIGN: Murphy's sign, jaundice, abdominal rebound tenderness.

DD: Myocardial infarct, peptic ulcer, pancreatitis, pneumonia, appendicitis, intestinal obstruction, pyelonephritis, hepatitis, intestinal cancer, pleurisy.

PHYS: 90% associated with gall stone in cystic duct. Bacterial infection possible.

Cholelithiasis (Gall stones)

TEST: WCC (H), S.bilirubin (H or N), ALP (VH), AST (H), ALT (H), S.amylase (N or H), BSP (H), S.GGT (H).

SIGN: Abdominal mass, Murphy's law.

DD: Hepatitis, hepatic malignancy, pancreatic carcinoma.

PHYS: Gall stones may pass asymptomatically. Only impacted stones cause symptoms and exert back pressure on the liver. They may cause minor trauma to the pancreas when low in the common bile duct.

Cholera

TEST: Faeces M/C/S (+), faeces specific antigen (+), S.electrolytes (AB), renal function tests (AB)

SIGN: Dehydration

DD: Other bacterial enteritis, viral enteritis, ulcerative colitis

Chondrocalcinosis

See Pseudogout

Choriocarcinoma

TEST: B.HCG (VH), S.placental lactogen (H), ultrasound (AB).

SIGN: Abnormal uterine bleeding.

DD: Hydatidiform mole, abortion, ectopic pregnancy.

PHYS: Usually follows a hydatidiform mole. Very rare.

Christmas Disease (Factor IX Deficit)

TEST: Clotting time (H), prothrombin consumption test (AB), thrombin time (N), partial thromboplastin time (H), bleeding time (N or H), prothrombin time (N).

DD: Other hereditary coagulation disorders, anticoagulant therapy.

PHYS: An hereditary lack of factor IX in the intrinsic blood clotting pathway.

See also Haemophilia A; von Willebrand's disease

Chronic Bronchitis

See Bronchitis, Chronic

Chronic Fatigue Syndrome

TEST: No specific diagnostic test available. FBC, ESR, CRP, LFT, S.creatinine, TFT and other tests considered justified by the physician to exclude any other cause of the symptoms should be performed

DD: See SYMPTOMS SECTION 1: Fatigue, Abnormal

See also SYNDROMES SECTION 6

Chronic Obstructive Airways Disease

See Bronchitis, Chronic

Ciguatera Poisoning

TEST: Detection of ciguatera toxin in suspect fish. No diagnostic tests available on patient

SIGN: Paraesthesia, lip numbness

DD: Other fish toxins; other causes of nausea, vomiting, diarrhoea and paraesthesia (See SYMPTOMS SECTION 1)

PHYS: Toxin found in larger reef fish, particularly the offal and nearby flesh

Cirrhosis, Hepatic

TEST: S.ALT (H), S.AST (H), S.ALP (H), S.bilirubin (H), U.bilirubin (H), S.albumin (L), S.GGT (H), WCC (L), Hb (L), S.gamma-globulin (H), S.IgG (H), S.IgM (H), S.sodium (L), S.cholesterol (H), prothrombin time (H), S.antimitochondrial antibodies (H), S.copper (H), ultrasound (AB), CT (AB), liver biopsy (AB).

SIGN: Cachexia, chloasma, clubbing of fingers, coffee grounds vomitus, hepatomegaly, pitting oedema, pleural effusion, shifting dullness (ascites), spider naevi, splenomegaly, fluid thrill (ascites), xanthelasma, xanthomatosis.

DD: Biliary tract obstruction by stone or neoplasm, hepatitis, haemochromatosis hepatoma, CCF, hepatic abscess, TB, lymphoma, metastatic carcinoma.

PHYS: The liver responds to chronic and recurrent abuse by fibrosing and scarring. Portal (Laennec's) and postnecrotic are the common forms of cirrhosis. Biopsy is the only definitive test.

Clostridial Myositis

See Gangrene, Gas

Coagulation Disorders

TEST: Hb, platelets, WCC, haematocrit, bleeding time, prothrombin time, platelet aggregation, APTT, fibrinogen, thrombin clotting time, factors.

PHYS: See PATHOLOGY SECTION 4 for interpretation.

See also Christmas Disease; Haemophilia

Coccidiomycosis

TEST: M/C/S of sputum, CSF, urine, cyst fluid, synovial fluid or biopsy specimen (+), specific serum complement fixation test (+), specific skin test (+ long term), chest x-ray (AB), ESR (H), CRP (H)
DD: Bacterial pneumonia, lung cancer, lymphomas
PHYS: Caused by the fungus *Coccidioides immitis*. Lungs usual primary site

Coeliac Disease (Non-tropical Sprue)

TEST: Faecal fat (+), S.endomysial antibodies (+), S.gliaden antibodies (H), S.fasting folate (L), small bowel biopsy (AB), S.albumin (L), S.cholesterol (L), HLA-B (+), HLA-DR3 (+), S.IgA (H or N), xylose absorption test (+), S.calcium (L), S.carotene (L), S.reticular cell antibodies (+), Hb (L), S.iron (L).
DD: Cystic fibrosis, Whipple's disease, disaccharide deficiency, other malabsorption syndromes.
PHYS: An intolerance to gluten in wheat and rye causes small intestinal changes that impair absorption from the gut.

Colic, Ureteric

See Nephrolithiasis

Colitis, Ulcerative

See Ulcerative Colitis

Colorectal Carcinoma

TEST: Lesion biopsy (+), S.CA 19-9 (H), S.CA 50 (H), S.CEA (H), faecal occult blood (+ or –), Hb (L or N), ESR (H or N), LFT (AB if metastases).
DD: Diverticulitis, ulcerative colitis, irritable bowel syn., polyposis coli, colonic torsion.
PHYS: Very common carcinoma. Presents with changed bowel habits, abdominal pain, melaena and anaemia.

Conjunctivitis, Infective

TEST: Swab M/C/S for bacteria, chlamydia and virus (+)
DD: Foreign body, chemical irritation, allergy, glaucoma, entropion

See also SYMPTOMS SECTION 1: Eye, Inflamed or Red

Conn Syndrome (Primary Hyperaldosteronism; Aldosteronism)

TEST: S.aldosterone (H), U.aldosterone (H), S.potassium (L), U.SG (L), S.sodium (H), S.pH (H), aldosterone/renin ratio (H).
SIGN: Hypertension, flaccid paralysis of legs.
DD: Essential hypertension, renal disease, excess liquorice ingestion.
PHYS: Due to hypersecretion of aldosterone from the adrenal gland, resulting in hypertension and electrolyte imbalances.

Connective Tissue Disease

See CREST Syndrome; Dermatomyosistis; Lupus Erythematosus, Systemic; Polymyositis; Rheumatoid Arthritis; Scleroderma; Sjögren Syndrome

Coronary Artery Disease

See Angina Pectoris

Cor Pulmonale (Pulmonary Hypertension)

TEST: PCV (H), arterial pO_2 (L), arterial pCO_2 (AB), chest X-ray (AB), ECG (large peaked P waves and other abnormalities), echocardiography (AB), nuclear angiocardiography (AB).
SIGN: Blue bloater, tachycardia, warm periphery, dyspnoea, jugular venous pressure, parasternal heave, 4th heart sound, hepatomegaly, diastolic murmur, peripheral oedema.
DD: CCF, ventricular failure, bronchiectasis, asthma, emphysema, lung fibrosis, lung cancer, pulmonary embolism, severe anaemia.
PHYS: Right ventricular dilation secondary to pulmonary hypertension which may be due to many different lung diseases.

CREST Syndrome

TEST: Centromere autoantibodies (+), ESR (H), CRP (H).
DD: Scleroderma, SLE, Sézary syn., carcinoid syn., porphyria cutanea tarda.
PHYS: Autoimmune disease. Form of scleroderma.

See also SYNDROMES SECTION 6: CREST Syndrome

Cretinism

TEST: S.free thyroxine (L), $S.T_4$ (L), S.TSH (H), PBI (L), LDH (H), CPK (H), S.cholesterol (H).
DD: Monogolism, nephritis, nephrosis, pituitary failure.
PHYS: Due to primary hypothyroidism (inadequate production of thyroid hormones) from congenital lack of the thyroid gland or iodine deficiency.

See also Hypothyroidism

Creutzfeldt Jakob Disease [CJD]

TEST: Electron microscopy of brain biopsy (+)
SIGN: Ankle clonus, ataxia
DD: Subacute combined degeneration of cord, multiple sclerosis, Friedreich's ataxia, tabes dorsalis, cerebellar lesions, posterior column lesions, metabolic disorders, alcohol abuse
PHYS: Initially a clinical diagnosis

Crohn's Disease (Regional Enteritis)

TEST: WCC (H), ESR (H), faecal occult blood (+ or –), Hb (N or L), S.albumin (N or L), S.calcium (L), intestinal biopsy history (AB), S.CRP (H).
SIGN: Abdominal mass, abdominal rigidity, abdominal rebound tenderness.

DD: Small bowel obstruction, amyloidosis,
         ulcerative colitis, intestinal carcinoma, sprue,
         appendicitis, lymphomas, TB, acute infectious
         enteritis, diverticulitis.
PHYS: Granulomatous response of the small intestine
         or colon to an unknown agent resulting in ulcer
         and fistula formation in the bowel.

Cryptogenic Fibrosing Alveolitis (Idiopathic Pulmonary Fibrosis)

TEST: ESR (H), Hb (N or L), S.total Ig (H),
         S.rheumatoid factor (+30%), chest x-ray (AB),
         radionuclide scan (AB), pulmonary function
         tests (AB), lung biopsy (AB).
SIGN: Clubbing, Cor pulmonale, cyanosis.
DD: Sarcoidosis, pneumoconiosis, TB, atypical
         pneumonia, haematological malignancy,
         chronic pulmonary hypertension, radiation
         damage.
PHYS: May occur in association with collagen vascular
         disorders. Aetiology unknown.

Cushing Syndrome (Adrenal Hyperplasia)

TEST: P.cortisol (loss of diurnal variation, levels
         generally H), S. and U.17-hydroxy steroids (H),
         S.electrolytes (AB), WCC (H), B.eosinphils (L),
         B.lymphocytes (L), B.neutrophils (H), U.glucose
         (+), GTT (AB).
SIGN: Exophthalmos, hypertension, moon face,
         buffalo hump, hirsutism, nail banding.
DD: Obesity, diabetes mellitus, hypertension,
         cirrhosis, steroid therapy
PHYS: Increased production of cortisol by adrenal
         gland due to excessive ACTH from the pituitary,
         results in a syndrome of truncal obesity,
         hypertension, malaise, oedema, hirsutism and
         osteoporosis.

See also SECTION 6

CVA

See Infarct, Cerebral

Cystic Fibrosis (Fibrocystic Disease)

TEST: Sweat chloride (H), intrauterine chorionic villus
         sampling (AB), specific PCR (+), S.pancreatic
         enzymes (L), B.immunoreactive trypsin (L),
         faecal fat (H).
SIGN: Salty taste to skin, clubbing of fingers, haemoptysis.
DD: Malnutrition, malabsorption syndromes, ileus,
         chronic bronchitis, emphysema, cirrhosis.
PHYS: Clinical syndrome characterised by fibrosis and
         cyst formation in the pancreas, steatorrhoea,
         electrolyte disturbances and pathological
         changes to the lungs. Transmitted as an
         autosomal recessive trait.

Cystinosis

See Fanconi Syndrome

Cystitis (Urinary bladder infection)

TEST: U.culture (+), U.microscopy (cells and bacteria),
         U.protein (+ or –), U.pH (AB), U.blood (+), WCC
         (H).
SIGN: Abdominal rebound tenderness.
DD: Pyelonephritis, nephrosis, diabetes mellitus,
         urinary neoplasm, beeturia, urinary calculus,
         urethral foreign body, prostatitis.
PHYS: Bacterial infection of the urinary bladder. May
         spread to kidneys.

Cytomegalovirus Infections

TEST: Specific complement fixing antibodies (RT),
         S.CMV IgG and S.CMV IgM (both + indicates
         current CMV infection, IgG+ and IgM– indicates
         previous infection), B.lymphocytes (AB), LFT
         (AB), Paul Bunnell (–).
DD: Infectious mononucleosis, toxoplasmosis,
         rubella, hepatitis, other viral infections,
         leukaemia, streptococcal pharyngitis,
         diphtheria, agranulocytosis.
PHYS: Often asymptomatic. Severe cogenital effects if
         infected during pregnancy.

de Quervain's Tenosynovitis

SIGN: Finkelstein's test
PHYS: Caused by repetitive wrist action

de Quervain's Thyroiditis

See Thyroiditis, de Quervain's Subacute

De Toni-Fanconi-Debré Syndrome

See Fanconi Syndrome

Deafness

SIGN: Rinne's test, Weber's test, labyrinth tests.

See also SYMPTOMS SECTION 1: Deafness

Dehydration

TEST: S.potassium (H), S.sodium (H), S.bicarbonate
         (L), S.chloride (L), S.osmolality (H), S.urea (H),
         U.SG (H), U.ketones (H), S.albumin (H),
         P.viscosity (H), PCV (H).
SIGN: Enophthalmos, hypotension, dry mucous
         membranes, poor skin turgor, oliguria.

Dengue Fever

TEST: S.dengue viral antigens (RT), S.dengue virus
         haemagglutination inhibition antibody (VH),
         WCC (N initially, L later), B. lymphocytes (L),
         immature neutrophils (H).
SIGN: Fever, photophobia, abdominal tenderness.
DD: Other viral, bacterial and rickettsial infections,
         leptospirosis, malaria.
PHYS: Viral infection spread by mosquitoes.

Depression, Endogenous (Affective depression)

TEST: Primarily a clinical diagnosis, but these investigations may also be useful: S.cortisol (H), dexamethasone suppression test (AB).

DD: Schizophrenia, organic brain syndromes, stress, neuroses, reactive situations, agoraphobia, phychoses, may be secondary to many chronic diseases.

PHYS: Often a subjective diagnosis, and elements include lowered mood, inability to concentrate, sleep disturbances, loss of interest, anxiety and varied somatic symptoms.

Dermatitis Herpetiformis

TEST: S.HLA-B8 (+), Hb (L), red cell folate (L), S.vit. B_{12} (L), skin biopsy immunofluorescence (AB), small intestine biopsy (AB), S.thyroid antibodies (+ or –), S.parietal cell antibodies (+ or –), S.antinuclear anitbodies (+ or –).

SIGN: Extensor surface pruiritic rash.

DD: Coeliac disease, psoriasis.

PHYS: Gluten dependent skin and intestinal lesions. Associated with autoimmune disorders of the thyroid, diabetes and pernicious anaemia.

Dermatitis, Atopic

See Eczema

Dermatitis, Contact

TEST: Skin biopsy (AB), patch testing (+)

DD: See SYMPTOMS SECTION 1: Rash

Dermatomyositis

TEST: ESR (H), S.CK (H), S.aldolase (H), S.LDH (H), U.creatinine (H), U.myoglobin (+), skin and/or muscle biopsy (AB) (soft tissue calcium deposits), electromyography (AB).

SIGN: Telangiectasia, erythema, oedema, V rash on neck/chest, Gottron's sign.

DD: Polymyalgia rheumatica, SLE, scleroderma, polyarteritis nodosa, malignancy.

PHYS: Up to 50% of cases associated with underlying neoplasia.

Diabetes Insipidus

TEST: U.SG (L), S.osmolality (H), S.ADH (L), S.glucose (N), S.sodium (H), S.creatinine (N), B.urea (L), fluid depletion test (AB).

DD: Psychogenic polydipsia, nephritis, diabetes mellitus, hyperparathyroidism.

PHYS: Pancreatic, renal and cerebral disease must be sought and excluded before diagnosis is made. May be temporary following head injury. Due to lack of vasopressin release from neurohypophysis, secondary to cerebral disease.

Diabetes Mellitus, Types One and Two

TEST: U. and B. glucose (H), GTT (AB), U.ketones (+), S.insulin (L type 1 diabetes), glycosylated Hb (H), S.glutamic acid decarboxylase antibodies (+type 1 diabetes, diabetic tendency), S.insulinoma associated 2 antibodies (+ or – type 1 diabetes, S.fructosamine (H), S.islet cell autoantibodies (+ type 1 diabetes).

SIGN: Ankle jerk and other reflexes, cachexia (severe), Argyll-Robertson pupils, Charcot's joints, hepatomegaly, hyperventilation (acidosis), large kidneys, Kussmaul's breathing, lens opacity (cataract), onycholysis, retinal exudates, retinal haemorrhages, xanthomatosis.

DD: Renal disease, pregnancy and stress can all cause glycosuria; polyglandular autoimmune syn.

PHYS: Complications include retinal damage, arterial disease, neuropathies, ketoacidosis, peripheral gangrene and coma.

Diabetic Ketoacidosis

TEST: S.glucose (H), U.glucose (H), S.sodium (L), S.chloride (L), S.potassium (H), S.magnesium (L), U.ketones (H), B.pH (L), S.bicarbonate (L), glycosylated Hb (H), S.osmolality (H).

DD: Gastrointestinal infections, causes of acute abdomen and/or dehydration.

PHYS: Gross hyperglycaemia due to lack of insulin causes massive fluid and electrolyte loss through the kidneys. Accumulating ketones leads to systematic acidosis and hypotension. Patient presents with polyuria, polydipsia, nausea, abdominal pain, dehydration, stupor and coma.

Diarrhoea

TEST: Faeces M/C/S (AB), faecal reducing substances (+ with lactose intolerance), S.potassium (L if dehydrated), S.osmolality (H if dehydrated), faecal occult blood (+ or –).

DD: Innumerable causes including bowel infections (viral, bacterial and amoebiasis), giardiasis, malabsorption syndromes, allergies, Crohn's disease, ulcerative colitis, diverticulitis, carcinoma, appendicitis, irritable bowel syndrome, diabetes, poisoning, drugs (eg. antibiotics).

PHYS: Any form of gut irritation or inflammation may lead to intestinal hurry.

DIC

See Disseminated Intravascular Coagulation

Diphtheria

TEST: Throat or nose culture (+), Schick test (+ in susceptible people), WCC (H).

SIGN: Mydriasis, pseudomembrane.

DD: Streptococcal URTI, Vincent's angina, glandular fever, leukaemia, thrush.

PHYS: Caused by *Corynebacterium diphtheriae*.
See also Pharyngitis

Disseminated Intravascular Coagulation [DIC]
TEST: B.platelets (L), B.fibrinogen (L), B.D-Dimer (+), B.erythrocytes (AB), B.fibrin degradation products (VH), APTT (H), prothrombin time (H)
SIGN: Purpura
DD: Snake bite, septicaemia, renal disease, intra-uterine fetal death, metastatic carcinoma, severe trauma, acute leukaemia
PHYS: Massive internal bleeding

Disseminated Lupus Erythematosus
See Lupus Erythematosus, Systemic

Disseminated Sclerosis
See Multiple Sclerosis

Diverticulitis
TEST: WCC (H), barium enema (AB), colonoscopy (AB).
DD: Appendicitis, ulcerative colitis, gastroenteritis, irritable bowel syn., colonic carcinoma.
PHYS: Inflammation of colonic diverticula.

Donavanosis
See Granuloma Inguinale

Down Syndrome (Mongolism, Trisomy 21)
TEST: Chromosome count (trisomy 21), intrauterine chorionic villus sampling (AB). Antenatal maternal tests that should be considered jointly: S.HCG (VH), S.alpha-fetoprotein (L), S.oestriol (L), neutrophil alkaline phosphatase (VH).
DD: Cretinism, other chromosome translocations.
PHYS: 47 chromosomes with triplicate chromosome 21.

Dracunculiasis (Guinea Worm Disease)
TEST: Abscess exudate microscopy (+), tissue biopsy microscopy (+), specific ELISA test (+).
SIGN: Subcutaneous tracks, blisters, abscess.
PHYS: Occurs in West and Central Africa, and South Central Asia.

See also Filariasis; Onchocerciasis

Drug Addiction
See Narcotic Addiction; Alcoholism

Duchenne Muscular Dystrophy
TEST: Specific PCR (+), S.CK (H), muscle biopsy (AB), electromyelogram (AB).
SIGN: Gower's manoeuvre, falls frequently, unable to run.

DD: Other hereditary muscle disorders, spinal cord disease or trauma, viral myositis, polymyositis, dystrophia myotonica, periodic paralysis, metabolic myopathies.
PHYS: Genetic disease of males.

Duodenal Ulcer
See Peptic Ulcer

Dwarfism
See Growth, Reduced

Dysentery, Bacillary
See Shigellosis

Dyskinesia, Tardive
TEST: None specific.
DD: Parkinson's disease, Huntington's chorea, Wilson's disease, Sydenham's chorea, thalamic or basal ganglia tumour, senile dyskinesia, schizophrenia, hypothyroidism, hyperthyroidism, other drugs (eg tricyclics, phenytoin, levodopa, oral contraceptive, antihistamines).
PHYS: Iatrogenic disease due to use of neuroleptic or psychotropic drugs.

See also SIGNS SECTION 2: Dyskinesia, Tardive

Echinococcosis
See Hydatid Cyst

Eclampsia and Pre-eclampsia
TEST: S.oestriol (determins fetal maturity), Hb (N), S.protein (L), S.uric acid (H), S.urea (N), U.M/C/S (RBC and casts), U.protein (+).
SIGN: Hypertension, pitting oedema, convulsions, intrauterine growth retardation, Chaussier's sign.
DD: Epilepsy, meningitis, intracranial tumour, stroke, essential hypertension, renal failure, intravenous lignocaine.
PHYS: A syndrome of hypertension, oedema, proteinuria and headache in pregnancy.

Ectopic Pregnancy
See Pregnancy, Ectopic

Eczema (Atopic Dermatitis)
TEST: S.IgE (H), B.eosinophils (H), RAST (+), skin allergen testing (+).
DD: Seborrhoeic dermatitis, contact dermatitis, psoriasis, miliaria, scabies, lichen simplex, SLE, zinc deficit, histiocytosis X.
SIGN: Subungal hyperkeratosis
PHYS: May be associated with asthma or hay fever. Chronic relapsing course common.

Embolism, Pulmonary
See Pulmonary Thromboembolism

Emphysema
TEST: Sputum microscopy (lymphocytes and polymorphs), sputum culture (+ with intercurrent infection), S.alpha$_1$-antitrypsin (L), B.pO$_2$ (L if severe), S.pH (L), RCC (H), PCV (H), chest x-ray (AB), repiratory function tests (AB).
SIGN: Barrel chest, Jacobsen-Holdsnedt phenomenon, papilloedema, pink puffer, thoracic tympany.
DD: Chronic bronchitis, asthma, silicosis, asbestosis, TB, sarcoidosis, lung cancer, bronchiectasis, CHF.
PHYS: Hyperinflation of the lung due to chronic bronchiolitis. Airway resistance is increased and respiratory effort greater.

See also Bronchitis, Chronic

Encephalitis, Japanese
See Japanese Encephalitis

Encephalitis, Viral
TEST: CSF virology (+), WCC (AB), B.neutrophils (H), CSF microscopy (cells +), CSF protein (H), CSF sugar (N), CSF pressure (N or H), S.CPK (H).
SIGN: Ankle clonus, choreiform movements, Kernig's sign, parkinsonian facies (lethargica), neck stiffness, resting tremor, convulsions, flaccid paralysis, reflexes abnormal.
DD: Febrile convulsion, meningitis, epilepsy, TB meningitis, cerebral abscess, cerebrovascular accident, CVA, CNS tumour, toxic encephalopathy.
PHYS: May be due to infection by one of many arboviruses. Only supportive therapy is available.

Endocarditis, Bacterial, Subacute [SBE]
TEST: B.culture (+), WCC (H), B.neutrophils (H), Hb (L-normocytic and normochromic), ESR (VH), C-RP (+), U.protein (+), S.Ig (H), U.blood (+), U.M/C/S (AB).
SIGN: Clubbing of fingers, retinal haemorrhages, splenomegaly (subacute), splinter haemorrhages, tachycardia, Janeway lesion.
DD: Rheumatic fever, SLE, periateritis nodosa, syphilis, lymphoma, brucellosis, TB, cardiac tumour or aneurysm, aortic aneurysm.
PHYS: Commonly occurs in previously damaged or abnormal hearts, particularly after rheumatic fever. Usually involves mitral or aortic valve. Insidious in onset with fever, petechiae, splenomegaly, anaemia and cardiac murmur.

Endometriosis
TEST: Laparoscopy (AB), ultrasound scan (AB or false N).
SIGN: Pelvic pain, backache, secondary dysmenorrhoea, infertility, dyspareunia, symptoms aggravated by menstruation, rectal bleeding.
DD: Pelvic inflammatory disease, ovarian cysts and neoplasms, uterine fibroids and myomas, bowel neoplasms.
PHYS: Ectopic deposits of endometrial tissue.

Enteritis, Regional
See Crohn's disease

Enteritis, Viral
SIGN: Dehydration.
DD: URTI, coryza, meningitis, septicaemia, coeliac disease, milk intolerance, other food allergies, haemolytic uraemic syn., pyloric stenosis, intussusception, appendicitis, Hirschsprung's disease.

Enterobiasis
See Pinworm

Epidemic Polyarthritis (Ross River fever)
TEST: S.specific antibody (RT), S.IgM (H), B.ESR (N).
SIGN: Maculopapular rash, fever.
DD: Influenza, rubella, dengue fever, Barmah forest virus.
PHYS: Epidemic arbovirus widespread in Australia and tropics. Spread by mosquito.

Epiglottitis
TEST: Blood clulture (+), WCC (AB)
DD: Tonsillitis, quinsy, croup, angioedema.
PHYS: If diagnosis suspect, do NOT examine or swab throat unless prepared to intubate, as epiglottic prolapse and asphyxia may occur.

Epilepsy, Idiopathic
TEST: None specific. Pathological cause must be excluded before diagnosis is made. Screening tests include: FBC, ESR, S.electrolytes, S.urea, U.M/C/S, liver function tests, S.calcium, S.phosphate, S.ALP, S.glucose, EEG, CT, screen for syphilis.
SIGN: Ankle clonus, Babinski's sign, convulsions, reflexes abnormal.
DD: Syncopal attacks, psychiatric disorders, subnormality, cerebral tumours, TB, diabetes, encephalitis, meningitis, syphilis, birth injury, phenylketonuria, hypocalcaemia, trauma, CVA, alcoholism, drugs, senility.
PHYS: Epilepsy describes recurrent convulsions due to many causes. Types include grand mal, petit mal, psychomotor, Jacksonian seizures, somatic and optic seizures.

Erythema Multiforme

TEST: Biopsy histology (AB or N), ESR (H), CRP (H).
SIGN: Papular rash, blistering rash, target lesions, itch.
DD: Urticaria, drug eruptions, toxic epidermal necrolysis, secondary syphilis, dermatitis herpetiformis, pemphigoid, pemphigus.
PHYS: Frequently follows *Herpes simplex* infection or sulfonamide drug use. May progress to Stevens-Johnson syn.

Erythema Nodosum

TEST: Skin biopsy (fatty atrophy), S.ASOT (H), throat culture (+ or –), WCC (AB), ESR (H).
DD: Bruising, erythema multiforme, Weber-Christian disease, thrombophlebitis, sarcoidosis, polyarteritis nodosa, metastatic neoplasia.
PHYS: Symptom complex that indicates underlying infection, systemic disease, toxic reaction. Characterised by painful red nodules on anterior aspect of shins.

Erythraemia

See Polycythaemia Rubra Vera

Factor IX Deficit

See Christmas Disease

Factor VIII Deficit

See Haemophilia

Failure to Thrive

TEST: Screening tests include: Faeces and U.M/C/S, WCC, TFT, B.urea, S.creatinine, bone age x-rays, chromosomal analysis, sweat test.
SIGN: Depends on cause, but may include muscular atrophy, blue sclera, bradycardia, cachexia, clubbing of fingers, Corrigan's sign, cardiac murmurs, exophthalmos, abnormal faeces, hepatomegaly, hydrocephalus, hypotonia, hypertonicity, intrauterine growth retardation, splenomegaly, muscular wasting, Santmyer swallow (puff reflex).
DD: Malnutrition, emotional deprivation, malabsorption syndromes, cystic fibrosis, chronic heart failure, endocrine disorders, Turner syn., chromosomal disorders, renal insufficiency, chronic infection, malignancies.
PHYS: Children who fail to gain weight for no obvious reason.

Fanconi's Syndrome

(De Toni- Fanconi-Débre Syndrome, Cystinosis)

TEST: U.phosphate (H), U.protein (+), WCC (cystine crystals in leukocytes), U.glucose (+), P.cystine (VH), S.pH (L), S.urate (H), S.phosphate (L), S.potassium (L).

DD: Congenital metabolic disorders, Wilson's disease, nephrotic syn., multiple myeloma, amyloidosis.
PHYS: Syndrome that occurs with proximal renal tubular dysfunction. Commonly due to cystine storage disease, but many other disease entities may produce this syndrome.

See also SYNDROMES SECTION 6:De Toni-Fanconi-Debré Syndrome

Felty Syndrome

TEST: S.rheumatoid factor (VH), LE cells (+), Hb (L or N), B.neutrophils (L), WCC (L), B.platelets (L or N).
SIGN: Splenomegaly.
DD: Rheumatoid arthritis, rheumatic fever, viraemia, leukaemia.
PHYS: Syndrome characterised by migratory polyarthritis, splenomegaly and leukopenia.

See also SYNDROMES SECTION 6: Felty Syndrome

Fetal Development

See Pregnancy, Progress

Fibrocystic Disease

See Cystic Fibrosis

Fibromyalgia

TEST: Nil specific. Differential diagnosis should be excluded by appropriate investigations.
SIGN: Widespread tender bony points.
DD: Polymyalgia rheumatica, rheumatoid arthritis, myopathies, hypothyroidism, hyperthyroidism, Addison's disease, metastatic carcinoma, Parkinson's disease, psychiatric conditions, alcoholism, narcotic or other drug withdrawal.
PHYS: Diffuse musculoskeletal pain and stiffness, widespread areas of local tenderness, fatigue.

Fibrosing Alveolitis, Cryptogenic

See Cryptogenic Fibrosing Alveolitis

Filiariasis

TEST: B.microscopy (+ microfilariae), B. specific filarial antibody (+ long term), S.IgE (H), B.eosinophils (H)
SIGN: Cyclical fever, chyluria, lymphoedema, pitting oedema.
DD: Thrombophlebitis, cellulitis, erysipelas, malignant lymphoedema, lymph node surgery
PHYS: Many different types of filaria including *Wuchereria bancrofti, Brugia malayi, Onchocerca volvulus* and *Loa loa*

See also Dracunculiasis; Onchocerciasis

Fits
See Epilepsy, Idiopathic

Flat Feet
SIGN: Windlass test.

Flu
See Influenza

Foetal Development
See Pregnancy, Progress

Food Poisoning
TEST: Suspect food sample culture and/or toxin assay (+), faeces M/C/S (+ or –). No specific patient tests available.
SIGN: Borborygmus
DD: Viral or bacterial enteritis, other causes of diarrhoea and vomiting (see SYMPTOMS SECTION 1)
PHYS: *Clostridium perfringens, Staphylococcus aureus* and *Bacillus cereus* most common causes

See also Botulism; Ciguatera Poisoning

Fracture
TEST: X-ray (AB), bone scan (AB). If pathological fracture is suspected tests that may be useful include – S.Ca, S.P., FBC, B.Hb, S.albumin, S.protein, protein electrophoresis, ESR, CRP, bone biopsy.
SIGN: Deformity, swelling, ecchymosis, impaired function, fracture blister, crepitus, hypermobility, Barford test (neck of femur).
DD: Dislocation, strain, sprain, cartilage trauma, ruptured tendon, ruptured ligament, severe bruising, sarcoma, osteomyelitis, Osgood-Schlatter's disease, osteoarthritis.

Fungal Skin Infection (Tinea)
TEST: Skin scraping M/C/S (+), skin biopsy (AB), Wood's light (Fluorescence in dark under UV light)
SIGN: Chip sign, subungal hyperkeratosis, nail discolouration, thickened nail, onycholysis.
DD: Psoriasis, eczema, atopic dermatitis, stasis dermatitis, pityriasis rosea, lichen planus, impetigo

Galactosaemia
TEST: RBC galactose-1-phosphate (VH), P.galactose (H), RBC galactokinase (L)
SIGN: Hepatomegaly, jaundice, mental retardation, cataract
DD: Liver disease, other disorders of carbohydrate metabolism.
PHYS: Inborn error of galactose metabolism.

Gall Stones
See Cholelithiasis

Gangrene, Gas (Clostridial Myositis)
TEST: Wound exudate, muscle biopsy or cervix discharge microscopy (Gram+ rods), anaerobic B.culture (+), WCC (VH), platelets (L), U.protein (+), RCC (L), U.blood (+), S.bilirubin (N or H).
SIGN: Tissue crepitations, jaundice, foul smell.
DD: Cellulitis, peritonitis, ruptured viscus, neoplasm.
PHYS: Rapidly spreading anaerobic infection of muscle tissue due to Clostridium sp., after penetrating trauma or abortion.

Gastric Ulcer
See Peptic Ulcer

Gastroenteritis
See Enteritis, Viral

Genital Herpes
See Herpes, Genital

German Measles
See Rubella

Giant Cell Arteritis (Temporal Arteritis)
TEST: ESR (VH), Hb (L), LFT (AB), artery biopsy (AB).
SIGN: Scalp tender.
DD: Polymyalgia rheumatica, migraine, temporomandibular joint disease.
PHYS: Inflammation of the temporal arteries. Optic artery involvement a severe complication.

Giardiasis
TEST: Faeces M/C/S (+)
SIGN: Abdominal bloating
DD: Other causes of diarrhoea and malabsorption (see SYMPTOMS SECTION 1)
PHYS: Intestinal infection by Giardia lamblia

Gingivostomatitis
See Vincent's Angina

Glands, Swollen and Inflamed
See Adenitis

Glandular Fever
See Infectious Mononucleosis

Glaucoma
TEST: Ocular tonometry (H), gonioscopy of anterior

chamber (AB), opthalmoscopy of optic disc (AB), visual fields (AB).
SIGN: Vision deterioration, rainbow halo, nausea, corneal oedema, dilated pupil, horizontal light test, swinging torch test.
DD: Different types of glaucoma must be differentiated (eg. open angle glaucoma, angle closure glaucoma, chronic forms of glaucoma, intermittent low pressure glaucoma, congenital glaucoma, secondary glaucoma), lens dislocation, trauma, uveitis, optic tumours, anterior chamber haemorrhage, corticosteroid damage to eye.
PHYS: An increase in intraocular pressure for many diverse reasons, sufficient to cause damage to the optic disc and retina. Early diagnosis essential to avoid long-term damage.

Glomerulonephritis, Acute
TEST: U.microscopy (cells and casts), Hb (L), S.urea (H), U.pH (acid), U.protein (+), ASOT (FT), ESR (H), S.creatinine (H), U.blood (+).
SIGN: Hypertension, pitting oedema, oliguria, tachycardia.
DD: Angioneurotic oedema, SLE, polyarteritis nodosa, subacute bacterial endocarditis, sarcoidosis, urinary tract infection, prostatitis, chronic renal disease, toxins.
PHYS: Immunological disorder resulting in generalised glomerular inflammation, and a subsequent failure in renal function. May follow an acute streptococcal infection.

Glomerulonephritis, Chronic
TEST: U.microscopy (casts and RBC), S.creatinine (H or N), Hb (L or N), U.protein (VH), S.urea (H or N), U.blood (+), S.albumin (L or N).
DD: Acute nephritis, pyelonephritis, multiple myeloma, amyloidosis, hypercalcaemia, SLE, periarteritis nodosa, subacute bacterial endocarditis.
PHYS: Collection of renal diseases that affect the glomerular tufts causing permanent damage. Includes nephrotic syn. and other chronic nephropathies.

Glycogen Storage Disorders
TEST: See SYNDROMES SECTION 6.
DD: Andersen syn., Cori syn., Hers syn., McArdle syn., Pompe syn., von Gierke syn.
PHYS: See under individual syndromes.

Gonadal Dysgenesis
See Turner's Syndrome

Gonorrhoea ('Clap')
TEST: Urethral, cervical, pharyngeal and rectal swabs, M/C/S (+), B.culture (N or +), U.protein (+ in male), VDRL and FTA (–).

DD: Male – NSU, prostatitis, cystitis, Reiter's disease, syphilis.
Female – thrush, trichomoniasis, NSU, leukorrhoea, cystitis, syphilis.
PHYS: Genital and/or oral infection by *Neisseria gonorrhoea*. Transmitted venereally. Swabs should be transported in Stuart's medium at body temperature. Smears also useful.

Goodpasture Syndrome
TEST: B.glomerular basement membrane antibodies (+), lung or renal biopsy (AB), sputum blood (+), sputum microscopy (haemosiderin laden macrophages), S.urea (H), S.creatinine (H), U.blood (+), U.protein (+).
DD: Bronchitis, pneumonia, TB, renal failure, nephrotic syn., glomerulonephritis.
PHYS: Syndrome of pulmonary haemorrhages and renal failure due to damaged basement membranes in the kidney and lungs.

See also SYNDROMES SECTION 6: Goodpasture Syndrome

Gout
TEST: S.urate (H), synovial fluid microscopy (urates present, fluid WCC (H), 24 hr. U.urates (L in underexcretors), ESR (H), WCC (H), S.creatinine (H).
DD: Osteoarthritis, pseudogout, rheumatoid arthritis, trauma, synovitis, cellulitis, osteomyelitis, sarcoid, multiple myeloma, psoriatic arthritis, Reiter syn., ankylosing spondylitis.
PHYS: Excess intake of purines and underexcretion of urates predisposes to high serum uric acid levels and crystal deposition in joints. A normal s.urate does not exclude gout as a diagnosis

Granuloma Inguinale (Donavanosis)
TEST: Tissue microscopy (Donovan bodies +).
SIGN: Papule or ulcer on genitals.
DD: Neoplasm, chancroid, syphilis, amoebiasis, lymphogranuloma venereum.
PHYS: Caused by *Calymmatobacterium granulomatis*.

Graves' Disease
See Hyperthyroidism

Growth, Reduced (Dwarfism)
TEST: Measurement of child siblings and parents, bone age x-rays, karyotyping. In addition following tests may be selected to exclude causative disease: Hb, FBC, ESR, electrolytes, urea, calcium, ALP, TFT, prolactin, growth hormone, pituitary x-ray, jejunal biopsy, ECG, respiratory function tests.

See also SYMPTOMS SECTION 1: Growth, Reduced

Guinea Worm Disease

See Dracunculiasis

Haemochromatosis

TEST: S.iron (H), PCR gene test (+),liver biopsy (+), S.ferritin (H), S.transferrin (H), marrow aspirate (+ for haemosiderin), S.iron binding capacity (L), U.haemosiderin (+), skin lesion biopsy (+ for haemosiderin), LFT (AB), HLA typing for family members..

SIGN: Heptatomegaly, cardiomegaly.

DD: Diabetes, hepatitis, hepatic carcinoma, cirrhosis, biliary tract obstruction, pancreatic tumour, CHF.

PHYS: Excessive deposits of iron in the body, particularly liver and skin. Inherited disorder of excessive iron absorption characterised by hepatomegaly, diabetes, cardiac failure and skin pigmentation.

Haemoglobinopathies

See Sickle Cell Disease; Thalassaemia Major; Thalassaemia Minor.
See also Haemoglobin in PATHOLOGY SECTION 4.

Haemophilia A (Factor VIII Deficit)

TEST: S.factor VIII (L), specific PCR (+), prothrombin time (N), bleeding time (N), clotting time (H or N), prothrombin consumption test (AB), tissue DNA probe (+), partial thromboplastin time (H), platelet count (N).

DD: Other hereditary coagulation disorders, von Willebrand's disease, vit. K deficit, anticoagulant or aspirin therapy, sprue, malnutrition, hepatic failure, leukaemia.

PHYS: Inherited X-linked recessive trait resulting in lack of factor VIII in the intrinsic blood clotting pathway.

See also Christmas Disease; von Willebraand's disease

Haemophilia, Vascular

See von Willebrand's Disease

Hand-Schuller-Christian Disease

TEST: Granuloma microscopy (foam cells present), B.eosinophils (VH), Hb (L), platelets (L), S.Cholesterol (N).

SIGN: Exophthalmos, polyuria, splenomegaly, hepatomegaly.

DD: Letterer-Siwe disease, histiocytosis X, diabetes insipidus, hepatic failure, lymphomas, hypogonadism, CCF.

PHYS: Excessive tissue retention of cholesterol forms foam cells in granulomatous lesions of skin, liver, bones and gut.

Hansen's Disease

See Leprosy

Hashimoto's Thyroiditis

See Thyroiditis, Hashimoto's

Hay Fever

See Allergic Rhinitis

Head Injury

TEST: X-ray skull and neck, CT, Hb, B.WCC, B.electrolytes, B.glucose, BUN, U.M/C/S. Results vary. See PATHOLOGY SECTION 4 for interpretation.

SIGN: CSF loss from ear or nose, pupil size and reaction, corneal reflex, gag reflex, tendon reflexes, joint flaccidity, neck stiffness, nystagmus, slurred speech, papilloedema, amnesia.

DD: Subarachnoid haemorrhage, stroke, subdural haemorrhage, intracranial tumour or abscess, meningitis.

Headache

TEST: The following tests may be considered in the investigation of intractable headache: Hb, FBC, ESR, antinuclear antibodies, CSF studies, temporal artery biopsy, cervical X-ray, temporomandibular joint X-ray, CT head and neck, MRI.

See also SYMPTOMS SECTION 1: Headache

Hepatic Metastases

TEST: S.GGT (H), S alpha-feto protein (H), ultrasound (AB), CT (AB).

SIGN: Hepatomegaly, jaundice, shifting dullness (ascites), fluid thrill (ascites).

DD: Other liver diseases, Hodgkin's disease.

PHYS: No specific test. Only positive result significant.

Hepatitis A (Acute Viral Infective Hepatitis)

TEST: S.IgM antiHAV (+), S.IgM (H), B.AST (H), B.ALT (VH), S.bilirubin (H), B.ALP (H), WCC (N or L), U.bilirubin (H), U.protein (+), U.urobilinogen (H early).

SIGN: Jaundice, hepatomegaly, splenomegaly.

DD: Hepatitis B, chronic active hepatitis. PLUS acute viral infections, infectious mononucleosis, dengue fever, Q fever, malaria, yellow fever, amoebiasis, drugs, toxins, leptospirosis, alcoholism, cirrhosis, biliary obstruction, pancreatic carcinoma, carotenaemia.

PHYS: Hepatic cell necrosis causes release of enzymes and bilirubin into blood. Viral infection of liver transmitted by food that causes severe damage and loss of function. Incubation period 2 to 6 weeks. Fulminant in 0.15% of cases. Does not cause hepatic malignancy. Vaccine available.

Summary of Viral Hepatitis Types				
Type	Transmission	Form	Tests	Prognosis
Hepatitis A	Faecal-oral	Acute Chronic	IgM antiHAV + up to 6 months after onset IgG antiHAV + 6 weeks to indefinite after onset	Good. Occasional relapse.
Hepatitis B	Sex, blood, mucous membranes, wounds	Acute Chronic	HbsAg + from onset to 4 months HBV-DNA + from onset to 1 month AntiHBc + from onset indefinitely HBeAg + from onset to 6 weeks Early –good prognostic sign DNA polymerase + from onset to 1 month IgM antiHBc rising titre from shortly after onset to 6 months, then rapid drop AntiHBe from 6 weeks indefinitely AntiHBs from 4 or 5 months indefinitely	Most good. 10% chronic 15% of chronic eventually fatal.
Hepatitis C	Blood	Acute Chronic	IgG antiHCV + AntiHCV + from 3 months after onset in 60%	50% chronic 20% cirrhosis
Hepatitis D	Sex, blood. Only with or after Hep. B	Acute & chronic	IgM antiHDV + from onset indefinitely IgG antiHDV + from onset indefinitely HDAg + from onset indefinitely	Often chronic Occasionally fulminant
Hepatitis E	Faecal-oral	Acute & chronic	IgM antiHEV + from onset for 1 to 2 years IgG antiHEV + from 3 weeks for 1 to 2 years	Good. Rarely fatal

Hepatitis B (Serum Hepatitis)

TEST: S.HBsAg (+ up to 4 months from onset), S.HBeAg (+ early), S.antiHBc (+ long-term), S.antiHBs (+ long-term from 3 months after onset), S.smooth muscle antibody (+ in chronic active form), S.IgG (H), S.IgM (H), B.AST (H), B.ALT (VH), S.bilirubin (H), B.ALP (H), beta$_2$-microglobulin (H), S.IgA (L or N), WCC (N or L), U.bilirubin (H).

SIGN: Jaundice.

DD: Hepatitis A. PLUS those listed under Hepatitis A above.

PHYS: Transmitted parenterally or sexually. Incubation period 1 to 6 months. Fulminant in 1% of cases. 10-20% develop chronic active infection. Risk of malignancy increased dramatically. Vaccine available.

Hepatitis C

TEST: S.antiHCV (+), S.ALT (H), LFT (AB).

SIGN: Jaundice.

DD: See Hepatitis A.

PHYS: Previously known as Non-A, Non-B Hepatitis. Parental, but not sexual, transmission. Incubation period 2- weeks. Fulminant form uncommon. 50% develop chronic infection, 20% develop cirrhosis. Probable increase in risk of malignancy. No vaccine available.

Hepatitis D

TEST: S.antiHDV (+), S.HBsAg (+), S.ALT (H), LFT (AB).

SIGN: Jaundice.

DD: See Hepatitis A.

PHYS: Caused by delta agent. Parenteral transmission to a patient who already suffers from Hepatitis B. Usually associated with IV drug abuse. Often severe, and may be associated with fulminant super infection. Aggravation of Hepatitis B chronicity common. Probably increases risk of hepatic malignancy. No specific vaccine once Hepatitis B already contracted, but may be prevented by vaccination before initial Hepatitis B infection.

Hepatitis E

TEST: S.antiHEV (+), LFT (AB).

SIGN: Jaundice.

DD: See Hepatitis A.

PHYS: Faecal-oral transmission in epidemics caused by contaminated water supply. Incubation period 3 to 9 weeks. May be fulminant, particularly in pregnant women. Does not cause chronic liver infection. Malignancy potential unknown. No vaccine available.

Hepatitis, Chronic Active Autoimmune

TEST: S.AST (H to VH), S.ALP (H), S.albumin (N to L), ESR (VH), prothrombin index (H), S.IgG (H), S. antinuclear antibodies (+), S.anti-smooth muscle antibodies (+), S.HLA-B8 (+), S.HLA DRw3 (+).

SIGN: Spider naevi, buffalo hump, moon facies, abdominal striae

DD: Chronic viral hepatitis, Wilson's disease,

alcoholic liver disease, cirrhosis, alpha$_1$-antitrypsin deficiency, sclerosing cholangitis

PHYS: Chronic, progressive. More common in young women. Aetiology unknown

Hepatolenticular Degeneration
See Wilson's Disease

Hepatoma
TEST: S.ALP (H), S.alpha$_1$-fetoprotein (+), S.CA 19-9 (H), S.calcium (H), ESR (H), WCC (H), B.glucose (L), S.copper (H), technetium^{99} liver scan (AB), liver biopsy (AB), ascitic fluid cytology (AB).

SIGN: Ascites, hepatomegaly, hepatic bruit, hepatic friction rub.

DD: Cirrhosis, chronic hepatitis, portal hypertension, focal nodular hyperplasia of liver, liver cell adenoma.

PHYS: Parenchymal tumour that often involves the vascular components of the liver and has a very poor prognosis.

Herpes Zoster
See Chickenpox; Shingles

Herpes, Genital
TEST: Lesion smear and culture for virus (+), S.HSV antibodies (+).

DD: Syphilis, scabies, shingles, impetigo, lymphogranuloma venereum, trauma, carcinoma, chancroid, erythema multiforme, vulvitis.

PHYS: Multiple, painful genital blisters that break down to ulcers. Incubation period 2 to 7 days.

Hip Dislocation
See Dislocated Hip

Hirsutism
TEST: The following tests may be considered in the investigation of hirsutism: S.testosterone, Hb, FSH, TFT, LH, DHEAS, 17 alpha-hydroxyprogesterone, prolactin, U.free cortisol, gonadal ultrasound.

See also SYMPTOMS SECTION 1: Hirsutism and Hypertrichosis

Histiocytosis X
TEST: Chest X-ray and CT (AB), lung biopsy (AB).

SIGN: Spontaneous pneumothorax.

DD: Tuberous sclerosis, neurofibromatosis, lymphangioleiomyomatosis.

PHYS: Manifests as Letterer-Siwe disease, eosinophilic granuloma and Hand-Schuller-Christian disease. Aetiology unknown.

Histoplasmosis
TEST: Sputum M/C/S (+ or −), bronchial lavage M/C.S (+), lung biopsy (AB), blood culture (+ or −), bone marrow M/C/S (+ or −), tissue microscopy (AB), S.specific antigen (+ long term) skin antigen test (+ long term), ESR (H), B.WCC (L), B.Hb (L), S.LDH (H), chest x-ray (AB)

DD: Chronic bronchitis, bronchiectasis, influenza, pneumonia, AIDS

PHYS: Often asymptomatic. Caught from bat or bird droppings. Caused by Histoplasma capsulatum

HIV
See Acquired Immune Deficiency Syndrome

Hives
See Urticaria

Hodgkin's Disease (Lymphoma)
TEST: Lymph node biopsy (+), bone marrow biopsy (AB), Hb (L or N), WCC (N or H), B.eosinophils (N or H), platelets (N or H), LFT (AB if hepatic involvement), ESR (H), S.fibrinogen (H), S.iron (L).

SIGN: Abdominal mass, cachexia, Pel-Ebstein phenomenon, adenitis.

DD: Infection, SLE, TB, syphilis, sarcoid, histiocytosis X, leukaemia, metastatic cancer, lymphangiomas.

PHYS: Painless, intermittent but progressive disease of lymphoid tissue including liver and spleen, resulting in cachexia and symptoms related to the anatomical areas involved.

Hookworm
See Roundworms, Intestinal

Huntington's Chorea
TEST: Specific PCR (+), intrauterine chorionic villus sampling (AB), CT (AB or N).

SIGN: Athetosis, choreiform movements, waddling gait.

DD: Senile chorea, psychoses, cerebellar degeneration, familial, tumours.

PHYS: Inherited disease caused by progressive degeneration of basal ganglia and the cortex.

Hydatid Cyst (Echinococcosis)
TEST: B.hydatid antibodies (90%+), B.eosinophils (H), sputum microscopy (+ with ruptured pulmonary cyst), hepatic scan (+).

SIGN: Hepatomegaly, jaundice.

DD: Hepatic or pulmonary tumour, TB, hepatic or pulmonary abscess, amoebiasis, allergies.

PHYS: Parasitism of liver or lung by Echinococcus granulosus in the larval stage. Usually due to ingestion of cysts from faeces of infected canines. Needle biopsy of mass contraindicated. Normal larval host is sheep. Skin Casoni test no longer performed

Hydatidiform Mole

TEST: S.HCG (VH), uterine ultrasound (AB), microscopy of curretings (+).
SIGN: Abdominal mass, abnormal vaginal bleed
DD: Ectopic pregnancy, miscarriage, uterine tumour
PHYS: Essential to follow patient with serial S.HCG for at least a year. Choriocarcinoma possible complication

Hyperaldosteronism, Primary
See Conn Syndrome

Hyperparathyroidism

TEST: S.calcium (H), S.phosphate (L), S.parathormone (H), S.ALP (H), U.calcium (H), U.phosphate (H).
DD: Metastatic carcinoma, sarcoidosis, hypervitaminosis D, hyperthyroidism, adrenal insufficiency, thiazide drugs, Paget's disease, osteoporosis, osteomalacia, multiple myeloma, osteosarcoma.
PHYS: Hypersecretion of parathyroid hormone due to adenomas, hyperplasia or carcinoma of the parathyroid results in hypercalcaemia, tissue calcification, renal calcification and bone resorption.

Hypertension, Essential

TEST: A pathological cause for hypertension should be excluded by selection from the following tests: U.M/C/S, Hb, B.urea, S.creatinine, S.electrolytes, S.uric acid, B.cholesterol, triglycerides, B.glucose, ECG, renal ultrasound, IVP. Additional tests if clinical suspicion of further pathology exists could include TFT, U.catecholamines, U.renin, dexamethasone suppression test. Echocardiography.
SIGN: Apex beat displacement, retinal arteriovenous nipping, exophthalmos (malignant), papilloedema, pulsus alternans, retinal exudates, retinal haemorrhages, Osler's phenomenon.
DD: Pathological causes include renal disease, renal artery stenosis, Cushing syn., Conn syn., phaeochromocytoma, toxaemia of pregnancy, aortic coarctation, ovarian tumours, porphyria, subarachnoid haemorrhage, lead poisoning, hormone therapy.
PHYS: Essential hypertension is high BP for which no pathological cause can be found. A pressure of 160/100 is associated with a threefold risk of mortality under 65 years.

Hyperthyroidism (Thyrotoxicosis) (Graves' Disease)

TEST: S.TSH (L), S.free thyroxine (H), total T_4 (H),

S.triiodothyronine (T_3) (H), S.anti-TSH receptor antibodies (+), isotopic studies (AB), U.calcium (H), U.creatinine (H), WCC (H), S.PBI (H), FTI (H), S.thyroid microsomal autoantibodies (+), S.thyrotropin receptor antibodies (+ or −)
SIGN: Abnormal reflexes, choreiform movements, bounding pulse, cachexia, exophthalmos, fasciculation, atrial fibrillation, hypertension, mydriasis, Pemberton's sign, onycholysis, spider naevi, systolic murmur, tachycardia, thyroid glitter, postural tremor, water-hammer pulse.
DD: Anxiety states, hepatic cirrhosis, myasthenia gravis, pheochromocytoma, thyroid neoplasia, CCF, atrial fibrillation, myocarditis, pericarditis, rheumatic fever, psychoses.
PHYS: Excessive release of thyroid hormones due to thyroid hyperplasia (Graves' disease), adenomas, goitre, ectopic thyroids or excessive thyroid medication. Produces exophthalmos, goitre, tremor, heat intolerance, sweating, palpitations, hyperactivity and emotional lability.

Hypervitaminosis A
See Carotenaemia

Hypoadrenocorticism
See Addison's Disease

Hypogonadism, Primary
See Turner Syndrome

Hypoparathyroidism

TEST: B.calcium (L), B.phosphate (H), U.calcium (L), U.phosphate (L).
SIGN: Chvostek's sign, lens opacity, obstetric hand (Trousseau's sign), twitching.
DD: Epilepsy, psychoses, hyperirritable musculature, Addison's disease, pernicious anaemia, hyperventilation, pseudohypoparathyroidism, polyglandular autoimmune syn.
PHYS: Deficient secretion of parathyroid hormone due to injury, surgery or idiopathic causes; resulting in hypocalcaemia and tetany.

Hypopituitarism

TEST: Hb (L), S.glucose (L), S.sodium (L), S.potassium (N), TFT (L), S.T_4 (L), S.17-hydroxy steroids (N or L), S.cortisol (L), S.ACTH (L), S.LH (L), S.FSH (L), S.testosterone (L), S.oestrogen (L).
SIGN: Cachexia, hypotension, muscular weakness.
DD: Gonadal failure, hypothyroidism, anorexia nervosa, Klinefelter syn., Addison's disease.
PHYS: Destruction of the anterior pituitary due to tumour, postpartum necrosis (Sheehan syn.), fibrosis, TB or aneurysm results in atrophy of gonads, thyroid and adrenal cortex.

Hypothyroidism (Myxoedema)

TEST: S.TSH (H), S.T$_4$ (L), S.free thyroxine (L), T$_3$ uptake (L), FTI (L), S.cholesterol (H), S.carotene (H), S.AST (H), S.LDH (H), S.CPK (H), S.uric acid (H or N), Hb (L or N).

SIGN: Hyporeflexia, bradycardia, hypotension, onycholysis, Pemberton's sign, pleural effusion, precocious puberty, shifting dullness (ascites).

DD: Pernicious anaemia, infantile cretinism, hypopituitarism, nephritis, uraemia, mongolism, psychoses.

PHYS: Lack of thyroid hormone from the thyroid gland due to Hashimoto's disease, surgery, drugs or congenital defects results in lowering of the metabolic rate.

Idiopathic Pulmonary Fibrosis

See Cryptogenic Fibrosing Alveolitis

IM

See Infectious Mononucleosis

Immunodeficiency

TEST: WCC, B.T cells, S.IgG, S.IgM, S.IgA, S.ASOT. Results vary. See PATHOLOGY SECTION 4 for interpretation.

SIGN: 8 or more minor infections a year.

PHYS: Immunodeficiency may be genetic, acquired or iatrogenic (eg. cytotoxic drugs, radiotherapy).

Impotence, Male

TEST: Screening tests include: S.LH, S.FSH, S.testosterone, S.prolactin, TFT, LFT, B.lipids, S.PSA, B.glucose, U.M/C/S, nocturnal penile tumescence measurement, corpora cavernosography, internal pudendal arteriography, brain CT scan (for pituitary tumour).

SIGN: Testicular size, knee and ankle reflexes, cremasteric reflex, pinprick and vibration sense in groin, peripheral pulses.

DD: See SYMPTOMS SECTION 1.

Incontinence of Urine

TEST: Screening tests include: U.M/C/S, IVP, urethroscopy, urinary flowmeter, urethral pressure measurement.

DD: See SYMPTOMS SECTION 1.

Infarct

See Myocardial Infarct; Pulmonary Thromboembolism; Infarct, Cerebral

Infarct, Cerebral (Stroke; Cerebrovascular Accident [CVA]; Cerebral Thrombosis)

TEST: Pathological investigations generally unrewarding. Lumbar puncture may be performed with caution in some patients: CSF pressure (<200mm H$_2$O), CSF blood (+ or N), CSF protein (H or N), CT (AB).

SIGN: Abnormal reflexes, ankle clonus, Babinski's sign, Brudzinski's sign, Cheyne-Stokes respiration, convulsions, dysdiadochokinesia, hypertonicity, hyperventilation or hypoventilation, intention tremor, Kernig's sign, neck stiffness, papilloedema, pronator sign, spastic paralysis.

DD: Cerebral tumours, trauma, subdural haematomas, cerebral infections, TB, cerebral abscess, hypoglycaemia, migraine.

PHYS: Due to arterial atherosclerosis, cerebral emboli, cerebral haemorrhage, severe hypotension, arterial spasm, cerebral hypoxia, cerebral thrombosis or arterial aneurysm.

See also Transient Ischaemic Attack

Infectious Mononucleosis [IM] (Glandular Fever)

TEST: Specific viral serology (+), rapid slide screen test (+), Paul Bunnell test (+), WCC (H), U.protein (+ or N), S.IgM (H), S.ALP (VH), S.AST (H), S.ALT (H), B.lymphocytes (H and AB forms).

SIGN: Splenomegaly, hepatomegaly, adenitis.

DD: Other viral and bacterial infections, diphtheria, hepatitis, rubella, toxoplasmosis, cytomegalovirus infection, encephalitis, leukaemia, lymphoma, aplastic anaemia, drug reactions.

PHYS: Infection with the Epstein-Barr virus causes a fever, adenitis, splenomegaly and pharyngitis. Specific antibody tests may not become positive for 10 to 14 days after start of symptoms.

Infertility, Female

TEST: To exclude pathological cause test: Hb, FTA, VDRL, Pap smear, vaginal swab M/C/S, U.FSH, S.LH, S.prolactin, S.progesterone, S.17beta-oestradiol, sperm antibodies, endometrial cytology. Essential to investigate male partner.

SIGN: Rubin test

PHYS: May be due to male factor, cervical factor, endometrial failure, corpus luteal failure, tubal factors, pituitary failure, ovarian factors, psychological causes, concurrent disease, coital failure.

See also SYMPTOMS SECTION 1: Infertility

Infertility, Male

TEST: To exclude pathological cause test: sperm count and quality, semen volume and color, semen microscopy, sperm antibodies, seminal fructose, S.FSH, S.LH, S.testosterone, S.prolactin, FTA, urethral swab M/C/S, testicular biopsy.

PHYS: May be due to infections, mumps, gonorrhoea,

leprosy, brucellosis, radiation, malnutrition, surgery, trauma.

See also SYMPTOMS SECTION 1: Infertility

Influenza (Flu)

TEST: Specific serum viral antibodies (+), complement fixation test (+), WCC (L), haemagglutination inhibition test (+), throat swab culture (+), U.protein (+ or –).

DD: Coryza, other viral or bacterial infections. Viral infection of the upper respiratory tract. A, B and C forms identifiable.

PHYS: Normally a clinical diagnosis. Investigate only if severe or early in course of epidemic

Insulinoma

TEST: P.insulin (H), C-Peptide suppression test (+), B.glucose (L).

SIGN: Signs of hypoglycaemia

DD: Diabetic medication abuse

PHYS: Tumours may be multiple.

Intussusception

TEST: Ba enema x-ray (AB).

SIGN: Dance's sign, abdominal pain, rectal bleeding or mucus, abdominal distension.

DD: Appendicitis, peritonitis, Meckel's diverticulitis, intestinal tumour.

Iron Deficiency Anaemia

See Anaemia, Iron Deficiency

Irritable Bowel Syndrome

TEST: To exclude other causes, test sigmoidoscopy, faeces M/C/S, FBC, S.electrolytes, B.urea, S.creatinine, LFT, rectal biopsy, barium enema, TFT.

SIGN: Mucus stools.

DD: Ulcerative colitis, bowel malignancy, bowel infection, diverticultis, colonic polyposis, haemorrhoids, Crohn's disease, anaemia, peptic ulcer, cholelithiasis.

PHYS: Primarily psychogenic in origin; diagnosis of exclusion.

Japanese Encephalitis

TEST: CSF anti-JE IgM (+), CSF lymphocytes (H), CSF neutrophils (H or N), CSF protein (H), EEG (AB).

SIGN: Convulsions, neck stiffness, Babinski's sign.

DD: Other acute encephalitis, cerebral malaria, cerebral abscess, amoebic meningitis, cerebral tumour.

PHYS: Caused by mosquito borne flavivirus throughout rural east and South Asia. Pigs are co-hosts.

Jaundice

See Anaemias; Cholecystitis; Cirrhosis; Hepatitis; Malaria; Pancreatitis; Yellow Fever
See also Carotenaemia
See also SYMPTOMS SECTION 1: Jaundice

Kala Azar (Visceral Leishmaniasis)

TEST: Spleen, liver or marrow biopsy (parasite isolated), specific immunological test (+), Hb (L), S.globulin (H), S.IgG (VH), WCC (L), platelets (L), B.monocytes (H), B.eosinophils (VL), ESR (H).

SIGN: Splenomegaly.

DD: Malaria, leukaemia, cirrhosis, TB, typhoid, histoplasmosis, brucellosis, schistosomiasis, septicaemia, trypanosomiasis, endocarditis.

PHYS: Infection by *Leishmania donovani* causes splenomegaly, hepatomegaly, fever and lymphadenopathy. Occurs in central Asia and Africa.

Keratoconjunctivitis Sicca

TEST: Slit lamp examination (AB).

SIGN: Schirmer's test.

DD: See Xerophthalmia in SYMPTOMS SECTION 1.

PHYS: May be associated with rheumatoid arthritis or Sjögren syn.

Kidney Disease

See Cystitis; Glomerulonephritis, Acute; Glomerulonephritis, Chronic; Nephrolithiasis; Nephrotic Syndrome; Pyelonephritis, Acute; Pyelonephritis, Chronic; Wilms' Tumour

Kidney Stones

See Nephrolithiasis

Klinefelter Syndrome

TEST: Chromosome count (XXY, XXYY or similar genotypes), sperm count (VL), U.gonadotrophins (H), FSH (H), S.LH (H or N), S.testosterone (L).

DD: Testicular trauma or surgery, radiation, chemotherapy, congenital hypogonadism.

PHYS: Genetic anomaly typified by small testes, gynaecomastia and infertility

See also SYNDROMES SECTION 6: Klinefelter Syndrome

Knee Injury

SIGN: McMurray sign, patellar tap, Apley's grind test, Lachman test.

DD: See Knee Pain in SYMPTOMS SECTION 1.

Korsakoff's Psychosis

See Wernicke-Korsakoff Syndrome

Kwashiorkor

TEST: S.albumin (L), S.protein (L), S.globulin (L or N), liver biopsy (fatty), Hb (L), BUN (L), S.potassium (L), B.cholesterol (L), S.ALP (L), S.amylase (L), S.lipase (L).

SIGN: Enophthalmos, cachexia, hepatomegaly, hypotension, ascites, pitting oedema.

DD: Chronic dysentery, TB, coeliac disease, pellagra, nephritis, worm infestations, marasmus, disseminated carcinoma, anorexia nervosa, terminal disease.

PHYS: Due to inadequate protein in diet, with presence of some carbohydrate.

Lassa Fever

TEST: Specific viral antigen (+), specific IgM (+), S.IgG (H), LFT (AB), B.urea (H), S.creatinine (H).

SIGN: Skin bleeding, mucous membrane bleeding, ascites, facial oedema.

DD: Viral and bacterial respiratory tract infections.

PHYS: West African viral haemorrhagic fever with high mortality rate, transmitted by rats.

Legionnaires' Disease

TEST: Sputum M/C/S (+), WCC (H), ESR (H), LFT (AB), U.protein (+), indirect fluorescent antibodies (+).

DD: Influenza, bronchitis, pneumonia, renal failure, Q fever, psittacosis, mycoplasma infection.

PHYS: Caused by *Legionella pneumophila*. Usually occurs in late summer in older people. Sensitive to erythromycin.

See also SECTION 5

Leishmaniasis, Visceral

See Kala Azar

Leprosy (Hansen's Disease)

TEST: Skin or lymph node biopsy microscopy (acid fast bacilli), lepromin test (+ or N).

SIGN: Charcot's joints, anaesthesia.

DD: Vitiligo, mycotic infections, SLE, psoriasis, scleroderma, motor neuron disease, yaws, leischmaniasis, neurofibromatosis, sarcoidosis, erythema nodosum.

PHYS: *Mycobacterium leprae* infection of skin and nerve tissue gives a mixed clinical picture that includes anaesthesia, gross skin lesions and deformities of hands, feet and face.

Leptospirosis

TEST: Specific serological test (+), blood or CSF M/C/S (+), WCC (AB), neutrophils (H), Hb (L or N), S.bilirubin (H or N), platelets (L), ESR (H),

U.protein (H), U.M/C/S (+), U.blood (+).

SIGN: Brudzinski's sign, Kernig's sign, neck stiffness.

DD: Meningitis, hepatitis, nephritis, influenza, septicaemia.

PHYS: Infection with Leptospira results in a two stage illness. Stage 1 is characterised by headache, myalgia, nausea and abdominal pain. Stage 2 presents with meningismus and fever.

Leukaemia, Acute

TEST: WCC (VH, occasionally L, immature cells common), marrow biopsy (AB), Hb (L), platelets (L), cytogenetics to classify type.

SIGN: Cachexia, hepatomegaly, splenomegaly, large kidney, retinal haemorrhages, Rinne's test, Roth's spots.

DD: Aplastic anaemia, infectious mononucleosis, Hodgkin's disease, lymphosarcoma, metastatic carcinoma, osteosarcoma.

PHYS: Excessive proliferation of white blood cells. Lymphatic and myeloblastic forms.

Leukaemia, Chronic Lymphatic (Lymphoblastic Leukaemia)

TEST: B.lymphocytes (VH), beta$_2$-microglobulin (H), WCC (VH), Hb (N or L), platelets (L), marrow biopsy (AB).

DD: Lymphosarcoma, infectious mononucleosis, infectious lymphocytosis, TB, syphilis, hyperthyroidism, SLE, toxoplasmosis, brucellosis, Hodgkin's disease, other chronic leukaemias.

PHYS: Progressive accumulation of small lymphocytes with pallor and lymph node enlargement.

Leukaemia, Chronic Myelocytic

TEST: WCC (VH), platelets (H), B.basophils (H), B.neutrophils and myelocytes (VH), beta$_2$-microglobulin (H), B.eosinophils (H), Hb (L), marrow biopsy (AB).

DD: Metastatic carcinoma, myelofibrosis, chronic infections, other chronic leukaemias.

PHYS: Proliferation of abnormal white cells resulting in lassitude, fever, splenomegaly and anaemia.

Lichen Planus

TEST: Skin biopsy (AB)

SIGN: Brittle nails

DD: Lichenified eczema, drug eruptions, psoriasis, secondary syphilis, pemphigus

PHYS: Cause unknown but may be autoimmune. Common drug precipitants include antimalarials, antituberculotics and heavy metals.

Listeriosis

TEST: B. culture (+), WCC (H).

DD: Influenza, septicemia.

PHYS: Caused by *Listeria monocytogenes* from poorly prepared or stored cheese, paté, etc.

Liver Disease
TEST: Screening tests include: S.bilirubin, S.AST, S.GGT, S.ALP, S.ALT.
PHYS: See PATHOLOGY SECTION 4 for test interpretation.

See also Cholecystitis; Cholelithiasis; Cirrhosis, Hepatic; Hepatic Metastases; Hepatitis; Malaria

Lockjaw
See Tetanus

Lumpy Jaw
See Actinomycosis

Lung Cancer (Bronchial Carcinoma)
TEST: Sputum microscopy (+), sputum culture (N), bronchial or node biopsy microscopy (AB), S.calcium (H with bony metastases), S.ACTH (H with oat cell form).
SIGN: Bronchial breathing, cachexia, clubbing of fingers, dull percussion note, Leser-Trelat sign, rhonchi, vocal fremitus.
DD: TB, bronchitis, pneumonia, sarcoidosis, secondary carcinoma, pituitary tumour, hyperpituitarism, thymoma, trauma.
PHYS: Presenting symptoms include haemoptysis, cachexia, finger clubbing, osteoarthropathy, hoarseness, cough and chest pain. Oat cell carcinomas may produce hormonal effects.

Lupus Erythematosus, Systemic [SLE] (Disseminated Lupus Erythematosus)
TEST: S.antinuclear antibodies (+), S.anti-DNA antibodies (+), S.HLA-DR3 (+), S.cardiolipin autoantibodies (+), S.histone autoantibodies (+ drug induced SLE), FANA (H), lupus anticoagulant antibodies (+), anti-Smith antibodies (H), B.LE cells (+), S.ANCA (H), S.complement C3 and C4(H), DNA Autoantibodies (+), S.ENA (H), Serum WCC (L), Hb (L), VDRL (false +), platelets (L), S.albumin (N or L), S.gamma-globulin (N or H), LFT (AB), Coombs' test (+), U.protein (+), ESR (H), CRP (N or H), synovial fluid WBC (H), S.complement (L), U.microscopy (+ casts, + blood).
SIGN: Alopecia, butterfly rash, choreiform movements, discoid rash, hypertension, large kidney, onycholysis, oral ulcers, photosensitivity, pleural effusion, splenomegaly, multiple system lesions.
DD: Rheumatoid arthritis, rheumatic fever, TB, scleroderma, glomerulonephritis, syphilis, Sjögren syn., dermatomyositis.
PHYS: Chronic inflammatory condition of skin, joints, kidneys and nervous system.

Lyme Disease
TEST: Specific IgM antibodies (+), S.IgG (H).
SIGN: Chronic migratory skin erythema, neck stiffness, lymphadenopathy.
DD: Other infectious diseases causing migratory arthralgia, fever and rashes.
PHYS: Tick transmitted spirochaetal infection most common in USA.

Lymphoblastic Leukaemia
See Leukaemia, Chronic Lymphatic

Lymphogranuloma Venereum (Chlamydial Infection)
TEST: Urine or swab PCR (+), urine or swab LCR (+), specific Chlamydia serology (+).
DD: Syphilis granuloma inguinale, carcinoma, genetal herpes, trauma, scabies, impetigo, chancroid, erythema multiforme.
PHYS: Transient, small painful or painless lesions of the genitals that are followed 2 to 6 weeks later by regional lymphadenopathy that may suppurate.

See also Chlamydia Infection

Lymphoma
See Hodgkin's Disease

Lymphoplasmacytoid Lymphoma
See Waldenström's Macroglobulinaemia

Malabsorption Syndromes
TEST: Screening tests include: B.FBC, S.albumin, faecal fat, S.cholesterol, S.calcium, S.phosphate, S.ALP, prothrombin time, S.carotene, Hb, S.iron, S.folic acid, S.electrolytes, S.glucose, S.vitamin B_{12}, faeces M/C/S.
DD: See SYMPTOMS SECTION 1
PHYS: Failure to thrive, muscle wasting, deformities, diarrhoea, anaemia, dehydration and ascites are some of the symptoms associated with a wide variety of malabsorption diseases. May be due to poor nutrition; gut, pancreatic, lymphatic or liver diseases; infections or drugs. See individual tests in PATHOLOGY SECTION 4 for interpretation .

Malaria
TEST: Blood smear microscopy (+), S.bilirubin (H), U.bilirubin (+), Hb (L), WCC (N or L), platelets (L), VDRL (false + or N), S.AST (H), S.ALT (H).
SIGN: Jaundice, cachexia, chloasma, hepatomegaly, splenomegaly.
DD: Typhus, amoebiasis, typhoid, relapsing fever, hepatitis, dengue fever, septicaemia, hypoglycaemia, meningitis, CNS lesions, pneumonia, viral infections, encephalitis, drugs, leptospirosis, schistosomiasis, lymphoma, leishmaniasis, Lassa fever.

PHYS: Infection of red blood cells by Plasmodium genus, injected by Anopheles mosquito that acts as a transmitter from host to host. Characterised by fevers, chills, malaise, splenomegaly and anaemia.

Malnutrition
See Kwashiorkor

Mastocytosis
TEST: U.histamine (H), S.tryptase (H), biopsy (AB)
SIGN: Darier's sign
DD: Urticaria, carcinoid tumour, angioedema
PHYS: Indolent mast cell hyperplasia

Measles (Morbilli)
TEST: Throat swab or blood culture (+), specific antibody test (RT), nephritis, WCC (L), nasal exudate microscopy (giant cells).
DD: Rubella, scarlet fever, roseola infantum, infectious mononucleosis, drug eruptions, secondary syphilis, allergies, other viral infections.
PHYS: Highly contagious viral infection characterised by rash and inflammation of conjunctivae and respiratory tract. Complications include otitis media, pneumonia and encephalomyelitis.

Measles, German
See Rubella

Melioidosis
TEST: Blood or sputum culture (+), S.IgM antibody test (+), indirect haemagglutination test (+), chest x-ray (AB).
DD: Pneumonia, bronchitis, septicaemia.
PHYS: Fulminating lung and blood infection of tropical regions (particularly South East Asia) caused by Pseudomonas pseudomallei.

Meningitis, Aseptic (Viral Meningitis)
TEST: CSF turbidity (clear), CSF cells (H), CSF M/C/S (−), CSF glucose (N), CSF protein (N or H), WCC (N or H).
SIGN: Neck stiffness, Kernig's sign, Brudzinski's sign.
DD: Bacterial or fungal meningitis, cerebral abscess, leptospirosis, TB, neurosyphilis, toxoplasmosis, leukaemia, malignancies, rabies, encephalitis.
PHYS: Acute infection of meninges due to virus or unknown cause. Runs a short, uncomplicated course with full recovery.

Meningitis, Bacterial
TEST: CSF M/C/S (+), CSF glucose (L), CSF turbidity (+), CSF cells (H-VH), CSF protein (H), blood culture (+ or −), S.LDH (H), WCC (H), U.protein (+), CSF pressure (H).

SIGN: Brudzinski's sign, Cheyne-Stokes respiration, Kernig's sign, neck stiffness, opisthotonus (spinal), papilloedema, Rinne's test.
DD: Aseptic meningitis, empyema, cerebral abscess, other febrile conditions, trauma, dehydration, TB, lead encephalopathy, drugs.
PHYS: Infection of meninges by Streptococcus pneumoniae, Neisseria meningitidis, Haemophilus influenzae or other bacteria causing fever, headache, lethargy, confusion, neck stiffness and nausea. Disseminated intravascular clotting a dangerous complication.

Menopause
TEST: U. and S.FSH (H), S.estradiol (L), S.LH (H), Pap. smear (AB), U.oestrogens (L), B.HGG (H), S.DHEA-S (L).
DD: Pregnancy, anxiety states, depression, hyperthyroidism, phaeochromocytoma, hypothyroidism, ovarian and uterine neoplasms.
PHYS: Due to cessation of ovarian function from age, surgery or irradiation.

Mercury Poisoning
TEST: B.mercury (H).
SIGN: Excess salivation, oedema of mucous membranes, ataxia, intention tremor, nail discolouration, cachexia, melaena.

Metastatic Carcinoma
See Hepatic Metastases

Migraine
TEST: None specific. Lumbar puncture and EEG may be indicated in some cases to exclude pathological cause.
SIGN: Vomiting, dysarthria, hemiparesis, neck stiffness.
DD: Cerebral tumour, cerebral abscess, trauma, meningitis, TB, neurosyphilis, metastatic carcinoma, temporal arteritis, toxins, drugs, hypertension, cluster headaches, glaucoma, sinusitis, dental causes, hysteria, muscle tension headaches.
PHYS: Paroxysmal headache causing nausea, visual disturbances and gut disturbances due to vascular alterations in the cerebrum. A brief vasoconstriction is followed by a prolonged vasodilation.

Mikulicz' Disease
See Sjögren Syndrome

Miscarriage
See Abortion, Recurrent

Mongolism
See Down Syndrome

Moniliasis
See Candidiasis

Mononucleosis, Infectious
See Infectious Mononucleosis

Morbilli
See Measles

Motor Neurone Disease
TEST: Brain CT (AB for bulbar form), myelogram (AB for amyotrophic lateral sclerosis), electromyography (AB with progressive muscular atrophy), nerve conduction studies (AB), muscle biopsy (AB).
SIGN: Fasciculation, hypotonia, muscle wasting, paradoxical reflexes.
DD: Extreme stress, cervical spondylosis, spinal tumour, polymyositis, poliomyelitis, pernicious anaemia, multiple sclerosis, brain stem tumour, metastatic carcinoma, hyperparathyroidism, hypophosphataemia, hyperthyroidism, heavy metal poisoning.
PHYS: Multifactorial disease with wide range of symptoms associated with motor nerve impairment.

MS
See Multiple Sclerosis

Multiple Myeloma
TEST: S.electrophoresis (abnormal spike), marrow aspirate (myeloma cells), Hb (L), beta$_2$-microglobulin (H), ESR (H), S.protein (H and AB), WCC (N), B.plasma cells (H), B.platelets (L), U.Bence-Jones protein (+), S.creatinine (H), S.calcium (H), S.globulin (VH), S.gamma-globulin (L excl. spike), S.urea (H), P.viscosity (H), S.anion gap (L), S.cyanocobalamin (L).
DD: Leukaemia, infection, renal failure, skeletal disease, sarcoma, secondary carcinoma, hyperparathyroidism, cirrhosis.
PHYS: Plasma cell neoplasia. Anaemia is due to bone marrow replacement. An abnormal gamma-globulin is found in serum and urine due to an immune response to abnormal plasma cells with suppression of normal gamma-globulin.

Multiple Sclerosis [MS] (Disseminated Sclerosis)
TEST: CSF protein (N or H), CSF cells (N or H), routine haematology (N), HLA-D3 (+), S.IgG (H), electrophysiological tests (AB), MRI (AB).

SIGN: Ankle clonus, peripheral reflexes abnormal, Babinski's sign, consensual reflex, nystagmus, papilloedema, flaccid or spastic paralysis, Rinne's test, scanning speech, intention tremor.
DD: Cerebral tumours, cerebral degeneration, cerebrovascular disease, motor neurone disease, cervical spondylosis, neurosyphilis.
PHYS: Demyelinating disorder of brain or cord giving wide variations in symptoms, signs, severity and prognosis.

Mumps
TEST: U. or saliva virus isolation (+), specific antibody titre (RT), WCC (H), S.amylase (H).
SIGN: Parotid adenitis.
DD: Parotitis, bacterial adenitis, lymphadenitis, obstructed salivary duct, quinsy, parotid tumours, meningitis, Mikulicz' disease, sarcoidosis.
PHYS: Acute, contagious viral infection of salivary glands, testes and pancreas.

Muscular Dystrophy
TEST: Muscle biopsy (AB), intrauterine chorionic villus sampling (AB), U.creatinine (H), S.CPK (H), S.AST (H), S.aldolase (H), electromyelography (AB).
SIGN: Peripheral reflexes, muscular atrophy, claw hand, fasciculation, hypotonia, flaccid paralysis, waddling gait, wrist drop, Gowers' manoeuvre.
DD: Orthopaedic anomalies, neurogenic diseases, polio, cretinism, gonadal disorders, Charcot-Marie-Tooth disease, polyneuritis.
PHYS: Inherited myopathies characterised by progressive, severe, muscular weakness. Many different subgroups.

Myasthenia Gravis
TEST: Response to cholinergic drugs (+), S.HLA-DR3 (+), S.anti-AChR (RT), electrophysiological studies (AB), S.skeletal muscle antibodies (+).
SIGN: Ptosis, flaccid paralysis.
DD: Hysteria, exhaustion botulism, peripheral neuropathy, polymyositis, amyotrophic lateral sclerosis, thymoma.
PHYS: Abnormal fatigue state, particularly in cranial and ocular muscles, that is reversed by cholinergic drugs.

Mycoplasma Infections
See Pneumonia

Myelocytic Leukaemia
See Leukaemia, Chronic Myelocytic

Myelofibrosis, Idiopathic
TEST: Bone marrow biopsy (AB), WCC (AB), B.Hb (L), B.platelets (H), S.folate (L), long bone x-ray (sclerosis).

SIGN: Splenomegaly, hepatomegaly
DD: Polycythemia rubra vera, chronic myelogenous leukaemia
PHYS: Caused by bone marrow fibrosis. Slow mid-life onset.

Myeloma, Multiple
See Multiple Myeloma

Myocardial Infarct
TEST: S.CK (H,12-72 hrs.), S.CK-MB factor (H, 4-48 hrs), S.troponin T (+ for 7 days), S.troponin I (+ for 7 days), S.AST (H, 18-72 hrs.), S.LDH (H, 1-7 days), S.ALT (H), WCC (H), ESR (H or N), S.aldolase (H). S.myoglobin (H, 15min-12 hrs), ECG (AB).
SIGN: Bradycardia, extrasystolic beats, atrial fibrillation, hypotension, gallop rhythm, pericardial friction rub, pleural effusion (late).
DD: Angina pectoris, pneumothorax, chest wall trauma, pulmonary thrombosis, oesophagitis, ischaemic heart disease, pericarditis, aortic aneurysm, pleurisy, neuralgia, Tietze syn., Bornholm disease, peptic ulcer, cholecystitis, pancreatitis, neuroses.
PHYS: Muscle necrosis causes release of enzymes into the blood stream. Any muscle trauma or major organ disease may cause elevation of enzyme levels. Enzyme levels peak at different times, as shown in the following graph:

Enzyme Levels Post-Myocardial Infarct

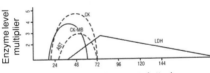

Hours after onset of attack

Myocarditis
TEST: B.culture (+), B.myocardial autoantibodies (+), WCC (AB), ESR (H), CRP (H), S.CK (H), S.CK-MB (H), S.troponin I (+), S.troponin T (+), myocardial biopsy M/C/S (+).
SIGN: Atrial fibrillation.
DD: All cardiac diseases, septicaemia, autoimmune diseases (eg. SLE, polyarteritis nodosa), drugs (eg. daunorubicin, adriamycin)
PHYS: Infection of the myocardium by virus, bacteria, protozoa or metazoa giving varied cardiac symptoms.

Myopathies
TEST: S.CK (H), U.myoglobin (+) ESR (H), CRP (H), S.Jo-1 antibodies (+) muscle biopsy (AB).
SIGN: Hypotonia.

DD: Alcoholism, autoimmune diseases (eg. SLE), sarcoidosis, electrolyte disturbances, hypothyroidism, Cushing syn., hereditary and acquired muscle dystrophies, drug reactions (eg. clofibrate, penicillamine)

Myxoedema
See Hypothyroidism

Narcolepsy
TEST: S.HLA-DR2 (+), sleep EEG (AB).
DD: Sleep apnoea, depression, schizophrenia, fugue states, CNS tumours, CNS infections, CNS trauma, anaemia, malnutrition, hepatic failure, renal failure, encephalopathies, allergies, hypothyroidism, hypoglycaemia, drugs (eg. alcohol, antidepressants, antihistamines).
PHYS: Disorder of excessive sleepiness in daytime.

Narcotic Addiction
TEST: B.analysis for specific drugs (+), LFT (AB).
SIGN: Sweating, restlessness, pinpoint pupils, piloerection ('gooseflesh'), needle tracking over veins, anxiety.
DD: Iatrogenic addition, alcoholism.
PHYS: Often use stories of migraine, renal colic, etc. to obtain drugs from doctors.

Nematode Infestations
See Roundworms, Intestinal; Trichinosis

Nephroblastoma
See Wilms' Tumour

Nephrolithiasis (Kidney Stones; Calculi, Renal)
TEST: U.protein (+), U.blood (+), U.microscopy (cells and crystals + or –), S.calcium (N or H), U.calcium (N or H), S.uric acid (N or H), calculi microscopy (determine type).
DD: Pyelonephritis, renal TB, renal tumour, renal infarct, appendicitis, peptic ulcer, cholecystitis, pancreatitis, peritonitis.
PHYS: Calculi of the urinary tract may be formed from calcium, oxalate, urate, or cystine. Cause acute pain if moving in ureter, or asympotomatic if stationary.

Nephrotic Syndrome
TEST: Renal biopsy (+), U.protein (VH), S.albumin (L), U.glucose (+), S.globulins [alpha$_1$ and gamma (L), alpha$_2$ and beta (H)], S.fibrinogen (H), S.cholesterol (H), S.triglycerides (H), U.microscopy (casts and cells), Hb (L).
SIGN: Pitting oedema, pleural effusion, shifting dullness, fluid thrill (ascites), hypertension.

DD: Glomerulonephritis, SLE, polyarteritis, amyloidosis, renal vein thrombosis, diabetes, myxoedema, multiple myeloma, malaria, toxins, drugs, neoplasms.

PHYS: Syndrome characterised by heavy urinary protein loss. Many causes, including those listed in DD above. May be idiopathic in children.

See also SYNDROMES SECTION 6: Nephrotic Syndrome

Niemann-Pick Disease

TEST: Tissue sphingomyelinase assay (AB), marrow biopsy (lipid filled macrophages).

SIGN: Convulsions, splenomegaly, hepatomegaly.

DD: Gaucher's disease, hyperglyceridaemia, cretinism.

PHYS: Excessive tissue storage of sphinogomyelin. Often inherited. Invariably fatal.

Nonspecific Urethritis [NSU]

TEST: Urethral or vaginal swab M/C/S (– or Chlamydiae +), VDRL (–), FTA (–).

DD: Gonorrhoea, syphilis, Reiter syn.

PHYS: Urethritis or vaginitis for which no specific cause can be demonstrated. Responds to tetracycline.

Obesity

TEST: Complications or pathological causes may be excluded by: S.cholesterol, S.triglycerides, TFT, DHEA-S, S.17-hydroxy steroids, S.insulin, B.glucose. For interpretation of these tests see PATHOLOGY SECTION 4.
Body Mass Index = Weight in kg/Height in m². Normal range: 20-25; <30: Obese; >40: Morbid obesity.

DD: Hypothyroidism, Cushing's disease, Stein-Leventhal syn., insulinoma.

PHYS: Excess adipose tissue may be due to excessive caloric intake, lack of exercise or the pathological causes listed in DD above.

Onchocerciasis

TEST: Skin snip microscopy (+), B.eosinophils (H), antifilarial complement fixing antibodies (+), Mazzotti test (+).

DD: Diabetes mellitus, uraemia, cirrhosis, eczema, other filariae.

PHYS: Filarial infection of skin, eye and lymph nodes. Endemic in central Africa, Arabia and Central America.

Orf

TEST: Electron microscopy of vesicle fluid (+), lesion microscopy (granulomatous reaction), specific complement fixing antibodies (+).

DD: Milkers' warts, anthrax, tularaemia, TB inoculation, cowpox.

PHYS: Disease of sheep and goats. Hard vesicles on hands and arms that break down to crusting sores.

Ornithosis
See Psittacosis

Osteitis Deformans
See Paget's Disease of Bone

Osteoarthritis

TEST: Synovial fluid microscopy WCC (H), cartilage fragments, ESR (N), WCC (N), bone scan (+). No specific tests.

SIGN: Heberden's nodes, Bouchard's nodes.

DD: Rheumatoid arthritis, haemochromatosis, neuropathies, ankylosing spondylitis, gonococcal arthritis, psoriasis, Reiter syn., rheumatic fever, fibrositis, sarcoidosis, Sjögren syn., brucellosis, TB, syphilis, diabetes, trauma, gout, haemophilia, scurvy, tumours, osteochondritis dessicans, drugs, leukaemia, etc.

PHYS: Degenerative joint disease, particularly involving major joints.

Osteomalacia (Rickets)

TEST: S.vit. D (L), B.calcium (N or L), S.25-hydroxy-vit. D (L), S.phosphate (L), S.parathyroid hormone (H), S.ALP (H), U.calcium (VL), faecal fat (H), U.phosphate (L), U.hydroxyproline/creatinine ratio (H).

SIGN: Chvostek's sign, frontal bossing, Trousseau's sign.

DD: Osteoporosis, Paget's disease, scurvy, cretinism, osteogenesis imperfecta, renal rickets, Fanconi syn., hyperparathyroidism, multiple myeloma.

PHYS: Softening of bone due to inadequate or ineffective levels of vit. D, resulting in reduced calcium absorption from the gut. Rickets is the infantile form.

Osteomyelitis

TEST: Bone or marrow biopsy M/C/S (+), ESR (H), B.culture (+ or –), WCC (H), Hb (N or L).

DD: Polio, rheumatic fever, myositis, sprains, fractures, Osgood-Schlatter's disease, Still's disease, septic arthritis.

PHYS: Infection of bone causing fever and localised bone pain.

Osteoporosis

TEST: S.calcium (N), S.phosphate (N), S.ALP (N), U.calcium (H or N), U.deoxypyridinoline (H), U.cross-linked N-telepeptides (H), U.hydroxyproline/creatinine ratio (H), dual

photon densitometry (AB), vertebral x-ray (AB).
DD: Cushing syn., multiple myeloma, hyperparathyroidism, osteogenesis imperfecta, metastatic carcinoma.
PHYS: Absence of normal quality of bone, rather than a bone disease. Blood tests unreliable. Diseases associated with osteoporosis include hyperthyroidism, hyperparathyroidism, Cushing syn., hypogonadism, rheumatoid arthritis, chronic renal and hepatic disease, multiple myeloma and malabsorption syndromes. Risk factors include early menopause, family history, corticosteroid use, smoking, excess alcohol, physical inactivity, low weight.

Osteosarcoma
See Bone Cancer

Otitis Media
TEST: Ear exudate M/C/S (+), WCC (H).
SIGN: Rinne's test.
DD: Otitis externa, mastoiditis, pharyngitis, laryngitis, dental disease, temporomandibular joint disorders, glue ear.
PHYS: Acute bacterial infection of middle ear causing pain, fever, hearing loss and discharge.

Otosclerosis
TEST: Audiometry (AB), Rinne's test (+ affected ear), Weber's test)+ affected ear).
SIGN: Itard Cholena's sign.

Ovarian Tumour
TEST: S.DHEA-S (H or N), S.CASA (+), ultrasound (AB), abdominal x-ray (AB), culdocentesis microscopy (AB), CA 5 (H), S.HCG (H), S.alpha-fetoprotein (H), D-Dimer (H).
SIGN: Pelvic mass, abdominal pain and tenderness, ascites.
DD: Uterine myomas, hydrosalpinx, diverticulitis, colonic tumours, pelvic kidney, metastatic carcinoma.
PHYS: Tumours have many forms from teratomas and cancer to follicle and corpus luteum cysts.

See also Ovarian Mass in SIGNS SECTION 2.

Paget's Disease of Bone (Osteitis Deformans)
TEST: S.ALP (VH), S.ACP (H), U.calcium (H), S.calcium (N), S.phosphate (N), U.deoxypyridinoline (H), U.cross-linked N-telopeptides (+), U.hydroxyproline (H), U.hydroxyproline/creatinine ratio (H).
DD: Metastatic carcinoma, hyperparathyroidism, multiple myeloma, osteosarcoma.
PHYS: Chronic, progressive disorder of bone causing gross bony deformities. Usually localised and asymmetrical.

PAN
See Polyarteritis Nodosa

Pancreatic Cancer
TEST: S.CA 19-9 (H), S.CA 50 (H), S.CEA (H), ultrasound (AB), CT (AB), ERCP (AB).
SIGN: Jaundice, migratory thrombophlebitis, splenomegaly.
DD: Pancreatitis, peptic ulcer, hepatitis, hiatus hernia.

Pancreatic Fibrosis
See Cystic Fibrosis

Pancreatitis
TEST: S.amylase (VH), S.lipase (H), S.trypsinogen (H), WCC (H), U.Amylase (H), BUN (H), U.glucose (N or H), B.glucose (N or H), S.bilirubin (N or H), S.calcium (L), S.albumin (L), S.potassium (L), U.protein (+), GTT (AB), S.ALP (H), Ultrasound (AB or N), CT (AB or N), ERCP (AB).
SIGN: Abdominal rigidity, abdominal rebound tenderness, pleural effusion.
DD: Peptic ulcer, biliary colic, renal colic, acute cholecystitis, small bowel obstruction, mesenteric thrombosis, dissecting aneurysm, peritonitis, myocardial infarct, porphyria, SLE, periarteritis nodosa.
PHYS: Acute inflammation of the pancreas due to gall stones, alcohol, trauma, infection, drugs, carcinoma, regional enteritis or idiopathic processes.

Paralysis Agitans
See Parkinson's Disease

Parathyroid Disease
See Hyperparathyroidism; Hypoparathyroidism

Parkinson's Disease (Paralysis Agitans)
TEST: None specific.
SIGN: Cogwheel rigidity, festination, hypertonicity, lead-pipe rigidity, parkinsonism, parkinsonian facies, resting tremor.
DD: Carbon monoxide poisoning, heavy metal poisoning, cerebral tumours, degenerative disease, alcoholism, drugs, encephalitis, arteriosclerosis.
PHYS: Insidiously progressive disease of unknown aetiology that produces a bland facies, tremor, rigidity and akinesia.

Pellagra
TEST: S.nicotinic acid (L), S.folic acid (L), Hb (L), S.riboflavine (L), S.vit. B_6 (L), S.vit. B_{12} (L).

DD: Sunburn, malabsorption syndromes, intestinal parasites, pernicious anaemia.
PHYS: Due to dietary deficit of niacin (nicotinic acid). Symptoms include anaemia, glossitis, malaise, diarrhoea and a red, blistering rash.

Pelvic Inflammatory Disease [PID]
TEST: Vaginal, cervical, urethral or endometrial swab M/C/S (+ or –), Pap smear (AB or N), ESR (H), WCC (H), CRP (H), laparoscopy (AB), hysterosalpingography (N or AB).
SIGN: Pelvic pain, secondary dysmenorrhoea, menstrual abnormalities, dyspareunia, infertility.
DD: Endometriosis, ovarian cysts and neoplasms, uterine fibroids and myomas, bowel neoplasms.
PHYS: May be preceded by acute intraperitoneal infection.

Pemphigoid
TEST: Skin biopsy microscopy (+), S.basement membrane autoantibodies (+), B.eosinophils (H), S.IgE (H), ESR (H)
DD: Pemphigus, contact dermatitis, exfoliative dermatitis, impetigo, urticaria, erythema multiforme

Pemphigus
TEST: Skin biopsy microscopy (+), S.intracellular cement substance antibodies (+), WCC (H), S.protein (VL), S.albumin (L), Hb (L), S.globulins (H), B.fibrinogen (H), S.sodium (L), S.chloride (L), ESR (H), S.calcium (L), S.potassium (N or H).
SIGN: Nikolsky sign
DD: Pemphigoid, contact dermatitis, exfoliative dermatitis, impetigo, urticaria, erythema multiforme.
PHYS: Skin disorder of unknown cause characterised by massive serum filled bullae and mucous membrane erosions.

Peptic Ulcer
TEST: Faecal blood (+ or –), Hb (N or L), ^{14}C breath test (+), CLO test (+), gastric acid release after histamine stimulation (H or N), S.Helicobacter pylori antibodies (+ or –).
SIGN: Abdominal rigidity (perforated), coffee grounds vomitus (penetrated), abdominal rebound tenderness.
DD: Peritonitis, pancreatitis, appendicitis, cholecystitis, pleurisy, myocardial infarct, pericarditis, oesophagitis, gastritis, intestinal carcinoma, Crohn's disease, TB, sarcoidosis, mesenteric adenitis, lymphoma, Zollinger-Ellison syn., drugs (eg NSAID, corticosteroids).
PHYS: Ulceration of the upper intestinal tract due to hypersecretion of acid and/or decreased tissue resistance.

Periarteritis Nodosa
See Polyarteritis Nodosa

Pericarditis, Infectious
TEST: B. culture (+ or–), WCC (H), pericardial biopsy microscopy (AB), cardiac enzymes (N), ECG (AB).
SIGN: Friction rub, gallop rhythm (constrictive), hepatomegaly, hypotension (constrictive), jugular venous pressure (constrictive), pleural effusion (constrictive), pulsus paradoxus (constrictive), shifting dullness (ascites), fluid thrill (ascites), atrial fibrillation.
DD: Trauma, myocardial infarct, SLE, rheumatic fever, allergies, drugs, neoplasms of heart and lung, sarcoma, pleurisy.
PHYS: Infection of the pericardium by virus, bacteria, (inc. TB) or mycoses causes effusion, pain and friction rub. May progress to cardiac failure with acute bacterial infections.

Peritonitis
TEST: Peritoneal aspirate M/C/S (+), WCC (H), S.electrolytes (AB).
SIGN: Abdominal rigidity, abdominal rebound tenderness, shifting dullness (ascites).
DD: Intestinal obstruction, acute cholecystitis, pelvic inflammatory disease, renal colic, gastrointestinal haemorrhage, ectopic pregnancy, mesenteric adenitis, acute urinary infections, biliary colic, peptic ulcer, SLE, appendicitis, pneumonia, porphyria, tabes dorsalis, familial Mediterranean fever, hysteria.
PHYS: Infection of the peritoneal cavity due to obstruction, infarct, neoplasia or inflammation of any hollow viscus; infection of viscera; idiopathic or iatrogenic causes.

Peritonsillar Abscess
See Quinsy

Pernicious Anaemia
See Anaemia, Pernicious

Pertussis (Whooping Cough)
TEST: Sputum or nasal swab M/C/S (+), sputum or nasal swab pertussis IgA antibodies (+ immediately), S.pertussis antibodies (+ later), WCC (H), B.lymphocytes (H).
DD: Coryza, influenza, tracheobronchitis, allergic bronchitis, pneumonia, cystic fibrosis, foreign body aspiration.
PHYS: Acute respiratory illness due to Bordetella pertussis that causes prolonged inspiratory effort and paroxysmal coughing.

Pheochromocytoma
TEST: U.HMMA (VH), U.catecholamines (H),

S.catecholamines (H), U.metanephrine (H).
SIGN: Hypertension, tachycardia, cardiomegaly.
DD: Essential hypertension, hyperthyroidism,
diabetes, psychoneuroses.
PHYS: Catecholamine producing tumour of the
sympathetic nerve tissue, usually in the adrenal
glands, causes marked hypertension that may
be episodic.

Pharyngitis
TEST: Throat swab M/C/S (+), viral serology (+ or –),
WCC (N or AB)
SIGN: Cervical adenitis
DD: Infectious mononucleosis, diphtheria, *Herpes
simplex* infection, Vincent's angina, leukaemia,
AIDS
PHYS: Bacterial, viral or rarely fungal infection of
pharynx

See also Diphtheria

Phenylketonuria [PKU]
TEST: B.phenylalanine (H)
SIGN: Skin hypopigmentation
DD: Other causes of mental retardation (see
SYMPTOMS SECTION 1)
PHYS: Congenital

PID
See Pelvic Inflammatory Disease

Pinworm (Enterobiasis)
TEST: Perineal skin scrapings microscopy (+), faecal
microscopy (+ or –).
DD: Perineal eczema, candidiasis, sweat rash,
haemorrhoids.
PHYS: Intestinal infection by *Enterobius vermicularis*.

Pituitary Disease
See Hypopituitarism

Pityriasis Versicolor
TEST: Skin scrapings (fungal +).
SIGN: Chip sign, depigmentation of skin, café-au-lait
spots.
DD: Pityriasis alba, eczema, vitiligo, leucoderma,
yaws.
PHYS: Superficial fungal infection of skin. Often
chronic, usually asymptomatic.

PKU
See Phenylketonuria

Plague, Bubonic (Black Death)
TEST: Blood or bubo M/C/S (+), WCC (H),
B.neutrophils (H), ESR (H), U.protein (+ or –).

DD: Tularaemia, malaria, lymphogranuloma
venereum, influenza, pneumonia, septicaemia.
PHYS: Infection of rats by *Yersinia (Pasteurella) pestis*,
transmitted to man by fleas.

Pleurisy
TEST: Pleural fluid M/C/S (+), pleural biopsy (AB)
SIGNS: Pleural and/or pericardial friction rub
DD: Bacterial or viral pleural or pulmonary infection,
pleurodynia (Bornholm disease), lung
carcinoma, subphrenic abscess, pulmonary
infarct, connective tissue disease (eg. SLE),
mesothelioma
PHYS: Inflammation and/or infection of the pleura.

Pleurodynia (Bornholm Disease)
TEST: Specific antibody titre (RT), throat swab and
viral isolation (+), WCC (N).
DD: May mimic all acute thoracic and abdominal
conditions.
PHYS: Coxsackievirus infection characterised by
sudden chest or abdominal pain.

Pneumonia
TEST: Sputum M/C/S (+), WCC (H), CRP (H), ESR (H),
B.culture (+ or –), cold agglutinins (+ with
mycoplasma), B.pO$_2$ (L or N), respiratory
function tests (AB), chest x-ray (AB).
SIGN: Bronchial breathing, crepitations, dull percussion
note, pericardial friction rub, hypoventilation,
whispering pectoriloquy, vocal fremitus.
DD: TB, psittacosis, Q fever, tularaemia, pulmonary
infarct, atelectasis, subphrenic abscess,
bronchogenic carcinoma, bronchitis.
PHYS: Acute infection of lungs due to *Streptococcus
pneumoniae, Haemophilus influenzae,
Klebsiella pneumoniae, Mycoplasma
pneumoniae* or other bacteria.

Pneumothorax, Spontaneous
TEST: Chest x-ray.
SIGN: Amphoric breathing, apex beat displacement,
cavernous breathing, coin test, hyperventilation
or hypoventilation, tracheal displacement,
thoracic tympany, vocal fremitus.
DD: Asthma, chronic bronchitis, trauma, TB,
pulmonary infarct, pleurodynia, pulmonary
abscess, emphysema, histiocytosis X.
PHYS: Lung rupture releases air into pleural space.
Due to trauma, disease or idiopathic causes.

Poliomyelitis
TEST: Throat or faecal virology (+), specific antibodies
(RT), WCC (N or H), CSF cells (H), CSF protein
(H), CSF sugar (N).
SIGN: Peripheral reflexes, ataxia, muscular atrophy,
fasciculation, heel-knee test, hypotonia, nose-
finger test, flaccid paralysis.

DD: Aseptic meningitis, Gullain-Barré syn., tick or snake bite paralysis, mumps, influenza, encephalitis, acute polyneuritis, porphyria, hysteria, spinal trauma or tumour, rabies, poisons (eg. arsenic).

PHYS: Contagious viral disease of CNS producing symptoms ranging from transient malaise to flaccid paralysis and death.

Polyarteritis Nodosa [PAN] (Periarteritis Nodosa)

TEST: Open biopsy of symptomatic site (+), WCC (H), B.eosinophils (H), ESR (H), S.CRP (H), S.ALP (H), U.protein and blood (+ or –), renal biopsy (AB).

SIGN: Hepatomegaly, splenomegaly, large kidney, hypertension, tachycardia, petechiae, cardiac arrhythmias, neurological lesions.

DD: Allergic angiitis, granulomatosis, rheumatoid arthritis, Goodpasture syn., SLE, syphilis, necrotising vasculitis, endocarditis, leptospirosis, transverse myelitis.

PHYS: Necrotic nodules form along major arteries, particularly at junctions. Secondary glomerulonephritis and liver involvement common. Aetiology unknown.

Polycystic Ovarian Syndrome

See Stein-Leventhal Syndrome

Polycythaemia (Rubra) Vera (Erythraemia)

TEST: Erythrocyte count (VH), absolute RBC volume (H), Hb (H), WCC (H), B.reticulocytes (H), P.erythropoietin (L), platelets (H), S.bilirubin (H), marrow biopsy (hyperplastic), hematocrit (H), neutrophil alkaline phosphatase (H).

SIGN: Splenomegaly, choreiform movements.

DD: Leukaemia, cardiopulmonary disease, hepatic disease.

PHYS: Chronic hyperplasia of red blood cells. Diverse symptomatology.

Polymyalgia Rheumatica

TEST: ESR (VH), CRP (H), Hb (L), S.ALP (N or H), technetium scan (AB).

DD: Rheumatoid arthritis, polymyositis, SLE, polyarteritis nodosa, ankylosing spondylitis, polychondritis, giant cell arteritis, viraemia, brucellosis, tuberculosis, malignancies, multiple myeloma, osteoarthritis, sarcoidosis, depression, psychogenic.

PHYS: Syndrome of muscle inflammation in the neck, shoulders and pelvis.

Polymyositis

TEST: S.CK (H), ESR (H), S.ANA (+), S.ENA (+), CRP (H), S.Jo-1 antibodies (+ in some forms), muscle biopsy (AB), electromyography (AB)

SIGN: Fasciculation, Gottron's sign

DD: SLE, dermatomyosistis, other connective tissue diseases

PHYS: Autoimmune connective tissue disease

See also SYMPTOMS SECTION 1: Paralysis and Muscular Weakness

Porphyria, Acute Hepatic

TEST: B.porphyrins (H), U.aminolevulenic acid and porpholbilinogen [Watson-Schwartz test] (VH), faecal porphyrin (H), RBC porphobilinogen deaminase (L), BSP retention test (H), S.sodium (L), FBC (N).

DD: All causes of acute abdomen, hyperthyroidism, eclampsia, hysteria.

PHYS: Faulty pyrole metabolism results in excessive secretion of porphyrins. Urine becomes dark brown on standing. Varied symptoms include acute abdominal pain. Aggravated by barbiturates and oral contraceptives.

Porphyria, Latent Hepatic (Porphyria Cutanea Tarda)

TEST: Faecal porphyrins (H), U.porphyrins (N).

DD: Skin lesions especially with exposure to sun.

PHYS: Dominant genetic disease aggravated by barbiturates and oral contraceptives.

Pre-eclampsia

See Eclampsia and Pre-eclampsia

Pregnancy, Antenatal Care

TEST: Investigations that should be carried out at first antenatal visit: FBC, Hb, blood group. Rh titres (if Rh–), rubella antibodies, S.RPR, S.Hepatitis B & C antibodies, U.M/C/S, Pap.smear. Investigations that may be appropriate to undertake at follow-up antenatal visits: Hb, rubella titre, Rh titres, U.M/C/S, B.glucose, GTT, S.oestriols, U.oestriols, HIV antibodies, genital swab M/C/S, S.alpha-fetoprotein, 'triple test' for Down syn. (older mothers), ultrasound, cardiotocography.

PHYS: See individual tests in PATHOLOGY SECTION 4.

Pregnancy Diagnosis

TEST: Immunology for HCG in urine (+), S.HCG (+).

SIGN: Areolar pigmentation, blue cervix and vagina, chloasma, Hegar's sign, spider naevi, bounding pulse, abdominal mass, pitting oedema (pre-eclampsia).

DD: Uterine tumours, pseudocyesis, uterine fibroids, hysteria, anorexia nervosa, other psychological and pathological causes of amenorrhoea.

PHYS: Blood and urine levels of HCG rise after the 25th day from conception (39th day from last period), and fall after 20 weeks.

See also Eclampsia and Pre-eclampsia

Pregnancy, Ectopic

TEST: B.HCG (+ or –), U.HCG (+ or –), ultrasound (AB), needle aspiration posterior vaginal fornix (old blood present).
SIGN: Golden's sign, vaginal bleeding, amenorrhoea.
DD: Hydatidiform mole, choriocarcinoma, normal pregnancy.

Pregnancy, Progress

TEST: Tests that may be used to monitor the health of the mother and fetus include: alpha-fetoprotein, amniotic fluid (steady drop between weeks 16 and 22 in normal pregnancy), serum (steady rise throughout normal pregnancy), S.oestriols (rise between weeks 30 and 40 in normal pregnancy), human placental lactogen (rises steadily from week 20 to 40), Lecithin-sphingomyelin ratio, amniotic fluid (H if fetal lung mature), phosphotidyl glycerol, amniotic fluid (present when fetal lungs mature); ultrasound scan; feto-maternal haemorrhage cytometry.
SIGN: Intrauterine growth retardation.
PHYS: See individual tests in PATHOLOGY SECTION 4.

See also Eclampsia and Pre-eclampsia

Progressive Systemic Sclerosis
See Scleroderma

Prostatic Carcinoma

TEST: S.prostate specific antigen (H), S.PSA free/total ratio (L), prostate biopsy (+), S.CK-BB (H), S.ALP (N or H), S.ACP (N or H), Hb (L).
SIGN: Prostatomegaly, poor urinary stream.
DD: Benign prostatic hyperplasia, urethral stricture, bladder tumour, neurogenic bladder, vesical stone.
PHYS: ACP is only increasd when neoplasia spreads beyond capsule of gland. Often presents as bladder outlet obstruction.

Prostatic Hypertrophy

TEST: S.prostate specific antigen titre (H or N), U.M/C/S (AB), U.blood (+ or –), BUN (H).
DD: Stricture, prostatic carcinoma, bladder, vesical stone.
PHYS: Prostatism causes poor urinary stream and may damage kidneys by chronic back pressure.

Pseudogout (Chondrocalcinosis)

TEST: Synovial fluid microscopy (calcium pyrophosphate crystals), synovial fluid WCC (H), S.uric acid (N), ESR (H), S.calcium (H or N).
DD: Gout, osteoarthritis, joint trauma, rheumatoid arthritis.
PHYS: Acute synovitis due to deposition of calcium salts in joint cartilage. May be associatd with hyperparathyroidism.

Psittacosis (Ornithosis)

TEST: Specific antibody titre (RT), blood or sputum culture (+), WCC (N or L), ESR (H), U.protein (+).
DD: Viral or bacterial pneumonia, TB, influenza, Q fever, histoplasmosis, typhoid, brucellosis, infectious mononucleosis, hepatitis.
PHYS: Infection by *Chlamydia psittaci* transmitted from birds.

Psoriasis

TEST: Skin biopsy (+)
SIGN: Nail discolouration, nail pitting, subungal hyperkeratosis, onychogryphosis, onycholysis, brittle nails, Auspitz's sign.
DD: Seborrhoeic dermatitis, intertrigo, moniliasis, lichen planus, Bowen's disease, discoid eczema, pityriasis rosea, lichen simplex, tinea corporis, drug reaction.
PHYS: Chronic, benign, erythematous, macular, pruritic skin disease.

Puberty, Delayed

TEST: S.testosterone (both sexes), S.oestrogen (female), S.LH, S.FSH, S.chorionic gonadotrophin (female), chromosomal analysis, X-ray wrists (bone age study), CT hypothalamus, ultrasound pelvis (female). See PATHOLOGY SECTION 4 for interpretation.
SIGN: Failure of menstruation or development of secondary sexual characteristics.
DD: Hypogonadism, hypothyroidism, Klinefelter syn., Turner syn., Noonan syn., orchitis, drug abuse, Prader-Willi syn.
PHYS: May be due to familial factors, malnourishment, chronic illness and vigorous physical activity (girls only). Careful physical examination essential.

See also SYMPTOMS SECTION 1: Puberty, Delayed

Pulmonary Fibrosis, Idiopathic
See Cryptogenic Fibrosing Alveolitis

Pulmonary Hypertension
See Cor Pulmonale

Pulmonary Thromboembolism (Pulmonary Infarct)

TEST: WCC (H), ESR (H), S.fibrin degradation products (H), S.bilirubin (H or N), S.LDH (H), S.fibrinogen (H), arterial pO_2 (L), technetium^{99} scan (AB), chest x-ray (unreliable), pulmonary angiography (AB).
SIGN: Dyspnoea, raised jugular venous pressure, pleural rub, hypotension.
DD: Myocardial infarct, bacterial pneumonia, asthma, pulmonary oedema, pericarditis,

atelectasis, pneumothorax, aortic aneurysm, tumours, pleurisy, acute upper adbominal disease, chest trauma.
PHYS: Due to blocking of small pulmonary arteries by detached thrombus or other foreign matter. May be caused by occult malignancy.

Pulmonary Valve Disease

TEST: Echocardiography (AB).
SIGN: INCOMPETENCE – Diastolic murmur, diastolic cardiac thrill.
STENOSIS – Jugular venous pressure, systolic murmur, systolic cardiac thrill.

PUO

See Pyrexia of Unknown Origin

Pyelonephritis, Acute

TEST: U.M/C/S (+), U.cells (H), U.blood (+), U.protein (H), Hb (L), WCC (N or H).
DD: All causes of acute abdomen, basal pneumonia, pancreatitis, urinary calculus.
PHYS: Pyogenic infection of the kidney.

Pyelonephritis, Chronic

TEST: Renal biopsy (+), U.M/C/S (white cells, culture + or –), U.blood (+ or –), U.casts (+), U.protein (+), S.sodium (L), Hb (L), B.urea (H), S.creatinine (H), U.SG (L).
DD: Urinary tract obstruction, nephrosis, TB, toxic nephropathies, urinary infections.
PHYS: Chronic inflammation of kidney due to repeated infection or toxic insult.

Pyrexia of Unknown Origin (PUO)

TEST: Tests that may be used rationally to assess possible causes of fever include: U.M/C/S, B.M/C/S, faeces M/C/S, CSF M/C/S, WCC, Hb, blood film, S.bilirubin, S.ALP, S.GGT, S.LD, S.AST, S.ANA, chest x-ray
DD: See Fever in SYMPTOMS SECTION 1.
PHYS: Undiagnosed fever that has been present for several weeks

Q Fever

TEST: Specific serological antibody test (RT), WCC (L).
DD: Viral pneumonia, hepatitis, brucellosis, TB, psittacosis.
PHYS: Acute, self-limiting Rickettsial infection often associated with pneumonitis.

See also Rickettsioses

Quinsy (Peritonsillar Abscess)

TEST: Throat swab M/C/S (+), WCC (AB), ESR (H), Paul Bunnell (–).

DD: Tonsillitis, infectious mononucleosis, pharyngitis, diphtheria, mumps, lymphoma, sialitis.
PHYS: Complication of acute tonsillitis.

Rabies

TEST: B.lyssavirus antibodies (+), skin or brain biopsy (rabies antigen +), salivary virology (+), CSF antibodies (H after 8 days).
SIGN: Hydrophobia, fever, opisthotonus, convulsions, neck stiffness, spasticity, tachycardia, flaccid paralysis, fasciculation.
DD: Tetanus, meningitis, cerebral space occupying lesion, hysteria, cerebral malaria, encephalomyelitis, polio, herpes, encephalitis.
PHYS: Post-exposure vaccination essential. Viral disease. Mortality 99%.

Reactive Arthritis

TEST: Tests to consider during investigation of the cause: B.culture, faeces M/C/S, urethra M/C/S, synovial fluid assay, S.HLA-B27, serological tests for Salmonella and Yersinia, S.uric acid, B.rheumatoid factor.
DD: Rheumatoid arthritis, gout, osteoarthritis, trauma.
PHYS: Reactive arthritis is any arthritis secondary to another disease, particularly enteric bacterial infections. Reiter'syn. and gonorrhoea may also be responsible. See PATHOLOGY SECTION 4 for interpretation of test results.

Rectal Carcinoma

See Colo-Rectal Carcinoma

Refsum Disease

TEST: S.phytanate (H)
SIGN: Cerebellar signs.
PHYS: Autosomal recessive disorder

Reiter Syndrome

TEST: WCC (H), HLA-B27 (+), urethral M/C/S (–), ESR (H), Hb (L), rheumatoid factor (–).
DD: Gonococcal arthritis, rheumatoid arthritis, ankylosing spondylitis, psoriatic arthritis.
PHYS: Disease of unknown aetiology characterised by arthritis, urethritis and conjuctivitis.

See also Reactive Arthritis
See also SYNDROMES SECTION 6: Reiter Syndrome

Relapsing Fever

TEST: Specific antibody test (+), B.microscopy (+), WCC (N or H), ESR (H), B.bilirubin (+), U.albumin (+ or –), U.blood (+ or –), S.IgG (H), S.IgM (H later).
DD: Malaria, typhus, dengue, influenza, smallpox, yellow fever, leptospirosis.

PHYS: Arthropod transmitted infection of human bloodstream by spirochetes of genus Borrelia.

Renal Calculi
See Nephrolithiasis

Renal Failure, Acute
TEST: B.urea (H), S.creatinine (H), creatinine clearance (L), Hb (L), B.WCC (AB), U.phosphate (H), B.pH (L), S.potassium (H), S.sodium (L), U.microscopy (AB), renal biopsy (AB).
DD: Urinary tract obstruction, acute glomerulonephritis, hepatorenal syn., collagen disease, renal artery obstruction.
PHYS: Syndrome of sudden decrease in glomerular filtration rate, oliguria and abnormal renal function.

Renal Failure, Chronic
TEST: S.creatinine (H), creatinine clearance (L), S.urate (Nor H), U.SG (L), S.sodium (AB, often H), S.potassium (N or H), S.bicarbonate (L), S.magnesium (L), S.calcium (L or N), S.phosphate (N or H), S.sulphate (H), S.protein (L), U.calcium (L), U.protein (+ or −), Hb (L), GTT (AB), S.glucose (N), S.triglycerides (H), S.ALP (H), B.pH (L), U.pH (L), BUN (H).
SIGN: Ankle clonus, Cheyne-Stokes respiration, exophthalmos, pericardial friction rub, Hess test, nail discolouration, Kussmaul's breathing.
DD: Glomerulonephritis, renal vascular disease, polycystic disease, pyelonephritis, drug nephropathy, congenital hypoplasia.
PHYS: Due to chronic damage to the kidneys caused by one or more of many factors.

Reye Syndrome
TEST: S.transaminases (H), S.ammonia (H), coagulation screen (AB), B.glucose (N or L).
DD: Infectious mononucleosis, hepatitis, encephalitis, meningitis.
PHYS: Flu-like illness followed by vomiting, cerebral signs, coma and death. Hepatomegaly common. Supportive therapy only available.

See also SYNDROMES SECTION 6: Reye Syndrome

Rheumatic Fever
TEST: S.ASOT (RT), S.CRP (H), ESR (H), WCC (H), Hb (L or N), throat swab M/C/S(+ or −), chest x-ray (N or AB), echocardiography (AB or N).
SIGN: Choreiform movements, subcutaneous nodules, erythema marginatum, arthritis, pericardial friction rub, cardiomegaly, hepatomegaly.
DD: Encephalitis, rheumatoid arthritis, osteomyelitis, endocarditis, TB, polio, SLE, meningitis, leukaemias, congenital heart disease, joint trauma, drug reaction.

PHYS: Initiated by group A haemolytic streptococcal infection. Frequently causes cardiac valvular deformities. Primarily a clinical diagnosis with major criteria being carditis, erythema, nodules, chorea, arthritis and fever. Minor criteria include fever, arthralgia, high ESR and/or CRP.

Rheumatoid Arthritis
TEST: Hb (L), ESR (H), S.CRP (H), rheumatoid factor (+ in 70%), S.ANA (H in 30%), S.HLA-DR4 (+), synovial fluid (AB), S.gamma-globulin (H), x-rays of hands and feet (AB).
SIGN: Boutonniére deformity, muscular atrophy, hepatomegaly, joint eythema, longitudinal nail ridging, spider naevi, splenomegaly (Felty syn.), splinter haemorrhages.
DD: Osteoarthritis, gout, chondrocalcinosis, SLE, psoriasis, gonorrhoea, sarcoidosis, ulcerative colitis, Reiter syn., Crohn's disease, malignancies, rheumatic fever, ankylosing spondylitis, viraemias, trauma.
PHYS: Chronic inflammation of synovial membranes (particularly in hands and feet), of unknown aetiology. Rheumatoid factor not diagnostic. Juvenile form known as Still's disease.

Rickets
See Osteomalacia

Rickettsioses
TEST: Specific complement fixation test (+), ELISA test (+), Weil-Felix reaction (+), S.IgM (H), S.IgG (H late), ESR (N), WCC (N).
DD: Typhus, measles, meningococcal infections, malaria, yellow fever.
PHYS: Transmitted by ticks and other insects. Types include scrub typhus, Q fever, Rocky Mountain spotted fever, etc.

Rocky Mountain Spotted Fever
See Rickettsioses

Rosacea
TEST: Skin biopsy (AB).
DD: Acne vulgaris, seborrheic dermatitis, lupus erythematosus.
PHYS: Aetiology unknown. Occurs in people of Celtic origin. Aggravated by sunlight.

Roseola Infantum
TEST: B.neutrophils (L), WCC (H).
DD: URTI, drug rash, measles, rubella, infectious mononucleosis.
PHYS: Very common, benign viral infection of children.

Ross River Fever
See Epidemic Polyarthritis

Roundworms, Intestinal (Nematode Infestations; Ascaris; Hookworm)

TEST: Faecal microscopy (eggs or worms), Hb (L), faecal blood (+ or –), LFT (N or AB), FBC (AB, depends on species).
SIGN: Cachexia, muscle pain (trichinosis), periorbital oedema (trichinosis), abdominal pain and tenderness, haemoptysis (ascariasis), urticaria, pruritus ani.
DD: Depends on infecting worm but includes: beriberi, nephrotic syn., bacterial gut infections, urticaria, all causes of acute abdomen, pneumonia.
PHYS: Nematodes that infect the gut include Strongyloides, threadworm, hookworm, toxocara (visceral larva migrans), ascaris and trichuriasis. Symptoms depend on species. Other nematodes may invade tissues.

See also Trichinosis

Rubella (German Measles)

TEST: Rubella IgG antibodies (RT), rubella IgM antibodies (+), WCC (L).
DD: Measles, infectious mononucleosis, roseola infantum, scarlet fever, drug rash, other viral infections.
PHYS: Acute, benign, infectious, viral infection. May cause severe congenital abnormalities in early pregnancy. Symptoms include rash, fever and cervical lymphadenitis.

Rubeola

See Measles

Salmonellosis

TEST: B. or faecal culture (+), specific agglutinins (RT), U.culture (– or +), WCC (N or L), faecal blood (+).
DD: Shigelloses, other enteric bacteria.
PHYS: Infection with one of the hundreds of types of Salmonella can cause acute diarrhoea, vomiting and abdominal pain. Typhoid and paratyphoid fevers are the commonest types.

See also Typhoid Fever

Salpingitis

See Pelvic Inflammatory Disease

Sarcoidosis

TEST: Lesion biopsy (+), Kveim test (+), S.angiotensin converting enzyme (H), tuberculin reaction (60%–), U.calcium (H), S.calcium (H or N), S.ALP (H), S.IgG (H), ESR (H), liver biopsy (AB), chest x-ray (AB).
SIGN: Clubbing of fingers, hepatomegaly, splenomegaly, skin lesions.
DD: TB, Hodgkin's disease, biliary cirrhosis, Crohn's ileitis, allergic alveolitis. May mimic any disease of the involved system.
PHYS: A multisystem granulomatous disorder of unknown aetiology, that may become widespread in almost any organ.

SBE

See Endocarditis, Bacterial, Subacute

Scarlet Fever (Streptococcal Throat)

TEST: Throat swab M/C/S (+), ASOT (RT), ESR (H), WCC (H).
SIGN: Circumoral pallor, strawberry tongue, tachycardia.
DD: Viral URTI, Vincent's angina, thrush, infectious mononucleosis, diphtheria, rubella, measles, drug eruptions, agranulocytosis, roseola infantum, Stevens-Johnson syn.
PHYS: Beta-haemolytic streptococcal infection of upper respiratory tract. Rash due to erythrogenic toxin.

Schistosomiasis

See Bilharzia

Scleroderma (Progessive Systemic Sclerosis)

TEST: S.ANA (+), S.ENA (+), ESR (H), Hb (L), S.iron (L), S.vit. B_{12} (L), B.LE cells (+), S.creatinine (N or H in advanced disease), S.gamma-globulin (H), U.protein (+ with renal involvement), S.rheumatoid factor (+), S.folate (L).
SIGN: Skin thickening, hypertension, telangiectasia.
DD: Rheumatoid arthritis, SLE, Raynaud's phenomenon, polycythaemia vera, progeria, myxoedema, porphyria cutanea tarda, lichen sclerosis, Werner syn., pulmonary fibrosis, amyloidosis, porphyria, other autoimmune diseases, malabsorption syndromes, all causes of dysphagia.
PHYS: Autoimmune disease of blood vessels and connective tissue causing organ fibrosis and vascular insufficiency.

Scrofula

TEST: See Tuberculosis, Pulmonary.
DD: Viral or bacterial lymphadenitis.
PHYS: Infection of cervical or mediastinal lymph nodes by *Mycobacterium tuberculosis.*

Scurvy

TEST: S.ascorbic acid (L), Hb (L).
SIGN: Bleeding gums, loose teeth, cachexia.
DD: Rickets, polio, rheumatic fever, osteomyelitis, osteoarthritis, haemorrhagic diseases, gingivitis.
PHYS: Due to inadequate vit. C (ascorbic acid).

Seizure

See Epilepsy, Idiopathic

Septic Arthritis

See Arthritis, Septic

Septicemia

TEST: B.cultures (+), U.M/C/S (N or +), wound swab M/C/S (N or +), WCC (AB), ESR (H), S.bicarbonate (AB).

DD: Other causes of shock, plague, meningitis, malaria, cardiac failure.

PHYS: 2 or 3 blood samples for culture must be taken before antibiotic therapy is started.

Serum Sickness

TEST: WCC (H), plasma cells (+ or –), ESR (N), U.Protein (+).

DD: Urticaria, bacterial infections, acute arthropathies, allergic diseases, gastroenteritis.

PHYS: Hypersensitive immune response to the injection of foreign serum protein.

Sexually Transmitted Disease [STD]

DD: **VIRUSES:** Human immunodeficiency virus (AIDS), human papilloma virus (genital warts), hepatitis A, hepatitis B, hepatitis C *Herpes simplex* (types 1 and 2), Epstein-Barr virus (glandular fever), cytomegalovirus, molluscum contagiosum.
BACTERIA: *Chlamydia trachomatis* (NSU, lymphogranuloma venereum), *Neisseria gonorrhoea, Treponema pallidum* (syphilis), *Haemophilus ducreyi* (chancroid), beta-haemolytic streptococcus, Calymmatobacterium granulomatis, *Mycoplasma hominis,* salmonella, shigella, *Ureaplasma urealyticum,* campylobacter.
FUNGI: *Candida albicans* (thrush).
PROTOZOA: *Giardia lamblia, Trichomonas vaginalis, Entamoeba histolytica.*
ARTHROPODS: *Pthiris pubis* (crabs), *Sarcoptes scabiei* (scabies).

See also Acquired Immune Deficiency Syndrome; Amoebiasis; Candidiasis; Chancroid; Cytomegalovirus Infections; Gonorrhoea; Granuloma Inguinale; Herpes, Genital; Infectious Mononucleosis; Lymphogranuloma Venereum; Nonspecific Urethritis; Syphilis; Trichomoniasis, Venereal; Warts, Ano-Genital

Sheehan's Disease

See Hypopituitarism

Shigellosis (Bacillary Dysentery)

TEST: Faeces M/C/S (+), faecal blood (+), S.electrolytes (AB), WCC (AB).

DD: Viral and bacterial enteritis, amoebic dysentery, salmonellosis, zoonotic infestations, ulcerative colitis, all causes of acute abdomen.

PHYS: Dysentery due to enteric infection by one of the many species of Shigella.

Shingles (Herpes Zoster; Varicella)

TEST: Vesicle smear (multinucleated giant cells and inclusion bodies), CSF pressure (H with cerebral involvement), CSF microscopy (monocytes with cerebral involvement).

DD: Pleurisy, pleurodynia, neuritis, radiculitis, peritonitis, disc lesion, *Herpes simplex,* urticaria, chickenpox.

PHYS: Unilateral, segmental infection of posterior root ganglions or cranial nerves by the virus *H. zoster,* resulting in pain and vesicular eruption in the affected nerve area.

See also Chickenpox

Sickle Cell Disease/Anaemia

TEST: Hb (L), blood film (AB ± target cells), specific PCR (+), reticulocyte count (VH), tissue DNA probe (+), S.iron (N or H), s.LDH (H), ^{51}Cr red cell survival (L), S.bilirubin (H), sodium metabisulfite screening test (+).

SIGN: **CHRONIC:** Scleral icterus, asthenia, normal spleen, negro.
ACUTE: Abdominal pain and rigidity, fever, bone pain, paralysis, convulsions.

DD: Other haemoglobinopathies, TB, genitourinary tumours, rheumatic fever, acute abdominal surgical conditions, sickle thalassaemia, HbF syn.

PHYS: Dominant hereditary disorder of negroes.

Sinusitis, Acute Bacterial

TEST: Nasal discharge M/C/S (+), WCC (H).

DD: Dental infection or abscess, infected tear sac, otitis media, neoplasm, cellulitis, influenza, meningitis, cerebral abscess, facial osteomyelitis.

PHYS: Causes facial pain, tenderness and swelling; fever and purulent nasal discharge.

Sjögren Syndrome (Mikulicz' Disease)

TEST: S.antinuclear antibodies (H), S.extractable nuclear antigen (H), S.HLA-DR3 (+), rheumatoid factor (+), Hb (L), WCC (L), ESR (H), B.eosinophils (H), S.gamma-globulin (H), salivary gland biopsy (AB).

DD: Rheumatoid arthritis, SLE, hepatobiliary disease, scleroderma, polymyositis, Hashimoto's disease, panarteritis.

PHYS: Autoimmune disease of women characterised by dry eyes, mouth and vagina. May effect mucous membranes of any organ.

See also SYNDROMES SECTION 6: Sjögren Syndrome

SLE

See Lupus Erythematosus, Systemic

Sleeping Sickness

See Trypanosomiasis

Smallpox (Variola)

TEST: Vesicular fluid microscopy (+), isolation of viral antigen in vesicle fluid (+), specific serum antibodies (+), WCC (H), U.protein (+).
DD: Chickenpox, meninococcaemia, typhus, erythema multiforme.
PHYS: Extremely contagious viral disease with high mortality, transmitted by droplet or contact. Wild cases entirely eradicated.

Smoking

TEST: S.carboxyHb (H), B.nicotine (H), S.cotinine (H).
PHYS: Life expectancy reduced 5 to 8 years.
increased risk of Lung cancer (x 10).
Myocardial infarct (x 2), Peptic ulcer (x 3).
Fracture of hip or vertebrae (x 4).
Mouth and throat cancer (x 8).
Emphysema and chronic bronchitis (x 12).
Bladder and cervix cancer
Infant low birth weight, respiratory infections in children of smokers.

Spherocytosis, Hereditary

TEST: B.smear (spherocytic white cells), RCC (L), MCV (L), MCHC (L), WCC (H), B.reticulocytes (H), platelets (H), Hb (L), bone marrow (AB), S.bilirubin (H), Coombs' test (–), osmotic fragility (H).
SIGN: Splenomegaly, jaundice, anaemia.
DD: Autoimmune diseases, haemolytic anaemia, drug abuse, alcoholism.
PHYS: Hereditary cell membrane defect that allows excess entry of sodium into cells.

Spinal Cord Lesions

SIGN: Ataxia, Babinski's sign, hypertonicity, Kernig's sign, peripheral reflexes, mass reflex, nose-finger test, spastic paralysis, heel-knee test, loss of proprioceptive sense (posterior column), Queckenstedt's test, Romberg's sign (posterior column).
DD: See SIGNS SECTION 2 for the interpretation of these clinical signs and the resultant differential diagnoses.

Sprue, Nontropical

See Coeliac Disease

Sprue, Tropical

TEST: Faecal fat (H), Hb (L), xylose absorption test (L),

B.megaloblasts (H), P.carotene (L), S.calcium (L), S.cholesterol (L).
SIGN: Foul greasy stools, cachexia.
DD: Coeliac disease, other malabsorption syndromes, bacterial enteritis, protozoan and helminthic enteritis.
PHYS: Intestinal disease due to nutritional deficiency and/or bacterial infection. Exact aetiology unknown.

Stein-Leventhal Syndrome (Polycystic Ovarian Syndrome)

TEST: S.testosterone (H), S.LH:FSH ratio (H), U.FSH (N), S.prolactin (H), S.oestrogen (N or L), U.17-ketosteroids (H).
SIGN: Oliogomenorrhoea, hirsutism.
DD: Follicular cysts, hypopituitarism, adrenal adenoma, Fröhlich syn., Chiari-Frommel syn., hyperthyroidism, oral contraceptives.
PHYS: Affects up to 5% of women.

See also SYNDROMES SECTION 6: Stein-Leventhal Syndrome

Sterility

See Infertility, Female; Infertility, Male

Still's Disease

See Rheumatoid Arthritis

Stomach Carcinoma

TEST: Biopsy cytology (+), Hb (L), S.folic acid (N or L), S.vit. B$_{12}$ (N or L), faecal occult blood (+ or –).
SIGN: Cachexia, coffee grounds vomitus, haematemesis, abdominal mass.
DD: Peptic ulcer, cholelithiasis, pancreatitis, gastritis, pancreatic neoplasm, coronary artery disease.
PHYS: Usually an adenocarcinoma or lymphoma. Symptoms include weight loss, pain and vomiting. Suspicion should be aroused when ulcers fail to heal.

Stones, Gall

See Cholelithiasis

Stones, Renal

See Nephrolithiasis

Streptococcal Throat

See Scarlet Fever

Stroke

See Infarct, Cerebral; Transient Ischaemic Attack

Subacute Bacterial Endocarditis
See Endocarditis, Bacterial, Subacute

Syphilis
TEST: Syphilis EIA (+), lesion fluid dark field microscopy (+), RPR (+), FTA (+), TPHA (+), Wassermann reaction (+). Cerebral syphilis – colloidal gold (AB), CSF lymphocytes (H), CSF protein (H).

SIGN: Argyll-Robertson pupil (tertiary), chloasma, frontal bossing (congenital), hepatomegaly, lens opacity (congenital), mydriasis (tertiary), slurred speech (GPI), postural tremor (GPI).

DD: Gonorrhoea, NSU, yaws, chancroid, lymphogranuloma venereum, herpes, neoplasm, drug eruptions, pityriasis rosea, nephritis. Tertiary syphilis may mimic a vast range of diseases.

PHYS: Complex venereal infection caused by the spirochete *Treponema pallidum*. Any organ or tissue of the body may be involved in the tertiary stage. Rational interpretation of test results is demonstrated in the following table:

SYPHILIS PATHOLOGY TEST RESULTS

Syphilis stage	Untreated RPR	FTA	Treated RPR	FTS
Early primary	–	–	–	–
Primary	+	+	–	–/+
Secondary	+	+	–	+
Early latent	+	+	–	+
Late latent	+	+	+	+
Tertiary	+	+	+	+
Quaternary	+/–	+/–	+/–	+/–

Systemic Lupus Erythematosus
See Lupus Erythematosus, Systemic

Systemic Sclerosis, Progressive
See Scleroderma

Tapeworms (Cestodes)
TEST: Faeces microscopy (+), specific skin test (+), complement fixation test (+), Hb (L).

DD: Pernicious anaemia, other enteric infestations, epilepsy.

PHYS: An often asymptomatic infection of the gut by one of numerous cestode species. Larval stages may infect brain, liver, lung, etc.

TB
See Tuberculosis, Pulmonary

Temporal Arteritis
See Giant Cell Arteritis

Testicular Cancer
TEST: S.alpha-fetoprotein (H), S.HCG (H), S.oestrogens (H or N).

SIGN: Gynaecomastia, virilisation.

DD: Hydrocoele, torsion, infection, teratoma, seminoma, metastases.

PHYS: Usually hormone producing and highly malignant.

Testicular Failure
See Infertility, Male

Tetanus (Lockjaw)
TEST: WCC (H), none specific.

SIGN: Peripheral reflexes, opisthotonus, risus sardonicus.

DD: Strychnine poisoning, acute CNS infections.

PHYS: *Clostridium tetani* infection of dirty, anaerobic wounds releases an exotoxin that causes severe muscle spasm. Prevented by active immunisation.

Thalassaemia Major
TEST: RBC (microcytic, hypochromic), specific PCR (+) Hb (VL), HbH (+ HbH thalassaemia), B.reticulocytes (H), B.target cells (+), tissue DNA probe (+), WCC (N or H), HbF (+), marrow biopsy (hyperplastic), S.bilirubin (H).

SIGN: Splenomegaly, hepatomegaly, south east Asian or Mediterranean origin.

DD: Other haemoglobinopathies, haemolytic anaemia.

PHYS: Congenital inability to produce adequate haemoglobin. Thalassaemia major is the homozygous form.

Thalassaemia Minor
TEST: RBC (H), Hb (L), HbH (+ HbH thalassaemia), MCV (L), MCHC (L), B.target cells (+), marrow biopsy (AB), tissue DNA probe (+).

SIGN: South east Asian or Mediterranean origin.

DD: Iron deficiency anaemia, haemoglobinopathies, sideroachrestic anaemia.

PHYS: Due to genetic defect, insufficient haemoglobin is produced. Thalassaemia minor is the heteroozygous form.

Threadworms
See Roundworms, Intestinal

Thromboanglitis Obliterans
See Buerger's Disease

Thrombophilia
TEST: FBC, prothrombin time, APTT, B.fibrinogen,

B.Antithrombin III, S.protein C, S.protein S,
S.lupus anticoagulant.
SIGN:	Skin necrosis.
DD:	Venous thrombosis from other causes.
PHYS:	Familial thrombophilia incidence 1:10,000.

Thrombosis, Cerebral
See Infarct, Cerebral

Thrombosis, Pulmonary
See Pulmonary Thromboembolism

Thrombosis, Venous
TEST:	Venography (AB), radioactive fibrinogen uptake
	test (+), ultrasound (AB), fibrin degradation
	products (H), serial dilution protamine sulfate
	test (+), S.antithrombin III (N or L),
	P.plasminogen (N or H), S.protein C (N or L),
	S.protein S (N or L), S.lupus anticoagulant (+ or
	–), impedance plethysmography (AB), doppler
	flow studies (AB).
SIGN:	Pitting oedema, Homan's sign.
DD:	Muscular strain or trauma, cellulitis, lymphatic
	obstruction, cardiac oedema, cirrhotic oedema,
	Baker's popliteal cyst.
PHYS:	Causes include immobilisation, post-operative,
	pregnancy, oestrogen supplementation (eg
	contraceptive pill), cardiac failure, renal failure,
	carcinoma, myeloproliferative disorders and
	phospholipid antibody syn. Pulmonary
	embolism is a possible dangerous complication.

See also SIGNS SECTION 2: Phlebitis

Thrush
See Candidiasis

Thyroid Carcinoma
TEST:	S.thyroglobulin (+), TFT (N), radionuclide
	scanning (AB), S.calcitonin (H or N). No
	definitive test.
DD:	Chronic thyroiditis, thyroid adenoma, goitre,
	thyroid cysts and nodules.
PHYS:	Insidious onset with painless swelling of gland.
	Open or needle biopsy essential if suspicious.

Thyroid Disease
*See Hyperthyroidism; Hypothyroidism; Thyroid
Carcinoma; Thyroid Nodules; Thyroiditis, de Quervain's
Subacute; Thyroiditis, Hashimoto's*

Thyroid Nodules
TEST:	TFT (see PATHOLOGY SECTION 4), thyroid
	scintiscanning, biopsy (open or needle),
	ultrasound
SIGN:	Nodule in thyroid gland
DD:	Thyroid cnacer, simple cyst, lymph node, goitre,

Hashimoto's disease, metastatic carcinoma,
lymphoma.
PHYS:	Important to make a definitive diagnosis of any
	thyroid lump

Thyroiditis, De Quervain's Subacute
TEST:	ESR (H), Hb (L), B.neutrophils (H or N), TFT
	(variable), S.thyroid binding immunoglobulins
	(H 40%), radionuclide scan (L uptake).
SIGN:	Thyrotoxic initially, hypothyroid later.
DD:	Other forms of thyroiditis, thyrotoxicosis,
	pharyngitis.
PHYS:	Painful, tender thyroid gland, often unilateral.

Thyroiditis, Hashimoto's
TEST:	S.antithyroglobulin (VH), S.antimicrosomal
	antibodies (VH), S.thyroxine (N or L), S.TSH
	(H), S.anti-thyroid peroxidase antibodies,
	thyroid biopsy (AB).
SIGN:	Goitre, hypothyroidism.
DD:	Thyroid adenocarcinoma, Grave's disease,
	polyglandular autoimmune syn.
PHYS:	Chronic autoimmune disease.

Thyrotoxicosis
See Hyperthyroidism

TIA
See Transient Ischaemic Attack

Tinea
See Fungal Skin Infection

Toxins
See Botulism; Ciguatera Poisoning; Tetanus

Toxocara Infection
See Visceral Larva Migrans

Toxoplasmosis
TEST:	Specific serum antibodies (RT), WCC (N),
	lymph node biopsy microscopy (+ or –),
	S.monocytes (H).
DD:	Lymphoma, infectious mononucleosis, TB,
	brucellosis, tularaemia, rickettsioses.
PHYS:	Infection by the protozoa *Toxoplasma gondii* of
	lymphatic tissue, brain, eyes, muscle, heart and
	lungs.

Trachoma
TEST:	Conjunctival scrapings M/C/S (+).
SIGN:	Arit's line, xerosis.
DD:	Viral or bacterial conjunctivitis, dacryocystitis,
	Parinaud syn.
PHYS:	Chlamydial infection of the conjunctiva.

Transient Ischaemic Attack [TIA]

TEST: No specific diagnostic test. Exclude other diagnoses and complications by: FBC, ESR, platelets, S.cholesterol, B.urea, S.electrolytes, B.glucose, syphilis screen, ECG, chest x-ray, CT, EEG, carotid duplex scan.

DD: Migraine, thromboembolism, epilepsy, CVA, raised intracranial pressure, cerebral trauma, cerebral tumours, cerebral haematoma, hypoglycaemia, hypotension, hypertension, polycythaemia, thrombocythaemia, anaemia, multiple sclerosis, psychogenic, transient global amnesia, vestibular disease, multiple sclerosis, alcoholism.

PHYS: Focal reduction in cerebral blood supply resulting in transient loss of function. Risk factors include hypertension, heart disease, smoking, hyperlipidaemia, diabetes, peripheral vascular disease, oral contraceptives. Significant risk of subsequent stroke.

Trichinosis (Trichiniasis)

TEST: Muscle biopsy (larvae), B.eosinophils (H), S.potassium (L), specific serological test (RT), specific skin test (+).

DD: Polymyositis, periarteritis nodosa.

PHYS: Acute tissue infection by the nematode *Trichinella spiralis*. Cysts form in muscle.\

See also Visceral Larva Migrans

Trichomoniasis, Venereal

TEST: Vaginal and/or urethral swab M/C (+ growth on special medium required).

DD: Candidiasis (thrush), gonorrhoea, other bacterial infections, leucorrhoea, urinary infection, prostatitis.

PHYS: Infection of vagina or urethra by *Trichomonas vaginalis*. Foul, foamy, yellow/green discharge may be present. 25% asymptomatic.

Tricuspid Valve Disease

TEST: Echocardiography (AB).

SIGN: **INCOMPETENCE:**Systolic murmur.
STENOSIS: Diastolic murmur, jugular venous pressure.

Trigeminal Neuralgia

DD: Infected tooth, poorly fitted artificial dentures, dental cyst, gingivitis, bruxism, migraine, temporal arteritis, sinusitis.

Trisomy 21

See Down Syndrome

Trypanosomiasis (Sleeping Sickness)

TEST: B. film microscopy (+), lymph gland biopsy (+), B.trypanosome antibodies (+), Hb (L), ESR (H),
S.globulin (H), S.protein (L), S.IgM (H), CSF M/C/S (AB), CSF pressure (H in cerebral forms), CSF protein (H in cerebral forms), CSF lymphocytes (H in cerebral forms).

DD: Malaria, kala azar, cerebral tumours and infections.

PHYS: Many types. Trypanosomes may infect blood stream, lymph nodes, heart, or brain.

Tubal Pregnancy

See Pregnancy, Ectopic

Tuberculosis, Pulmonary [TB]

TEST: Tuberculin test (+), PCR (+), sputum M/C/S (+), lymph node biopsy (+), Hb (L), ESR (H), WCC (H), sputum blood (+), chest x-ray (AB), bronchopsy (AB), lung biopsy (AB).

SIGN: Amphoric breathing, bronchial breathing, cachexia, cavernous breathing, chloasma, crepitations, dull percussion note, pericardial friction rub, geographic tongue, hepatomegaly, whispering pectoriloquy, pleural effusion, shifting dullness (peritoneal), splenomegaly, tracheal displacement, thoracid tympany (cavitation), vocal fremitus.

DD: Any pulmonary disease, carcinoma of lung, sarcoidosis.

PHYS: *Mycobacterium tuberculosis* infection of the lung causes variable pulmonary symptoms. Secondary infection of other organs possible.

Tularaemia

TEST: B.culture (+), specific skin test (+), S.specific antibody (RT), S.IgM (H), S.IgG:IgM radio (>2), WCC (N).

SIGN: Adenitis, inoculation site papule or ulcer.

DD: Rickettsial infections, cat-scratch disease, infectious mononucleosis, meningococcal infections, fungaemia.

PHYS: Arthropod or water borne infection. Occurs only in northern hemisphere, but not in UK. Zoonotic infection. Vaccine available in USSR.

Turner Syndrome (Gonadal Dysgenesis, XO Syndrome)

TEST: Chromosome count (45X [XO], or other mosaics), U.FSH (H), U.17-ketosteroids (L).

SIGN: Webbing of neck, infantile sexual characteristics, cardiac anomalies.

DD: Noonan syn., delayed menarche, anorexia nervosa, genital tract abnormalities, hypopituitarism, adrenal or thyroid disease.

PHYS: Delayed menarche usual presenting symptom. Congenital primary hypogonadism due to lack of second X chromosome.

See also SYNDROMES SECTION 6: Turner Syndrome

Typhoid Fever (Enteric Fever)

TEST: B.culture (+), faecal culture (+), U.culture (+), Hb

(L), WCC (L), Widal antibody test (RT).
SIGN: Dicrotic pulse, diarrhoea, splenomegaly.
DD: Septicaemia, TB, viral infections, Q fever, psittacosis.
PHYS: Caused by *Salmonella typhi*.

See also Salmonellosis

Typhus, Epidemic Louse Borne

TEST: Specific serological test (RT), Weil-Felix test (+), Rickettsiae isolation from blood by animal inoculation (+), WCC (AB), U.protein (+), U.blood (+).
SIGN: Brudzinski's sign, Kernig's sign, neck stiffness, fever, maculopapular rash.
DD: Any febrile illness.
PHYS: Rickettsial infection spread by body lice in conditions of overcrowding and poor hygiene.

Ulcer, Peptic

See Peptic Ulcer

Ulcerative Colitis

TEST: Rectal biopsy (+), WCC (H), platelets (H), Hb (L, hypochromic, microcytic), faecal blood (+), prothrombin time (H), ESR (H), S.potassium S.albumin (L).
DD: Infectious colitis, irritable bowel syn., diverticulitis, amoebiasis, colonic infarct, colonic tumour, Crohn's disease, ischaemic colitis, purgative abuse.
PHYS: Unpredictably recurrent, inflammatory disease of colon causing diarrhoea.

Ulnar Nerve Paralysis

SIGN: Froment's sign.
DD: Axillary or cervical nerve lesion, cerebrovascular accident.

Undulant Fever

See Brucellosis

Uraemia

See Renal Failure, Acute; Renal Failure, Chronic

Urethritis, Nonspecific

See Nonspecific Urethritis

Urinary Infection

See Cystitis; Pyelonephritis, Acute; Pyelonephritis, Chronic

Urticaria (Hives)

TEST: B.eosinophils (H), S.allergen specific IgE (H), ESR (H or N), provocation tests (+).

DD: Contact dermatitis, dermographia, insect bites, scabies.
PHYS: Erythematous, macular, pruritic skin eruption secondary to allergen exposure.

Valve Disease, Heart

See Aortic Valve Disease; Mitral Valve Disease; Pulmonary Valve Disease; Tricuspid Valve Disease

Varicella

See Chickenpox

Variola

See Smallpox

Vascular Haemophilia

See Von Willebrand's Disease

Venereal Disease [VD]

See Sexually Transmitted Disease

Venous Thrombosis

See Thrombosis, Venous

Vestibular Disease

TEST: Electronystagmography (AB
SIGN: Caloric tests, nystagmus, Unterberger's test.
PHYS: Due to disorders of the labyrinth in the inner ear

Vincent's Angina (Gingivostomatitis)

TEST: Lesion smear and/or biopsy microscopy (fusospirochaetal forms seen), WCC (H).
DD: Diphtheria, streptococcal or staphylococcal infection, malignant neutropenia, herpangina.
PHYS: Ulceration of the mouth and lips due to either Fusobacterium and/or *Borrelia vincentii*. Usually secondary to poor hygiene or malnutrition.

Viraemia (Viral Infections)

TEST: Specific serological test (RT), virus isolation from blood (+), B.neutrophils (L). Other tests and results depend on specific virus.
DD: Bacterial, zoonotic and rickettsial infections; allergic, drug and toxic reactions.
PHYS: Viruses are intracellular, crystalline, molecular particles that can cause diverse illnesses in humans. Sera taken several days or weeks apart necessary to detect rising titre.

See also Viral Serology in PATHOLOGY SECTION 4

Visceral Larva Migrans (Toxocariasis)

TEST: B.eosinophils (VH), S.globulins (H), S.toxocara antibodies (+), skin lesion biopsy (AB)

DD: *Ancyclostoma, Trichinella, Strongyloides
        stercoralis* and other nematodes
PHYS: Usually caused by *Toxocara canis*, but may also
        be due to *Toxocara cati*. Caused by nematodes
        that are normally parasitic for other species

Vitamin B₁₂ Deficit

See Pernicious Anaemia

Vitamin C Deficit

See Scurvy

Vitamin D Deficit

See Osteomalacia

von Willebrand's Disease (Vascular Haemophilia)

TEST: Bleeding time (H, VH after aspirin), collagen
        binding assay (AB), PTT (H), factor VIII (L),
        P.von Willebrand factor (VL), platelets (N),
        prothrombin time (N).
DD: Haemophilia, Christmas disease, Glanzmann
        syn., macroglobulinaemia, other
        coagulopathies.
PHYS: Due to lack of factor VIII and poor platelet
        adhesiveness.

See also Christmas Disease; Haemophilia A

Waldenström's Macroglobulinaemia (Lymphoplasmacytoid Lymphoma)

TEST: Hb (L), B.lymphocytes (AB), marrow biopsy
        (AB), S.IgM (H), S.viscosity (H), S.protein (H)
SIGN: Splenomegaly, purpura
DD: Chronic lymphocytic leukaemia, multiple myeloma
PHYS: Malignant disease of B.lymphocytes

Warts, Ano-Genital

TEST: Smear microscopy (+), biopsy (+).
DD: Condyloma accuminata, skin tags, piles, hymen
        fragments.
PHYS: Caused by human papilloma virus (HPV).
        Incubation period up to 12 months. Increased
        risk of cervical cancer. Venereal transmission
        with 60% infectivity. Non-sexual transmission
        possible.

Wegener's Granulomatosis

TEST: S.anti-neutrophil cytoplasmic antibodies (+),
        ESR (H), CRP (H).
DD: Lymphoma, sarcoidosis, polymorphic
        reticulocytosis.
PHYS: Uncommon, but 80% mortality.

Wernicke-Korsakoff Syndrome (Korsakoff Psychosis)

TEST: S.thiamine (L), B.alcohol (H or N).

DD: Other cerebral and psychiatric disease.
PHYS: Chronic alcohol abuse and dietary vit. B₁
        insufficiency leads to cerebral lesions.

Whooping Cough

See Pertussis

Wilms' Tumour (Nephroblastoma)

TEST: Hb (AB), WCC (H), U.albumin (+), U.blood (+ or
        –), ESR (VH), S. albumin (L), S.appha₂ globulin
        (H).
DD: Other renal tumours, nephrotic syn., urinary
        infections, urinary calculi.
PHYS: Rapidly growing and metastasising embryonal
        tumour of the kidney in children.

Wilson's Disease (Hepatolenticular Degeneration)

TEST: S.copper (AB), S.ceruloplasmin (L), U.copper (H).
SIGN: Ankle clonus, athetosis, nail discolouration,
        parkinsonian facies, postural tremor, Kayser-
        Fleischer ring.
DD: Other liver diseases, Parkinson's disease.
PHYS: Familial disorder involving metabolism of
        copper, basal ganglia disease and liver
        cirrhosis.

Worms

See Pinworm; Roundworms, Intestinal; Tapeworms

XO Syndrome

See Turner Syndrome

Yaws

TEST: Lesion exudate dark field microscopy (+), FTA
        (+), VDRL (+), treponema inhibition test (+).
SIGN: Ulcerating papules, lymphadenitis.
DD: PATHOLOGY SECTION 4 – identical to
        syphilis, but easily clincally differentiated.
        Tropical ulcers, traumatic ulcers, impetigo,
        secondary syphilis, leischmaniasis.
PHYS: Cutaneous infection in conditions of poor
        hygiene by *Treponema pertenue*.

Yellow Fever

TEST: Specialised virus isolation and serological tests
        (+). S.albumin (H), S.bilirubin (H), WCC (L),
        U.protein (H), U.bilirubin (H).
SIGN: Tachycardia or bradycardia, jaundice,
        hypotension, coffee grounds vomitus.
DD: Leptospirosis, hepatitis, carbon tetrachloride
        poisoning, malaria, typhoid fever, dengue fever,
        influenza.
PHYS: Acute viral disease, endemic in equatorial Africa
        and America, transmitted by mosquitoes.

Zollinger-Ellison Syndrome

TEST: S.gastrin (H), S.calcium (H), basal stomach acid
output (H).

DD: Other causes of peptic ulceration.

PHYS: Gastrin secreting tumour of pancreas,
duodenum or elsewhere, causes very high
levels of gastric acid secretion in stomach,
which leads to repeated acute peptic ulceration.

*See also SYNDROMES SECTION 6: Zollinger-Ellison
Syndrome*

Zoster

See Chickenpox, Shingles

SECTION FOUR
PATHOLOGY

THE INTERPRETATION OF PATHOLOGY TESTS

FORMAT

Test Name, Test Substance [Abbreviation](Alternate Name) [Abbreviation]

RI: Reference interval (or value), and units. Système Internationale (SI) units are used where possible. (Alternative units are in brackets). 90% of the population have results that lie within this range.

IND: Indications. The suspected diseases and conditions in which the test is indicated.

INT: Interpretation of the results. The diseases, conditions, syndromes etc. that should be considered with results that vary from the reference interval (eg: HIGH, LOW, V.LOW). With a history, examination and possibly other tests (in some instances, other tests that should be considered are in brackets after the diagnosis followed by a ?), a definite diagnosis may be made from the differential diagnoses suggested.

PHYS: The basic physiology of the test, to enable the significance to be better understood.

See also Other Relevant Tests

Abbreviation
See Test Name

Please Note:
Reference intervals for tests vary considerably between laboratories, particularly with enzyme tests. When available, reference intervals supplied by the testing laboratory should be used.

3-Hydroxybutyrate, Plasma
See Hydroxybutyrate, Plasma

4-Hydroxy-3-Methoxy Mandelic Acid, Urine [HMMA] (Vanillylmandelic Acid) [VMA]
RI: 10–35 µmol/day (1.8–7.1 mg/day) (<2.5 µg/mg creatinine)
IND: Severe hypertension
INT: V.HIGH – Phaeochromocytoma (catecholamines?)
       HIGH – Neuroblastoma, some foods (eg. caffeine, bananas), drugs (eg. salicylates)
PHYS: Urinary catecholamines and their metabolites (eg. HMMA) are increased 10–100 times in the presence of phaeochromocytoma. Catecholamines increase BP markedly. For 3 days before test avoid meat, fish, poultry and gelatin

See also Metanephrine, Urine

5-Aminolaevulinate, Urine
RI: <40µmol/L
       <3.8mmol/mol creatinine
IND: Prophyria (B.porphyrins?)
INT: HIGH – Acute attack of acute intermittent porphyria, lead poisoning, type 1 tyrosinaemia

---

5 HIAA
See 5-Hydroxyindole Acetic Acid, Urine

5-Hydroxyindole Acetic Acid, Urine [5 HIAA]
RI: 10–80 µmol/24 hours (2–10 mg/24 hours)
IND: Malabsorption syndromes
INT: HIGH – Sprue, (S.gliaden A/B?), gluten intolerance, carcinoid syn.
PHYS: Patients with malabsorption often have abnormalities in tryptophan metabolism. 5 HIAA is a tryptophan metabolite, and its urinary level is increased with excessive tryptophan breakdown. For 3 days before test avoid alcohol, avocado, banana, eggplant, coffee, tea, pineapple, plum, tomatoes, walnuts and drugs (eg. imipramine, paracetamol, MAOIs, phenothiazines)

See also Vitamin D, Serum

---

^{14}C Breath Test
See Carbon–14 Urea, Breath

17-Hydroxy Steroids, Serum
See Steroids, 17-Hydroxy, Serum

25-Hydroxyvitamin D, Blood
RI: 45–150 nmol/L
IND: Osteomalacia, rickets
INT: LOW – Poor diet, malabsorption syndromes, lack of sun exposure, chronic liver disease, chronic renal disease, hyperthyroidism, anticonvulsant therapy
       HIGH – Vit. D intoxication
PHYS: 25-Hydroxyvitamin D is essential for absorption of calcium from gut

---

AAT
See Alpha$_1$-Antitrypsin, Serum

ACE
See Angiotensin Converting Enzyme, Blood

Acetaminophen
See Paracetamol

Acetone, Serum
RI: 0.05–0.35 mmol/L (0.3–2 mg/100 mL)
IND: Diabetes, coma
INT: HIGH – Diabetic acidosis (glucose?)
PHYS: Intracellular carbohydrate starvation in diabetes inhibits the citric acid cycle and the metabolism of ketone bodies

---

Acetone, Urine
RI: Negative
INT: POSITIVE – Diabetic acidosis

Accetylator Status, Blood or Urine
RI: >70% drug excreted in acetylated form
IND: Risk of drug toxicity
INT: LOW – Slow acetylator, potential to develop drug toxicity
PHYS: Caffeine or sulphonamide used as test drug, and urine or serum collected 6 hours later. Slow acetylators may become rapidly toxic when given drugs that are excreted in acetylated form (eg. sulphas, isoniazid, procainamide, hydralazine)

Acetylcholine Receptor Antibody
See Anti-Acetylcholine Receptor Antibody Titre, Serum

Acetylcholinesterase, Amniotic Fluid [AChE]
RI: Second trimester <9 U/L
       Third trimester <7 U/L
IND: Suspect fetal neural tube defect
INT: HIGH – Significant risk of neural tube defect (eg. spina bifida, anencephaly, microcephaly) (AFP?)
PHYS: Experimental, but economic and reliable screening test. Small numbers of false positives may occur

---

AChE
See Acetylcholinesterase, Amniotic Fluid

Acidified Serum Test, Blood (Ham Test)

RI: Negative
IND: Haemolytic anaemia
INT: POSITIVE – paroxysmal nocturnal
       haemoglobinuria, congenital dyserythropoietic
       anaemia
PHYS: Washed red cells incubated with fresh acidified
       serum. Lysis positive

Acidosis

See Base excess; Bicarbonate, Serum; Lactate, Blood;
pH, Serum

Acid Phosphatase, Total, Serum [ACP]

RI: 2.3–5.7 U/L (0.5–4 KAU)
IND: Prostatic disease
INT: HIGH – Prostatic carcinoma (PSA?), acute
       myelocytic leukaemia (FBC?)
PHYS: Phosphatase is present in high concentration in
       the prostate gland. It is released only when
       carcinoma spreads beyond the gland capsule. It
       may be high after rectal examination

ACLA

See Cardiolipin Autoantibodies, Blood

ACTH

See Adrenocorticotrophic Hormone, Plasma

Activated Partial Thromboplastin Time, Plasma [APTT]

RI: 30–45 seconds
IND: Coagulation disorders
INT: HIGH – Heparin therapy, coagulopathy
       requiring further investigation
PHYS: Nonspecific test measuring numerous factors
       except numbers VII and XIII

See also other tests listed under Coagulation Screen

Activated Protein C Resistance, Serum [APC Resistance]

RI: Negative (>2.2)
IND: Recurrent thromboembolism
INT: POSITIVE (<2.0) – Familial thrombobophilia
PHYS: Inherited resistance to anticoagulant action of
       activated protein C resulting in removal of a
       check on the clotting mechanism. Ratio of
       clotting time with and without activated protein C
       is measured

Acute Phase Reactants

See C-Reactive Protein; Erythrocyte Sedimentation Rate

Addis Count

See White Cell Count, Urine

Adenosine Deaminase, Red Blood Cell

RI: Refer to laboratory
IND: Immunodeficiency
INT: LOW – Severe immunodeficiency due to lack of
       adenosine deaminase

ADH

See Antidiuretic Hormone, Serum

Adrenal Cell Antibodies, Serum [AdCA]

RI: Absent
IND: Addison's disease
INT: PRESENT – Addison's disease

Adrenaline

See Catecholamines, Urine

Adrenocorticotrophic Hormone, Plasma [ACTH]

RI: 10–80 ng/L (0–0.5 mU/100 mL, 2.2–17.8
       pmol/L). Morning reading
IND: Pituitary disease
INT: LOW – Pituitary insufficiency, extrapituitary
       Cushing's disease
       HIGH – Cushing's disease of pituitary origin
       (P.cortisol?), adrenal insufficiency, pituitary
       adenoma, oat cell carcinoma of lung
PHYS: ACTH stimulates production of all adrenal
       cortical hormones. Produced in the pituitary
       gland. Specimen should be taken between 8
       and 10 am. Rapid assessment and special
       transportation required

AFP

See Alpha-Fetoprotein, Amniotic Fluid;
Alpha-Fetoprotein, Serum

Alanine Amino Transferase, Serum [ALT] (Alanine Transaminase Glutamic Pyruvic Transaminase) [SGPT]

RI: 3–40 U/L
IND: Liver or heart disease
INT: V.HIGH – Acute hepatitis (bilirubin, Ig?), liver
       necrosis
       HIGH – Obstructive jaundice (AST?), chronic
       hepatitis, neoplastic liver disease, cirrhosis,
       myocardial infarct (LDH, CPK?), infectious
       mononucleosis, Reye syn., viraemia, alcohol
       ALT > AST – Extrahepatic obstruction, acute
       hepatitis
       ALT < AST – Cirrhosis, intrahepatic neoplasm,
       haemolytic jaundice, alcoholic hepatitis
       LOW – Renal failure, vit. B_6 deficiency
PHYS: Liver tissue is rich in the transferases of the
       Kreb's cycle, as are the heart, kidney and
       muscle. ALT more liver specific than AST

See also Aspartate Amino Transferase, Serum

Albumin Concentration Gradient, Ascitic Fluid/Serum

RI: No difference
Difference between serum albumin and ascitic fluid albumin measured
IND: Ascites
INT: < 11 g/L – Exudative ascites (i.e. malignancy, peritoneal inflammation)
> 11 g/L – Transudative ascites (i.e. liver disease, cirrhosis, portal hypertension)
PHYS: Ascitic fluid protein concentration depends on the relative permeability to protein and serum of the vascular bed from which the ascites arises

Albumin, Serum

RI: 35–55 g/L (45–55%)
IND: Liver disease. Guide to prognosis
INT: LOW – Hepatic necrosis, hepatitis (LFT?), hepatic cirrhosis, malnutrition, malabsorption, nephrotic syndrome, systemic infections, chronic inflammation, autoimmune diseases, CCF, overhydration, glomerulonephritis, protein losing enteropathy, leukaemia, Wilm's tumour, burns, pregnancy, elderly.
HIGH – Shock, dehydration, prolonged tourniquet during venepuncture, steroid therapy.

See also Serum-Ascites Albumin Gradient

Albumin, Urine

RI: <15mg/day
IND: Renal disease
INT: HIGH – Urinary tract infection, diabetic nephropathy, nephrotic syndrome, glomerulonephritis, renal failure, pregnancy-induced hypertension
PHYS: Sensitive test for early renal damage in diabetes. Radio-immunoassay

Albumin-Globulin Ratio

RI: 1 – 2.2
IND: Liver disease
INT: HIGH – Liver damage (LFT?)
PHYS: In liver disease there is a hypoalbuminaemia which lowers plasma osmotic pressure and causes ascites. At the same time gamma-globulins rise, increasing the ratio between the two

Albumin Gradient, Serum-Ascites

See Serum-Ascites Albumin Gradient

Alcohol

See Ethanol, Serum

Aldolase, Serum

RI: 1–8 IU/L (1–8 U/mL)
IND: Suspected major organ damage
INT: HIGH – Myocardial infarct (CPK, LDH?), muscular dystrophies, haemolytic anaemia (Hb?), metastatic prostatic carcinoma (ACP, PSA?), leukaemia (FBC?), acute pancreatitis (amylase?), hepatitis
PHYS: Destruction of tissue results in the release of aldolase into the serum. It is present in all tissues. Creatine phosphokinase is a better test

Aldosterone, Plasma

RI: 100–400 pmol/L (0.003–0.01 µg/100 mL)
IND: Hypertension
INT: HIGH – Adrenocortical adenoma (K?), oedema, malignant hypertension, diuretic therapy, congestive cardiac failure, pregnancy
LOW – Adrenocortical insufficiency (S.E., S.urea?), diabetic nephropathy, renal failure (S.creatinine?), drugs (eg. ACE inhibitors, beta-blockers, NSAID, cyclosporin, triamterene)
PHYS: Aldosterone secretion by the adrenal cortex is controlled by volume receptors, angiotensin II, potassium concentration, and minimally by ACTH. Take sample in morning after rest. High aldosterone/renin ratio in adrenal disease. High aldosterone and renin in renal disease

See also Renin, Plasma

Aldosterone, Urine

RI: 8–33 nmol/24 hours (6–16 µg/24 hours)
IND: Adrenal gland investigation, hypertension
INT: HIGH – Adrenocortical adenoma, cirrhosis, nephrosis, ascites, CCF, toxaemia of pregnancy, malignant hypertension (VMA?)
PHYS: Excess secretion of aldosterone by the adrenal cortex causes hypertension and hypokalaemia

Alkaline Phosphatase, Neutrophils

INT: V.HIGH (in mother) – Down syn.
HIGH – Polycythaemia rubra vera (B.erythrocytes?)
PHYS: Use in combination with maternal S.HCG, S.AFP and S.oestriol levels

Alkaline Phosphatase, Serum [ALP]

RI: Adult male 15–130 U/L
Adult female 15–115 U/L
Bone isoenzyme 10–20%
Liver isoenzyme 40–60%
Child 70–300 U/L
IND: Bone and liver disease
INT: V.HIGH – Hepatic duct blockage, metastatic carcinoma of liver
HIGH – Bone metastases, osteomalacia, rickets (Ca, vit. D?), myositis ossificans, Paget's disease of bone (ACP?), hyperparathyroidism, hepatitis (LFT?), primary biliary cirrhosis, prostatic carcinoma, pancreatic disease, recent fracture, children with rapid bone growth, late pregnancy, breastfeeding
LOW – Hypothyroidism (T_4?), hypophosphatasia, growth retardation, zinc deficiency

PHYS: Alkaline phosphatase is present in high concentrations in growing bone and bile. Normal levels do not exclude hepatic disease

Alkalosis

See Base excess; Bicarbonate, Serum; pH, Serum

Allergen Specific Immunoglobulin E

See Radioallergosorbent Test, Serum

Alpha₁-Antitrypsin, Faeces [AAT]

RI:　　<1.5mg/g dry weight
　　　　Clearance <12.5mL/d
IND:　　Protein losing enteropathy
INT:　　HIGH – Protein losing enteropathy
PHYS:　Blood loss into intestine may give false high

Alpha₁-Antitrypsin, Serum [AAT]

RI:　　1.8–3.6 g/L
IND:　　Liver disease, lung disease
INT:　　HIGH – Cirrhosis (LFT?), cholestasis, hormone excess, many infections
　　　　LOW – Hepatic necrosis (LFT?), severe protein loss, emphysema, congenital
PHYS:　Glycoprotein synthesised in liver that inhibits trypsin and other proteases

Alpha₁-Microglobulin, Urine

RI:　　<15mg/L
　　　　<1.5g/mol creatinine
IND:　　Renal tubular disease
INT:　　HIGH – Fanconi syn. (S. & U.phosphate?), nephrotic syndrome (U.protein?), nephrotic syndrome (U.protein?), other renal tubular disorders
PHYS:　Immunoassay

Alpha-Fetoprotein, Amniotic Fluid [AFP]

RI:　　16 weeks gestation 8–24 µg/L
　　　　18 weeks gestation 7–23 µg/L
　　　　20 weeks gestation 3–16 µg/L
IND:　　Monitoring pregnancy
INT:　　DROP – Normal pregnancy
　　　　RISE – Fetal distress (L–S ratio?), neural tube defect, congenital nephrotic syn., twins
　　　　V.LOW – Down syn. (see INVESTIGATIONS SECTION 3)
PHYS:　Level should slowly drop throughout middle trimester of pregnancy

See also Oestriols, Plasma

Alpha-Fetoprotein, Serum [AFP]

RI:　　Non-pregnant < 12 µg/L
　　　　Pregnant – rises throughout up to 50 µg/L or more at term
IND:　　Liver disease, monitoring pregnancy, gonadal cancer

INT:　　V.HIGH, PREGNANT – Down syn. [trisomy 21], neural tube defect
　　　　HIGH – Hepatic carcinoma, colon carcinoma, stomach carcinoma, hepatitis, cirrhosis, other hepatic diseases, gonadal teratoma, testicular carcinoma, embryonal carcinoma, steady rise in normal pregnancy
　　　　LOW – Drop in late pregnancy indicates fetal distress
PHYS:　Normal plasma protein in fetus which drops to very LOW levels after birth. Excess in non-pregnant adult indicates serious disease

Alpha Subunit, Glycoprotein Hormones, Serum

RI:　　Male: <0.6 IU/L
　　　　Female:　Premenopausal: <1.0 IU/L
　　　　　　　　 Post menopausal: <2.0 IU/L
　　　　　　　　 Pregnant: <2.5 IU/L
IND:　　Pituitary tumour
INT:　　HIGH – Hormone secreting pituitary tumour
PHYS:　Some pituitary tumours secrete only alpha subunit of glycoprotein hormone (eg. LH, TSH, FSH) rather than complete hormone

ALT

See Alanine Amino Transferase, Serum

Aluminium, Serum

RI:　　<400 nmol/L
　　　　Toxic >2000 nmol/L
IND:　　Renal dialysis
INT:　　HIGH – Renal failure, dialysis encephalopathy, medications
PHYS:　Contamination of specimen may occur easily

Amikacin, Blood

See Aminoglycosides, Blood

Amino Acids, Urine

RI:　　Units mmol/mol creatinine
　　　　Alanine　　　　　　< 100
　　　　3-Amino-butyric acid　< 25
　　　　Arginine　　　　　　< 20
　　　　Citrulline　　　　　< 5
　　　　Glutamine　　　　　< 150
　　　　Glycine　　　　　　< 350
　　　　Histidine　　　　　< 400
　　　　Isoleucine　　　　< 10
　　　　Leucine　　　　　　< 10
　　　　Lysine　　　　　　< 100
　　　　Methionine　　　　< 10
　　　　Ornithine　　　　　< 10
　　　　Phenylalanine　　　< 20
　　　　Serine　　　　　　< 100
　　　　Taurine　　　　　　< 300
　　　　Tyrosine　　　　　< 20
　　　　Threonine　　　　　< 30
　　　　Valine　　　　　　< 10

IND: Suspected metabolic disease
INT: ALL HIGH – Premature infant, Hartnup disease
Arginine HIGH – Arginase deficiency syn.
Citrulline HIGH – Hyperornithinaemia-
hyperammonaemia-hypercitrullinuria syn.
Glycine HIGH – Nonketotic hyperglycinaemia,
familial iminoglycinuria
Histidine HIGH – Histidinaemia
Leucine and isoleucine HIGH – Maple syrup
urine disease, other rare conditions of organic
acid metabolism
Methionine HIGH – Homocystinuria
Ornithine HIGH – Gyrate atrophy of the choroid
and retina, hyperornithinaemia-
hyperammonaemia-hypercitrullinuria syn.
Phenylalanine HIGH – Phenylketonuria
Tyrosine HIGH – Richner-Hanhart syn. (see
SYNDROMES SECTION 6), tyrosinosis
MIXED PATTERN – Fasting, infection
Others HIGH – Usually rare inherited errors of
metabolism
PHYS: Changes in urinary concentration of certain
amino acids can be used to detect metabolic
diseases
Chromatographic process

See also Cystine, Urine

Aminoglycosides, Blood

RI: Amikacin – peak 25–30mg/L, trough <10mg/L
Gentamicin – peak 5–8 mg/L, trough <2mg/L
Tobramycin – peak 5–8mg/L, trough <2mg/L
Vancomycin – trough 5–10mg/L
IND: Monitoring of antibiotic dose
INT: Adjust dosage as appropriate
PHYS: Peak measure taken 6 hours after once daily
dosage, trough immediately before next dose.
Toxicity if levels above exceeded, ineffective
dose if peak doses too low. Vancomycin peaks
not accurate for dosage management

5-Aminolaevulinate, Urine
See numerical entries at beginning of this section

Amiodarone, Serum

RI: Therapeutic range 1.5–3.9 µmol/L (1.0–2.5 mg/L)
IND: Amiodarone treatment
PHYS: Elimination half life 40 days. Measure drug
levels only 3 months after dosage adjustment

Amitriptyline, Serum

RI: Therapeutic range 60–240 µg/L (150–880 nmol/L)
PHYS: Several weeks may be required to reach steady
state due to long half-life

Ammonia, Serum [NH$_3$]

RI: < 50 mmol/L (< 90 µg/100 mL)
IND: Liver disease
INT: HIGH – Hepatic insufficiency (bilirubin?),

portacaval shunt, high protein diet, organic
acidaemia, gastrointestinal tract bleeding,
methicillin or spironolactone therapy, Reye
syn., genetic hyperammonaemia, transient in
neonate
PHYS: Serum ammonia is derived from the
putrefaction of food in the bowel by bacteria,
and from protein metabolism

Amoeba Antibodies, Serum

RI: Absent
IND: Extraintestinal amoebiasis
INT: POSITIVE – Hepatic amoebiasis in past
RISING TITRE – Recent hepatic infection
PHYS: Gut infections do not cause antibody reaction.
Test will remain positive for many years

Amylase, Serum

RI: 30–180 U/L (Racial differences)
IND: Pancreatic disease
INT: HIGH – Acute pancreatitis (aldolase, lipase?),
cancer of the pancreas, mumps, salpingitis,
perforated duodenal ulcer, sialectasis, hepatic
disease, ruptured ectopic pregnancy,
dissecting aortic aneurysm, small bowel
obstruction
LOW – Hepatitis, toxaemia of pregnancy,
pancreatic insufficiency
PHYS: Amylase is produced in the pancreas and
salivary glands. Excess is produced in
inflammation, or is forced into the serum by
pancreatic duct blockage

Amylase, Urine

RI: 170–2000 U/L (Racial differences)
(0.8–80 u/mmol creatinine) (<17 IU/L)
IND: Pancreatitis
INT: HIGH – Pancreatitis
PHYS: Urinary amylase is raised with the same
conditions as serum amylase. Useful in late
presentation of pancreatitis, as levels remain
high for 7 days after serum amylase drops

ANA
See Antinuclear Autoantibodies, Fluorescent, Blood

Anabolic Steroids, Urine

RI: Absent
IND: Detection of steroid use
INT: POSITIVE – Use of anabolic steroids in
previous days or weeks
PHYS: Rate of metabolism and clearance from urine
depends on individual characteristics, type of
steroid and dose

Anaemia
See Haemoglobin

ANCA
See Anti-Neutrophil Cytoplasmic Antibodies, Serum

Androgens
See Testosterone, Serum

Androstenedione, Serum
RI: Males 1.7–5.2 nmol/L (0.05–0.29 µg/100mL)
Females 1.7–7.0 nmol/L (0.05–0.35 µg/100mL)
Prepubertal < 2 nmol/L (<0.05 µg/100mL)
Postmenopause 1.7–4.5 nmol/L
IND: Female hirsutism
INT: HIGH – Hirsutism, virilising tumours, congenital adrenal hyperplasia, polycystic ovarian syndrome, acne, premature baldness, pubertal status
PHYS: Collect sample mid-morning. Immunoassay

ANF
See Antinuclear Autoantibodies, Fluorescent, Blood

Angiotensin Converting Enzyme, Blood [ACE]
RI: 11–40 U/L (higher levels in children)
IND: Suspect sarcoidosis
INT: HIGH – Sarcoidosis, tuberculosis, leprosy, silicosis, asbestosis, cirrhosis, diabetes mellitus, alcoholism, hyperthyroidism, Gaucher's disease
LOW – Drugs (eg. ACE inhibitors)
PHYS: Good measure of sarcoid disease activity

Angiotensin II, Plasma
RI: 5–35 pmol/L (5–35 ng/L)
IND: Hyperaldosteronism
INT: HIGH – Hyperaldosteronism
PHYS: Collect in heparin at mid-morning. Unstable hormone requiring immediate blood separation. Must rest for 12 hours before test, and be off all drugs for one month. Angiotensin II controls aldosterone production from the adrenal glands

Anion Gap, Serum
RI: 8–16 mmol/L
IND: Electrolyte imbalance
INT: HIGH – Metabolic acidosis, diabetic ketoacidosis (GTT?), renal failure, lactic acidosis, methanol ingestion, salicylate overdose, hepatic failure, alcoholism, magnesium deficiency, starvation
LOW – Hypoalbuminaemia, liver disease, multiple myeloma, hypercalcaemia
PHYS: Anion gap = cations $(Na^+ + K^+)$ – anions $(Cl^- + HCO_3^-)$. Gap is made up of phosphate, sulfate, protein, pyruvate, lactate and other ions. If all elements are considered, gap is zero

ANS
See Anti-Smith Antibodies, Serum

Anti-Acetylcholine Receptor Antibody Titre, Serum [Anti-AChR]
RI: –0.5 to +0.5 nmol/L
IND: Myasthenia gravis
INT: HIGH – Myasthenia gravis
PHYS: Specific antibody for myasthenia gravis that is elevated in 80% of cases

Antibodies, Specific
See Immunoglobulin Antibodies, Specific, Serum

Anticardiolipin Antibodies, Blood
See Cardiolipin Autoantibodies, Blood

Anti-Centromere Antibodies
See Centromere Autoantibodies, Blood

Anti-Deoxyribonuclease-B Titre, Serum [Anti-DNAse B]
RI: 0–340 (varies widely between labs)
IND: Rheumatic fever
INT: HIGH – Streptococcal pyoderma, rheumatic fever (ASOT?), nephritis
PHYS: Antibody to extracellular enzyme of group A Streptococci. Persists for longer than ASOT

See also Anti Streptolysin O Titre

Anti-Deoxyribonucleic Acid Titre, Serum [Anti-DNA]
RI: <100 IU/mL)
IND: Connective tissue disease
INT: HIGH – SLE (ANA?), rheumatoid arthritis
PHYS: Used in association with other tests to diagnose and follow course of SLE. Does not rise in drug induced SLE

See also ANCA, Serum; Andi-DNA, Serum; Anti-Smith Antibodies, Serum; Cardiolipin Autoantibodies, Blood; Complement C3 and C4; DNA Autoantibodies; ENA, Serum; Histone Autoantibodies, Blood; HLA-DR3, Serum; LE Cells, Blood; Lupus Anticoagulant Antibody, Serum

Antidiuretic Hormone, Serum [ADH] (Vasopressin, Serum) [AVP]
RI: 0.4–2.4 pg/mL
IND: Disorders of urine production
INT: HIGH – Syndrome of inappropriate ADH secretion, central diabetes insipidus
LOW – Nephrogenic diabetes insipidus
PHYS: Diurnal variation in level, maximum in early hours of morning, minimum in early afternoon

See also Osmolality, Serum

Anti-Double Stranded DNA Antibodies, Serum [Anti-dsDNA]
RI: <7 IU/L

IND: Inflammatory joint disease, suspect SLE
INT: HIGH – Systemic lupus erythematosus
PHYS: Highly selective for SLE, but antibodies are not present in all patients with SLE. Levels vary with disease activity and can be used to assess patient response to treatment

ANTI-dsDNA

See Anti-Double Stranded DNA Antibodies, Serum

Anti-Factor XA, Plasma [AntiXa]

RI: Therapeutic range 0.3–0.5 U/mL
IND: Monitoring of low molecular weight heparin dosage
INT: Adjust dosage depending on results
PHYS: Not used routinely for patients on low molecular weight heparin

Anti-Gliaden Antibodies, Serum

See Gliaden Antibodies, Serum

Anti-Glutamic Acid Decarboxylase Antibodies, Serum [Anti-GAD]

RI: Negative
IND: Diabetes mellitus
INT: POSITIVE – Insulin dependent diabetes mellitus
PHYS: High incidence of positive results in association with autoimmune thyroid disease and diabetes, particularly early in course of disease. Test currently experimental, but may find use in mainstream medicine in diagnosis of some types of autoimmune disease

Anti-Histone Antibodies

See Histone Autoantibodies, Blood

Antimicrobial Antibodies, Serum or CSF

RI: Absent
IND: Check for cause or type of infection
INT: POSITIVE – Present or recent infection with specific microbe
PHYS: Test is specific for a particular infective agent. Only a limited number of microbes (and their diseases) can be checked. Tests available include those for Brucellosis, Chlamydia, Coxiella (Q fever), Coxsackie virus, Cytomegalovirus, Echoviruses, Epstein-Barr virus (infectious mononucleosis), hepatitis A, hepatitis B, hepatitis C, *Herpes simplex*, Legionnaires disease, Leptospirosis, measles, mumps, *Mycoplasma pneumoniae*, Ross River fever, rubella, salmonellosis and toxoplasmosis

Anti-Microsomal Antibodies

See Thyroid Microsomal Autoantibody Titre, Serum

Antimitochondrial Antibodies, Serum

See Mitochondrial Autoantibodies, Serum

Anti-Neutrophil Cytoplasmic Antibodies, Serum [ANCA]

RI: Negative
IND: Vasculitis
INT: POSITIVE – SLE, vasculitis, Churg-Strauss syn., Wegener's granulomatosis
PHYS: Titres fluctuate with severity of disease

See also LE Cells, Blood; Lupus Anticoagulant Antibody, Serum

Antinuclear Autoantibodies, Fluorescent, Blood [ANA] (Antinuclear Factor) [ANF]

RI: 0–25 IU/mL (titre 0–10)
IND: SLE and other connective tissue diseases
INT: V.HIGH – SLE, scleroderma
        HIGH – Autoimmune conditions (eg: rheumatoid arthritis, Felty syn., Sjøgren syn., dermatopolymyositis, vasculitis, juvenile chronic polyarthritis, mixed connective tissue disease), thyroid disease (eg: Hashimoto's thyroiditis, Graves disease), malignancy, (eg: lymphoma, leukaemia, some solid tumours), liver disease (eg: chronic active hepatitis, cirrhosis, hepatitis B, chronic liver disease), lung diseases (eg: pneumoconioses, asbestosis, idiopathic pulmonary fibrosis, fibrosing alveolitis, primary pulmonary hypertension, TB), haematological disorders (eg: pernicious anaemia, idiopathic thrombocytopenic purpura), parasitic diseases (eg: malaria), subacute bacterial endocarditis, myasthenia gravis, leprosy, relatives of SLE patients, pregnancy, some elderly people, drugs [eg. hydralazine, procainamide]
PHYS: Tested by indirect immunofluorescence of nuclei in tissue substrates. Homogenous pattern in SLE and Sjøgren syn. Peripheral pattern uncommon but occurs in 10% of SLE patients. Speckled pattern in SLE, scleroderma, other connective tissue diseases and up to 20% of normal elderly women

See also LE Cells, Blood; Lupus Anticoagulant Antibody, Serum

Anti-Skeletal Muscle Antibodies, Serum [SKM]

RI: Negative
IND: Myasthenia gravis (anti-AChR?)
INT: POSITIVE – Myasthenia gravis
PHYS: Specific tissue autoantibody

Anti-Smith Antibodies, Serum [ANS]

RI: Negative
IND: SLE
INT: POSITIVE – SLE (33% of cases)
PHYS: More vasculitis and less renal disease in this form of SLE

See also LE Cells, Blood; Lupus Anticoagulant Antibody, Serum

Anti-Smooth Muscle Antibodies, Serum [SMA]

RI: Negative
IND: Hepatic disease
INT: POSITIVE – Chronic active hepatitis, primary biliary cirrhosis, infectious mononucleosis, disseminated carcinoma, SLE, viral hepatitis, other infections, other autoimmune diseases
PHYS: Specific tissue autoantibody

Antistreptolysin O Titre [ASOT]

RI: 0–300 IU/mL (<200 Todd units/mL) [varies widely between labs]
IND: Severe infections
INT: HIGH – Haemolytic streptococcal infection, rheumatic fever
PHYS: Persons infected with beta-haemolytic Streptococci often develop antibodies against the haemolysin O produced by Streptococcus. This antibody inhibits haemolysis of red cells by a standardised Streptococcus haemolysin

See also Anti-Deoxyribonuclease-B Titre

Antithrombin III, Blood [AT III]

RI: 80–120% (0.77–1.20 U/mL)
IND: Unusual venous thromboses
INT: LOW (< 60%) – Congenital (autosomal dominant) AT III deficit, dysfunctional AT III, familial thrombophilia
PHYS: AT III inhibits clotting by preventing conversion of fibrinogen to fibrin, and also acts on factors IX, X, XI and XII

Anti-Thyroglobulin Antibody, Serum

See Thyroglobulin Antibody, Serum

Anti-Thyroid Peroxidase Antibodies, Serum

RI: <35 U/mL
IND: Thyroid disease
INT: HIGH – Inflamed thyroid gland, Hashimoto's thyroiditis, other autoimmune conditions affecting the thyroid

Anti-TSH Receptor Antibodies, Serum [TRAB]

RI: Negative
IND: Thyroid disease
INT: POSITIVE – Graves' disease, thyrotoxicosis
PHYS: TRAB are the autoantibodies that bind to the TSH receptor and activate it, causing the excess production of thyroid hormones in Graves' disease

AntiXa

See Anti-Factor Xa, Plasma

APC Resistance

See Activated Protein C Resistance, Serum

Apolipoproteins, Serum [Apo]

RI: ApoA1 1.0–1.8g/L, ApoB 0.8–1.6g/L
IND: Atherosclerosis
INT: LOW – Increased risk of atherosclerosis
PHYS: Immunoassay. May be measured as an alternative to HDL and LDL

See also High Density Lipoprotein Cholesterol, Blood; Low Density Lipoprotein Cholesterol, Blood

APTT

See Activated Partial Thromboplastin Time, Plasma

Arbovirus Antibodies, Specific

See Immunoglobulin Antibodies, Specific, Serum

Arsenic, Urine [As$_2$O$_3$]

RI: 0–0.1 mg/L (< 3 µmol/day)
IND: Suspected arsenic poisoning
INT: HIGH – Arsenic poisoning

Ascitic Fluid

See Paracentesis Fluid

Ascorbic Acid, Serum

See Vitamin C

ASOT

See Antistreptolysin O Titre

Aspartate Amino Transferase, Serum [AST] (Aspartate Transaminase) (Glutamic Oxaloacetic Transaminase) [SGOT]

RI: 8–40 IU/L
IND: Liver disease
INT: V.HIGH – Obstructive jaundice, acute hepatitis (bilirubin, lg ?)
HIGH – Cirrhosis, myocardial infarct (LDH, CPK?), intrahepatic neoplasm, haemolytic jaundice, trauma, Reye syn., muscular dystrophy, trauma, alcoholism, some anaesthetics, vigorous exercise, paracetamol overdose, haemolysis or refrigeration of sample
LOW – Renal failure, vit. B$_6$ deficiency
PHYS: AST is widely distributed with high concentrations in liver, heart, muscle and kidney. Rises to a peak 36 hours after infarct, and returns to normal after 3–4 days

See also Alanine Amino Transferase, Serum

Aspergillus Precipitins, Serum

RI: Absent
IND: Asthma triggered by aspergillosis
INT: PRESENT – Allergic bronchopulmonary aspergillosis
PHYS: Does not diagnose invasive aspergillosis

AT III
See Antithrombin III, Blood

Autoantibodies
*See Antinuclear Autoantibodies, Fluorescent, Blood;
Anti-Skeletal Muscle Antibodies, Serum; Anti-Smith
Antibodies, Serum; Anti-Smooth Muscle Antibodies,
Serum; Anti-Thyroid Peroxidase Antibodies; Basement
Membrane Autoantibodies, Blood; Cardiolipin
Autoantibodies, Blood; Centromere Autoantibodies,
Blood; Extractable Nuclear Antigen Autoantibodies,
Serum; Glomerular Basement Membrane
Autoantibodies, Blood; Histone Autoantibodies, Blood;
Intercellular Cement Substance Autoantibodies, Blood;
Intrinsic Factor Autoantibodies, Blood; Islet Cell
Autoantibodies, Blood; Mitochondrial Autoantibodies,
Serum; Myocardial Autoantibodies, Blood; Ovarian
Autoantibodies, Blood; Parietal Cell Autoantibodies,
Serum; Reticular Cell Autoantibodies, Serum; Thyroid
Microsomal Autoantibody Titre, Serum*

Autohaemolysis Test, Blood
RI: Lysis at 48 hours with added glucose < 0.9%.
Lysis at 48 hours without added glucose 0.2–2.0%
IND: Red cell disorders
INT: HIGH WITHOUT GLUCOSE – Hereditary
spherocytosis, other red cell membrane
congenital defects
HIGH WITH AND WITHOUT GLUCOSE –
Pyruvate kinase deficiency, disorders of red cell
glycolysis
PHYS: Competence of cell membrane and glucose
metabolism affects degree of red cell lysis

AVP
See Antidiuretic Hormone, Serum

B Cell Lymphocytes, Blood
RI: $0.06–0.60 \times 10^9$/L
IND: Leukaemia
INT: CD20 HIGH – Acute lymphoblastic leukaemia
PHYS: Follicular dendritic cell

See also T Cell Lymphocytes, Blood

B$_2$M
See Beta–2 Microglobulin, serum

B$_{12}$
See Cyanocobalamin, Serum

Barbiturates, Serum
RI: Zero
IND: Overdosage, control of therapy
INT: HIGH – Overdosage
PHYS: Coma over 90–170 µmol/L (higher with
phenobarbitone). Plasma half-life 2–6 days

Barmah Forest Virus Antibodies, Serum
See Immunoglobulin Antibodies, Specific, Serum

Base Excess, Arterial Blood
RI: +3 to –3 mmol/L
IND: Metabolic disorders
INT: HIGH – Metabolic alkalosis, respiratory acidosis
LOW – Metabolic acidosis, respiratory alkalosis
PHYS: Collected in sealed, heparinised syringe

Basement Membrane Autoantibodies, Blood (Pemphigoid Autoantibodies)
RI: Negative
IND: Blistering skin diseases
INT: POSITIVE – Pemphigoid
PHYS: Immunofluorescent test. Titre does not
correlate with disease severity

Basophils, Blood
RI: $<0.1 \times 10^9$/L (10–100/µL) (0.1–1.0%)
IND: To determine nature of infection or blood disease
INT: V.HIGH – Chronic myeloid leukaemia,
myelofibrosis, polycythaemia vera, urticaria,
pigmentosa
HIGH – Chronic inflammation, myxoedema,
ulcerative colitis, allergic reactions, some
viraemias, splenectomy
LOW – Steroid therapy, stress, pregnancy,
hyperthyroidism, some infections

Bence-Jones Proteins, Urine
RI: Nil
IND: Myelomatoses
INT: PRESENT – Multiple myeloma, renal damage,
macroglobulinaemia, plasmacytoma,
autoimmune diseases
PHYS: Light chains of abnormal immunoglobulins are
easily filtered through kidney into urine

Beta HCG
See Chorionic Gonadotrophin, Human, Beta, Serum

Beta-2 Microglobulin, Serum [β_2M]
RI: Adults 0.8–2.5 mg/L; >65 years 0.8–3.0 mg/L
IND: Multiple myeloma, suspected AIDS
INT: HIGH – AIDS (HIV ?), multiple myeloma, chronic
lymphocytic leukaemia, acute monoblastic
leukaemia, hepatitis B, Epstein-Barr virus and
cytomegalovirus infections, sarcoid,
rheumatoid arthritis, Sjøgren syn., Crohn's
disease, renal failure
PHYS: Raised in early stage of AIDS, and increases
with worsening immune dysfunction. Useful
prognostic marker in lymphoproliferative
disorders

Beta-2 Microglobulin, Urine

RI: < 0.5 mg/L (< 40 µg/mmol creatinine)
IND: Renal dysfunction
INT: As for Beta-2 Microglobulin, Serum, plus:
HIGH – Renal damage [eg. from cytotoxic drugs, heavy metal poisoning, NSAID overdose, aminoglycosides], glomerulonephritis
PHYS: Globulin excreted in renal tubulo-interstitial disorders

Bicarbonate, Serum $[HCO_3^-]$

RI: 24–32 mmol/L (24–32 mEq/L)
IND: Acid-base imbalance
INT: HIGH (Respiratory Acidosis) – Underventilation of lungs (VC, FEV_1?)
HIGH (Metabolic Alkalosis) – Bicarbonate therapy, potassium depletion (K?), vomiting, pyloric stenosis, gastric aspiration, late salicylate poisoning, Cushing syn., diuretics, antacids, steroid therapy
LOW (Respiratory Alkalosis) – Hyperventilation, hysteria, altitude sickness, excess artificial respiration
LOW (Metabolic Acidosis) – Starvation, diarrhoea, liver failure, dehydration, early salicylate poisoning, diabetes mellitus (glucose?), anuria, severe renal disease, ureterocolic anastamosis
PHYS: The bicarbonate level is dependent upon removal of carbon dioxide from the blood as well as the amount of acid or base formed in or added to the body

Bilirubin, Serum

RI: Total 1–20 µmol/L (0.1–1.1 mg/100 mL)
Direct (conjugated) 1–6 µmol/L (0.1–0.4 mg/100 mL)
Indirect 2–13 µmol/L (0.2–0.7 mg/100 mL)
Neonate 17–170 µmol/L (1–10 mg/100 mL)
IND: Liver disease, anaemia
INT: HIGH DIRECT & INDIRECT – Hepatitis (Ig, ALT, AST?), bile duct blockage, gall stones, toxic reactions, Gilbert's disease, malignancy, cirrhosis (LFT?), Dubin-Johnson syn.
HIGH INDIRECT ONLY – Haemolytic disease, haematoma resorptions
HIGH IN NEONATE – Physiological jaundice, haemolytic disease, spherocytosis, sickle cell anaemia, birth trauma, hepatitis, hypothyroidism, prematurity, biliary atresia, choledocal cyst, starvation, meconium ileus, Crigler-Najjar syn., drugs
PHYSIOLOGICAL JAUNDICE (infants) – Clinical icterus is not apparent in infants until S.bilirubin is >5 mg/100 mL, but in older children is apparent clinically when S.bilirubin is > 2 mg/100 mL
PHYS: Haemoglobin destruction gives bilirubin, which is conjugated in the liver and excreted in the bile. Any overload or blockage of this system raises levels. The direct van den Bergh reaction reads conjugated bilirubin. The graph shows progressive changes in serum bilirubin levels

Changes in Serum Bilirubin Levels in the Neonate

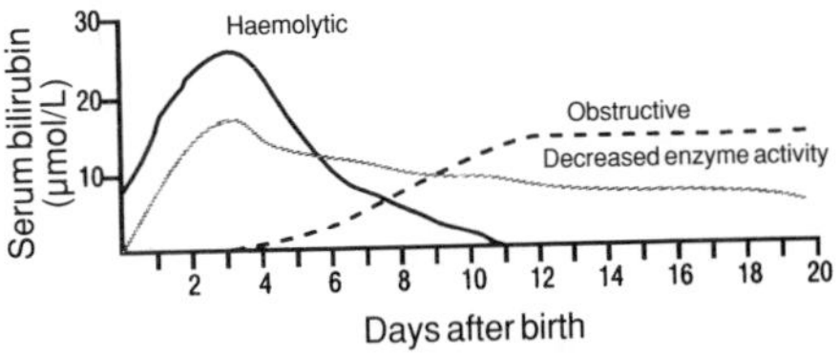

due to haemolytic jaundice, obstructive jaundice (eg. biliary atresia, cystic fibrosis, galactosaemia) and decreased liver enzyme activity (eg. prematurity, Gilbert's disease, physiological disorders, viral infections, Crigler-Najjar syn., breastfeeding)

Bilirubin, Urine

RI: Nil
IND: Liver disease
INT: PRESENT – Jaundice due to conjugated hyperbilirubinaemia
ABSENT WITH CLINICAL JAUNDICE – Jaundice due to unconjugated hyperbilirubinaemia, hypervitaminosis A
PHYS: Unconjugated bilirubin is lipid soluble, and cannot appear in urine. Conjugated bilirubin is water soluble. In hypervitaminosis A, jaundice is not due to bilirubin, but carotene

See also Bilirubin, Serum

Bismuth, Serum

RI: < 20 nmol/L
IND: Bismuth poisoning (eg. bismuth subcitrate medication)
INT: < 48 nmol/L – Nontoxic level
48–240 nmol – Intermediate range, possible toxicity
> 240 nmol – Toxic

Blast Cells, Blood

RI: Nil
IND: Noted on routine blood film
INT: PRESENT – Marrow infiltration, carcinoma, leukaemia, sarcoma
PHYS: Most primitive form of white cell. Further investigation essential when found in peripheral blood

Bleeding Time

RI: 1–7 minutes
IND: Coagulation disorders
INT: HIGH – Drugs (eg. aspirin, NSAIDs), thrombocytopenia, thromboasthenia (platelets?), haemophilia, Christmas disease, von Willebrand's disease, Bernard-Soulier syn., Glanzmann syn.
PHYS: Normal with anticoagulant therapy (eg. heparin, warfarin). Measures platelet function

Blood Gases
See Carbon Dioxide, Blood; Oxygen, Blood

Blood Group
RI: Types – A (A1 & A2), AB, B, O
        Rhesus factor:
        Rh+ (87%) (genotype cDe,CDe, CDE)
        Rh– (13%) (genotype cde, cdE)
        Rh± (rare) (genotype Cde)
        Other factors – M, N, S, s, U
        Familial factors – Kell, Duff, Lewis, Kidd, etc.
IND: Blood transfusion, presurgery, medicolegal,
        precautionary
INT: Blood type and factors determine which blood a
        patient should receive. In emergency: O– is
        universal donor, AB+ is universal recipient.
        Parentage can be determined within limits by
        comparing grouping and other blood factors
        (particularly M and N) of parents and child

Blood Volume
RI: 60–80 mL/kg
        Mean values: Male 4,500 mL,
        Female 3,600 mL
PHYS: Measured by dye or radioisotope dilution
        methods. Increased 40% in pregnancy

Blood, Faecal, Occult
See Occult Blood, Faeces

Blood, Urine
See Haematuria

Bone Marrow
See Marrow Cells, Bone

Bone Mineral Density [BMD]
RI: T score above –1
IND: Osteoporosis
INT: BELOW –2.5 – Osteoporosis requiring treatment
        –1 to –2.5 – Borderline, retest in 2 yrs, institute
        prevention with HRT or calcium
PHYS: Dual photon densitometry measures bone
        density at wrist and interpreted as a T score
        variation from young normal mean

Breast Milk Analysis
RI: **Colostrum** (1–5 days postpartum)
        Energy 239 kJ/100 mL (57 calories/100mL)
        Total protein 1460–6800 mg/100 mL
        Lactose 1100–7900 mg/100 mL
        Amino acids 700–4000 mg/100 mL
        Total fats 2740–3180 mg/100 mL
        Total solids 10–16 g/100 mL
        Sodium 26–135 mEq/L
        Iron 0.02–0.05 mg/100 mL
        Transition Milk (5–10 days postpartum)
        Energy 264 kJ/100 mL (63 calories/100mL)
        Total protein 1270–1890 mg/100 mL
        Lactose 6100–6700 mg/100 mL
        Amino acids 600–1000 mg/100 mL
        Total fats 2730–5180 mg/100 mL
        SG 1.034–1.036
        Total solids 10.5–15.5 g/100 mL
        Sodium 19–53 mEq/L
        Iron 0.04–0.07 mg/100 mL
        Mature Milk (15+ days postpartum)
        Energy 272 kJ/100 mL (65 calories/100mL)
        Total protein 730–2000 mg/100 mL
        Lactose 4900–9500 mg/100 mL
        Amino acids 900–1600 mg/100 mL
        Total fats 1340–8290 mg/100 mL
        SG 1.026–1.037
        Total solids 10.3–17.5 g/100 mL
        Sodium 6–43 mEq/L
        Iron 0.02–0.09 mg/100 mL
IND: Infant feeding problems, failure to thrive
INT: Abnormal results indicate inadequate or
        inappropriate lactation

Breath test, Carbon-14 Urea
See Carbon -14 Urea Breath Test

Brucellosis Antibodies, Serum
See Immunoglobulin Antibodies, Specific, Serum

Buccal Smear
INT: Microscopic examination of cells from the
        buccal mucous membrane enables the sex of
        the individual to be determined. The presence of
        a Barr body on the nucleus indicates female, its
        absence indicates male.

See also Oestrogens, Urinary

BUN
See Urea, Blood

Bunnell, Paul
See Paul Bunnell Test

^{14}C Breath Test
See numerical entries at beginning of this section

C3 and C4
See Complement, Serum

Ca
See Calcium, Ionised, Blood; Calcium, Corrected, Serum; Calcium, Serum; Calcium, Urine

CA
See Cancer Associated Antigens, Serum

Cadmium, Serum

RI: < 0.04 µmol/L
IND: Industrial exposure in battery, electroplating, paint, plastic & ceramic factories; copper, lead or zinc smelting
INT: HIGH – Excessive exposure
PHYS: May accumulate in food chain, particularly in shellfish

Caeruloplasmin, Serum

RI: 1.5–3.5 mmol/L (0.2–0.47 g/L)
IND: Copper deficiency
INT: HIGH – Pregnancy, hyperthyroidism (ETR?), infection, aplastic anaemia, (FBC, Hb?), acute leukaemia, liver cirrhosis
        LOW – Wilson's disease
PHYS: Serum copper is 95% bound to caeruloplasmin

Calcitonin, Plasma

RI: < 27 pmol/L (< 100 ng/L)
IND: Thyroid and parathyroid disease
INT: HIGH – Thyroid carcinoma, primary hyperparathyroidism, phaeochromocytoma, Cushing syn., multiple neuromas, carcinoid tumour
PHYS: Collect specimen mid-morning. Polypeptide hormone involved in regulation of calcium and bone metabolism

Calcium, Corrected, Serum

RI: 2.15–2.55 mmol/L
IND: As for Calcium, Serum
INT: As for Calcium, Serum
PHYS: Calculated by an algorithm that corrects artefacts due to hypoalbuminaemia and hyperalbuminaemia

Calcium, Ionised, Blood

RI: 1.14–1.30 mmol/L
IND: Investigation of abnormal S.calcium
INT: HIGH – Hyperparathyroidism (Nordin test?), early malignancy, sarcoidosis, vit. A toxicity, vit. D toxicity, milk-alkali syn., other causes of hypercalcaemia
        NORMAL IONISED, HIGH TOTAL SERUM CALCIUM – Chronic alkalosis (i.e. from vomiting, steroids or diuretics)
        NORMAL IONISED, LOW TOTAL SERUM CALCIUM – Protein binding anomaly, chronic acidosis, hypoalbuminaemia
        LOW – Hypoparathyroidism, vit. D deficiency, dietary insufficiency, other causes of hypocalcaemia
PHYS: The ionised calcium fraction alone interacts with cell membranes and transport systems, and is responsible for clinical signs and symptoms of hypo- or hypercalcaemia. Any variation from normal range highly significant

See also Calcium, Serum

Calcium, Serum [Ca]

RI: 2.2–2.7 mmol/L (9–10.8 mg/100 mL)
IND: Renal, bone and parathyroid disease
INT: HIGH – Parathyroid overactivity (P, PTH?), osteolytic tumours, hypervitaminosis A, hypervitaminosis D, vit. D sensitivity, excess Ca absorption, lymphomas, sarcoidosis (S.ACE?), other neoplasias, hypophosphatasia, dehydration, hyperalbuminaemia, renal tubular acidosis, thyrotoxicosis (TSH?), von Recklinghausen's disease of bone, excess milk ingestion, multiple myeloma, Paget's disease of bone, hyperthyroidism, milk-alkali syn., adrenal insufficiency, acute rhabdomyolysis, prolonged immobilisation, parenteral nutrition, infancy, postmenopause, familial benign hypercalcaemia (U.Ca?), prolonged application of tourniquet during collection, transient effect in 4%, drugs (eg. thiazide diuretics, lithium, tamoxifen)
        LOW – Lack of vit. D, chronic illness, hypoparathyroidism (P?), renal failure, insensitivity to vit. D, renal rickets, nephrotic syn., hypoalbuminaemia, rhabdomyolysis, acidosis, acute pancreatitis, hypomagnesaemia, di George syn., pregnancy, hyperventilation
PHYS: The absorption of calcium is dependent on vit. D which is obtained by sun irradiation of a skin cholesterol. The amount of calcium added to or removed from bone depends on calcitonin which is secreted by the parathyroid glands. Fasting sample required. Use of tourniquet during venesection may cause false high result.

See also Calcium, Corrected, Serum; Calcium, Ionised, Blood

Calcium, Urine [Ca]

RI: 2.5–7.5 mmol/day
IND: Parathyroid or bone disease
INT: HIGH – Hyperparathyroidism, high serum calcium, osteoporosis
        LOW – Renal failure, nephrotic syn.
PHYS: Strongly affected by diet

See also Calcium, Serum

Calculi, Renal

See Renal Calculi

Cancer Associated Antigens, Serum (Carbohydrate Antigens) [CA]

RI: < 30 U/mL; mean 12.9 U/mL; peak 6 U/mL
IND: Detection or monitoring of certain cancers
INT: CA 15–3 HIGH – Metastatic breast cancer (70%+), localised breast cancer (10%+). False positive with hepatic failure
        CA 19–9 HIGH – Pancreatic cancer (80%+), bile duct cancer (66%+), stomach cancer (50%+), hepatoma (50%+), colorectal cancer (25%+). False positive with cirrhosis, cholangitis, pancreatitis

CA 50 HIGH – Pancreatic cancer (75%+), colorectal cancer (45%+).
False positive with pancreatitis
CA 125 HIGH – Epithelial ovarian cancer (85%+), endometrial cancer. False positive with endometriosis
CA 195 – Pancreatic cancer (85%+), gastrointestinal cancer
CA 549 – Breast cancer (50%+), lung cancer, colon cancer, prostate cance. False positive with endometriosis, hepatic disease, ovarian disease

PHYS: A reading above 30 U/mL highly suspicious of carcinoma. Any reading above the mean should be regarded suspiciously and repeated to check for rising values. Used for following course of carcinoma and for screening in patients with family history of carcinoma. Radio-immunoassay using monoclonal antibodies

See also Squamous Cell Carcinoma Associated Antigen; Vasoactive Intestinal Peptide

Cancer Associated Serum Antigen, Serum [CASA]

RI: Negative
IND: Ovarian cancer
INT: POSITIVE – Epithelial ovarian cancer (75%+), colon cancer, uterine cancer, cervix cancer, breast cancer. False positive possible in late pregnancy

Carbamazepine, Serum (Tegretol)

RI: Therapeutic range 20–50 µmol/L (6–12 µg/mL)
IND: Carbamazepine therapy
INT: Adjust dosage to keep serum level within therapeutic range
PHYS: Carbamazepine is used for epilepsy and trigeminal neuralgia. Sample prior to next dose

Carbohydrate Antigens

See Cancer Associated Antigens, Serum

Carbohydrate-Deficient Transferrin, Blood

RI: Varies between laboratories
IND: Alcoholism
INT: HIGH – Chronic alcoholism, carbohydrate-deficient glycoprotein syndrome
PHYS: Immunoassay. Very reliable test for chronic alcoholism with regular ingestion of .>50g alcohol/day. Negative result does not exclude diagnosis

Carbon Dioxide, Blood [pCO₂]

RI: 25–30 mmol/L (25–30 mEq/L) (combining power 45–65% vol.)
pCO_2 4.6–6.0 kPa (42 ± 4 mmHg)
IND: Pulmonary or vascular insufficiency
INT: HIGH – Hypoxia due to poor air entry, poor lung function, or poor circulation. Higher values far

The Relation Between Blood CO_2 and ventilation

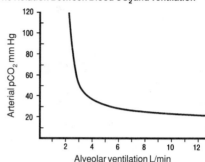

more significant than slightly raised values, as relationship between alveolar ventilation and pCO_2 is not linear (see graph)

See also Bicarbonate, Serum

Carbon-14 Urea, Breath (^{14}C Breath Test)

RI: Negative
IND: Peptic ulcer
INT: POSITIVE – Confirms presence of *Helicobacter pylori* as causative agent of peptic ulcer
PHYS: A small amount of radiolabelled urea is swallowed on an empty stomach. After 15 minutes, samples of breath carbon dioxide are collected into hyamine solution. ^{14}C activity is measured by liquid scintillation counting and results expressed using the following formula:–

$$\frac{\%\ administered\ dose}{mmol\ CO_2\ trapped}\ X\ \ weight\ in\ Kg.$$

High levels are positive

See also CLO Test; Helicobacter pylori Antibodies

Carboxyhaemoglobin B, Serum

RI: 0.5–1.5% of Hb
IND: Determine smoking status
INT: HIGH – Smoker, inhalation of exhaust fumes

See also Nicotine, Serum; Cotinine, Serum

Carcinoembryonic Antigen, Serum [CEA]

RI: 0–2.5 µg/L
IND: Colorectal carcinoma, monitoring cancer therapy
INT: HIGH – Colorectal cancer, gastric cancer, thyroid cancer, breast cancer, lung cancer, cervix cancer, seminoma, pancreatic cancer, hepatomas, cirrhosis, heavy smokers
PHYS: Produced by tumours of endodermal tissue. False positives common. Useful to follow progress of cancer therapy

See also Cancer Associated Antigens, Serum

Cardiac Enzymes
See Aldoase, Serum; Aspartate Amino Transferase, Serum; Creatine (Phospho) Kinase, Serum; Lactate Dehydrogenase, Serum; Serum; Myoglobin, Serum; Troponin T, Serum

Cardiolipin Autoantibodies, Blood [ACLA] (Anticardiolipin Antibodies)
RI: Absent
IND: Autoimmune disease
INT: PRESENT – SLE, phospholipid antibody syndrome, other autoimmune diseases, thromboembolic disorder, serious infection
PHYS: ELISA test. Antibodies may be IgG or IgM class.

See also ANA, Serum; ANCA, Serum; Anti-DNA, Serum; Anti-Smith Antibodies, Serum; Complement C3 and C4; DNA Autoantibodies; ENA, Serum; Histone Autoantibodies, Blood; HLA-DR3, Serum; LE Cells, Blood; Lupus Anticoagulant Antibody, Serum

Carnitine, Plasma
RI: Free: 30–70 µmol/L
       Total: 40–80 µmol/L
IND: Myopathies
INT: LOW – Carnitine deficiency states may cause myopathy (including heart) and hypoglycaemia
PHYS: Carnitine deficiency may be due to reduced intake, impaired synthesis, renal disease or acidaemia

Carotene, Serum
RI: 0.93–3.7 µmol/L
IND: Icterus, malabsorption
INT: HIGH – Carotenaemia due to excessive intake of papaya, carrots, pumpkin, etc., hypothyroidism, hyperlipidaemia
       LOW – Tropical sprue, fat malabsorption

CASA
See Cancer Associated Serum Antigen, Serum

Casoni's Test
RI: Negative
IND: Hydatid disease (Echinococcosis)
INT: POSITIVE – hydatid disease, false positive possible
PHYS: Superseded skin test. Blood hydatid antibody test more reliable

See also Hydatid Antibodies, Blood

Casts, Urine
See White Cell Count, Urine

Catecholamines, Plasma
RI: Adrenaline < 0.3 nmol/day
       Noradrenaline < 2.5 nmol/day
       Dopamine < 0.5 nmol/day

IND: Severe hypertension
INT: ADRENALINE & NORADRENALINE HIGH – Phaeochromocytoma
       DOPAMINE HIGH – Neuroblastoma
PHYS: Relax patient for 30 min. after insertion of IV canula to allow catecholamines to return to base state

See also Catecholamines, Urine; Clonidine Suppression Test

Catecholamines, Urine
RI: Adrenaline < 80 nmol/day (0.11–0.52 mnol/L)
       Noradrenaline < 780 nmol/day (1.27–2.81 nmol/L)
       Dopamine < 3500 nmol/day
IND: Hypertension
INT: ALL HIGH – Phaeochromocytoma (HMMA?), drugs (eg. methyldopa)
       DOPAMINE HIGH – Ganglioneuroma, neuroblastoma
       LOW – Failure (or damaged) adrenal medulla
PHYS: Adrenaline and noradrenaline are the catecholamines produced in the adrenal medulla. Excesses are produced by the organ of Zuckerkandl and other areas of the medulla in phaeochromocytoma

See also Catecholamines, Plasma; Clonidine Suppression Test

CD Types, Lymphocytes
See T Cell Lymphocytes, Blood

CEA
See Carcinoembryonic Antigen, Serum

Centromere Autoantibodies, Blood
RI: Absent
IND: CREST syn.
INT: PRESENT – CREST syn. (see SYNDROMES SECTION 6)
PHYS: Highly accurate test for this syndrome

Cerebrospinal Fluid, Cells
RI: Neutrophils 0/µL
       Lymphocytes 0–5/µL
       Erythrocytes 0–5/mL (higher with traumatic tap)
IND: CNS disease
INT: HIGH (25–2000 – predominantly lymphocytes) – Viral encephalitis, TB, syphilis, brain abscess, polio, trauma, toxoplasmosis, subdural or cerebral haemorrhage, brain tumour, multiple sclerosis, alcoholism, uraemia
       V.HIGH (> 2000 – predominantly polymorphonuclear leucocytes) – acute bacterial meningitis

Cerebrospinal Fluid, Colour
RI: Clear
IND: CNS trauma or infection

INT: YELLOW – Old haemorrhage, very high protein
RED – Recent haemorrhage, traumatic tap
CLOUDY – High cell count

Cerebrospinal Fluid, Glucose
See Glucose, CSF

Cerebrospinal Fluid, Immunoglobulins
See Immunoglobulin G, CSF

Cerebrospinal Fluid, Lactate
See Lactate, CSF

Cerebrospinal Fluid, Pressure
RI: Horizontal adult 70–200 mm H_2O
Horizontal child < 100 mm H_2O
Horizontal infant < 80 mm H_2O
IND: Brain disease
INT: HIGH – Viral meningitis or encephalitis,
subdural haemorrhage, subarachnoid
haemorrhage, alcoholism
V.HIGH – Bacterial meningitis, syphilis, TB,
cerebral haemorrhage, toxoplasmosis

Cerebrospinal Fluid, Protein
See Protein, CSF

Cerebrospinal Fluid, Specific Gravity
See Specific Gravity, CSF

Cerebrospinal Fluid, Volume
RI: 100–140 mL

Ceruloplasmin
See Caeruloplasmin, Serum

Cervical Smear
See Papanicolaou Smear, Cervix

Chlamydia Detection
See Immunoglobulin Antibodies, Specific, Serum; Ligase Chain Reaction, Urine; Polymerase Chain Reaction, Blood

Chloride, CSF [Cl⁻]
RI: 120–130 mmol/L (700–750 mg/100 mL)
IND: Meningitis
INT: LOW – Acute meningeal infections, TB

Chloride, Serum [Cl⁻]
RI: 97–108 mmol/L
IND: Water, electrolyte imbalance, renal disease
INT: LOW – Dehydration, salt losing nephropathy,
diuretics, chronic or severe diarrhoea,

alcoholism (GGT?), vomiting, cystic fibrosis
HIGH – Salt water drowning, excess ingestion,
dehydration, renal tubular acidosis, diarrhoea,
excess purging, ureterosigmoidoscopy, biliary
drainage, idiopathic
PHYS: The level of Cl⁻ is directly dependent on the level
of Na

Chloride, Sweat [Cl⁻]
RI: 4–50 mmol/L (4–50mEq/L)
IND: Malabsorption
INT: HIGH – Fibrocystic disease
PHYS: Sweat collected on electrolyte-free gauze pads
or by iontophoresis

Chloride, Urine [Cl⁻]
RI: 100–200 mmol/L/day (as NaCl)
IND: Little clinical value
INT: Varies with diet, acid-base balance, electrolyte
and water balance

Chlorpromazine, Serum (largactil)
RI: 0.16–0.94 umol/L
Toxic >2.4umol/L
IND: Chlorpromazine therapy
INT: Adjust dosage to keep serum levels within
therapeutic range
PHYS: Used in treatment of psychoses, schizophrenia
and sever agitation. Sample prior to next dose

Cholesterol, Serum
RI: 2.2–6.5 mmol/L (<5.5 mmol/L recommended)
(150–250 mg/100 mL)
Neonate 0.2–4 mmol/L
IND: Obesity, hypertension, heart disease
INT: HIGH – Hypercholesterolaemia (HDL:LDL
ratio?), familial, hypothyroidism (ETR, TSH?),
diabetes mellitus (glucose?), nephrotic syn.,
chronic hepatitis, cirrhosis, lipaemia, porphyria,
protein deficit, hypergammaglobulinaemia,
anorexia nervosa, elderly, pregnancy
LOW – Acute hepatitis, Gaucher's disease,
hyperthyroidism, acute infections (FBC?),
uraemia, myocardial infarct, malnutrition, familial
PHYS: Level determined by metabolic functions that
are influenced by diet and heredity. 70% of
cholesterol occurs as low density lipoproteins.
No alcohol for 72 hours and no food for 12 hours
before test

See also Triglycerides, Serum; High Density Lipoprotein Cholesterol, Blood

Cholinesterase, Serum
RI: Significant variation between labs
IND: Scoline apnoea in anaesthesia
INT: LOW – Scoline (suxamethonium) apnoea,
familial tendency to scoline apnoea,
organophosphate poisoning, liver disease
SLIGHTLY LOW – Pregnancy

PHYS: Cholinesterase essential for metabolism of
        scoline. Lack causes prolongation of scoline
        effect. Synthesised in liver

See also Cholinesterase, RBC

Cholinesterase, Red Cell

RI: Significant variation between labs
ND: Insecticide poisoning
NT: LOW – organophosphate or carbamate poisoning
PHYS: Levels slowly return to normal with cessation of
        exposure

See also Cholinesterase, Serum

Chorionic Gonadotrophin, Human, Beta, Serum [HCG]

RI: < 10 IU/L (non-pregnant)
ND: Pregnancy, gonadal carcinoma
NT: 20–100 IU/L – 1–2 weeks postconception,
        menopause (LH?)
        100–6000 IU/L – 3–4 weeks postconception, 3rd
        trimester of pregnancy, embryonal carcinoma,
        choriocarcinoma, testicular carcinoma
        6000–30,000 IU/L – Increases between weeks
        7 and 30 of pregnancy, then decreases
        >30,000 IU/L – Increased risk of Down syn. (see
        INVESTIGATIONS SECTION 3)
PHYS: Secreted by the trophoblast to stimulate and
        maintain the corpus luteum. Rises to a peak at
        10 weeks gestation, then slowly declines.
        Reliable only 10 days after conception as cross
        reacts with LH. Also acts as a reliable marker to
        certain gonadal tumours

Chorionic Gonadotrophin, Human, Urine [HCG]

RI: < 30 IU/day
ND: Pregnancy
NT: HIGH – Pregnant, seminomas,
        choriocarcinoma, hydatidiform mole
PHYS: Peak level at 10 weeks pregnancy

Chorionic Villus Sampling

ND: Suspected congenital disease
NT: Abnormal results may be obtained in Down syn.,
        haemoglobinopathies, cystic fibrosis, Huntington's
        chorea, haemophilia, Christmas disease, X-linked
        muscular dystrophy, some metabolic disorders.
        Fetal sex may also be determined
PHYS: Sample of chorionic villi from placenta obtained
        antenatally by needle aspiration through
        abdominal wall, under ultrasound guidance,
        between the 9th and 12th week of pregnancy.
        Tissue obtained may be subjected to
        chromosome, DNA or enzyme analysis

Chromosomes

RI: 22 pairs + 1 pair sex chromosomes (X, Y)
ND: Genetic abnormalities, sex determination
NT: 47 – Down syn. (Trisomy 21)

        XXY – Klinefelter syn.
        XO – Turner syn.
        Many other abnormalities known
PHYS: Cells (blood lymphocytes, bone marrow,
        amniotic fluid, chorionic villi) from the patient
        grown in culture have mitosis arrested by
        colchicine. Examination under microscope
        determines chromosome pattern and numbers

Chymotrypsin, Faecal

RI: > 75 µg/g
IND: Pancreatic disease
INT: LOW – Impaired pancreatic function
PHYS: Screening test only

CK

See Creatine (Phospho) Kinase, Serum

Cl⁻

See Chloride, CSF; Chloride, Serum; Chloride, Sweat;
Chloride, Urine

CLO Test (Campylobacter Like Organism Test)

RI: Negative
IND: Peptic ulcer
INT: POSITIVE – Helicobacter pylori present
PHYS: Test for urease on stomach biopsy specimen

See also Carbon-14 Urea Breath Test; Helicobacter
pylori antibodies

Clonazepam, Serum (Rivotril)

RI: Therapeutic range 60–150 nmol/L (25–75 µg/L)
IND: Clonazepam therapy
INT: Adjust dosage to keep serum levels within
        therapeutic range
PHYS: Clonazepam is used in treatment of epilepsy.
        Sample prior to next dose

Clonidine Suppression Test, Blood

RI: 50% drop in plasma adrenaline and
        noradrenaline (catecholamines0 within 3 hours
IND: Phaeochromocytoma diagnosis
INT: LESS THAN 50% DROP IN
        CATECHOLAMINES – Phaeochromocytoma,
        other catecholamine producing tumour
PHYS: Test performance criteria
        – relaxed lying patient with IV line
        – baseline plasma for catecholamines collected
        – 300 ug clonidine given orally
        – plasma for catecholamines collected hourly
          for 3 hours

See also Catecholamines, Plasma; Catecholamines, Urine

Clotting Time

RI: < 10 minutes
IND: Bleeding disorders

INT: HIGH – Anticoagulant therapy, lack of blood clotting factors
PHYS: Covers intrinsic and common pathway from factor XII to fibrinogen. Screening test for bleeding disorders

Cluster Differentiation Antibodies, Lymphocytes
See T Cell Lymphocytes, Blood

CO$_2$
See Carbon Dioxide, Blood

Coagulation Screen
See Activated Partial Thromboplastin Time; Anti-Factor Xa, Plasma; Antithrombin III, Blood; Clotting Time; Factor VIII, Blood; Factor XIII Screen, Blood; Fibrin Degradation Products, Blood; Fibrinogen, Blood; Platelet Count, Blood; Protein C, Plasma; Prothrombin Time; Thrombin Clotting Time; von Willebrand Factor, Plasma

Cold Agglutins, Blood
RI: Low titre
IND: Pneumonia
INT: HIGH TITRE – Mycoplasma pneumonia, infectious mononucleosis, lymphoid neoplasms, viral disease, syphilis
PHYS: Test for antibodies that react to cause haemolysis at low temperatures (i.e. 4°C) *in vitro*. Haemolysis due to fixation of complement (C3) to surface of erythrocytes

Collagen Binding Assay, von Willebrand Factor, Serum
See von Willebrand Factor, Plasma

Collagen Crosslink Fragments, Serum
See Deoxypyridinoline, Urine

Complement, Serum [C3 and C4]
RI: C3 0.83–1.7 g/L
           C4 0.19–0.59 g/L
IND: SLE
INT: LOW – SLE, rheumatoid arthritis, other connective tissue diseases, cirrhosis, urticaria, splenectomy, pneumococcal infection, Neisseria infection
           HIGH – Anaphylaxis
PHYS: Useful for following progress of SLE. C4 levels more sensitive. C3 levels drop only in severe disease

See also Cold Agglutins, Blood; LE Cells, Blood; Lupus Anticoagulant Antibody, Serum

Complete Blood Examination
See Full Blood Count

Coombs' Test (Direct Antiglobulin Test)
RI: Negative
IND: Haemolytic anaemia, jaundice, blood transfusion
INT: DIRECT POSITIVE – Autoimmune haemolytic anaemia, SLE, chronic lymphatic leukaemia, lymphosarcoma, Hodgkin's disease, cytomegalovirus infection, incompatible blood transfusion
           DIRECT WEAK POSITIVE – Rheumatoid arthritis, ulcerative colitis, drugs (eg. penicillin, methyldopa)
           INDIRECT POSITIVE – Excess serum antibody from autoimmune haemolytic anaemia
PHYS: Haematological agglutination test to detect abnormal plasma protein (often IgG) attached to red blood cells. Detected by Coombs' serum, which is an animal anti-human Ig antibody

Copper, Serum [Cu]
RI: 11–22 µmol/L (70–140 µg/100 mL)
IND: Liver disease, Wilson's disease
INT: HIGH – Wilson's disease (early stage), anaemia, infection, cirrhosis, hepatoma
           LOW – Wilson's disease (late stage), major malabsorption disorders
PHYS: 95% bound to caeruloplasmin, 5% bound to albumin

See also Caeruloplasmin, Serum

Copper, Urine
RI: < 1.2 µmol/day
IND: As for Copper, Serum
INT: As for Copper, Serum

Coproporphyrins, Urine
RI: 0–240 nmol/day (0–161 µg/24 hours)
INT: HIGH – Porphyria, hereditary coproporphyria, barbiturates, salicylates

Cortisol, Serum
RI: Morning – 130–770 nmol/L (5–28 µg/100 mL)
           Evening – < 390 nmol/L (< 14 µg/100 mL)
           Midnight – < 220 nmol/L (< 8 µg/100 mL)
IND: Cushingoid
INT: HIGH – Cushing syn., oral contraceptives, obesity, stress, drugs (eg. hormones), depression, pregnancy
           NO RESPONSE TO IV TETRACOSACTRIN – Addison's disease
PHYS: Specimen normally taken at 9 am. Stimulation and suppression tests essential when significant rises in levels should occur with tetracosactrin and insulin

See also Dexamethasone Suppression Test; Synacthen Stimulation Test

Cortisol, Urine, Free
RI: 97–330 nmol/day

IND: Cushingoid
INT: HIGH – Cushing syn., hormone therapy
PHYS: 24 hour collection essential. No fluctuation with short-term stress

Cotinine, Serum or Urine

RI: 0 mg/L
IND: Determination of smoking status
INT: HIGH – Smoker
PHYS: 5% of nicotine metabolises to cotinine

See also Nicotine, Serum; Carboxyhaemoglobin B, Serum

C-Peptide Suppression Test, Blood

RI: B.C-peptide <0.4nmol/L (1.2µg/L) when patient hypoglycaemic (B.glucose <2.2mmol/L)
IND: Insulinoma
INT: HIGH – Insulinoma
PHYS: Autonomous source of endogenous insulin prevents fall of C-peptide to below RI result in hypoglycaemic patient

CPK

See Creatine (Phospho) Kinase, Serum

C-Reactive Protein, Serum [CRP]

RI: <5 mg/L (<5 µg/mL)
IND: Inflammation
INT: HIGH – Inflammation, tissue injury, rheumatoid arthritis, infections, pneumonia, myocardial infarct, widespread malignancy, breast cancer, acute gout, ankylosing spondylitis, rheumatic fever, SLE, thromboembolism, bacterial meningitis, polyarteritis nodosa, inflammatory bowel disease
PHYS: Found in certain patients with tissue inflammation, damage or necrosis. Released from most tissue under stress. Nonspecific test, but usually indicates organic disease. More sensitive than ESR

See also C-reactive Protein, Ultrasensitive, Serum

C-Reactive Protein, Ultrasensitive, Serum

RI: Variations in CRP as low as 0.1mg/L measured
IND: Unstable angina
INT: RISING LEVELS – Poor prognosis for angina, increasing tissue damage in other organs
PHYS: Slowly increasing levels associated with increasing myocardial tissue damage even though total level of CRP may be quite low

See also C-Reactive Protein, Serum; Troponin, Serum

Creatine (Phospho) Kinase, Serum [CK or CPK]

RI: Male 60–280 IU/L
         Female 30–190 IU/L
IND: Suspected myocardial infarct
INT: HIGH – Myocardial infarct (LDH, AST?, troponin

T?), muscle dystrophies, polymyositis, pulmonary embolus, seizures, postoperative, myocarditis, muscle trauma (eg. seizures, exercise, IM injection)
PHYS: CK rises 3–5 hours after myocardial infarct. Returns to normal in 2–3 days. Heart and skeletal muscle is rich in this enzyme, which converts ADP into ATP + creatine

See also Creatine Kinase Isoenzymes, Serum

Creatine Kinase Isoenzymes, Serum

RI: CK-MB ratio < 6%
         MB factor < 10 U/L (<5% total CK, <0.6µg/L)
         MM factor 96% of total CK
         BB factor rarely detected
IND: Myocardial infarct
INT: CK-MB ratio and MB factor HIGH – Myocardial infarct (troponin T?), myocarditis
         Total CK and MM factor HIGH – As in CK above
         BB factor HIGH – Cerebral damage
PHYS: MB factor is 4% of skeletal muscle CK, but 40% of CK in cardiac muscle. MM factor makes up rest of CK, except in brain, where significant amounts of BB factor (which is very short lived in serum) occurs

Creatine Kinase Isoforms, Serum

RI: CK-MM3 – Absent
         CK-MM1/CK-MM3 ratio – <1.5
         CK-MB2 – <1U/L
         CK-MB2/CK-MB1 ratio – <1.5
IND: Myocardial infarct
INT: HIGH – Myocardial infarct (troponin T?), myocarditis
PHYS: Very early test for myocardial damage, but difficult to measure

Creatinine, Serum

RI: 0.06–0.11 mmol/L (0.6–1.5 mg/100 mL)
IND: Renal disease
INT: HIGH – Acute or chronic renal insufficiency (urea, K?), urinary tract obstruction, hypertension, chronic glomerulonephritis, diabetic nephropathy, polycystic kidneys, reflux nephropathy, SLE, acute muscle wasting, elderly, toxins, large intake of meat or vit. C, drugs (eg. analgesics, NSAIDs)
         LOW – Pregnancy, chronic muscle wasting
PHYS: Creatinine is excreted by filtration through the glomerulus; retention is an indication of glomerular insufficiency. Abnormal results (up or down) may be caused by high blood glucose or bilirubin, or by the drug cefoxitin

See also Urea, Blood

Creatinine, Urinary Clearance

RI: Male 1.2–2.35 mL/second (70–140 mL/minute)
         Female 1.2–2.16 mL/second (70–130 mL/minute) (Corrected for surface area)

IND: Renal function test
INT: HIGH – Muscular dystrophies, myositis,
myasthenia gravis, starvation, hyperthyroidism
LOW – Renal insufficiency (urea?),
hypothyroidism, amyotonia congenita
PHYS: Creatinine is excreted solely by the kidney.
Excess is produced in states of elevated
catabolism. Values decrease with age

Creatinine, Urine

RI: Male: 8–18 mmol/day
Female: 5–16 mmol/day
Child; 0.07–0.19 mmol/d/Kg
IND: As for Creatinine, Urinary Clearance
INT: As for Creatinine, Urinary Clearance

Cross-Linked Fibrin Derivatives

See D-Dimer, Blood

Cross-Linked N-Telopeptides, Urine

See N-Telopeptides, Cross-Linked, Urine

CRP

See C-Reactive Protein, Serum

Cryoglobulin, Serum

RI: Absent
IND: Immune disorders
INT: PRESENT – Infection (eg. hepatitis C),
myeloma, lymphoma, SLE, other immune
complex disorder
PHYS: Cryoglobulin precipitates at 4°C and redisolves
at 37°C

Crystals, Urine

RI: Phosphate crystals common in alkaline urine.
Oxalate crystals common in acid urine. Uric acid
crystals occur in high uric acid excretors and
some normal people
INT: Little clinical significance

CSF

See individual entries under Cerebrospinal Fluid

Cu

See Copper, Serum; Copper, Urine

Cyanocobalamin, Serum

See Vitamin B$_{12}$

Cystine, Urine

RI: 0.04–0.8 mmol/day
IND: Cystinuria
INT: HIGH – Fanconi syn., cystinuria, other
aminoacidurias

PHYS: 24 hour collection essential

Cytogenetics

PHYS: FISH (Fluorescent in situ hybridisation) can be
used to label a specific gene on a chromosome
with a fluorescent dye to detect a large number
of genetically determined conditions including
Angelman syn., Di George syn., Down Syn.,
Miller Dieker syn., Prader Willi syn., Smith
Magenis syn., Trisomy syn., Turner syn.,
Williams syn., retinoblastoma tendency etc.

*See SYNDROMES SECTION 6, for interpretation of
syndromes above*

Cytomegalovirus Antibodies, Serum

See Immunoglobulin Antibodies, Specific, Serum

D-Dimer, Blood (Cross-Linked Fibrin Derivatives)

RI: Negative or < 0.2 mg/L
IND: Thromboembolic disorders
INT: POSITIVE (high titre) – Venous or arterial
thrombosis (eg. deep vein thrombosis,
disseminated intravascular coagulation)
PHYS: Measures breakdown products of cross linked
fibrin. Correlates with, but more specific than,
Fibrin Degradation Products (see separate entry)

Dehydroepiandrosterone Sulfate, Blood [DHEA-S]

RI: Male or female neonate 4.4–9.2 µmol/L
(1670–3600 ng/mL)
Male adult 5.3–9.0 µmol/L (2000–3400 ng/mL)
Female child 0.1–1.5 µmol/L (100–600 ng/mL)
Female adult 2.0–9.0 µmol/L (820–3380 ng/mL)
Female pregnant 1.0–3.0 µmol/L (230–1170
ng/mL)
Female postmenopausal 0.1–1.5 µmol/L
(100–600 ng/mL)
IND: Test of gonadal function
INT: LOW – Pubertal failure, gonadal failure
HIGH – Ovarian or testicular tumours,
polycystic ovary, Stein-Leventhal syn., adrenal
tumour or hyperplasia
PHYS: Androgen that is precursor to testosterone.
Fasting specimen required

Dengue Fever Antibodies, Serum

See Immunoglobulin Antibodies, Specific, Serum

Densitometry, Bone Mineral

See Bone Mineral Densitometry

Deoxypyridinoline, Urine [DPyd]

RI: Male 2.5–5.0 nmol DPyd/mmol creatinine
Female 3.0–5.5 nmol DPyd/mmol creatinine

IND: Bone resorption
INT: HIGH – Chronic hypogonadism, osteoporosis (densitometry?), Paget's disease, hyperthyroidism, primary hyperparathyroidism, chronic hepatic disease, chronic renal disease, vitamin D deficiency, rheumatoid arthritis, corticosteroid therapy
PHYS: When bone is broken down by resorptive processes, collagen breakdown products are released into the blood and excreted in urine. DPyd is one of these products. Enzyme-linked immunosorbant assay (ELISA)

Dexamethasone Suppression Test

RI: U.17-hydroxycorticosteroids < 3.5 mg/day on 2nd day of test
IND: Cushing syn.
INT: HIGH – Cushing syn., endogenous depression
PHYS: Dexamethasone 0.5 mg is given every 6 hours for 2 days, and U.17-hydroxysteroids are measured on 2nd day

Diabetes Autoantibodies
See Glutamic Acid Decarboxylase Antibodies, Serum; Insulinoma Associated 2 Antibodies, Serum

Diazepam, Serum (Valium)

RI: Therapeutic range 400–1500 µg/L (0.7–5.3 umol/L)
IND: Diazepam therapy
INT: Adjust dosage to keep levels within therapeutic range
PHYS: Half-life 2–8 hours. Sample prior to next dose

Digoxin, Serum (Lanoxin)

RI: Therapeutic range 1–2.6 nmol/L (0.8–2 ng/mL) Toxic > 2.6 nmol/L (> 2 ng/mL)
IND: Digoxin therapy
INT: Adjust dosage to keep levels within therapeutic range
PHYS: Sample 8 hours after dose

Dilantin, Serum
See Phenytoin Sodium, Serum

Direct Antiglobulin Test
See Coombs' Test

DNA Autoantibodies, Blood

RI: < 10 U/mL
IND: SLE
INT: V.HIGH – SLE (ENA?)
HIGH – Rheumatoid arthritis, chronic active hepatitis, lupoid hepatitis
PHYS: Radio-immunoassay on fasting blood sample, specific for double stranded DNA

See also LE Cells, Blood; Lupus Anticoagulant Antibody, Serum

DNA Probes, Tissue (Gene Mapping)

RI: Absent
IND: Congenital diseases
INT: POSITIVE – Presence of specific congenital disease
PHYS: The range of DNA probes available is rapidly increasing. Those currently available include tests for alpha- and beta-thalassaemia, sickle cell disease, haemophilia, Duchenne muscular dystrophy, cystic fibrosis, neurofibromatosis, Huntington's chorea, polycystic kidney disease, phenylalanine hydroxylase deficiency, myotonic dystrophy, fragile X syn., X-linked retinitis pigmentosa, Leber's optic atrophy, alpha1-antitrypsin deficiency, X-linked hydrocephalus, Friedreich's ataxia, fructose intolerance. Chorionic villi may be used as the tissue sample in antenatal diagnosis. May identify identical twins

Dohle Bodies, Neutrophils

RI: Absent
IND: PRESENT – Bacterial infection. Occasionally seen in viral infections, neoplasia, cytotoxic therapy, necrosis, pregnancy
INT: Routinely reported if found on blood film microscopy

Dopamine
See Catecholamines, Urine

DPyd
See Deoxypyridinoline, Urine

Dual Photon Densitometry
See Bone Mineral Density

Effective Thyroxine Ratio [ETR]

RI: 0.93–1.06 (93–106%)
IND: Thyroid disease
INT: LOW – Hypothyroidism
HIGH – Hyperthyroidism

See also Thyroxine, Free, Serum

Electrolytes
See Anion gap, serum; Bicarbonate, serum; Chloride, serum; Magnesium, serum; Potassium, serum; Sodium, serum

Electrophoretic Pattern of Plasma [EPP]

RI: Albumin 35–55 g/L
Globulin 20–39 g/L
Fibrinogen 2–4 g/L
INT: See entries for individual plasma proteins

ENA
See Extractable Nuclear Antigen Autoantibodies, Serum

Endomysial Antibodies, Serum
RI: Absent
IND: Coeliac disease
INT: PRESENT – Coeliac disease, dermatitis herpetiformis
PHYS: 10% false positive, but more sensitive than Gliaden Antibodies

See also Gliaden Antibodies, Serum

Enolase, Serum
See Neurone Specific Enolase, Serum

Eosinophils, Blood
RI: Adult: 0.05–0.4 x 10⁹/L (50–400/mm³) (1–5%)
Child: 0.1–1.4 x 10⁹/L (100–1400/mm³)
Neonate: <2.0 x 10⁹/L (<2000/mm³)
IND: Determining nature and course of infection. Part of FBC
INT: V.HIGH – Carcinoma, eosinophilic leukaemia, hydatid disease
HIGH – Allergy (IgE?), hay fever, asthma, eczema, infectious mononucleosis (monocytes?), psoriasis, scabies, polyarteritis nodosa, Hodgkin's disease, intestinal or hepatic worms, serum sickness, rheumatoid arthritis, dermatitis herpetiformis, polyarteritis nodosa, irradiation, pemphigoid, pemphigus,Churg-Strauss syn., Job-Buckley syn., Loeffler syn., drugs (eg. penicillin, aspirin, sulphonamides, gold, carbamazepine, iodides)
LOW – Acute bacterial infections, hydrocortisone therapy

Epilim, Serum
See Sodium Valproate, Serum

EPP
See Electrophoretic Pattern of Plasma

Epstein-Barr Virus
See Infectious Mononucleosis

Erythrocyte Count, Blood (Red Blood Cell Count) [RBC] [RCC]
RI: Male 4.5–6.5 x 10¹²/L
Female 3.9–5.6 x 10¹²/L
IND: Haematological disorders
INT: **Abnormal number**
HIGH – Polycythaemia rubra vera, thalassaemia trait, renal disease (eg. tumours, cysts, transplant), dehydration, hypoxia, high altitudes, congenital heart disease, some lung diseases, hepatoma, Cushing syn., Gaisböck

syn., idiopathic, smoking, diuretic therapy
LOW – Haemolytic anaemia, malignancy, chronic disease, aplastic anaemia, dilution by IV fluids, pregnancy
Abnormal forms
SPHEROCYTES – Hereditary, immune haemolytic anaemia (Coombs' test?), severe burns, *Clostridium welchii* septicaemia
ELLIPTOCYTES – Hereditary, iron deficiency anaemia (Fe?)
SICKLE CELLS – Sickle cell disease
SPUR CELLS – Severe hepatic disease
TARGET CELLS – Liver disease
BURR CELLS – Renal disease
FRAGMENTED RBC – Disseminated intravascular coagulation, renal disease, Bassen-Kornzweig syn.
PHYS: RBC carry Hb. Reticulocytes are the immature form

See also Haemoglobin; Mean Corpuscular Volume; Reticulocytes, Blood;

Erythrocyte Count, Urine (Red Blood Cell Count, Urine)
See Haematuria

Erythrocyte Sedimentation Rate, Blood [ESR]
RI: Child 0–20 mm/hour (Westergren method)
Male 0–10 mm/hour
Female 0–20 mm/hour
Elderly male 0–20 mm/hour
Elderly female 5–45 mm/hour
Algorithm for calculating mean ESR in elderly:–
Male mean ESR = Age in years/2
Female mean ESR = (Age in years + 10)/2
IND: May indicate hidden infection, inflammation or neoplasia.
INT: V.HIGH – Collagen diseases (eg. myeloma, polymyositis), Mycoplasma infection, leukaemia (FBC?), myelomatosis, myocardial infarct
HIGH – Pregnancy, bacterial & viral infections (FBC?), localised acute suppurations, some neoplasms, TB, Hodgkin's disease, SLE, polymyalgia rheumatica, temporal arteritis, subacute bacterial endocarditis, anaemia, hyperfibrinogenaemia, hyperbilirubinaemia, thyroiditis, rheumatoid or reactive arthritis, Reiter's disease, Sjögren syn., vasculitis, dermatomyositis, rheumatic fever, Crohn's disease, sarcoidosis, amyloidosis, end stage renal failure, drugs (eg. oral contraceptives, hydralazine, procainamide), obesity, smoking, idiopathic
FALSE LOW – Polycythaemia, sickle cells, hypochromic microcytic anaemia, congenital heart disease, technical errors, drugs (eg. NSAIDs, corticosteroids, clofibrate)
PHYS: Two methods of determination:
Wintrobe – fall of level of cells against plasma in fine tube held vertically for 1 hour

Westergren – more complex, but more accurate ESR depends on the concentration of macromolecules in plasma, especially fibrinogen. ESR faster with macromolecules present. Non specific and inappropriate screening test

See also C-Reactive Protein, Serum; Spherocytes, Blood

Erythropoietin, Plasma

RI: 3–16 mIU/L
ND: Erythrocyte abnormalities
INT: LOW – Polycythemia rubra vera, chronic renal failure
HIGH – Secondary erythrocytosis, most anaemias
PHYS: Differentiates primary from secondary erythrocytosis

ESR

See Erythrocyte Sedimentation Rate, Blood

Ethanol, Serum [C_2H_5OH]

RI: Zero
IND: Suspected alcohol intoxication
INT: 0.05 g/100 mL (11 mmol/L) – Legally liable in some States
0.08 g/100 mL (17 mmol/L) – Stuperose
0.3–0.5 g/100 mL (66–110 mmol/L) – Comatose
> 0.5 g/100 mL (> 110 mmol/L) – Potentially fatal
PHYS: Ethanol is absorbed from the stomach and metabolised by the liver. In unchanged form, it is excreted from the kidneys at a fixed rate

Ethosuximide, Serum (Zarontin)

RI: Therapeutic range 280–700 µmol/L (40–100 µg/mL)
IND: Ethosuximide therapy
INT: Adjust dosage to keep serum levels within therapeutic range
PHYS: Ethosuximide is used to treat epilepsy. Sample prior to next dose

ETR

See Effective Thyroxine Ratio

Extractable Nuclear Antigen Autoantibodies, Serum [ENA]

RI: Titre < 10
IND: Connective tissue disease
INT: PRESENT – Raynaud's phenomenon, SLE (ANA?), scleroderma, Sjögren syn., rheumatoid arthritis, other connective tissue diseases
PHYS: Several subtypes of ENA are specific to different connective tissue diseases (DNA antibodies?)

Factor 1

See Fibrinogen, Blood

Factor V Leiden Mutation, Serum

See Activated Protein C Resistance, Serum

Factor VIII, Blood

RI: Very wide variation in normal levels. Assay of the molecular components of factor VIII (a and c) may give a more accurate diagnosis, but interpretation is difficult and false positives and negatives occur. Consult with your local haematologist
IND: Haemophilia, von Willebrand's disease
INT: Diagnosis of these diseases and the carrier state may be determined with careful analysis. Increased in pregnancy

Factor XIII Screen, Plasma

RI: Insoluble in urea
IND: Congenital bleeding disorders
INT: SOLUBLE IN UREA – Factor XIII deficiency
PHYS: Plasma clot incubated for 12 hours in strong urea solution

Faecal Fat

See Fat, Faecal

Faecal Occult Blood

See Occult Blood, Faeces

FANA

See Antinuclear Autoantibodies, Fluorescent, Blood

Fat, Faecal

RI: < 21 g/3 days (< 60 mmol/3 days)
IND: Cachexia
INT: HIGH – Malabsorption syn., tropical sprue, afferent loop syn., coeliac disease, chronic pancreatitis, cystic fibrosis, lactose (milk) intolerance, short bowel syn., inadequate bile salts

FBC

See Full Blood Count

FDP

See Fibrin Degradation Products

Fe

See Iron, Serum; Iron, Urine

Ferritin, Serum

RI: Male 20–320 µg/L
Female 15–300 µg/L
Neonate 50–350 µg/L

IND: Iron deficiency and excess states
INT: LOW – Iron deficit, anaemia, chronic disease (eg. rheumatoid arthritis, renal failure), dialysis
HIGH – Haemochromatosis, infection, overtransfusion, leukaemia, chronic inflammation, haemolysis, megaloblastosis, autoimmune diseases, iron overload
V.HIGH – Hodgkin's disease, acute and chronic hepatic disease, neoplasia
PHYS: Sensitive measure of total body iron by radio-immunoassay. Results usually lower in women. Normal result does not exclude iron deficiency

See also Iron, Serum

Fetal Haemoglobin

See Haemoglobin F, Fetal

Fetomaternal Haemorrhage Testing, Blood [FMH]

RI: Nil
IND: Rh – pregnancy
INT: HIGH – Fetomaternal haemorrhage present
PHYS: Flow cytometry test using monoclonal antibodies. Determines dose of Anti-D immunoglobulin necessary. Proportion of fetal antibody labelled RBC in mother's blood counted

FEV$_1$

See Forced Expiratory Volume in 1 Second

Fibrin Degradation Products, Blood [FDP]

RI: 0–10 µg/mL
IND: Coagulation disorders
INT: V.HIGH – Disseminated intravascular coagulation, abruptio placentae
HIGH – Venous thrombosis (thrombophlebitis), liver disease, bacterial infections, carcinomas, hyperfibrinolytic syn., haemolytic-uraemic syn., pulmonary embolism, pre-eclampsia, intrauterine fetal death, snake bite, stress
PHYS: Breakdown products of clots

See also D-Dimer, Blood

Fibrin Degradation Products, Urine

RI: Mean 0.25 µg/mL
IND: Renal disease
INT: HIGH – Disseminated intravascular coagulation, polycystic kidney disease, hydronephrosis, lupus nephritis, proliferative glomerulonephritis, renal transplantation, haemolytic-uraemic syn.
PHYS: Useful for following progress of renal disease or transplant rejection

See also D-Dimer, Blood

Fibrin Derivatives

See D-Dimer, Blood

Fibrinogen, Blood (Factor 1)

RI: 2–6 g/L
IND: Blood clotting anomalies
INT: LOW – Defibrination syn., Waterhouse-Friderichsen syn., endotoxic shock, abruptio placentae, intrauterine fetal death, amniotic fluid embolism, disseminated intravascular coagulation
HIGH – Nephrotic syn., Hodgkin's disease, pemphigus, pulmonary embolism, pregnancy
PHYS: Fibrinogen is involved in the first stage of the blood clotting cycle

See also tests listed under Coagulation Screen

FISH

See Cytogenetics

Fluid Deprivation Test, Urine Osmolality

RI: > 800 mOsmol/kg
IND: Polyuria
INT: Urine Osmolality Under Test Conditions

After dehydration	After desmopressin	Diagnosis
<300 mOsm/Kg	>800 mOsm/Kg	Cerebral diabetes insipidus
<300 mOsm/Kg	<300 mOsm/Kg	Nephrogenic diabetes insipidus
>800 mOsm/Kg	<800 mOsm/Kg	Normal or polydipsia

PHYS: Test used to determine presence of diabetes insipidus, and the cause of the disease. From 08.00 am, patient is banned from all fluid intake for 8 hours, but dry food is permitted. No coffee, tea, caffeine or smoking in preceding 12 hours is permitted. Patient is weighed regularly to assess degree of dehydration. Urine is passed hourly, and both volume and osmolality are measured. Desmopressin 2 µg IMI is administered at 4.30 pm, and patient is then allowed to take fluids, but only 50% more than amount passed during preceding 12 hours. Urine is collected for further 16 hours to measure osmolality

Fluorescent Antinuclear Antibodies

See Antinuclear Autoantibodies, Fluorescent, Blood

Fluorescent In-situ Hybridisation

See Cytogenetics

Fluorescent Treponemal Antibodies [FTA]

RI: Negative. Results are expressed as a titre (dilution of serum at which test is still positive)
IND: Sexually transmitted disease
INT: POSITIVE – Syphilis, yaws

PHYS: Antibodies specific for *Treponema pallidum* are detected in serum by adding fluorescein labelled anti-human gamma globulin. Antibodies form in the serum after infection with *T. pallidum*, and remain for many years to dormant infection in aqueous humour, CSF, etc. Thus the test may remain positive for many years after successful treatment. RPR & TPHA are better screening tests

See also Rapid Plasma Reagin Test, Serum; Treponema Pallidum Haemagglutination Test, Serum
See also iNVESTIGATIONS SECTION 3: Syphilis investigation chart

FMH
See Fetomaternal Haemorrhage

Foetal Haemoglobin
See Haemoglobin F, Fetal

Folate, Red Blood Cells
RI: 225–800 µg/L
IND: Anaemia
INT: LOW – Elderly, infancy, poor diet, pregnancy and lactation, alcoholism, scurvy, kwashiorkor, tropical sprue, coeliac disease, malabsorption syndromes, Crohn's disease, partial gastrectomy, congestive cardiac failure, septicaemia, Whipple's disease, scleroderma, chronic haemolytic anaemias, carcinoma, multiple myeloma, leukaemia, myelofibrosis, TB, psoriasis, haemodialysis, active liver disease, malaria, prematurity, drugs (eg. barbiturates, oral contraceptive, trimethoprim, tetracyclines, nitrofurantoin, primidone, methotrexate)
FALSE LOW – Severe vit. B_{12} deficiency
FALSE NORMAL – Blood transfusion, reticulocytosis
HIGH – Excess daily intake
PHYS: Indication of total body folate. Less affected by diet. Stored primarily in liver

Folate, Serum
RI: 3.6–20 µg/L (7–40 nmol/L)
IND: Anaemia
INT: As for Folate, Red Blood Cells
PHYS: Serum folate reflects folate absorption in past week only

Folic Acid, Red Blood Cell Concentration
RI: > 318 nmol/L (> 140 ng/mL)
IND: Anaemia
INT: LOW – Chronic alcoholism, oral contraceptives, anticonvulsants, malnutrition, sprue, sickle cell anaemia, cytotoxic drugs, pregnancy, malabsorption syndromes

Folic Acid, Serum
RI: 9.1 – 57 nmol/L (4 – 25 ng/mL)
IND: Anaemia
INT: LOW – Chronic alcoholism, oral contraceptives, anticonvulsants, malnutrition, spure, sickle cell anaemia, cytotoxic drugs, pregnancy, malabsorption syndromes
PHYS: Essential for metabolism of cell nuclear materials. Low levels cause megaloblastic anaemia

Follicle Stimulating Hormone, Serum [FSH]
RI: Prepubertal 0–3 IU/L
Adult female 1–9 IU/L
Female at ovulation 10–30 IU/L
Postmenopausal 40–200 IU/L
Adult male 1–5 IU/L
IND: Infertility
INT: LOW – Infertile (both sexes)
V.HIGH – Gonadal absence, failure or disease. Normally rises at mid-cycle in ovulating female
FSH <<LH – Stein-Leventhal syn.
PHYS: Pituitary hormone that acts with LH to stimulate ovulation and spermatogenesis. Feedback control by gonadal hormones

See also Luteinising Hormone, Serum

Forced Expiratory Volume in 1 Second [FEV₁]
RI: 84% ± 7%
Male 3.5 ± 1.5 L
Female 2.5 ± 1.0 L
IND: Test of airway resistance
INT: LOW – Asthma or other lung disease (VC?)
PHYS: FEV_1 is the percentage of vital capacity expelled by forced expiration in 1 second. Reduced by airway narrowing, by spasm or secretions. Measured by a spirometer

Free Thyroxine Index [FTI]
RI: 17–50
IND: Thyroid dysfunction
INT: HIGH – Hyperthyroidism (T_3, T_4?)
LOW – Hypothyroidism (T_3, T_4?)
PHYS: $FTI = T_4 \times T_3$ uptake/100

Free Thyroxine Total [Free T₄]
See T_4 Serum (Total Thyroxine)

Fructosamine, Serum
RI: Adult 200–290 µmol/L
Child 200–260 µmol/L
Pregnant 200–250 µmol/L
IND: Diabetes control
INT: HIGH – Poorly controlled diabetes mellitus
PHYS: Randomly timed specimens can give a good indication of control of diabetes, without reference to absolute blood glucose levels or

dietary intake. Measure of integrated glucose concentration over preceding 10–15 days, and of glycosylated serum proteins

See also Glycosylated Haemoglobin, Blood

Fructose, Seminal Fluid

RI: 3.5–28 mmol/L
IND: Infertility
INT: LOW – Ejaculatory duct obstruction, vesiculitis, Leydig cell deficiency (common at puberty), polyzoospermia, seminal vesicle obstruction
PHYS: Fructose is the energy source for sperm. Low levels cause reduced sperm motility

FSH

See Follicle Stimulating Hormone, Serum

FTA

See Fluorescent Treponemal Antibodies

FTe

See Testosterone, Free, Serum

FTI

See Free Thyroxine Index

Full Blood Count

This includes the following investigations: Haemoglobin; White Cell Count; MCV; MCH; MCHC; Haematocrit

G-6-PD

See Glucose 6-Phosphate Dehydrogenase, Serum

GAD

See Glutamic Acid Decarboxylase Antibodies, Serum

Galactokinase, Red Blood Cells

RI: 18–40mU/g Hb
IND: Juvenile onset cataract, galactosaemia
INT: LOW – genetic deficiency, increased risk of cataract
PHYS: Radiometric assay. Familial

See also Galactose, Plasma

Galactose, Plasma

RI: < 1.0 mmol/L
IND: Galactosaemia
INT: HIGH – Galactosaemia, galactose-1-phosphate deficiency

See also Galactokinase, RBC; Galactose-1-Phosphate, RBC

Galacto-1-Phosphate, Red Blood Cells

RI: <170 nmol/g Hb
IND: Galactosaemia
INT: V.HIGH (>500 nmol/g Hb) – Galactosaemia
       HIGH – Galactosaemia on galactose free diet
PHYS: Used to both diagnose and monitor severity of galactosaemia

See also Galactokinase, RBC; Galactose, Plasma

Gamma Glutamyl Transpeptidase (Transferase), Serum [Gamma GT or GGT or SGGT]

RI: Male < 45 U/L
       Female < 30 U/L
IND: Liver disease
INT: V.HIGH – Alcoholism, liver metastases, liver abscess, hepatic granuloma, obstructive biliary disease
       HIGH – Pancreatitis, myocardial infarct, hepatitis, fatty liver, cirrhosis, obesity, anorexia nervosa, porphyria, some renal diseases, renal carcinoma, drugs (eg. tricyclic antidepressants, phenytoin, barbiturates, paracetamol overdose)
PHYS: Hepatic and renal enzyme, released with tissue damage

See also Liver Function Tests

Gastric Cell Autoantibodies, Serum

See Parietal Cell Autoantibodies, Serum

Gastric Fluid Assay, Acid Output

RI: 0–6 mEq/hour (24–29 mEq/L)
       After histamine stimulation:
       Males 10–40 mEq/hour
       Females 5–30 mEq/hour
IND: Peptic ulceration
INT: HIGH – Peptic ulcer tendency
       LOW AFTER HISTAMINE – Pernicious anaemia, postvagotomy
PHYS: Patients with duodenal ulcers have higher numbers of acid secreting parietal cells than normal

Gastric Fluid Assay, pH (Gastric Fluid Acidity)

RI: 0.9–1.5
INT: HIGH – Pernicious anaemia, (Vit.B_{12}?), postvagotomy
       LOW – Peptic ulcer tendency

Gastrin, Serum

RI: < 50 pmol/L (<90 ng/L)
IND: Peptic ulceration
INT: HIGH – Gastric outlet obstruction, renal failure, short bowel syn., antral hyperplasia and ulceration, pernicious anaemia, atrophic gastritis, gastric cancer, postvagotomy, phaeochromocytoma

V.HIGH (> 250 pmol/L) – Zollinger-Ellison syn. (gastrinomas)

Genetics
See Cytogenetics

Gentamicin, Blood
See Aminoglycosides, Blood

GFR
See Glomerular Filtration Rate

GGT
See Gamma Glutamyl Transpeptidase, Serum

GHb
See Glycosylated Haemoglobin, Blood

Glandular Fever
See Infectious Mononucleosis

Gliaden Antibodies, Serum (Anti-Gliaden Antibodies)
RI: < 25
IND: Coeliac disease, diet compliance
INT: HIGH – Coeliac disese, 2% false positive rate
PHYS: ELISA assay of serum IgG and IgA anti-gliaden (gluten) antibodies. Antibodies return to normal when a strict gluten free diet followed

See also Endomysial Antibodies, Serum

Globulin, Serum
RI: Total 20–35 g/L (24–60%)
     alpha₁ 2–4 g/L (3–7%)
     alpha₂ 4–8 g/L (5–11%)
     beta 6–10 g/L (9–18%)
     gamma 6–15 g/L (9–23%)
     A clotted specimen of blood is required
IND: Liver disease
INT: TOTAL LOW – Malnutrition, lymphatic leukaemia, immunodeficiency
     alpha₁ LOW – Nephrotic syn.
     gamma LOW – Nephrotic syn., multiple myeloma, lymphosarcoma, leukaemia, Bruton's syn., steroid therapy
     TOTAL HIGH – Cirrhosis (bilirubin?), chronic hepatitis, hepatoma, malaria, SLE (LE cells?), bile duct obstruction, typhus, multiple myeloma, elderly, AIDS (HIV antibodies?)
     alpha₁ HIGH – Oestrogen therapy, pregnancy
     alpha₂ HIGH – Acute infections (albumin?), myocardial infarct, trauma, nephrotic syn., Wilms' tumour
     beta HIGH – Hypercholesterolaemia, cirrhosis, nephrotic syn., pregnancy, hypothyroidism

gamma HIGH – Infection, Sjögren syn., other connective tissue diseases, cirrhosis, myeloma, lupus erythematosus
PHYS: Electrophoresis is used to separate the various protein fractions and a pattern similar to the normal one below emerges.

Typical Electrophoretic Pattern of Globulin Fractions

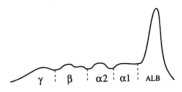

$$\text{GFR (mL/min)} = \frac{(140 - \text{age in years}) \times \text{weight in Kg.}}{814 \times \text{plasma creatinine in mmol/L}}$$

Glomerular Basement Membrane Autoantibodies, Blood
RI: Absent
IND: Goodpasture syn.
INT: PRESENT – Goodpasture's syn.
PHYS: Radio-immunoassay

Glomerular Filtration Rate [GFR]
RI: Units: mL/minute/1.73 m²
     Male, 20 years 117–170
     Male, 50 years 96–138
     Male, 70 years 70–110
     Female, 20 years 104–158
     Female, 50 years 90–130
     Female, 70 years 70–114
     Pregnancy – Add 20%
IND: Renal disease
INT: LOW – Renal failure
PHYS: GFR decreases by 1 mL/minute/year above age 35 years. Measured by variable means including insulin clearance, creatinine clearance (see separate entry), urea clearance (see separate entry) and radiopharmaceuticals. It may also be estimated using the following equation:–

Multiply by 0.85 for females. Accurate over the range 10 to 100 mL/minute. Not valid in pregnant, obese or oedematous patients

Glucagon, Plasma
RI: 25–250µg/L
IND: Abnormal presentations of diabetes
INT: HIGH – Glucagonoma tumour of the pancreas, diabetes mellitus, some acute illnesses
PHYS: Not a diagnostic test for glucagonoma unless clinical signs present. Overnight fast before test

Glucose, Blood

RI: 3.5–6 mmol/L (60–100 mg/100 mL)
     (Fasting whole blood specimen)
IND: Diabetes
INT: HIGH – Diabetes mellitus [>7.0 fasting
     diagnostic] (GTT?), infection (WCC?),
     hyperthyroidism (ETR?), hyperpituitarism,
     adrenal cortical excess, hepatic disease
     (LFT?), acromegaly, phaeochromocytoma,
     Leschke syn., Prader-Willi syn., Reaven syn.,
     Turner syn., polyglandular autoimmune syn.,
     hypokalaemia, burns, steroid therapy, recent
     meal
     LOW – Vomiting, diarrhoea, insulinoma,
     hyperinsulinism, adrenal insufficiency,
     hypopituitarism, Addison's disease,
     hypothyroidism (ETR?), severe hepatic disease
     (LFT?), hepatoma, alcoholism (GGT?), post-
     gastrectomy, von Gierke syn., Hers syn., Reye
     syn., unpreserved blood specimen, drugs (eg.
     insulin, laxatives, hypoglycaemic agents
     diuretics)
PHYS: Glucose in adequate levels is essential for
     normal body functions. Its level is controlled by
     the insulin released by the Islets of Langerhan in
     the pancreas. No food for 12 hours before test

Glucose, CSF

RI: 2.1–4 mmol/L (40–100 mg/100 mL)
IND: Cerebral disease
INT: LOW – Bacterial meningitis (chloride and
     protein, CSF?), TB, syphilis, insulin
     HIGH – Postinfectious encephalitis, tumours,
     uraemia, diabetic coma

Glucose, Urine

RI: Absent
IND: Diabetes
INT: POSITIVE – Diabetes mellitus, pregnancy,
     physical stress, congenital renal glycosuria,
     Fanconi syn., galactosaemia, alkaptonuria
PHYS: Glucose levels in urine only proportional to that
     of serum provided no renal disease present

Glucose 6-Phosphate Dehydrogenase, Serum [G-6-PD]

RI: 6.0–11.0 U/gHb
     Several systems of measurement
     Varies between labs
IND: Anaemia
INT: LOW – Normal in some Mediterranean
     Caucasians and some Asians, hereditary
     defect, drug induced haemolytic anaemia,
     drugs (eg. aspirin, primaquine, dapsone,
     nitrofurantoin)
PHYS: A lack of G-6-PD or its inactivation by drugs
     leads to anaemia. The enzyme may be lacking
     genetically

Glucose Tolerance Test [GTT]

RI: 75 g of glucose is given orally. The blood sugar
     level should not exceed 8 mmol/L (140 mg/100
     mL) after 30 minutes, and should return to normal
     within 2 hours. No sugar should appear in the urine
IND: Diabetes
INT: V.HIGH (> 11 mmol/L) – Diabetes mellitus
     HIGH (8–11 mmol/L) – Latent diabetes
     (impaired glucose tolerance), pregnancy
     (additional obstetric care required), chromium
     deficiency
PHYS: Diabetic (and potential diabetic) patients do not
     produce adequate insulin to clear glucose from
     serum rapidly. Test may be impaired by diuretics,
     steroids, lithium, phenytoin, phenothiazines

Glutamic Acid Decarboxylase Antibodies, Serum [GAD]

RI: <0.9 U/mL
IND: Diabetes
INT: HIGH – Type one diabetes mellitus, potential to
     develop type one diabetes mellitus, autoimmune
     thyroid disease
PHYS: Present in 70% of type one diabetics, and
     frequently in first degree relatives of patients,
     and others at risk of developing the disease.
     More commonly raised in early stages of
     disease

Glutamic Oxaloacetic Transaminase, Serum [SGOT]

See Aspartate Amino Transferase, Serum

Glutamic Pyruvic Transaminase, Serum [SGPT]

See Alanine Amino Transferase, Serum

Glutamine, Plasma

RI: 450–750 µmol/L
IND: Hyperammonaemia
INT: HIGH – Genetic hyperammonaemia

Glycated Haemoglobin, Blood, Total Non-labile [HbA$_1$]

RI: < 13% of Hb
IND: Diabetic management
INT: HIGH – Above average normal glucose level (ie.
     diabetes, poorly controlled diabetic,
     noncompliance with therapy)
PHYS: Alternative to Glycosylated Haemoglobin A$_{1c}$
     (see below). Integrated measure of diabetic
     control over preceding 2–3 months

Glycosylated Haemoglobin, Blood [GHb or HbA$_{1c}$]

RI: 5–9% of Hb as HbA$_{1c}$
IND: Diabetic management
INT: HIGH – Above average normal glucose level (ie.

diabetes, poorly controlled diabetic, noncompliance with therapy)
FALSE HIGH – Uraemia, beta thalassaemia
FALSE LOW – Haemolytic anaemia, blood loss
PHYS: Glucose reacts with and attaches to Hb nonenzymatically. Index of compliance and efficacy of treatment as life cycle of erythrocyte is about 3 months. Should not be used in under this time for change of therapy. Inaccurate in conditions of shortened RBC lifespan (eg. haemolytic disease, blood loss)

See also Glycated Haemoglobin, Blood, Total Non-labile

Growth Hormone, Serum

RI: Adult < 0.3 pg/mL,
Child > 1 pg/mL
IND: Growth abnormalities
INT: LOW – Dwarfism
HIGH – Gigantism, acromegaly, stress
PHYS: Growth hormone stimulates growth of all non-endocrine tissue. Produced by the anterior pituitary. Fasting specimen required. Insulin and glucose stress testing gives more accurate interpretation

GTT

See Glucose Tolerance Test

Haematocrit

See Packed Cell Volume

Haematuria (RBC in Urine)

RI: < 1000 RBC/mL (< 1 RBC/HPF)
ND: Urinary tract and renal disease
INT: HIGH – Glomerulonephritis, cystitis, prostatitis, urinary calculi, urinary tract neoplasms, renal papillary necrosis, trauma, foreign body, coagulopathies, TB, schistosomiasis, hydronephrosis, renal infarct, malignancy, hypertension, polycystic disease, nephrotic syn., SLE, PAN, haemolytic-uraemic syn., amyloidosis, Goodpasture syn., congenital haematuria, leukaemia, exercise stress, drugs (eg. cyclophosphamide, warfarin, heparin, aspirin, carbidopa, phenytoin, metronidazole, phenothiazines)
FALSE POSITIVE ON DIPSTICK TEST – Iodine contamination, oxidising agents in container, haemoglobinuria, myoglobinuria, peroxidase action of bacteria if sample not fresh
FALSE NEGATIVE ON DIPSTICK TEST – High urinary nitrate, high urinary vit. C
PHYS: Causes of red urine that may be confused with haematuria include beetroot, urates, pyridium, phenindione, porphyria, phenolphthalein, vegetable dyes, haemoglobinuria

See also SYMPTOMS SECTION 1: Haematuria and Red Urine

Haemoglobin, Blood [Hb]

RI: Male 135–180 g/L (13.5–18 g/dL)
Female 115–165 g/L (11.5–16.5 g/dL)
Neonate 170–220 g/L (17–22 g/dL)
Infant 110–125 g/L (11–12.5 g/dL)
Child 120–140 g/L (12–14 g/dL)
Pregnancy 110–150 g/L (11–15 g/dL)
IND: Anaemia
INT: LOW – Acute or chronic blood loss, deficient RBC production (iron, copper, cobalt, vit. B_{12} or folic acid deficiencies), bone marrow failure (aplastic or sideroblastic anaemia), excess RBC destruction, thalassaemia, sickle cell anaemia, chronic disease (cancer, arthritis), renal disease, liver disease, coeliac disease, many types of carcinoma, rheumatoid arthritis, myxoedema, protozoal infections, autoimmune diseases, pregnancy, analgesic nephropathy, elite athletes
HIGH – Haemosiderosis, polycythaemia rubra vera, haemochromatosis, smoking, diuretics
FALSE HIGH – Hyperlipoproteinaemia, hyperbilirubinaemia, very high WCC
PHYS: The Hb in RBC is essential for the transport of oxygen to the tissues. Measured by photometry

See also Iron, Serum; Mean Corpuscular Haemoglobin; Mean Corpuscular Haemoglobin Concentration; Mean Corpuscular Volume; Copper, Serum; Cyanocobalamin, Serum

See also investigations listed under Full Blood Count

Haemoglobin, Glycated

See Glycated Haemoglobin, Blood, Total Non-labile

Haemoglobin, Glycosylated

See Glycosylated Haemoglobin, Blood

Haemoglobin, Oxygen Affinity, Blood

RI: p50 O_2 – 3.4–3.8 kPa (25–29 mmHg)
IND: Erythrocytosis, abnormal oxygen transport
INT: LOW – Haemoglobinopathy causing increased oxygen affinity, decreased release of oxygen to tissues
HIGH – Decreased oxygen affinity, increased release of oxygen to tissues
PHYS: p50 O_2 is the partial pressure of oxygen at which Hb is 50% saturated

Haemoglobin, Urine

See Haematuria

Haemoglobin A$_2$, Blood [HbA$_2$]

RI: 1.5–4% of total Hb
IND: Suspect thalassaemia
INT: HIGH – Thalassaemia trait

Haemoglobin F, Fetal [HbF] (Kleihauer Test)

RI:	At birth 10.5–14 mmol/L (17–22.5 g/100 mL)
	Adult < 1% of total Hb (negative Kleihauer test)
IND:	Anaemia and blood abnormalities
INT:	HIGH – Marrow overactivity, transplacental
	haemorrhage
PHYS:	Normal Hb found in the fetus and during early
	infancy. Its formation may continue abnormally
	in infancy as a result of any type of anaemia that
	causes marrow overactivity

Haemoglobin H, Blood [HbH]

RI:	Negative
IND:	Thalassaemia
INT:	POSITIVE – HbH Thalassaemia major or minor
	(Haemoglobin H disease)
PHYS:	Care in preparing sample essential, as HbH
	tends to precipitate out of red cell lysates easily.
	HbH in affected patients may vary from 5 to 40%
	of total Hb

Haemoglobin M, Blood [HbM]

RI:	Absent
IND:	Chronic cyanosis
INT:	PRESENT – Inherited methaemoglobinaemia

Haemoglobin S, Blood [HbS]

RI:	Absent
IND:	Haemolytic anaemia
INT:	PRESENT – Sickle cell anaemia, some types of
	thalassaemia

Haemosiderin, Urine

RI:	Absent
IND:	Chronic anaemia
INT:	PRESENT – Intravascular haemolysis
PHYS:	Haemoglobin degraded to haemosiderin in
	kidney

Haemoximetry

See Carbon Dioxide, Blood; Carboxyhaemoglobin B, Serum; Haemoglobin, Oxygen Affinity, Blood; Methaemoglobin, Blood; Oxygen, Blood; Sulphaemoglobin, Blood

Ham Test

See Acidified Serum Test

Haptoglobin, Blood

RI:	0.3–2 g/L
IND:	Hemolysis, inflammation
INT:	LOW – Severe intravascular haemolysis,
	megaloblastic anaemia, liver disease (LFT?),
	congenital
	HIGH – Most acute inflammatory conditions
	(ESR?), biliary obstruction, pregnancy,
	steroids, oestrogen supplements

	FALSE NORMAL – Acute pancreatitis
PHYS:	An alpha$_2$-globulin that binds free Hb in blood
	stream

Hb

See Haemoglobin, Blood

HbA$_1$

See Glycated Haemoglobin, Blood, Total Non-labile

HbA$_{1c}$

See Glycosylated Haemoglobin, Blood

HbF

See Haemoglobin F, Fetal

HbH

See Haemoglobin H, Blood

HbM

See Haemoglobin M, Blood

HbS

See Haemoglobin S, Blood

HCG

See Chorionic Gonadotrophin, Human, Beta, Serum; Chorionic Gonadotrophin, Human, Urine

HCO$_3^-$

See Bicarbonate, Serum

HDL

See High Density Lipoprotein Cholesterol, Blood

Heaf Test

See Tuberculin Skin Test

Heavy Metals

See Arsenic; Cadmium; Copper; Lead; Manganese; Mercury

Heinz Bodies, Blood

RI:	Absent
IND:	Anaemia
INT:	PRESENT – Intravascular haemolysis, post-
	splenectomy, G-6-PD deficiency, haemo-
	globinopathies, drug or chemical exposure
PHYS:	Heinz bodies created by oxidation of Hb. Seen
	by microscopy as red cell inclusions

Helicobacter pylori Antibodies, Serum

RI: Negative
IND: Peptic ulcer
INT: POSITIVE – Presence of H. pylori in stomach highly likely
PHYS: H. pylori implicated in the causation of peptic ulcers and can be eradicated by triple therapy (eg. bismuth subcitrate, metronidazole, tetracycline)

See also Carbon-14 Urea Breath Test; CLO Test

Hepatitis A, Serum Antigens and Antibodies

RI: Nil
IND: Hepatitis, jaundice
INT: IgM anti-HAV POSITIVE – Hepatitis A
PHYS: See INVESTIGATIONS SECTION 3

See also Immunoglobulin Antibodies, Specific, Serum

Hepatitis B, Serum Antigens and Antibodies

RI: Nil
IND: Suspected hepatitis B, persons engaged in an at risk lifestyle
INT: See graph below
Viral antigens
Hepatitis B surface antigen (HBsAg)
Hepatitis B e antigen (HBeAg)
Viral antibodies
Hepatitis B surface antibody (anti-HBs)
Hepatitis B core antibody (anti-HBc)
Hepatitis B e antibody (anti-HBe)
PHYS: For as long as HBsAg is detectable, the patient's blood and other bodily fluids are infectious for hepatitis B. The presence of HBeAg indicates very rapid viral replication. The presence of antiHBs signifies recovery or successful immunisation with seroconversion

Hepatitis B with Seroconversion and Resolution

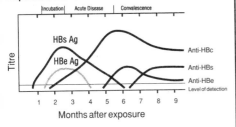

Hepatitis B Chronic Carrier – No Seroconversion

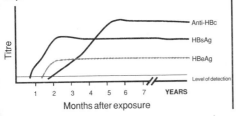

See also Immunoglobulin Antibodies, Specific, Serum

Hepatitis C, Serum Antigens and Antibodies

See INVESTIGATIONS SECTION 3: Hepatitis C
See also Immunoglobulin Antibodies, Specific, Serum

Hepatitis D, Serum Antigens and Antibodies

See INVESTIGATIONS SECTION 3: Hepatitis D

Hepatitis E, Serum Antigens and Antibodies

See INVESTIGATIONS SECTION 3: Hepatitis E

Herpes Simplex Antibody, Serum [HSV]

RI: Negative
IND: Genital herpes
INT: POSITIVE IgG – Current or previous infection
POSITIVE IgM – Current infection
PHYS: Separate antibody tests for type one and two Herpes simplex available from most laboratories

See also Immunoglobulin Antibodies, Specific, Serum

Hess Test

See SIGNS SECTION 2: Hess Test

Hexosamine, Serum

RI: 80–125 mg/100 mL
IND: Suspected tissue damage. Poor wound healing
INT: HIGH – Presence of inflammatory reaction
PHYS: Rises to a peak 3 days after tissue injury, and returns to normal after 7–10 days. Essential for wound healing

5 HIAA

See 5-Hydroxyindole Acetic Acid, Urine with numerial entries at beginning of this section

High Density Lipoprotein Cholesterol, Blood [HDL]

RI: Male 0.9–2.0 mmol/L
Female 1.0–2.2 mmol/L
IND: Obesity, high total cholesterol
INT: LOW – Increased risk of atherosclerosis and coronary artery disease, Reaven syn., pregnancy
HIGH – Lower risk of atherosclerosis
PHYS: Ratio of total cholesterol:HDL cholesterol is best prognostic marker. Should not exceed 4.5; the higher the ratio, the poorer the prognosis

See also Apolipoproteins, Serum

Histidyl-tRNA Synthetase Antibodies, Serum

See Jo-1 Antibodies, Serum

Histocompatibility Antigen

See HLA-B27, Serum; HLA-DR2, Serum; HLA-DR3, Serum; HLA-DR4, Serum

Histone Autoantibodies, Blood

RI: Absent
IND: SLE
INT: PRESENT – Drug induced SLE

See also LE Cells, Blood; Lupus Anticoagulant Antibody, Serum

HIV-1 RNA

See HIV Viral Load, Serum

HIV Antibody, Serum (Human Immunodeficiency Virus Antibody) (HTLV-3 Antibody)

RI: Negative
IND: High risk individuals; possible exposure to HIV
INT: POSITIVE – AIDS, lymphadenopathy syn., exposure to HIV
PHYS: May be positive in subclinical, potential and dormant cases of AIDS. Test is for presence of antibody, not the presence of HIV. May take <= 3 months from contact to become positive

See also INVESTIGATIONS SECTION 3: Acquired Immune Deficiency Syndrome

HIV Viral Load, Serum [HIV-1 RNA] (Human Immunodeficiency Virus-1 RNA)

RI: Method dependent
IND: Monitoring progress of HIV infection
INT: RISING LEVEL – Increasing HIV activity
     DECREASING LEVEL – Good response to treatment

HLA-B27, Serum (Human Leucocyte Antigen Histocompatibility Antigen)

RI: Negative
IND: Rheumatic diseases
INT: POSITIVE – Ankylosing spondylitis, Reiter's disease, juvenile chronic polyarthritis, postinfective arthritis, inflammatory bowel disease, acute anterior uveitis, 5% of normal people, of prognostic significance in children
PHYS: Large percentage of false negatives possible. Useful for matching donors in organ transplantations

HLA-DR2, Serum (Human Leucocyte Antigen Histocompatibility Antigen DR2)

RI: Negative
IND: Sleep disorders
INT: POSITIVE – Narcolepsy (99% of sufferers), 25% of normal population

HLA-DR3, Serum (Human Leucocyte Antigen Histocompatibility Antigen DR3)

RI: Negative
IND: Autoimmune diseases
INT: POSITIVE – SLE, Sjögren's syn., Addison's disease, chronic hepatitis, coeliac disease, myasthenia gravis, Grave's disease
PHYS: Expensive and performed in specialised laboratories only

See also LE Cells, Blood; Lupus Anticoagulant Antibody, Serum

HLA-DR4, Serum (Human Leucocyte Antigen Histocompatibility Antigen DR4)

RI: Negative
IND: Arthritis
INT: POSITIVE – Rheumatoid arthritis

HMMA

See 4-Hydroxy-3-Methoxy Mandelic Acid, Urine

Homocysteine, Serum

RI: 0.5–2.2 nmol/mL
IND: Family history of myocardial or cerebral infarct
INT: HIGH – Homocysteinaemia, atherosclerosis, increased risk of myocardial or cerebral infarct
PHYS: Cystathionine beta-synthase deficiency causes congenital atherosclerosis. Detected by measuring homocysteine which is an abnormal metabolite. Metabolic pathway may be additionally stressed by methionine loading

Homogentisic Acid, Urine

RI: Negative
IND: Alkaptonuria
INT: PRESENT – Alkaptonuria
PHYS: Increasing levels diagnostic

Homovanillate, Urine [HVA] (4-Hydroxy-3 Methoxyphenylacetate)

RI: Adult <5.5 umol/nmol creatinine
    Considerable variation between labs
IND: Brain tumours
INT: HIGH – Neuroblastoma, ganglioneuroma
PHYS: Serial levels useful in monitoring progress of tumour

HSV Antibodies

See Herpes Simplex Antibodies, Serum

HTLV-3 Antibody, Serum

See HIV Antibody, Serum

Human Chorionic Gonadotrophin

See Chorionic Gonadotrophin, Human, Beta, Serum; Chorionic Gonadotrophin, Human, Urine

Human Leucocyte Antigen

See HLA-B27, Serum; HLA-DR2, Serum; HLA-DR3, Serum; HLA-DR4, Serum

Human Placental Lactogen

See Placental Lactogen, Human, Serum

HVA

See Homovanillate, Urine

Hydatid Antibodies, Blood

RI: Absent
IND: Hydatid disease
INT: PRESENT – Past or current hydatid infection
PHYS: Test remains positive long term after infection

Hydrogen Ion

See pH, Serum

4-Hydroxy-3-Methoxy Mandelic Acid, Urine [HMMA]

See numerical entries at beginning of this section

Hydroxybutyrate, Plasma

RI: <1.2mmol/L
IND: Metabolic acidosis
INT: HIGH – Ketosis, poorly controlled diabetes mellitus, starvation, alcoholism, hyperinsulinism
PHYS: More accurate measure of acidosis than ketones

See also ketones, Blood

17-Hydroxy Steroids, Serum

See Steroids, 17-Hydroxy, Serum

5-Hydroxyindole Acetic Acid, Urine [5 HIAA]

See numerical entries at beginning of this section

Hydroxyproline, Urine

RI: <35mmol/mol creatinine/2 hours
IND: Assessment of bone resorption
INT: HIGH – Osteoporosis, Paget's disease of bone, bone cancer
PHYS: Timed two hour urine collection after overnight fast. No gelatin (eg. meat, jelly, ice cream) for 24 hours before test

Hydroxyproline/Creatinine Ratio

RI: <0.02
IND: Pathological fractures, postmenopause
INT: HIGH – Paget's disease of bone, hyperparathyroidism, osteomalacia, hyperthyroidism, postmenopausal osteoporosis, renal fracture, severe fracture
PHYS: Measure of bone resorption and calcium loss. Calcium supplementation lowers ratio postmenopausally

25-Hydroxyvitamin D, Blood

See numerical entries at beginning of this section

IA2

See Insulinoma Associated 2 Antibodies, Serum

IBC

See Iron Binding Capacity, Total, Serum

Ig

See Immunoglobulins, Serum

IGF-1, Serum (Somatomedin C)

RI: Under 10 years – 0–18nmol/L
       10 to 15 years – 15–90nmol/L
       15 to 25 years – 25–60nmol/L
       25 to 40 years – 10–50nmol/L
       Over 40 years – 5–30nmol/L
IND: Acromegaly
INT: HIGH – Acromegaly (growth hormone?), gigantism
       LOW – Laron dwarfism, protein malnutrition
PHYS: Results vary markedly with age, as shown in the graph below

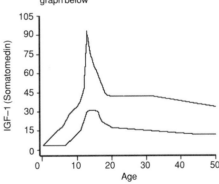

Immunoglobulin G, CSF [IgG]

RI: Adult 5–45 mg/L
       Child 8–64 mg/L
IND: Meningitis
INT: HIGH – Viral infection

Immunoglobulin, Antibodies, Specific, Serum

RI: Negative
IND: Many bacterial, viral, rickettsial and fungal diseases. Examples include Barmah Forest virus, brucellosis, Chlamydia, cytomegalovirus,

Dengue fever, Entamoeba, Histolytica, Epstein-Barr virus, hepatitis A, B & C, *Herpes simplex*, HIV, hydatid, influenza, Legionella, Leptospira, Lyme disease, measles, mumps, Mycoplasma, parvovirus, Q fever, Ross River fever, rubella, Salmonella, Shigella, Streptococci, Strongyloides, syphilis, Toxoplasma, typhus

INT: IgG & IgM NEGATIVE – No exposure or too early to detect in acute phase
IgG ANTIBODY POSITIVE, IgM ANTIBODY NEGATIVE – Past exposure to infective agent
IgG & IgM POSITIVE – Current or recurrent infection
IgG ANTIBODY NEGATIVE, IgM ANTIBODY POSITIVE – Very early acute phase or false positive IgM

PHYS: Most infective agents create antibodies within 2 weeks of infecting an individual, but syphilis, Q fever and Legionella may take up to 2 months. For immune status, only IgG needs to be tested

Immunoglobulin Postinfection Profile

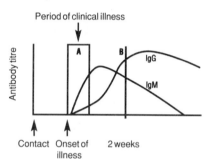

A Collect serum for acute stage antibodies
B Collect serum for IgM antibodies

$$INR = \frac{\text{Patient prothrombin time}}{\text{Control prothrombin time}}$$

$$PI = \frac{\text{Control prothrombin time}}{\text{Patient prothrombin time}} \times 100$$

Immunoglobulins, Serum [Ig]

RI:

	Adult	10yrs	5yrs	1yr
IgA	0.6–3.7	0.5–2.4	0.2–1.5	0.1–1.1
IgG	6.5–16	6.0–16	4.6–12	3.5–12
IgM	0.5–2.8	0.5–2.4	0.4–2.0	0.4–2.7
IgE	<100	<200	<60	<15

Units for IgA, IgG, IgM are g/L
Units for IgE are IU/mL

IND: Liver disease, paraproteinaemia

INT: ALL HIGH – Acute viral hepatitis
IgA and IgG HIGH – Laennec's cirrhosis
IgG HIGH – Chronic acute hepatitis, viral infection, myelomatosis, SLE, Lassa fever
IgM HIGH – Primary biliary cirrhosis, viral infection, trypanosomiasis, nephrotic syn., Waldenström's macroglobulinaemia

IgA HIGH – Buerger's disease
IgE HIGH – Extrinsic asthma, atopic eczema, allergic rhinitis (RAST?), allergic conjunctivitis, aspergillosis, parasitic diseases, myeloma, bullous pemphigoid, Job-Buckley syn.
IgA LOW – Intestinal disease, respiratory infections, drugs (eg. phenytoin, penicillamine)
IgM LOW – Septicaemia
IgG LOW – Nephrotic syn., hypogammaglobulinaemia, infancy
IgE LOW – Hypogammaglobulinaemia
ALL LOW – Bruton syn.

PHYS: Immunoglobulins possess antibody activity. They are composed of two heavy (A, G, M, D or E) and two light chains. They form part of the gammaglobulin protein factor. Significant number of false high and low results with IgE

See also Bilirubin, Serum;Alanine Amino Transferase, Serum; Aspartate Amino Transferase, Serum; Radioallergsorbent Test, Serum

Infectious Mononucleosis Screen, Serum (Epstein-Barr Virus; Glandular Fever)

RI: Negative
IND: Suspect infectious mononucleosis
INT: POSITIVE – Infectious mononucleosis
PHYS: Specific agglutination test

See also Paul Bunnell Test; Immunoglobulin Antibodies, Specific, Serum

Influenza Antidbodies, Serum

See Immunoglobulin Antibodies, Specific, Serum

INR

See International Normalised Ratio – Prothrombin

Insulin, Plasma

RI: < 19 mIU/L (< 0.9 µg/L) fasting
50–130 mIU/L 1 hour after 75 g glucose
< 100 mIU/L 2 hours after 75 g glucose
IND: Diabetes mellitus, insulinoma
INT: LOW AFTER GLUCOSE – Diabetes due to lack of insulin, malnutrition
HIGH – Diabetes due to tissue unresponsiveness to insulin, insulinoma, Reaven syn., pregnancy
PHYS: Insulin essential for the uptake and utilisation of glucose by tissue. Collected after 15 hour fast and during GTT

See also Glucose, Blood

Insulinoma Associated 2 Antibodies, Serum [IA2]

RI: <0.75 U/mL
IND: Diabetes
INT: HIGH – Type one diabetes mellitus, potential to develop type one diabetes mellitus
PHYS: Present in up to 60% of type one diabetics, and frequently in first degree relatives of patients and others at risk of developing the disease

Intercellular Cement Substance Autoantibodies, Blood (Pemphigus Autoantibodies)

RI: Absent
IND: Blistering rash
INT: PRESENT – Pemphigus, extensive burns, skin drug reactions
PHYS: Regular measurement of titre can be used to follow disease activity

International Normalised Ratio – Prothrombin [INR] (Prothrombin Ratio)

RI: 0.9–1.1
IND: Control of anticoagulant therapy
INT: Modify dose of warfarin to maintain ratio within desired therapeutic range
1.5–2.5 – transient ischaemic attacks, CVA, atrial fibrillation
2.0–3.0 – Deep venous thromboses, pulmonary embolism, heart valve disease, transplanted animal heart valves, cardiomyopathy, myocardial infarct, postoperative prophylaxis (eg. after hip replacement)
2.5–3.5 – Mechanical heart valves

Intrinsic Factor Autoantibodies, Blood

RI: Absent
IND: Anaemia
INT: PRESENT – Pernicious anaemia
PHYS: Negative result does not exclude diagnosis

See also Cyanocobalamin, Serum

Iron, Marrow Transit Time

RI: Mean 3.5 days
IND: Iron deficiency anaemia

Iron, Serum [Fe]

RI: Male 12–35 µmol/L
Female 10–28 µmol/L
IND: Anaemia
INT: LOW – Iron deficiency anaemia (MCV, MCHC?), dietary deficiency, chronic inflammation, malabsorption, chronic bleeding, infections, Hodgkin's disease, chronic inflammatory disorders, malignancy, elderly, bleeding peptic ulcer, bleeding haemorrhoids, bowel cancer, coeliac disease, menorrhagia, gastrectomy, pregnancy, scurvy, trauma, elite athletes
HIGH – Other anaemias, gastrointestinal bleeding (faecal blood?), liver necrosis, haemochromatosis, haemosiderosis, beta-thalassaemia, alcoholism (GGT?), iron therapy
PHYS: Iron is essential for the formation of Hb. Iron is actively absorbed in the duodenum. Its absorption may be reduced by phosphates and sprue. Collect specimen in morning to avoid false low reading

See also Ferritin, Serum; Haemoglobin, Blood; Iron Binding Capacity, Total, Serum

Iron, Urine [Fe]

RI: 50–400 µg/24 hours
INT: Variation from normal is rare

Iron Binding Capacity, Total, Serum [IBC, TIBC]

RI: Male 45–70 µmol/L (250–380 µg/100 mL)
Female 44–74 µmol/L (245–400 µg/100 mL)
IND: Anaemia
INT: HIGH – Late pregnancy, iron deficiency anaemia (transferrin?)
LOW – Chronic infection, rheumatoid arthritis, cancer, liver cirrhosis, nephrotic syn., haemochromatosis
PHYS: The total iron binding capacity is related to plasma transferrin levels

Iron Clearance, Blood

RI: Half-life 60–140 minutes
IND: Iron deficiency anaemia

Iron Studies

	Iron	IBC	Transferrin Sat.	Ferritin
Iron deficit	L	H	L	L
Iron excess	H	N	H	H
Acute phase response	L	L	L	H

See also Ferritin, Serum; Iron, Serum; Iron Binding Capacity; Transferrin Saturation

Iron Turnover, Blood

RI: 70–140 µmol/L/day
IND: Iron deficiency anaemia

Iron Utilisation, Blood

RI: 70–80% per fortnight
IND: Iron deficiency anaemia

Islet Cell Autoantibodies, Blood

RI: Absent
IND: Diabetes mellitus
INT: PRESENT – Type I (insulin dependent) diabetes mellitus, close relatives of diabetic patients, other autoimmune diseases (false positive)
PHYS: Titre decreases slowly after initial onset of disease. May predict potential to develop diabetes mellitus

Isoenzymes

See Lactate Dehydrogenase Isoenzymes, Serum; Creatine Kinase Isoenzymes, Serum

Jo-1 Antibodies, Serum (Histidyl-tRNA Synthetase Antibodies)

RI: Negative
IND: Polymyositis

INT: POSITIVE – Polymyositis with interstitial lung disease and thrombocytopenia
PHYS: Defines a specific subset type of polymyositis

K+
See Potassium, Serum; Potassium, Urine

Ketones, Blood
RI: 0.02–0.5 mmol/L (0.1–3 mg/100 mL)
INT: See Ketones, Urine

See also Hydroxybutyrate, Plasma

Ketones, Urine
RI: Nil
IND: Diabetes mellitus
INT: HIGH – Diabetic ketoacidosis (B.glucose?), urinary tract infection (U.M/C/S?), starvation, vomiting, dehydration, general anaesthesia, strenuous exercise, cold exposure
PHYS: Ketones formed in liver are normally completely metabolised. Altered carbohydrate metabolism causes accumulation and appearance in urine

Kidney
See Renal Function Tests; Renal Calculi

Kleihauer Test
See Haemoglobin F

Kveim Test, Skin (Kveim-Siltzbach Test)
RI: Negative
IND: Sarcoidosis
INT: POSITIVE – Sarcoidosis
PHYS: Heat treated suspension of spleen sarcoidosis extract is injected intradermally. Site biopsied 1 month later; 80%show sarcoid-like lesions. 5% false positive

Lactate, Blood (L-Lactate, Blood)
RI: Venous blood 0.3–1.3 mmol/L
Arterial blood 0.3–0.8 mmol/L
IND: Metabolic disorders
INT: HIGH – Lactic acidosis, diabetes mellitus, congestive cardiac failure, hypoxia, shock, other metabolic disturbances
PHYS: Fasting blood sample necessary

Lactate, CSF
RI: 1.2–2.8mmol/L
IND: Meningitis
INT: HIGH – Bacterial and cryptococcal meningitis, severe cerebral hypoxia
PHYS: levels do nit rise with viral meningitis. Very early sign in bacterial meningitis

Lactate Dehydrogenase, Serum [LD or LDH]
RI: 120–230 U/L
IND: Myocardial infarct
INT: HIGH – Myocardial infarct (CK, AST?), tissue necrosis, muscle damage, RBC destruction (Hb?), kidney damage (S.creatinine), malignancy, pulmonary infarct, infectious hepatitis (LFT?), other hepatic diseases, polycythaemia rubra vera, pernicious anaemia, seminoma, muscular dystrophy, paracetamol overdose, haemolysed blood specimen
PHYS: LDH is present in all cells, and is released from them when they are damaged. Rises over 3–4 days after damage, and declines to normal over following 5–7 days

Lactate Dehydrogenase Isoenzymes, Serum
RI: $LDH_1 < 65$ IU/L
$LDH_2 < 120$ IU/L,
$LDH_3 <785$ IU/L
$LDH_4 < 20$ IU/L
$LDH_5 < 20$ IU/L
IND: Raised total LDH, myocardial infarct, liver disease
INT: LDH_1 & LDH_2 HIGH – Heart, kidney, brain or erythrocyte damage or disease
LDH_3 HIGH – Lung, pancreas, adrenal, spleen, thymus, lymph node or leucocyte damage or disease
LDH_4 & LDH_5 HIGH – Skeletal muscle or liver damage or disease
PHYS: Human serum contains 5 distinct isoenzymes of LDH which differ from each other in their electrophoretic mobility and their tissue source

Lactogen, Human Placental
See Placental Lactogen, Human, Serum

Lactose Tolerance Test
RI: Rise in B.glucose < 1.0 mmol/L after lactose challenge
IND: Food intolerance, diarrhoea
INT: B.GLUCOSE RISES > 1.0 mmol/L – Lactose intolerance, false positive result
PHYS: 50 g of lactose given to patient who has fasted overnight. B.glucose measured at 30 minute intervals for 3 hours. Rise in B.glucose indicates low or absent lactase activity. False positive rate about 25%

Lanoxin, Serum
See Digoxin, Serum

Largactil, Serum
See Chlorpromazine, Serum

Latex Agglutination, Blood
RI: 0–60 IU/mL
IND: Connective tissue disease

NT: V.HIGH – Rheumatoid arthritis (FANA, CRP, rheumatoid factor?), Sjögren's syn.
        HIGH – SLE, polyarteritis, polymyositis, liver disease, viral infection, 5% of normal people
HYS: More sensitive for rheumatoid arthritis than rheumatoid factor, but more false positives. Normal levels do not exclude rheumatoid arthritis. Agglutination of specifically sensitised latex particles measured

ATS
See Long Acting Thyroid Stimulator Antibody, Serum

CR
See Ligase Chain Reaction, Urine

D or LDH
See Lactate Dehydrogenase, Serum

DL
See Low Density Lipoprotein Cholesterol, Blood

E Cells, Blood (Lupus Erythematosus Cells)
RI: Absent
ND: Autoimmune disease
NT: PRESENT – SLE (ANA?), scleroderma, rheumatoid arthritis, chronic active hepatitis
HYS: Normal leucocytes incubated with the serum of a patient with SLE gain homogeneous mass that stains purple with Romanowsky stain. The mass is altered nuclear material, the cell is an LE cell. May be found in other diseases of disordered immunity

See also ANA, Serum; ANCA, Serum; Anti-DNA, Serum; Anti-Smith Antibodies, Serum; Cardiolipin Autoantibodies, Blood; Complement C3 and C4; DNA Autoantibodies; ENA, Serum; Histone Autoantibodies, Blood; HLA-DR3, Serum; Lupus Anticoagulant Antibody, Serum

Lead, Plasma [Pb]
RI: < 1.2 µmol/L (< 30 µg/100 mL)
NT: 1.3–1.9 µmol/L – Retest adults three monthly, risk of mental damage in children
        1.9–2.4µmol/L – Retest adults monthly, check sources of exposure
        2.4µmol/L – Remove adults from exposure, treat children with aggressive elimination
HYS: 95th. percentile for whole population is <0.8µmol/L

See also Lead, Urine

Lead, Urine
RI: 5–105 µg/24 hours (< 0.5 µmol/L) (< 0.25 µmol/day)
ND: Lead poisoning
NT: HIGH – Lead poisoning
HYS: May be caused by ingestion (eg. old paint battery workers) or inhalation (eg. exhaust fumes from leaded petrol) of lead. Treated with EDTA. Pregnant and breast feeding women should not work with lead

See also Lead, Plasma

Lecithin-Sphingomyelin Ratio, Amniotic Fluid [L-S Ratio]
RI: < 2:1
IND: Assessment of fetal maturity
INT: HIGH (> 2:1) – Fetal lung mature
        LOW (< 2:1) – Fetal lung not mature (P.oestriols?)
PHYS: Lecithin from the fetal lung is produced in increasing quantities in relation to sphingomyelin after 34 weeks of gestation

See also Alpha-Fetoprotein, Amniotic Fluid; Alpha-Fetoprotein, Serum; Oestriols, Plasma; Phosphatidyl Glycerol, Amniotic Fluid

Legionella Antibodies, Serum
See Immunoglobulin Antibodies, Specific, Serum

Leptospira Antibodies, Serum
See Immunoglobulin Antibodies, Specific, Serum

Leucocytes
See White Cell Count, Blood; White Cell Count, Urine

LFT
See Liver Function Tests

LH
See Luteinising Hormone, Serum

Ligase Chain Reaction, Urine [LCR]
RI: Negative
IND: Sexually transmitted or pelvic inflammatory disease, cervicitis, conjunctivitis
INT: POSITIVE – Chlamydia trachomatis infection
PHYS: May also be applied to a swab from affected area

Lipase, Serum
RI: 0.2–1.5 IU/L
IND: Pancreatic disease
INT: HIGH – Acute pancreatitis (amylase?), pancreatic duct obstruction
PHYS: Pancreatic lipase is released into the blood with pancreatic damage. Remains elevated for longer than amylase in pancreatitis

Lipids, Total Plasma
RI: After fasting 12 hours, 400–600 mmol/L
IND: Obesity, hypertension
INT: HIGH – Hyperlipidaemia, atherosclerosis, diabetes, hypothyroidism
PHYS: Specific type of hyperlipidaemia is determined

by measuring the cholesterol and triglyceride components of the total plasma lipids

Lipoproteins

See Apolipoproteins, Serum; High Density Lipoprotein Cholesterol, Blood; Low Density Lipoprotein Cholesterol, Blood; Very Low Density Lipoprotein Cholesterol, Blood

Lithium, Serum

RI: Therapeutic range 0.5–1 mmol/L
IND: Lithium therapy
INT: Adjust dosage to keep serum levels within therapeutic range
PHYS: Sample 12 hours after last dose

Liver Function Tests [LFT]
PHYS:

Summary of Liver Function Test Abnormalities

DISEASE	ALT	AST	GGT	ALP
Viral hepatitis	+++	+++	++	N/+
Drug induced hepatitis	++	++	++	N/+
Chronic active hepatitis	++	++	++	+
Infectious mononuc. hepatitis	+	+	++	N
Primary biliary cirrhosis	+	+	+++	++
Alcoholic cirrhosis	N	+	+++	N/+
Intrahepatic cholestasis	++	++	++	++
Extrahepatic cholestasis	+	+	+++	+++
Hepatoma	N/+	+	++	+

See Albumin, Serum; Alkaline Phosphatase, Serum; Alanine Amino Transferase, Serum; Aspartate Amino Transferase, Serum; Gamma Glutamyl Transpeptidase, Serum; Bilirubin, Serum; Immunoglobulins, Serum; Protein, Serum, Total

L-Lactate Blood
See lactate, Blood

Long Acting Thyroid Stimulator Antibody, Serum [LATS]

RI: Negative
IND: Thyroid disease
INT: POSITIVE – Hyperthyroidism
PHYS: May be normal in up to 40% of cases of thyrotoxicosis

See also other Thyroid Function Tests

Low Density Lipoprotein Cholesterol, Blood [LDL]

RI: <3.0 mmol/L
IND: High total cholesterol
INT: HIGH – Increased risk of arteriosclerosis, heart disease and cerebrovascular disease (HDL?)
PHYS: Ratio between LDL and HDL important

See also Apolipoproteins, Serum

L-S Ratio
See Lecithin-Sphingomyelin Ratio, Amniotic Fluid

Lung Function Tests
See Forced Expiratory Volume in 1 Second; Vital Capacity, Lungs; Peak Expiratory Flow Rate

Lupus Anticoagulant Antibody, Serum (Lupus Inhibitor)

RI: Nil
IND: Suspected SLE, recurrent abortions
INT: POSITIVE – SLE, recurrent thromboembolism, other autoimmune diseases, neoplasia, recurrent abortions, antiphospholipid syn. (see SYNDROMES SECTION 6)
PHYS: Autoantibody to cardiolipin which inhibits intrinsic and extrinsic clotting pathways

See also ANA, Serum; ANCA, Serum; Anti-DNA, Serum; Anti-Smith Antibodies, Serum; Cardiolipin Autoantibodies, Blood; Complement C3 and C4; DNA Autoantibodies; ENA, Serum; Histone Autoantibodies, Blood; HLA-DR3, Serum; LE Cells, Blood

Lupus Erythematosus Cells
See LE Cells, Blood;
See also INVESTIGATION SECTION 3: Lupus Erythematosus, Systemic

Luteinising Hormone, Serum [LH]

RI: Prepubertal 1–3.4 IU/L
Male 2–9 IU/L
Female 2–20 IU/L
Ovulating female 10–50 IU/L
Postmenopausal 30–200 IU/L
Results and units vary between labs
IND: Menstrual disorders, infertility
INT: LOW – Infertile, hypogonadism
HIGH – Ovulation, precocious puberty, Stein-Leventhal syn. (FSH?)
LH >>FSH – Imminent ovulation, impeded ovulation, polycystic ovarian syn. (Stein-Leventhal syn.).
PHYS: Released from the pituitary gland under regulation by the posterior hypothalamus. Responsible for ovulation and corpus luteum formation in the female, and stimulates Leydig cells and production of androgens in the testes

See also Follicle Stimulating Hormone, Serum

Lyme Disease Antibodies, Serum
See Immunoglobulin Antibodies, Specific, Serum

Lymphocytes, Blood

RI: 1.5–3.5 x 10^{9}L (1,500–3,500/mm^3) (20–40%)
IND: Infection, blood disorders
INT: HIGH (normal forms) – Chronic infection, TB,

syphilis, pertussis, infectious lymphocytosis, chronic lymphocytic leukaemia
HIGH (abnormal forms) – Infectious mononucleosis (P. Bunnell?), measles, acute lymphatic leukaemia, cytomegalovirus, toxoplasmosis, rubella, hepatitis, brucellosis, typhoid fever, bacterial endocarditis, serum sickness, other viral infections
LOW – Stress, trauma, haemorrhage (Hb?), gross infection, Hodgkin's disease, AIDS, irradiation, TB, cytotoxic drugs, elderly
HYS: Lymphocytes migrate freely between lymph glands and blood. They enter the blood stream via the thoracic duct. Antigenic challenge produces an increase in the number of specific small normal form lymphocytes

ymphocytye CD Types
ee T Cell Lymphocytes, Blood

yssavirus Antibody Enzyme Immunoassay, ierum
I: Negative (<0.5 IU/L)
ID: Rabies exposure
IT: POSITIVE – Rabies, other lyssavirus infections, post-vaccination for rabies
HYS: Numerous lyssavriuses exist that cause rabies and similar diseases (eg: Australian bat lyssavirus infection)

lacrocytosis
iee Mean Corpuscular Volume

lagnesium, Faeces [Mg]
I: <45mmol/L (<15mmol/d)
ID: Unexplained diarrhoea
IT: HIGH – Abuse of laxatives containing magnesium, hypomagnesaemia due to gut loss of Mg

lagnesium, Serum [Mg]
I: 0.7–1.0 mmol/L (1.7–2.3 mg/100 mL)
       Neonate 0.6–0.9 mmol/L
ID: Renal disease
IT: HIGH – Chronic renal failure
       LOW – Renal tubular defects, chronic alcoholism, hyperaldosteronism, hepatic cirrhosis, malabsorption syn., diarrhoea, parathyroidectomy, diabetic ketoacidosis, malnutrition, alcoholism, vomiting, prolonged intravenous therapy, drugs (eg. diuretics, amphotericin, gentamicin, laxatives, cisplatin, cytotoxics)
HYS: Magnesium is an important intracellular cation that is filtered by the kidneys. Low levels can cause cardiac arrhythmias. Co-factor to at least 300 body enzymes

lagnesium, Urine [Mg]
I: 2.5–8.0 µmol/day (20–180 mg/day)

INT: LOW – Malabsorption syn., severe body fluid loss, alcoholism, diabetic acidosis, hepatic cirrhosis, primary aldosteronism, chronic renal failure

Manganese, Blood
RI: 140–220 nmol/L
IND: Manganese poisoning
INT: HIGH – Manganese poisoning
PHYS: Beware of sample contamination

Manganese, Urine
RI: <3µmol/L
IND: Manganese poisoning
INT: HIGH – Manganese poisoning

Mantoux Test
See Tuberculin Skin Test

Marrow Cells, Bone
RI: Sideroblasts 40–60%
       Neutrophils 7–30%
       Eosinophils 0.5–4%
       Basophils 0–0.7%
       Lymphocytes 3–17%
       Myeloblasts 0.5–5%
       Metamyelocytes 13–30%
       Megakaryocytes 0–3%
       Plasma cells 3–5%
       Monocytes 0.5–5%
       Normoblasts 7–32%
       Myelocytes 5–22%
       Promyelocytes 1–8%
       Pronormoblasts 1–8%
       Reticular cells 0.1–2%
       Note: Adult values only for all above
IND: Abnormal peripheral blood smear
INT: ABNORMAL – Agranulocytosis, aplastic anaemia, haemolytic anaemia, leukaemias, osteogenic sarcoma, cytotoxic and immunosuppressive drugs, myelomatosis, Hodgkin's disease, myeloproliferative disorders, visceral leishmaniasis
       SIDEROBLASTS LOW – Iron deficiency
PHYS: For further details consult a more detailed text

MCH
See Mean Corpuscular Haemoglobin

MCHC
See Mean Corpuscular Haemoglobin Concentration

MCV
See Mean Corpuscular Volume

Mean Corpuscular Haemoglobin [MCH]
RI: Adult: 27–31 pg
       Child: 24–30 pg

Neonate: 24–34 pg
IND: Anaemia
INT: LOW – Iron deficiency (Fe?), chronic blood loss, sprue, achlorhydria, pregnancy, thalassaemia, sideroblastic anaemia, megaloblastic anaemia
HIGH – Pernicious anaemia (vit.B$_{12}$?), folic acid deficiency, starvation, reticulocytosis (FBC?), hypothyroidism (ETR?), aplastic anaemia
PHYS: Useful to determine type of anaemia
MCH = Hb/RBC

Mean Corpuscular Haemoglobin Concentration [MCHC]

RI: 300–340 g/L (30–34%) (18.6–21.2 mmol/L)
IND: LOW – Iron deficiency (Fe?), blood loss, pregnancy, thalassaemia, anaemias of chronic disease, sideroblastic anaemia
NORMAL – Other anaemias
PHYS: In iron deficiency, there is less Hb in each RBC
MCHC = Hb/PCV

Mean Corpuscular Volume [MCV]

RI: Adult 80–96 fL (80–96 cubic microns)
Child 73–89 fL (73–89 cubic microns)
Neonate 85–106 fL (85–106 cubic microns)
IND: Anaemia
INT: V.LOW – Iron deficiency (Fe, MCHC?), chronic blood loss, pregnancy, chronic disease (eg. rheumatoid arthritis)
LOW (microcytosis) – Acute blood loss, haemolytic anaemia, bone marrow neoplasia, sideroblastic anaemia, thalassaemia trait, elderly
HIGH (macrocytosis) – Pernicious anaemia (vit. B$_{12}$), alcoholism, folic acid deficiency, sprue, starvation, reticulocytosis, aplastic anaemia, hypothyroidism, liver disease, hyperlipidaemia, scurvy, sideroblastic anaemia, leukaemia, megaloblastic anaemia, chronic respiratory failure, myelomatosis, cytotoxic drugs
PHYS: Useful to determine type of anaemia
MCV = PCV/RBC

Measles Antibodies, Serum

See Immunoglobulin Antibodies, Specific, Serum

Melaena

See Occult Blood, Faeces

See also SYMPTOMS SECTION 1: Melaena and Rectal Bleeding

Mercury, Urine [Hg]

RI: < 0.2 µmol/day
IND: Mercury poisoning
INT: HIGH – Mercury poisoning, Minamata disease

Metadrenalines, Urine

See Metanephrine, Urine

Metanephrine, Urine (Metadrenalines, Urine)

RI: < 5 µmol/day (age dependent)
IND: Hypertension
INT: HIGH – Phaeochromocytoma, neuroblastoma ganglioneuroma, drug interference
PHYS: Metabolite of catecholamines excreted in urine

Methaemoglobin, Blood

RI: < 1% of total Hb
Infants < 1.5% of total Hb
IND: Cyanosis
INT: HIGH – Poisoning by oxidant drugs (eg. sulfonamides, nitrates, nitrites, aniline dye)
PHYS: Poison causes haemolysis and cyanosis

Mg

See Magnesium, Serum; Magnesium, Urine

Microalbumin

See Albumin, Urine

Microcytosis

See Mean Corpuscular Volume

Microglobulin, Beta-2

See Beta-2 Microglobulin, Serum

Milk, Breast

See Breast Milk Analysis

Mitochondrial Autoantibodies, Serum [AMA]

RI: Negative
IND: Liver disease
INT: HIGH – Primary biliary cirrhosis (?LFT), chronic active hepatitis

Monocytes, Blood

RI: 0.2–0.8 x 10^9/L (200–800/mm^3) (4–8%)
IND: Infection
INT: LOW – Chronic infection, brucellosis, subacute bacterial endocarditis, malaria, rickettsial infection, cytotoxic drugs
HIGH – TB, some acute and chronic bacterial infections, carcinoma, acute monocytic leukaemia, glandular fever, malaria, Hodgkin's disease, splenectomy
PHYS: Helps to determine the nature and course of infection

Myocardial Autoantibodies, Blood

RI: Absent
IND: Myocarditis
INT: PRESENT – Dressler syn. (see SYNDROMES SECTION 6), postcardiotomy syn., autoimmune myocarditis, cardiac surgery,

cardiac infarct, heart trauma
HYS: Nonspecific test of myocardial damage

yoglobin, Serum

: Male < 70 µg/L
 Female < 50 µg/L
D: Myocardial infarct
T: HIGH – Myocardial infarct
HYS: Rises within 2–4 hours of an infarct. Should not be used as a late marker, as it is rapidly cleared from blood stream

yoglobin, Urine

: Absent
D: Muscle damage, haemoglobinuria
T: PRESENT – Any significant muscle trauma, rhabdomyolysis, electric shock, snake bite, myopathies, hypokalaemia
HYS: Insensitive test, not able to detect most myocardial infarcts. May be used to differentiate confusion with Hb in urine

ysoline, Serum
ee Primidone, Serum

a+
ee Sodium, Serum; Sodium, Urine

AP
ee Neutrophil Alkaline Phosphatase, Blood

eonatal Screen
HYS: Screening tests for galactosaemia (P.galactose), phenylketonuria (B.phenylalanine), cretinism (hypothyroidism – S.TSH) and cystic fibrosis (B.trypsin)

eurone Specific Enolase, Serum
: <12µg/L
D: Monitoring specific cancers
T: RISING LEVEL – Progress of small cell lung carcinoma or neural crest tumour
HYS: Not a screenign or diagnostic test

eutrophil Alkaline Phosphatase, Blood [NAP]
: 30–180. See Phys
D: Abnormal blood film
T: HIGH WCC, HIGH NAP – Bacterial infection, other causes of reactive leucocytosis
HIGH WCC, LOW NAP – Chronic leukaemia
HIGH RCC, HIGH NAP – Polycythaemia rubra vera
HIGH RCC, LOW NAP – Other causes of erthrocytosis
U.Hb, HIGH NAP – Haemolytic anaemia, hypoplastic anaemia

U.Hb, LOW NAP – Paroxysmal nocturnal haemoglobinuria
PHYS: 100 neutrophils in capillary blood film examined by microscopy. Dye intensity of cells compared, and scored on a basis of 0 for no dye, 1 for light dye, 2 for medium dye, 3 for heavily dyed, and 4 for very heavily dyed. Score added, to give a NAP value between 0 and 400. Test useful for differentiating cause of high WCC or high RCC

Neutrophils, Blood

RI: Adult: 2.1–7.5 x 10^9/L (2,100–7,500/mm^3) (40–60%)
Child: 1.6–9.0 x 10^9/L (1,600–9,000/mm^3)
Neonate: 4.5–12 x 10^9/L (4,500–12,000/mm^3)
IND: Infection
INT: V.HIGH – Pneumococcal pneumonia, lung abscess, disseminated carcinoma
HIGH (neutrophilia) – Bacterial infections, rabies, actinomycosis, some viral infections (eg. Herpes zoster), severe inflammation anywhere in body (eg. infarction, arthritis, dermatitis), haemorrhage, haemolysis, malignancy, myeloproliferative disease, splenectomy, pregnancy, burns, trauma, physical stress, drugs (eg. lithium, corticosteroids)
LOW (neutropenia) – Viral infection (eg. infectious mononucleosis, HIV), severe bacterial infection (eg. pneumonia, cellulitis, septicaemia), typhoid, hepatitis, TB, brucellosis, aspergillosus, starvation, vit. B$_{12}$ and folic acid deficiencies, acute leukaemia, lymphosarcoma, aplastic anaemia, Gaucher's disease, SLE, rheumatoid arthritis, haemodialysis, myelodyspasia, hypersplenism, Chediak-Higashi syn., Diamond-Blackfan syn., Felty syn., irradiation, drugs (eg. cytotoxics, NSAID, sulphonamides, captopril penicillin)
HYPERSEGMENTATION – Renal disease, vit. B$_{12}$/folate deficit, cytotoxic iron deficit, sideroblastic anaemia, leukaemia, hereditary, very high neutrophil count
PHYS: Rate of entry of neutrophils to circulation can be increased by certain stimuli. Once reserves in marrow are depleted, blood levels may drop markedly

See also Basophils, Blood; Monocytes, Blood; Eosinophils, Blood

Neutrophil Cytoplasmic Antibodies, Serum
See Anti-Neutrophil Cytoplasmic Antibodies, Serum

Nicotine, Serum
RI: < 0.006 mg/L
IND: Determination of smoking status
INT: HIGH – Smoker, passive smoker
PHYS: Plasma half-life of nicotine averages 40 minutes

See also Carboxyhaemoglobin B, Serum; Cotinine, Serum

Nicotinic Acid, Serum
See Vitamin B₃

Nitrite, Urine
RI: Negative
IND: Cystitis
INT: POSITIVE – Urinary tract infection (eg.
          Pseudomonas), chronic renal failure
PHYS: Certain bacteria, when in high concentration in
          urine, metabolise nitrates in urine to nitrites,
          thus indicating their presence

Noradrenaline
See Catecholamines, Urine

Nordin Test, Blood and Urine
RI: Phosphate excretion 0.06–0.2 mmol/L or
        glomerular filtrate
        Index of phosphate excretion –0.16 to +0.16
IND: Abnormal calcium levels. Hyperparathyroidism
INT: HIGH – Excessive parathyroid hormone
        activity, hyperparathyroidism, PTH excreting
        adenoma
PHYS: Tested in conjunction with serum and urine
        calcium and phosphate, and renal function tests

Nortriptyline, Serum
RI: Therapeutic range 60–240 µg/L (150–880
        nmol/L)
PHYS: Several weeks may be required to reach steady
        state due to long half-life

N-Telopeptides, Cross-Linked, Urine [Ntx]
RI: Negative
IND: Osteoporosis
INT: POSITIVE – Osteoporosis (hydroxyproline?),
        Paget's disease, malignancy, inflammatory
        disease, steroid therapy
PHYS: Ntx is a fragment of bone collagen which is
        released with bone resorption

Occult Blood, Faeces
RI: Negative
IND: Suspected gut bleed
INT: See table below

CHEMICAL TEST	IMMUNO CHEMICAL	INTERPRETATION
Positive	Negative	Upper gastrointestinal bleed (eg: oesophageal varices, gastric or duodenal ulcer etc.)
Positive	Positive	Lower gastrointestinal bleed (eg: rectal carcinoma, polyps, ulcerative colitis etc.)
False Positive	Negative	Certain foods (see Physiology below)

PHYS: Chemical test detects haem molecule, while
        immunochemical test detects only intact Hb,
        allowing differentiation between upper and
        lower gastrointestinal tract bleeds. No red mea
        cauliflower, broccoli, turnips, bananas or
        radishes for 3 days before test as these may
        interfere with chemical test. Three tests on
        consecutive days are necessary

See also SYMPTOMS SECTION 1: Melaena and Recta
Bleeding

Oestradiol, 17-beta, Plasma
RI: Male < 300 pmol/L (< 82 ng/L)
        Female follicular stage 180–1500 pmol/L
        (50–400 ng/L)
        Female luteal phase 400–800 pmol/L (120–20
        ng/L)
        Menopausal < 200 pmol/L (< 55 ng/L)
IND: Ovulatory status
INT: LOW – Anovulatory, prepubertal,
        postmenopausal

Oestriols, Plasma
RI: 32 weeks 145–800 nmol/L
        34 weeks 170–1040 nmol/L
        36 weeks 230–1400 nmol/L
        38 weeks 300–1560 nmol/L
        40 weeks 350–1600 nmol/L
IND: Suspect fetal welfare
INT: Repeated tests necessary, single test of little
        value. The level should rise steadily as the
        pregnancy progresses. If no rise noted, or level
        drop, fetal distress is likely (L-S ratio, AFP?).
        Low level may be due to Down syn. (see
        INVESTIGATIONS SECTION 3)
PHYS: Oestriols are produced by a chain of processes
        starting in the fetal adrenal, and progressing
        through the fetal liver and the placenta before
        entering the maternal circulation. Steroids and
        ampicillin may depress values

See also Lecithin-Sphingomyelin Ratio, Amniotic Fluid

Oestrogens, Urinary
RI: See table below (units: µg/24 hours)

Oestrogen	Male	Female menstruating	Female postmenopaus
Oestrone	0–5	5–20	0.3–2.4
Oestradiol	0–5	2–10	0–1.4
Oestriol	0–10	5–30	2.2–7.5

IND: Menstrual status, infertility, sex determination
INT: HIGH (female) – Hormone therapy
        HIGH (male) – Feminisation
        LOW – Infertile
PHYS: Oestrogens stimulate ovulation and the
        development of secondary sexual
        characteristics

Osmolality, Serum

RI: 280–300 mmol/kg water
IND: Water imbalance
INT: HIGH – Hyperglycaemia, uraemia, salicylate
         overdose, alcohol, hypernatraemia, diabetes
         insipidus, dehydration
         LOW – Hyponatraemia, water overload,
         pregnancy
PHYS: Plasma osmolality is well controlled by electrolytes
         and other small molecules. Proteins are significant

Osmolality, Urine

RI: 500–800 mmol/kg
         12 hour water deprivation > 800 mmol/kg
         Fluid overload < 100 mmol/kg
IND: Renal disease
INT: Result compared with serum osmolality (above)
         to separate renal causes of polyuria from
         extrarenal causes of polyuria

Osmotic Fragility of Red Blood Cells

RI: 0.40–0.45% saline before incubation
         0.47–0.60% saline after 24 hour incubation
IND: Spherocytosis
INT: HIGH – Hereditary spherocytosis, autoimmune
         haemolytic anaemia

Ovarian Autoantibodies, Blood

RI: Absent
IND: Ovarian disease
INT: PRESENT – Autoimmune ovarian disease,
         Addison's disease

Oxalate, Urine

RI: 0.22–0.44 mmol/day
IND: Recurrent renal calculi
INT: HIGH – Calcium oxalate renal stone formers,
         congenital
PHYS: 24 hour collection essential. Varies with diet

Oxygen Affinity of Haemoglobin

See Haemoglobin, Oxygen Affinity, Blood

Oxygen, Blood [pO₂]

RI: **Arterial**
         97% pO_2 10–13 kPa (75–100 mmHg)
         Venous
         60–85% pO_2 5–9.5 kPa (40–70 mmHg)
IND: Pulmonary disease
INT: LOW – Hypoxia due to poor air entry, poor lung
         function or poor circulation (eg. high
         altitude, pulmonary fibrosis, pulmonary
         oedema, emphysema, A-V shunt, brain stem
         damage, chronic obstructive airways disease,
         neuromuscular defects)

See also Carbon Dioxide, Blood; Forced Expiratory
Volume in 1 Second; Vital Capacity, Lungs

Oxygen Saturation, Arterial Blood

RI: > 95%

P

See Phosphorus, Inorganic, Serum

Packed Cell Volume [PCV] (Haematocrit)

RI: Adult male 40–54%
         Adult female 36–47%
         Child 32–42%
IND: Haematological disorders
INT: HIGH – Polycythaemia rubra vera, dehydration
         LOW – Anaemia (Hb, FBC?), pregnancy
PHYS: A blood specimen is centrifuged and the
         percentage of packed cells to plasma in the tube
         is measured

Papanicolaou Smear, Cervix

RI: Normal
IND: Routine every 12–36 months for all sexually
         active women
INT: ATYPICAL CELLS – Smear should be repeated
         in 3–6 months
         CIN 1 DYSPLASIA – Colposcopy advised with
         repeat smears frequently
         CIN 2 DYSPLASIA – Colposcopy and punch
         biopsy followed by appropriate treatment and
         follow-up
         CIN 3 CARCINOMA IN SITU – Definitive
         treatment necessary (eg. cone biopsy) and
         careful follow-up
         INVASIVE CARCINOMA – Definitive treatment
         essential (eg. hysterectomy, irradiation)
PHYS: Vaginal infections often also reported on
         smears. CIN is an index of cervical
         intraepithelial neoplasia

Paracentesis Fluid (Ascitic Fluid; Peritoneal Fluid)

RI: Colour – clear
         Red blood cells – nil
         White blood cells – nil
IND: Ascites
INT: **Colour**
         STRAW – Cirrhosis, infection, neoplasm,
         cardiac failure
         PINK/RED – Neoplasm, TB, pancreatitis
         WHITE – Lymphatic obstruction, infection
         Red blood cells
         FEW – Cirrhosis, infection, neoplasm
         NUMEROUS – Pancreatitis, TB, neoplasm,
         traumatic tap
         White blood cells
         <250 x 10⁶/L – Cirrhosis, neoplasm, cardiac
         failure
         >250 x 10⁶/L – Infection, TB, pancreatitis

See aslo Serum-Ascites Albumin Gradient

Paracetamol, Blood (Acetaminophen)

RI: Toxic > 1300 µmol/L (195 mg/L) four hours after ingestion
IND: Assessment of overdose
PHYS: Liver damage and death can result from overdose. Serum levels can rise for 4 or more hours after ingestion

Parathormone, Serum [PTH], (Parathyroid Hormone)

RI: 1.0–7.0 pmol/L whole molecule PTH
<100pmol/L (<100 ng/L) mid-molecule PTH
10–65 ng/L P-intact parathyroid hormone
IND: Parathyroid disease
INT: HIGH – Hyperparathyroidism (S.Ca, S.phosphate?), osteomalacia (S.Ca, S.phosphate?), renal failure, vitamin D deficiency, pregnancy, anticonvulsant therapy
PHYS: Parathormone maintains extracellular fluid calcium concentration

Parathyroid Hormone

See Parathormone, Serum

Parietal Cell Autoantibodies, Serum (Gastric Cell Autoantibodies, Serum)

RI: Negative
IND: Pernicious anaemia
INT: POSITIVE – Pernicious anaemia, chronic atrophic gastritis, autoimmune endocrinopathies, thyroid disease
PHYS: Specific tissue autoantibody

Paul Bunnell Test

RI: Titre up to 1:128
IND: Infectious mononucleosis
INT: HIGH – Infectious mononucleosis (glandular fever)
PHYS: Patients with infectious mononucleosis develop a high titre of sheep cell agglutinating antibodies. Obsolete test

See also Infectious Mononucleosis Screen, Serum; Immunoglobulin Antibodies, Specific, Serum

Pb

See Lead, Plasma;Lead, Urine

pCO₂

See Carbon Dioxide, Blood

PCR

See Polymerase Chain Reaction, Blood

PCV

See Packed Cell Volume

Peak Expiratory Flow Rate

RI: See table below :–

Correlation of Peak Flow Rate with Patient Height

Height (cm)	Peak flow rate (L/min)
120	160–320
140	310–480
160	480–630
180	620–780

IND: Respiratory distress
INT: LOW – Asthma, chronic obstructive airways disease, emphysema

See also GENERAL INFORMATION: Respiratory Function Tests

Pemphigoid Autoantibodies, Serum

See Basement Membrane Autoantibodies, Serum

Pemphigus Autoantibodies

See Intercellular Cement Substance Autoantibodies, Blood

Pericardial Fluid

RI: protein >25g/L: Exudate
Protein <25g/L: Transudate
IND: Pericardial effusion
INT: EXUDATE – infection (eg. TB), malignancy
TRANSUDATE – Congestive cardiac failure, cirrhosis, nephrotic syn., Meigs syn., hypothyroidism

Peritoneal Fluid

See Paracentesis Fluid

Pertussis IgA Antibodies, Nasopharyngeal Secretions

RI: Absent
IND: Suspected pertussis
INT: POSITIVE – Recent or current pertussis infection
Phys: Result positive early in infection, but short lasting. Serum pertussis IgA antibodies increase late, and persist long term, but only occur with infection, not vaccination

pH, Faeces

RI: Meconium 5.7–6.4
Breastfed infant 4.0–7.0
Cows' milk fed child 5.0–7.5
Adult 6.0–8.0
IND: Malabsorption syndromes
INT: LOW – Lactose malabsorption syn., disaccharide deficiency, some bacterial gut infections

pH, Serum

RI: 7.36–7.44 (42–36 mmol/L)

Outside range 6.8–8 (130–15 mmol/L) causes death
IND: Acid-base imbalance
INT: LOW – Acidosis (high SI units) –
Underventilation of lungs (VC, FEV$_1$, CO$_2$?), shock, severe diarrhoea, starvation, diabetes mellitus (glucose?), anuria, uraemia, renal disease (BUN, creatinine?), ureterocolic anastomosis
HIGH – Alkalosis (low SI units) –
Hyperventilation, hysteria, altitude sickness, vomiting, salicylate overdose, Cushing syn.
PHYS: pH of blood determined by level of bicarbonate (indirectly CO$_2$) and other electrolytes

See also Carbon Dioxide, Blood

pH, Urine

RI: 4.6–8.0 (mean 6.0)
IND: Urinary tract infection
INT: Varies with diet
LOW – Acidic – Bacterial infections, particularly Escherichia coli
HIGH – Alkaline – Bacterial infections (particularly Proteus sp.), renal tubular acidosis, urinary alkalinising drugs
PHYS: Proteus splits urea to give ammonia and thus an alkaline reaction

Phenobarbitone, Serum (Phenobarbital)

RI: Therapeutic range 65–170 μmol/L (15–40 μg/mL)
IND: Control of therapy
INT: Adjust dosage to keep levels within therapeutic range
PHYS: Phenobarbitone is used to control epilepsy. Half-life 50–140 hours. Sample prior to next dose

Phenylalanine, Blood

RI: 40–120 μg/mL)
IND: Screening and monitoring of PKU
INT: HIGH – Phenylketonuria (PKU), hyperphenylalanaemia

Phenytoin Sodium, Serum (Dilantin)

RI: Therapeutic range 40–80 μmol/L (10–20 mg/L)
IND: Phenytoin therapy
INT: Adjust dosage to keep levels within therapeutic range
PHYS: Phenytoin is used to treat epilepsy. Sample prior to next dose. Peak 8 hours after administration

Phosphate Excretion, Urine
See Nordin Test, Blood and Urine

Phosphate, Serum

RI: 0.79–1.40 mmol/L (2.4–4.5 mg/100 mL)

IND: Bone disease
INT: LOW – Elderly male, primary hyperparathyroidism (S.ALP?), renal tubular acidosis, osteomalacia (S.ALP?), poor diet, alcoholism (GGT), severe burns, starvation, gout, pregnancy, prolonged IV therapy, drugs (eg. diuretics, insulin)
HIGH – Elderly female, severe illness, renal disease, acidosis, sample haemolysis
V.HIGH – Hypoparathyroidism, renal rickets
PHYS: Should be compared with S.calcium level

Phosphate, Urine

RI: 10–40 mmol/day
IND: Parathyroid and bone disorders
INT: HIGH – Renal tubular disorders, hyperpara-thyroidism, osteomalacia, hypercalcaemia
PHYS: Excess levels of parathyroid hormone will cause phosphate excretion

Phosphate Threshold, Urine

RI: 0.8–1.35 mmol/L
IND: Renal disease
INT: HIGH – Proximal tubule damage, primary hyperparathyroidism, drugs affecting phosphate resorption
PHYS: After fasting overnight, the patient passes urine in the morning, drinks 200 mL of water, and passes urine again 2 hours later, at which time the blood sample is also drawn. The ratio of phosphate clearance to creatinine clearance is then calculated thus:–

$$\frac{\text{Phosphate clearance}}{\text{Creatinine clearance}} = \frac{\text{U. phosphate x P. creatinine}}{\text{U. creatinine x P. phosphate}}$$

The resulting threshold is read from a standard nomogram

Phosphatidyl Glycerol, Amniotic Fluid

RI: Present
IND: Determination of fetal lung maturity
INT: ABSENT – Fetal lungs not mature
PHYS: More reliable than lecithin-sphingomyelin ratio in diabetic mothers

See also lecithin-Sphingomyelin Ratio, Amniotic Fluid

Phosphorus, Inorganic, Serum [P]

RI: 0.9–1.5 mmol/L (3–4.5 mg/100 mL)
IND: Bone and kidney disease
INT: HIGH – Renal insufficiency, hypoparathyroidism (Ca?), hypervitaminosis D
LOW – Hyperparathyroidism, hypovitaminosis D, rickets (Ca, vit. D?), osteomalacia, steatorrhoea, renal tubular insufficiency (BUN, creatinine?), insulin therapy, postprandial state
PHYS: The concentration of inorganic phosphate is influenced by parathyroid gland function, intestinal absorption, renal function, bone metabolism and nutrition. Diurnal variation

Phytanate, Serum

RI: 3-11µmol/L
IND: Peroxisomal diseases
INT: HIGH - Zellweeger disease, Refsum disease, very high intake of dairy products

Placental Lactogen, Human, Serum

RI: Variable
IND: Pregnancy monitoring
INT: STEADY RISE – Normal pregnancy
V.HIGH – Choriocarcinoma, small cell carcinoma of lung

Plasma Cells, Blood

RI: Absent (Unit: no./mm^3)
IND: Reported if found on FBC
INT: FEW – Infection, serum sickness
MANY – Multiple myeloma

Plasma Protein

See Protein C, Plasma; Protein S, Plasma

Plasminogen, Plasma

RI: 50–150%
IND: Thromboembolism
INT: LOW – Infants, liver disease
HIGH – Pregnancy, contraceptive pill use, elderly, Negroes
PHYS: High levels associated with increased risk of thromboembolism

Platelet Count, Blood

RI: 150–450 x 10^9/L (150,000–450,000/mm^3)
IND: Bleeding disorders
INT: HIGH (thrombocytosis) – Myelofibrosis, chronic leukaemia, polycythaemia rubra vera, essential thrombocythaemia
LOW NUMBER, NORMAL TYPE (thrombocytopenia) – Marrow suppression or infiltration, carcinoma, myeloma, cytotoxic drugs, infections, megaloblastic anaemia, SLE, acute leukaemia, disseminated intravascular coagulation, haemolytic-uraemic syn., massive transfusion, autoimmune diseases, hypersplenism, rheumatoid arthritis, Fanconi syn., HELLP syn., sticky platelet syn., Wiskott-Aldrich syn., alcohol, viral or bacterial infections (eg. rubella, infectious mononucleosis), idiopathic, congenital, post-transfusion, drugs (eg. quinidine, quinine, heparin, aurothiomalate, NSAIDs)
NORMAL NUMBER, ABNORMAL TYPE (thromboasthenia) – Glanzmann's disease
LOW NUMBER, ABNORMAL TYPE – May-Hegglin anomaly
PHYS: Platelets are essential for blood clotting

See also Fibrinogen, Blood; Clotting Time

Platelet Function Analysis, Blood

RI: Collagen epinephrine aperture – 82 to 150 secs.
Collagen ADP aperture – 42 to 110 secs.
IND: Suspected bleeding disorder
INT: HIGH – Abnormal platelet function, aspirin or other anticoagulant use, inherited platelet function disorders
PHYS: Whole blood sample passed under high shear stress through different apertures in a biochemically activated membrane and time to clot formation and aperture blockage measured. Test within 5 hours of collection

Platelet Survival, Blood

RI: 8–10 days
IND: Thrombocytopenia
INT: LOW – Immune thrombocytopenia, hypersplenism, other causes of platelet destruction
PHYS: Radioactive platelets injected, and sampled after 30 minutes and 2 hours, then at daily intervals

Pleural Fluid

RI: Protein >25g/L: Exudate
Protein <25g/L: Transudate
IND: Pleural effusion
INT: EXUDATE – Infection (eg. TB, pneumonia), malignancy
TRANSUDATE – Congestive cardiac failure, cirrhosis, nephrotic syn., Meigs syn., hypothyroidism

Polycythaemia

See Haemoglobin, Blood; Erythrocyte Count, Blood; Packed Cell Volume

Polymerase Chain Reaction, Blood [PCR]

RI: Negative
IND: Certain infectious and other diseases
INT: POSITIVE – Specific results for selected diseases. Range of diseases increasing regularly. Examples include Charcot-Marie-Tooth disease, cystic fibrosis, Duchenne muscular dystrophy, fragile X syn., haemophilia, hepatitis C, haemochromatosis, Huntington's chorea, sickle cell disease, thalasaemia trait, tuberculosis and *Chlamydia trachomatis*
PHYS: Very specific and sensitive test

Porphobilinogen, Urine

RI: <10µmol/L
IND: Porphyria
INT: HIGH – Acute intermittent porphyria, porphyria variegata, hereditary coproporphyria
PHYS: Only positive when symptoms present

Porphobilinogen Deaminase, RBC

RI: 500–800 mU/L

IND: Porphyria
INT: LOW – Acute intermittent porphyria, asymptomatic genetic defect for porphyria
PHYS: Useful for detecting asymptomatic carriers

Porphyrins, RBC

RI: <900nmol/L
IND: Porphyria
INT: HIGH – Childhood protoporphyria, erythropoietic porphyria, lead poisoning, iron deficiency
PHYS: Differentiates above forms of porphyria from porphyria cutanea tarda and porphyria variegata. Blood sample must be protected from light

Porphyrins, Faeces

RI: Absent
IND: Latent porphyria variegata
INT: PRESENT – Porphyria variegata, gastrointestinal disorders

Porphyrins, Urine

RI: Absent
IND: Acute porphyria variegata
INT: PRESENT – Acute porphyria, liver disease, alcoholic cirrhosis, lead poisoning infections, anaemia, CCl_4 poisoning

See also Coproporphyrins, Urine

Potassium, Serum [K+]

RI: 3.5–5.2 mmol/L
IND: Renal or gut disease. Electrolyte imbalance. Diuretic therapy
INT: HIGH – Acute renal failure (creatinine?), anuria, uraemia, Addison's disease (P.cortisol?), haemolysed blood sample, acidosis, hypoaldosteronism, massive trauma, sepsis, vigorous exercise, excess intake, drugs (eg. digoxin, ACE inhibitors, NSAIDs, triamterine, amiloride, spironolactone)
LOW – Vomiting, diarrhoea, ulcerative colitis, malabsorption syn., colonic adenomas, excessive purgatives, renovascular disease, diabetes mellitus, Conn syn. (bicarbonate?), Cushing syn., oat cell carcinoma of lung, ureterocolic anastomosis, familial periodic paralysis, dietary deficiency, renal tubular acidosis, alkalosis, Liddle syn. (see SYNDROMES SECTION 6), secondary aldosteronism, drugs (eg. diuretics, steroids, laxatives, insulin, sympathomimetics)
PHYS: Potassium is lost from the kidneys and colon; it is readily absorbed from the gut. 95% is intracellular

See also Anion Gap, Serum

Potassium, Urine [K+]

RI: 30–90 mmol/day

INT: HIGH – Diuretic therapy, excess parenteral potassium therapy

Prealbumin, Serum (Transthyretin, Serum)

RI: 185–320mg/L.
IND: Protein malnutrition
INT: NORMAL - Good protein nutrition. LOW – Poor nutrition, septicaemia, adult respiratory distress syndrom, abscesses. HIGH – Renal insufficiency, steroid therapy.
PHYS: Prealbumin has a half life of one to two days, making it a good marker of nutritional adequacy. Acts as a transporter of thyroxine, so hypothyroidism may interfere with results

Primidone, Serum (Mysoline)

RI: Therapeutic range 22–50 µmol/L (5–12 µg/mL)
IND: Primidone therapy
INT: Adjust dosage to keep serum levels within therapeutic range
PHYS: Sample prior to next dose. Very variable half-life. Metabolises to phenobarbitone

Procainamide, Serum

RI: Therapeutic range 17–40 µmol/L (4–11 µg/mL)
IND: Procainamide therapy
INT: Adjust dosage to keep serum levels within therapeutic range
PHYS: Procainamide is used to control cardiac arrhythmias. Half-life 3–5 hours. Sample immediately before next dose

Progesterone, Serum

RI: Female luteal phase 7–70 nmol/L
Female follicular phase 2–4.5 nmol/L
Male and postmenopause < 2 nmol/L
IND: Ovulatory status
INT: Increases throughout pregnancy to peak at 36 weeks
PHYS: Levels should be taken before and after expected ovulation time for best results

Prolactin, Plasma

RI: Female 3–25 µg/L (< 600 mU/L)
Male 2–15 µg/L (< 450 mU/L)
IND: Female infertility, galactorrhoea
INT: HIGH – Pituitary tumours or hyperplasia, suprasellar tumours, cerebral trauma, hypothyroidism, renal failure, sarcoidosis, pregnancy, Stein-Leventhal syn., premenstrual tension, stress, drugs (eg. phenothiazines, antidepressants, antihistamines), caffeine
PHYS: Hormone produced in anterior lobe of pituitary that helps control menstrual cycle and lactation. High levels cause sterility, amenorrhoea, galactorrhoea

Prostate Specific Antigen, Serum [PSA]

RI: < 4 µg/L
IND: Prostatic disease
INT: HIGH – Prostatic cancer, benign prostatic hypertrophy, prostatitis
PHYS: Significant false positive and false negative results. Not a screening test. Used for assessing progress of disease rather than diagnosis

See also Prostate Specific Antigen Free/Total Ratio

Prostate Specific Antigen Free/Total Ratio, Serum

RI: >25%
IND: Prostate disease
INT: LOW – Prostate cancer
PHYS: Only appropriate to use when PSA >4µg/L

Prostatic Acid Phosphatase

See Acid Phosphatase, Total, Serum

Protein C, Plasma

RI: 50–150%
IND: Thrombosis
INT: LOW – Recurrent thromboses, skin necrosis with warfarin, familial thrombophilia
PHYS: Protein C degrades coagulation factors V and VII. An autosomal dominant lack causes recurrent severe thromboses, that may commence as a neonate

Protein S, Plasma

IND: Thrombosis
INT: LOW – Recurrent thromboses, familial thrombophilia
PHYS: Co-factor of Protein C. Lack is an autosomal dominant trait

Protein, CSF

RI: Adult 0.1–0.4 g/L
Child < 0.2 g/L
Infant < 0.3 g/L
IND: CNS disease
INT: V.HIGH – Bacterial meningitis (Cl-, glucose, CSF?), TB, meningitis, toxoplasmosis, premature infant
HIGH – Syphilitic meningitis (FTA?), polio, traumatic tap, cerebral haemorrhage, brain tumour, neonate

Protein, Serum, Total

RI: 60–80 g/L
Neonate 45–75 g/L
INT: LOW – Nephrotic syn., chronic renal failure, malnutrition, child under 5 years, severe liver disease, overhydration, protein losing enteropathy

HIGH – Alcoholism (GGT?), dehydration, multiple myeloma, lymphoma, autoimmune diseases, chronic liver disease, chronic infection, prolonged tourniquet during venepuncture
PHYS: Raised if plasma (which contains fibrinogen) instead of serum assayed

See also Albumin, Serum; Globulin, Serum; Fibrinogen, Blood

Protein, Urine

RI: < 0.07 g/L (< 0.15 g/day)
IND: Renal disease
INT: HIGH – Glomerular disease, cystitis, pyelonephritis, toxaemia of pregnancy, hypertension, SLE, nephrotic syn., ureteric stone, renal tract tumour, diabetes mellitus, congenital tubal disorders, Wilson's disease, sarcoidosis, analgesic nephropathy, congestive cardiac failure, renal transplant rejection, amyloidosis, myelomatosis, Alport syn., fever, strenuous exercise, emotional stress, prolonged bed rest
PHYS: Damage to the glomeruli increases their permeability and allows plasma protein to escape into the urine. Bleeding within tract often causes test for protein to be positive

See also Bence-Jones Proteins, Urine

Prothrombin Index [PI]

RI: 90–110. Therapeutic range 40–60
IND: Bleeding disorders, anticoagulant therapy
INT: LOW – Bleeding disorders (fibrinogen?), anticoagulants
PHYS: Test obsolete. replaced by INR

See also International Normalised Ratio

Prothrombin Ratio [INR]

See International Normalised Ratio – Prothrombin

Prothrombin Time [PT]

RI: 12–16 seconds
Therapeutic range 20–30 seconds
IND: Bleeding disorders
INT: LONG – Lack of fibrinogen, prothrombin, factors V, X, or VII. Liver disease, anticoagulant therapy, vit. K deficit
PHYS: Tissue factor (brain extract), calcium chloride, and test plasma are incubated and compared to a control. The time for clotting is noted

See also tests listed under Coagulation Screen

PSA

See Prostate Specific Antigen, Serum

PTH
See Parathormone, Serum

Pyruvate, Blood
RI: 0.03–0.10 mmol/L
ND: Liver disease
NT: HIGH – Thiamine deficiency, cirrhosis, other
        severe liver diseases, hypoxia
PHYS: When compared to serum lactate result, may
        assist in determining cause of lactic acidosis

Pyruvate Kinase, Serum
RI: International standard not established. Traces
        usually present
ND: Chronic anaemia and haemolysis
NT: LOW – Pyruvate kinase deficiency anaemia
PHYS: Low levels are associated with an autosomal
        recessive disorder that results in chronic
        haemolytic anaemia from birth

Q Fever Antibodies, Serum
See Immunoglobulin Antibodies, Specific, Serum

Quinidine, Serum
RI: Therapeutic range 6–15 µmol/L (2–5 µg/mL)
ND: Quinidine therapy
NT: Adjust dosage to keep serum levels within
        therapeutic range
PHYS: Quinidine is used in cardiac disease. Half-life
        4–7 hours. Sample prior to next dose

Rabies Antibodies
See Lyssavirus Antibody Enzyme Immunoassay

Radioallergosorbent Test, Serum [RAST]
RI: Negative or < 0.69 kU/L
IND: Allergies
INT: POSITIVE or HIGH – Allergy to test substance
        (IgE?)
PHYS: Suspect allergen is introduced and serum
        samples are tested at intervals thereafter. Both
        false negative and positive results possible

Rapid Plasma Reagin Test [RPR] Venereal Disease Research Laboratory Test [VDRL]
RI: Negative
IND: Sexually transmitted disease
INT: POSITIVE – Syphilis (FTA?), yaws
PHYS: Non specific serological test for syphilis that
        detects presence of reagin, not a specific
        antitreponemal antibody. Becomes negative
        some years after successful treatment

See also Fluorescent Treponemal Antibodies; Syphilis
Enzyme Immunoassay, Serum; Treponema pallidum
Haemagglutination, Serum

See also INVESTIGATIONS SECTION 3: Syphilis
investigation chart

RAST
See Radioallergosorbent Test, Serum

RBC
See Erythrocyte Count, Blood

RCC
See Erythrocyte Count, Blood

Red Blood Cell Count, Blood
See Erythrocyte Count, Blood

Red Blood Cell Count, Urine
See Haematuria

Red Blood Cell Fragility, Osmotic, Blood
RI: Saline concentration causing 50% lysis in fresh
        blood 4.0–4.5 g/L (68–82 mmol/L)
        Saline concentration causing 50% lysis in
        stored blood 4.6–5.9 g/L (84–100 mmol/L)
IND: Haemolytic anaemia
INT: HIGH FRAGILITY – Spherocytosis, hereditary
        haemolytic anaemias
        LOW FRAGILITY – Thalassaemia, liver
        disease, iron defiency
PHYS: Results not diagnostic. Not a commonly used
        test

Red Blood Cell Mass, Blood
RI: Males 25–35 mL/kg
        Females 20–30 mL/kg
IND: Polycythaemia
INT: HIGH – Polycythaemia
PHYS: Measured using radioisotope labelled red cells.
        Inaccurate with splenomegaly

Red Blood Cell Survival, Blood
RI: Red cell half-life 25–33 days
IND: Haemolysis
INT: LOW – Indication of severity of haemolysis
PHYS: Measured by measuring survival of red cells
        labelled with radioactive ^{51}Cr

Reducing Substances, Faeces
RI: Negative
IND: Malabsorption, diarrhoea
INT: POSITIVE – High dose vit. C, Crohn's enteritis,
        short bowel syn., gastroenteritis, maldigestion
        of sugars, drugs (eg. levodopa)
PHYS: Screening test. Keep faeces refrigerated at 4°C
        or test promptly. Reducing substances are
        electron donating chemicals, eg. glucose

Renal Calculi

IND: Renal lithiasis
INT: CALCIUM OXALATE – 40% sole ingredient,
      85% partial ingredient. Causes include excess
      soft drinks, oxalate foods (eg. silverbeet,
      rhubarb, chocolate, nuts) but often idiopathic
      CALCIUM PHOSPHATE – 2% sole ingredient,
      35% partial ingredient. Causes include primary
      hyperparathyroidism, hypercalcaemia, distal
      renal tubular acidosis, idiopathic
      URIC ACID – 10% sole ingredient, 30% partial
      ingredient. Causes include hyperuricaemia,
      aciduria
      CYSTINE – Rare. Cause is usually familial
      amino aciduria
      MAGNESIUM AMMONIUM PHOSPHATE – 2%
      of stones. Caused by chronic urinary infection
PHYS: Stone collected by sieving urine after symptoms
      of ureteric calculus present, or analysis of
      urinary gravel when present

Renal Function Tests

See Urea, Blood; Creatinine, Urinary Clearance;
Glomerular Filtration Rate; Creatinine, Serum; Renal
Calculi; Urate, Plasma

Renin, Plasma

RI: Varies markedly between labs, patient
      preparation, posture, etc.
IND: Secondary hypertension
INT: LOW RENIN, HIGH ALDOSTERONE –
      Mineralocorticoid abnormality, Conn syn.
      HIGH RENIN, HIGH ALDOSTERONE – Renal
      abnormality
PHYS: Must be performed in conjunction with
      aldosterone studies

See also Aldosterone, Plasma

Renin Activity, Urine

RI: 1.3–4.0 ng/mL/hour
IND: Aldosteronism, secondary hypertension
INT: LOW – Primary aldosteronism, adrenal
      adenoma, adrenal hyperplasia
      HIGH – Secondary hyperaldosteronism

Resin Uptake of T_3

See T_3 Uptake of Resin

Respiratory Function Tests

See Peak Expiratory Flow Rate; Vital Capacity, Lungs;
Forced Expiratory Volume in 1 Second

See also GENERAL INFORMATION: Respiratory
Function Tests

Reticulocytes, Blood

RI: 0.5–1.5% of RBC (10–100 x 10^9/L)
      Infants 2–6%

IND: Anaemia
INT: HIGH – Increased rate of RBC formation due to
      haemorrhage, haemolysis, treatment of
      pernicious anaemia, iron therapy in iron
      deficiency anaemia
PHYS: Reticulocytes are immature red blood cells (RBC)

See also Erythrocyte Count, Blood

Reticulum Cell Autoantibodies, Serum [RCA]

RI: Absent
IND: Autoimmune disease
INT: POSITIVE – Coeliac disease, Crohn's disease,
      gluten sensitive enteropathies, dermatitis
      herpetiformis, IgA deficiency, other systemic
      autoimmune diseases

Reverse T_3, Serum

RI: 0.12–0.54 nmol/L

Rheumatoid Factor, Serum [RF] (Rose-Waaler Test; Rheumaton Titre)

RI: Titre < 16 (< 40 IU/mL)
IND: Arthritis
INT: HIGH – 75% of adults with rheumatoid arthritis
      have rheumatoid factor. RF is present in many
      adults without rheumatoid arthritis. Higher titres
      are more significant prognostically. Other
      causes include SLE, scleroderma, other
      connective tissue disease, chronic active
      hepatitis, sarcoid, myelomatosis, chronic
      infection, neoplasia, infectious mononucleosis,
      TB, fibrosing alveolitis, brucellosis, parasitic
      infiltrations, leprosy, subacute bacterial
      endocarditis, syphilis, malaria
      V.HIGH – Sjögren syn.
PHYS: Rheumatoid factor is a macroglobulin that
      circulates in plasma in combination with gamma
      globulins. Agglutination of sensitised latex
      particles or sheep RBC indicates presence of RF

Riboflavine, Plasma

See Vitamin B_2

Rickettsial Serology

See Weil-Felix Reaction

Ristocetin Cofactor

See von Willebrand Factor, Plasma

Rivotril

See Clonazepam, Serum

Rose-Waaler Test

See Rheumatoid Factor, Serum

Ross River Fever Antibodies, Serum

See Immunoglobulin Antibodies, Specific, Serum

RPR

See Rapid Plasma Reagin Test, Serum

Rubella Antibodies, Serum

IND: To determine immune state, particularly in early
pregnancy

INT: TITRE < 10 – Not immune (no previous infection
or vaccination)
TITRE 10–20 – Previous infection or
vaccination, subclinical reinfection possible
TITRE > 20 – Immune

PHYS: Once infected with rubella (actively or
passively), antibody levels rise permanently
and reinfection is not possible. Subsequent
subclinical infections do not result in viraemia.
Infection in early pregnancy may lead to fetal
abnormalities, particularly deafness

See also Immunoglobulin Antibodies, Specific, Serum

SAAG

See Serum-Ascites Albumin Gradient

Salicylates, Serum

RI: Therapeutic range 1.0–2.5 mmol/L (15–35
mg/100 mL)
Toxic > 2.5 mmol/L (> 35 mg/100 mL)

IND: Overdose, control of salicylate therapy

INT: Adjust dosage to keep serum levels within
therapeutic range

PHYS: Sample prior to next dose

SCC Associated Antigen

See Squamous Cell Carcinoma Associated Antigen

Schilling Test

IND: Vit. B_{12} deficiency

INT: ABNORMAL 1st. STAGE – Regional enteritis,
lymphomas
ABNORMAL 2nd. STAGE – Lack of intrinsic
factor, terminal ileal disease, pernicious
anaemia, total gastrectomy
ABNORMAL 1st AND 2nd STAGE, NORMAL
3rd STAGE – Blind loop syn., scleroderma,
multiple small bowel diverticula, ileal bacterial
overgrowth

PHYS: Carried out in three stages: 1. without intrinsic
factor; 2. with intrinsic factor; 3. after antibiotics.
Vitamin B_{12} is absorbed in the ileum. This may
be prevented by damaged ileal receptor sites, a
lack of intrinsic factor or conditions that allow
bacteria to take up vitamin B_{12} ahead of the
ileum. Now superseded by other tests

See also Cyanocobalamin, Serum

Selenium, Blood/Plasma

RI: Blood: 1.21–2.5 umol/L
Plasma: 0.7–1.3µmol/L

IND: Dietary deficiency

INT: LOW – Dietary selenium deficiency, Keshan
disease (form of cardiomyopathy), Kaschin-
Beck disease (arthropathy/myopathy)

PHYS: Common problem with parenteral feeding

Semen Analysis

RI: Volume 2.5–10 mL (average 4 mL)
Number of sperm > 20,000,000/mL
Motility > 70%
Morphology > 60% normal forms
Viscosity – Compared against standard
Colour – Cream
Leucocytes < 15/HPF
Erythrocytes – nil
Hb – nil

IND: Infertility

INT: LOW VOLUME, COUNT OR MOTILITY –
Infertile
MORPHOLOGY > 70% ABNORMAL – Infertile,
mumps orchitis, poor nutrition, drugs, radiation,
excess local heat, surgery, vas deferens
infection, cryptorchidism, germinal aplasia,
pituitary or thyroid hormone defects
VISCOSITY LOW – Urine contamination
VISCOSITY HIGH – Defective prostate function
COLOUR WHITE – Infection
COLOUR CLEAR – Low sperm count
COLOUR RED – Trauma, malignancy, renal
damage, prostate damage
LEUCOCYTES HIGH – Prostatitis, urethritis,
epididymitis, orchitis
ERYTHROCYTES OR Hb HIGH – Trauma,
genital tract malignancy, renal damage

PHYS: Measured by direct microscopy or automatic
analyser of sperm obtained by masturbation
immediately prior to examination

Seminal Fructose

See Fructose, Seminal Fluid

Serotonin, Platelets

RI: <5.4nmol/10^9 platelets

IND: Carcinoid syndrome

INT: HIGH – Carcinoid syn.

PHYS: Blood or serum serotonin may also be
measured, but platelet levels more accurate.
Must be assayed immediately after venepuncture

Serum-Ascites Albumin Gradient [SAAG]

RI: 11g/L

IND: Diagnosing cause of ascites

INT: HIGH – (>11g/L) – Portal hypertension,
cirrhosis, alcoholic hepatitis, extensive hepatic
metastases, advanced hepatic failure, cardiac
causes

LOW (<11g/L) – TB peritonitis, peritoneal carcinoma or metastases, pancreatitis, bile leak

PHYS: SAAG Correlates with portal pressure. SAAG = ascitic fluid ablumin – serum albumin

See also Paracentesis Fluid

Sex Determination
See Buccal Smear; Oestrogens, Urinary

SG
See Specific Gravity

SGGT
See Gamma Glutamyl Transpeptidase, Serum

SGOT
See Aspartate Amino Transferase, Serum

SGPT
See Alanine Amino Transferase, Serum

Sickle Cells, Blood
RI: Absent
IND: Anaemia
INT: PRESENT - Sickle cell anaemia, sickle cell trait
PHYS: May be combined with HbC disease, HbD disease, beta thalassaemia. Triggers include deoxygenation, dehydration, acidosis, hypothermia. Almost invariably occurs in Negroes. Seen on routine blood film

Skeletal Muscle Autoantibodies, Serum [SKM]
See Anti-Skeletal Muscle Antibodies, Serum

SKM
See Anti-Skeletal Muscle Antibodies, Serum

SMA
See Anti-Smooth Muscle Antibodies, Serum

Smear Test
See Papanicolaou Smear, Cervix

Smith Antibodies
See Anti-Smith Antibodies, Serum

Smooth Muscle Autoantibodies, Serum [SMA]
See Anti-Smooth Muscle Antibodies, Serum

Sodium, Faeces [Na+]
RI: <45mmol/L
IND: Diarrhoea
INT: HIGH – Secretory diarrhoea (eg. cholera)

Sodium, Serum [Na+]
RI: 135–145 mmol/L
IND: Fluid/electrolyte imbalance
INT: LOW (hyponatraemia) – Over hydration, acute or chronic diarrhoea, salt losing nephropathy, hypothyroidism, fresh water drowning, hyperglycaemia, Addison's disease, hypopituitarism, acute renal failure, syndrome of inappropriate ADH secretion, infection, carcinoma, cirrhosis, ascites, congestive cardiac failure, cystic fibrosis, severe burns, excess sweating, prolonged storage of sample, drugs (eg. diuretics, tricyclic antidepressants, carbamazepine, phenothiazines, clofibrate) HIGH (hypernatraemia) – Dehydration, salt water drowning, uraemia, diabetes insipidus, hyperaldosteronism, excess salt intake, mechanical ventilation
PHYS: The level of serum sodium regulates body water volumes. Dehydration may be due to lack of water or lack of salt (sodium)

See also Anion Gap, Serum

Sodium, Urine [Na+]
RI: 40–200 mmol/day (40–200 mEq/day)
INT: HIGH – Addison's disease, chronic nephritis

Sodium Valproate, Serum (Epilim)
RI: Therapeutic range 300–600 µmol/L (40–85 µg/mL)
IND: Sodium valproate therapy
INT: Adjust dosage to keep serum levels within therapeutic range
PHYS: Valproate is used to treat epilepsy. Sample prior to next dose

Somatomedin C, Serum
See IgF-1, Serum

Specific Gravity, CSF
RI: 1.003–1.009

Specific Gravity, Plasma
RI: 1.050–1.060

See also Specific Gravity, Serum

Specific Gravity, Serum [SG]
RI: 1.025–1.029
IND: Determine status of hydration
INT: HIGH – Dehydration
       LOW – Water intoxication, Addison's disease, heat stroke, sodium depletion, excess antidiuretic hormone due to oat cell carcinoma of lung
PHYS: Plasma volume rises or falls with water excess or loss, while content of protein remains

relatively stable, thus altering the specific gravity

Specific Gravity, Urine [SG]

RI: 1.003–1.030
IND: Renal disease
INT: HIGH – Diabetes mellitus (glucose?)
LOW – Diabetes insipidus, pituitary lesions, renal damage due to hypercalcaemia and hypokalaemia, renal failure
PHYS: High in diabetes mellitus due to sugar in urine. Low in pituitary lesions due to low antidiuretic hormone secretion. Patient unable to lower SG after heavy water load in renal failure and Addison's disease

Sperm Antibodies, Serum or Seminal Fluid

RI: Absent
IND: Infertility, vasectomy reversal
INT: POSITIVE – Sperm survival unlikely
PHYS: Positive result would indicate cause for infertility. Vasectomy reversal unlikely to be successful if result positive

Sperm Count

See Semen Analysis

Spherocytes, Blood

RI: Nil
IND: May be found on routine blood smear
INT: PRESENT – Hereditary spherocytosis, autoimmune haemolytic anaemia, alcoholism, HbC disease, drug induced (eg. methyldopa) haemolytic anaemia, severe viraemia, neoplasia
PHYS: RBC have a defective membrane that is highly permeable to sodium, so they become swollen and fragile

Sputum, Microscopy of Gram Stained Smear

IND: Lung infection
INT: **Moderate numbers**
GRAM-POSITIVE OR NEGATIVE COCCI – Normal flora
GRAM-POSITIVE OR NEGATIVE BACILLI – Normal flora
Large numbers
GRAM-POSITIVE DIPLOCOCCI – Pneumococcal infection
GRAM-POSITIVE COCCI IN CLUSTERS – Staphylococcal infection
GRAM-NEGATIVE PLEOMORPHIC COCCOBACILLI – Haemophilus infection
GRAM-NEGATIVE BACILLI – Coliform or Pseudomonas infection, excessive normal flora
PHYS: Acute lung infections are best diagnosed by culture and sensitivity of responsible organism. Information from microscopy may be useful in immediate selection of antibiotic agent while awaiting culture result

Squamous Cell Carcinoma (SCC) Associated Antigen, Serum

RI: Negative
IND: Monitoring organic SCC, detecting organic SCC in patients with family history
INT: POSITIVE – > 60% SCC of lung, cervix, head & neck; < 20% other lung cancers; false positive common

See also Cancer Associated Antigens, Serum

Steroids, 17-Hydroxy, Serum

RI: Male 13 + or – 6 µg/100 mL
Female 15 + or – 6 µg/100 mL
IND: Measured in adrenocortical inhibition tests
INT: HIGH – Adrenal cortex overactivity
LOW – Addison's disease
PHYS: 17-Hydroxy steroids are produced in the adrenal gland

See also Dehydroepiandrosterone Sulphate, Blood

Stones, Renal

See Renal Calculi

Sugar

See Glucose, Blood; Glucose, CSF; Glucose, Urine

Sulfate, Serum

RI: 50–150 µmol/L
IND: Renal disease
INT: HIGH – Renal failure

Sulphaemoglobin, Blood

RI: Absent
IND: Cyanosis
INT: PRESENT – Haemolysis from exposure to sulphonamides, dyes, other oxidants

Sweat Chloride

See Chloride, Sweat

Synacthen Stimulation Test

RI: > 100% rise in S.cortisol after ACTH injection
IND: Addison's disease
INT: LOW – Addison's disease, adrenal cortical insufficiency
PHYS: An initial S.cortisol reading is taken. A short acting ACTH preparation is given IM and a further specimen for S.cortisol is taken 30 minutes later

Synovial Fluid Clarity

RI: Transparent
IND: Arthritis
INT: TRANSLUCENT – Inflammatory arthritis
OPAQUE – Septic arthritis

PHYS: Clarity decreases with presence of white cells

Synovial Fluid Colour

RI: Colourless to straw
IND: Arthritis
INT: PALE YELLOW – Noninflammatory arthritis
YELLOW – Inflammatory arthritis
YELLOW/BROWN – Septic arthritis

Synovial Fluid Crystals

RI: Nil
IND: Arthritis
INT: URATE CRYSTALS – Gout (uric acid?)
CALCIUM PYROPHOSPHATE CRYSTALS – Pseudogout
PHYS: Crystals deposit in cartilage and periarticular structures when in high serum concentration

Synovial Fluid Mucin

IND: Joint disease
INT: LOW – Gout, pseudogout, rheumatoid arthritis
V.LOW – Acute bacterial arthritis

Synovial Fluid Viscosity

RI: High
IND: Joint disease
INT: LOW – Osteoarthritis, SLE, trauma
V.LOW – Rheumatoid arthritis, gout, infection

Synovial Fluid White Cell Count

RI: < 200/mL
IND: Arthritis
INT: HIGH (> 1500) – Osteoarthritis, SLE, trauma
V.HIGH (> 15,000) – Gout, pseudogout, rheumatoid arthritis
EXTREMELY HIGH (> 50,000) – Septic arthritis, severe gout, rheumatoid arthritis

Syphilis IgG Enzyme Immunoassay, Serum [Syphilis EIA]

RI: Negative
IND: Sexually transmitted disease
INT: POSITIVE – Syphilis (RPR, TPHA?)
PHYS: Very sensitive for Treponema pallidum antibodies, but does not show disease status

T Cell Lymphocytes, Blood

RI: CD3 Mature T Cells – 0.8–2.4 x 10^9/L
CD4 T Helper Cells – 0.5–1.6 x 10^9/L
CD8 T Suppressor Cells – 0.2–1.0 x 10^9/L
CD16 Natural Killer Cells – 0.07–0.6 x 10^9/L
IND: Immunodeficiency
INT: LOW – Immune deficiency (IgG?), AIDS (HIV?), neoplasms, leukaemia, chemotherapy
CD16 LOW – Immunocompromised, cancer, Chediak-Higashi syndrome
PHYS: CD4 – macrophages
CD8 – nerves, splenic sinusoids

(CD = Cluster Differentiation antibodies)
T lymphocytes are responsible for a significant proportion of the body's immunological defence

T_3 Uptake of Resin [T_3 RU] (T_3 Uptake of Monoagglutinated Albumin)

RI: 22–35%
IND: Thyroid dysfunction
INT: HIGH – Hyperthyroid (T_4?), nephrotic syn., Graves' disease, drugs (eg. phenytoin, aspirin)
LOW – Hypothyroid (T_4?), pregnancy, oral contraceptives, chronic liver disease, drugs (eg. propranolol, phenytoin)
PHYS: Indirect measure of thyroxine binding protein. Largely superseded by other thyroid function tests

See also Triiodothyronine, Free, Serum;
Triiodothyronine, Total, Serum

T_4, Serum (Total Thyroxine)

RI: 64–160 nmol/L (5–13 µg/100 mL)
IND: Thyroid dysfunction
INT: LOW – Hypothyroidism(T_3?), nephrotic syn., chronic disease, drugs (eg. aspirin, steroids, frusemide, diazepam, lithium, sulfamethoxazole/trimethoprim)
HIGH – Hyperthyroidism (T_3?), pregnancy, Graves' disease, severe infections, hyperemesis, high altitudes, familial, acute psychiatric conditions, stress, drugs (eg. oral contraceptives, amiodarone, amphetamines)
PHYS: Direct measure of total circulating thyroxine

See also Thyroxine, Free, Serum

Tegretol, Serum

See Carbamazepine, Serum

Testosterone, Free, Serum [FTe]

RI: Female 16–40 years – 3–12 pmol/L
Female 40+ years – 2–10 pmol/L
Male 16–40 years – 60–130 pmol/L
Male 41–70 years – 40–100 pmol/L
Male 70+ years – 30–90 pmol/L
IND: Female hirsutism, sexual dysfunction
INT: As for Testosterone, Serum

Testosterone, Serum

RI: Male 12–34 nmol/L
Female 0.4–3.6 nmol/L
Prepubertal 0.4–0.7 nmol/L
IND: Sexual dysfunction
INT: LOW – Male hypogonadism, panhypopituitarism, male climacteric, delayed puberty, Addison's disease, sterility
HIGH – Virilising adrenal tumour, Stein-Leventhal syn. (see SYNDROMES SECTION 6), pregnancy
PHYS: Oestrogen therapy may raise testosterone level also

See also Dehydroepiandosterone Sulfate, Blood

Testosterone/Epitestosterone Ratio, Urine

RK: <6
ND: Testosterone doping in sport
NT: HIGH - Extra testosterone injected or taken as an aid to sporting performance
PHYS: Both testosterone and epitestosterone are synthesised by the testes. If extra testosterone is added ratio will be abnormal

Theophylline, Serum

RI: Therapeutic range 55–110 µmol/L (10–20 mg/L)
ND: Theophylline therapy
NT: Adjust dosage to keep levels within therapeutic range
PHYS: Theophylline is used for relief of bronchial spasm. Half-life 3–9 hours. Sample 4 hours after dose. Clinical effects may be observed at levels below the therapeutic range

Thiamine, Blood

See Vitamin B$_1$

Thrombin Clotting Time, Plasma

RI: 10–15 seconds
ND: Coagulation disorders
NT: HIGH – Low fibrinogen levels, heparin therapy

See also tests listed under Coagulation Screen

Thrombocytes

See Platelet Count, Blood

Thromboplastin Time

See Activated Partial Thromboplastin Time, Plasma

Thrombotest

RI: Therapeutic range 8–12% ± 3%
ND: Anticoagulant therapy
NT: Adjust anticoagulant dosage to keep levels in therapeutic range
PHYS: Outdated by prothrombin time against a standard reference thromboplastin. Measures overall clotting activity

Thyroglobulin Antibody, Serum (Anti-Thyroglobulin Antibody)

RI: <40 U/mL
ND: Thyroid disease
NT: HIGH – Hyperthyroidism (25% of cases), autoimmune thyroiditis, thyroid carcinoma

See also other Thyroid Function Tests

Thyroglobulin, Serum

RI: <38µg/L
IND: Thyroid inflammation or cancer
INT: HIGH – Thyroiditis, thyroid cancer, intrinsic thyrotoxicosis
PHYS: Used to check for recurrence of thyroid cancer after total thyroidectomy

Thyroid Antibodies, Serum

See Anti-Thyroid Peroxidase Antibodies, Serum; Thyroglobulin Antibody, Serum; Thyroid Microsomal Autoantibody Titre, Serum

Thyroid Function Tests

PHYS:

Parameter	Hyper-thyroidism	1° Hypo-thyroidism	2° Hypo-thyroidism
FTI	H	L	L
T$_4$ total	H	L	L
T$_4$ free	H	L	L or N
T$_3$ total	H	L or N	L or N
T$_3$ free	H	L or N	L or N
TSH	L	H	N or L

L = low H = high N = normal

See Anti-TSH Receptor Antibodies, Serum; Long Acting Thyroid Stimulator Antibody, Serum; Thyroglobin Antibody, Serum; Thyroid Microsomal Autoantibodies, Serum; Thyrotropin Receptor Antibody Serum; Thyroxine, Free, Serum; Free Thyroxine Index; T$_4$, Serum; Effective Thyroxine Ratio; Triiodothyronine, Free, Serum; Triiodothyronine, Total, Serum; T$_3$ Uptake of Resin

Thyroid Function Test Interpretation

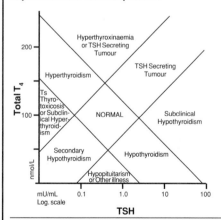

Thyroid Microsomal Autoantibodies, Serum (Anti-Microsomal Antibody Titre)

RI: <100
IND: Thyroid disease
INT: HIGH – Hashimoto's thyroidisis, hyperthyroidism

See also other Thyroid Function Tests

Thyroid Stimulating Hormone, Plasma [TSH]

RI: 0.2–4.0 µU/mL
IND: Thyroid disorders
INT: HIGH – Hypothyroidism, autoimmune thyroid disease, iodine deficiency goitres
LOW – Excess hormone replacement
LOW AFTER 200 µg TRF IMI – Steroid therapy, primary hyperthyroidism
PHYS: Produced in anterior pituitary. 200 µg IMI of thyrotropin releasing factor normally causes a rise of TSH to 2 x initial level

Thyrotropin Receptor Antibody Serum

RI: Negative
IND: Thyroid disease
INT: POSITIVE – Some cases of hyperthyroidism

See also other Thyroid Function Tests

Thyrotropin Releasing Hormone Stimulation Test

RI: See table
IND: Thyroid disease
INT: See table :

Status	Base TSH	TSH after TRF	Base T_4	T_4 after TRF
Normal	N	H	N	H
Hyperthyroidism	L	L	H	H
Primary hypothyroidism	H	VH	L	L
Secondary hypothyroidism	N or L	N or L	L	L

N = normal H = high VH = very high L = low

PHYS: Blood specimens for basal TSH and T_4 thyroxine taken. 200 µg of TRF is given rapidly IV. Further samples for TSH testing are taken 20 and 60 minutes after injection

See also T_4, Serum; Thyroid Stimulating Hormone

Thyroxine, Free, Serum (Free T_4)

RI: 10–25 pmol/L (0.8–2.0 ng/100 mL)
IND: Thyroid gland dysfunction
INT: HIGH – Hyperthyroidism, thyroiditis, stress, drugs (eg. frusemide, amiodarone, amphetamines)
LOW – Hypothyroidism, pregnancy, elderly, drugs (eg. phenytoin)
PHYS: Measures the level of thyroxine affecting the cell. Varied by steroid therapy

See also T_4, Serum

Thyroxine, Total

See T_4, Serum

Thyroxine Index

See Free Thyroxine Index

TIBC

See Iron Binding Capacity, Total, Serum

Tobramycin, Blood

See Aminoglycosides, Blood

Toxoplasma Antibodies, Serum

See Immunoglobulin Antibodies, Specific, Serum

TPHA

See Treponema pallidum Haemagglutination Test, Serum

TRAB

See Anti-TSH Receptor Antibodies, Serum

Transaminases and Transferases

See Aspartate Amino Transferase, Serum; Alanine Amino Transferase, Serum

Transferrin, Plasma

RI: 1.7–3.5 g/L
IND: Anaemia
INT: LOW – Haemochromatosis, iron supplements
HIGH – Iron deficiency anaemia (IBC?)
PHYS: A globulin that transfers iron from the reticuloendothelial system to red cell precursors, and carries iron in the blood stream

See also Carbohydrate-Deficient Transferrin, Blood; Transferring Saturation, Serum

Transferrin Saturation, Serum

RI: 25–50%
IND: Anaemia, haemochromatosis
INT: LOW – Iron deficiency anaemia, iron depletion
HIGH – Increased iron stores, haemochromatosis
PHYS: Substantial circadian and diurnal variation

See also Iron, Serum; Iron Binding Capacity; Transferrin, Plasma

Transthyretin, Serum

See Prealbumin, Serum

Treponema pallidum Haemagglutination, Serum [TPHA]

RI: Negative
IND: Sexually transmitted disease
INT: POSITIVE – Syphilis (active, latent or treated), yaws

PHYS: Less sensitive than FTA, and does not disappear with treatment

See also Fluorescent Treponemal Antibodies; Rapid Plasma Reagin Test, Serum
See also INVESTIGATIONS SECTION 3: SYPHILIS INVESTIGATION CHART

TRF

See Thyrotropin Releasing Hormone Stimulation Test

Triglycerides, Serum

RI: < 2.3 mmol/L (< 200 µg/100 mL) after 12 hour fast
ND: Obesity, heart disease
NT: LOW – malnutrition
      HIGH – Increased risk of ischaemic heart disease and atherosclerosis, familial, nephrotic syn., chronic renal failure, diabetes mellitus, hypothyroidism, Cushing syn., pancreatitis, hypopituitarism, acromegaly, glycogen storage disease, alcohol, pregnancy, drugs (eg. oral contraceptives, steroids)
PHYS: Triglycerides also known as VLDL (very low density lipoproteins). Hypertriglyceridaemia may be familial or associated with diabetes and other metabolic disorders. No alcohol for 72 hours and no food for 12 hours before test

See also Cholesterol, Serum

Triiodothyronine, Free, Serum (Free T$_3$)

RI: 4–8 pmol/L
IND: Thyroid disease
INT: LOW – Hypothyroidism, sick euthyroid syn.
      HIGH – Thyroiditis
PHYS: Only drops late in hypothyroidism

Triiodothyronine, Total, Serum (Total T$_3$)

RI: 0 to 5 years: 1.6–3.3 nmol/L
      5 to 10 years: 1.5–3.0 nmol/L
      > 10 years: 1.5–2.7 nmol/L
IND: Thyroid disease
INT: HIGH – T$_3$ thyrotoxicosis, hyperthyroidism
PHYS: More sensitive test for hyperthyroidism than free thyroxine (free T$_4$)

See also T$_3$ Uptake of Resin

'Triple Test' Antenatal Investigation for Down Syndrome, Serum

PHYS: Results of S.alpha-fetoprotein, S.HCG and S.Oestriol tests are compared to give an indication of risk for Down syn., in foetus. See individual tests for further information

Troponin I, Serum

RI: <0.6ug/L
IND: Myocardial damage
INT: HIGH – Myocardial infarct (CK?), myocarditis, myocardial trauma,

      VERY HIGH (>2ug/L) – High risk of death from existing MI within 30 days
PHYS: Positive within 4 hours of pain onset in myocardial infarct. Remains for at least 7 days. Very specific immunoassay. Odds ratio for death from MI increases rapidly with higher Troponin I levels.

Troponin T, Serum

RI: Negative (<0.2µg/L)
IND: Myocardial damage
INT: POSITIVE – Myocardial infarct (CK?), unstable angina, myocarditis, myocardial trauma, renal failure.
PHYS: More sensitive than CK. 80% positive within 4 hours, and 99% within 6 hours, of pain onset in myocardial infarct. Remains for at least 7 days. Very specific immunoassay

Trypanosome Antibodies, Blood

RI: Negative
IND: Sleeping sickness
INT: POSITIVE – Trypanosomiasis (sleeping sickness), Chaga's disease
PHYS: False positive results common. CSF and lymph node aspirate can also be used for test

Trypsin, Immunoreactive, Blood

RI: Nil
IND: Neonatal screen for cystic fibrosis
INT: HIGH – Cystic fibrosis, acute pancreatitis
PHYS: Determined by radio-immunoassay. Trypsin present in blood up to a level of 1.9 mg/mL is inhibited and undetectable. Cystic fibrosis levels appear to drop after one month of age as trypsin inhibitors increase in blood

Tryptase, Serum

RI: <2u/L
IND: Anaphylaxis
INT: HIGH – Anaphylaxis, severe allergy, mastocytosis
PHYS: Tryptase released by mast cell degeneration. False negative possible

TSH

See Thyroid Stimulating Hormone, Plasma

Tuberculin Skin Test (Mantoux Test)

RI: Negative
IND: Tuberculosis screening
INT: POSITIVE (> 10 mm indurated area) – Past or present tuberculosis
      DOUBTFUL (5–9 mm indurated area) – Recent TB infection, cross-sensitivity to other mycobacteria, allergy
      NEGATIVE (< 5 mm indurated area) – TB not likely

PHYS: Tuberculin antigen is administered intracutaneously by multiple puncture (Heaf test) or by scratch (Mantoux test). Standardised serums are used, and skin reactions measured

Tumour Markers
See Cancer Associated Antigens, Serum

Typhoid Antibodies
See Widal Test

Urate, Plasma (Uric Acid)
RI: Male 0.24–0.42 mmol/L (3.2–8.1 mg/100 mL)
      Female 0.17–0.36 mmol/L (2.2–7.1 mg/100 mL)
IND: Acute arthritis
INT: HIGH – Gout (urate,), toxaemia of pregnancy, leukaemia (FBC?), polycythaemia, renal failure (S.creatinine?), myeloma, lymphoma, other malignancies, prolonged pyrexia, hypothyroidism, hyperlipidaemia, starvation, psoriasis, viraemia, alcoholism (GGT), fasting, haemolytic anaemia, rhabdomyolysis, acidosis, lead poisoning, Lesch-Nyhan syn., idiopathic, drugs (eg. thiazides, other diuretics, salicylates, cytotoxics, lead)
      LOW – Acute hepatitis (LFT?), probenecid or allopurinol therapy, Fanconi syn., renal tubular disease, syndrome of inappropriate ADH secretion, diuresis, pregnancy
PHYS: Uric acid is an end product of purine metabolism, and is excreted by the kidney. Gout is a metabolic disease characterised by increased levels of uric acid, and crystals of this are deposited in joints. Results are raised by thiazide diuretics, lowered by salicylates, methyldopa and phenylbutazone

Urate, Urinary 24 Hour Excretion
RI: < 3.6 mmol/day (< 600 mg/day)
IND: Gout
INT: HIGH – Urate overproduction type of gout
      LOW – Urate underexcretion type of gout (uric acid?), renal disease
PHYS: Test after 5 days on low purine diet. Overproduction treated with allopurinol or similar drug, underexcretion with uricosuric drug

Urea, Blood [BUN]
RI: 3.2–8.0 mmol/L (20–45 mg/100 mL)
      Neonate 1.7–5.3 mmol/L
IND: Renal disease
INT: HIGH – Renal insufficiency (S.creatinine?), nephritis, urinary tract obstruction, dehydration (SG?), intestinal bleeding, shock, CCF, excess protein catabolism, diabetic nephropathy, polycystic kidney disease, reflux nephropathy, adrenal insufficiency (17-hydroxy steroids?), dehydration, elderly, drugs (eg. analgesics, NSAIDs)
      LOW – Hepatic failure (LFT?), nephrosis,

cachexia, diabetes insipidus, pregnancy, over-hydration, diuresis, kwashiorkor, low protein diet
PHYS: Renal damage prevents urea excretion. Excretion of urea load is a good test of renal function. Results are affected by methyldopa, indomethacin, propranolol, etc. BUN varies directly with protein intake, and inversely with the rate of excretion of urea. S.creatinine a more reliable estimate of renal function

Urea, Breath
See Carbon-14 Urea, Breath

Urea, Urine
RI: 420–720 mmol/day
INT: HIGH – Blood urea high, excess protein intake
      LOW – Renal insufficiency

See also Urea, Blood

Urea Nitrogen, Blood [BUN]
See Urea, Blood

Urease, Breath
See Carbon-14 Urea, Breath

Uric Acid, Serum
See Urate, Plasma

Urinary Urate
See Urate, Urinary 24 Hour Excretion

Urine, Blood
See Haematuria

Urine Acidification Test
RI: Adult: pH ≤5.3
      Child: pH<5.5
      Ammonium >35μmol/min/m^2
IND: Renal tubular acidosis
INT: pH HIGH – Distal renal tubular acidosis
      pH NORMAL – Metabolic acidosis, proximal tubular acidosis
      AMMONIUM LOW – Proximal tubular acidosis
PHYS: One hour urine specimen collected from acidotic patient (acidosis is induced if necessary). Blood gases confirm acidosis

Urine Casts
See White Cell Count, Urine

Urine Colour
RI: Light yellow and clear ('straw')
INT: RED – Blood, myoglobin, drugs (eg. rifampicin,

phenindione), foods (eg. beetroot, berries)
DARK YELLOW – Dehydration
BROWN – Bilirubin, urobilinogen, porphyria (changes colour when left to stand)
BLUE GREEN – Drugs (eg. amitriptyline)
CLOUDY – Leucocytes (eg. infection), salts (eg. urates, phosphates), refrigeration and time (precipitation of salts)

Urobilinogen, Faeces

RI: 68–474 µmol/day (40–280 mg/day)
IND: Liver disease
INT: HIGH – Excess bilirubin production, haemolytic anaemia
       LOW – Antibiotics, hepatobiliary disease, bile duct obstruction, infant
PHYS: Averaged over 4 day collection

Urobilinogen, Urine

RI: < 4.23 µmol/day (0–2.5 mg/day) (0.1–1.0 Ehrlich units/100 mL)
IND: Liver disease
INT: HIGH – Parenchymal liver disease, haemolytic anaemia
PHYS: Bacteria convert bilirubin to urobilinogen

Valium, Serum

See Diazepam, Serum

Valproate

See Sodium Valproate, Serum

Vancomycin, Blood

See Aminoglycosides, Blood

Vanillylmandelic Acid

See 4-Hydroxy-3-Methoxy Mandelic Acid, Urine

Varicella Zoster Antibody, Serum

RI: Negative
IND: Detection of past exposure to Varicella zoster
INT: PRESENT - Past infection with chickenpox or shingles
PHYS: used in immunocompromised patients. Not for diagnosis of current infection

Vasoactive Intestinal Peptide, Serum

RI: Negative
IND: Following progress of certain cancers
INT: POSITIVE – Some cases of bronchogenic lung cancer, pancreatic islet cell cancer, neuroblastoma, thyroid medullary cancer, phaeochromocytoma; occasionally in shock, cirrhosis, hepatic failure

See also Cancer Associated Antigens, Serum

Vasopressin

See Antidiuretic Hormone

VC

See Vital Capacity, Lungs

VDRL [Venereal Disease Research Laboratory Test]

See Rapid Plasma Reagin Test, Serum

Very Low Density Lipoprotein Cholesterol, Blood [VLDL]

RI: < 1 mmol/L
IND: Hypercholesterolaemia
INT: HIGH – Reaven syn.

Viral Serology

See Immunoglobulin, Specific, Serum

Viscosity, Plasma

RI: 1.6–1.9 mPa.s (1.52–1.72 centipoise)
IND: Thrombosis
INT: HIGH – Hyperviscosity syn., multiple myeloma, Waldenström, macroglobulinaemia, polycythaemia rubra vera, acute leukaemia, chronic myeloid leukaemia, rheumatoid arthritis, acute inflammation, dehydration, hypothermia
       LOW – Overhydration, IV fluids
PHYS: A high viscosity may be a precipitant of venous thrombosis

Vital Capacity, Lungs [VC]

RI: Units: Litres (L)
       See table below:–

Reference Intervals, Vital Lung Capacity

Age (years)	Male	Female
20–50	3 – 6L	2 – 4.5L
>50	2.5 – 5.5L	1.9 – 4L

IND: Pulmonary disease
INT: LOW – Inadequate pulmonary ventilation due to asthma, bronchitis, TB, bronchiectasis, pneumonia, surgery, etc.
PHYS: Vital capacity is the maximum volume of gas that can be expired after maximal inspiration

See also Forced Expiratory Volume in 1 Second

Vitamin A, Plasma

RI: 0.7–2.8 µmol/L
IND: Malnutrition, eye disease
INT: HIGH – Excess ingestion of vit. A, carotenaemia
       LOW – Xerophthalmia, keratomalacia, photophobia, night blindness, malnutrition
PHYS: Vit. A is vital in retinal pigment. Found in fish oil, milk and eggs, vegetables

Vitamin B₁, Blood (Thiamine)

RI: Mean values:
Male 8.9µg/100mL
Female 7.6 µg/100mL
IND: Malnutrition
INT: LOW – beriberi, Wernicke syn.
PHYS: Thiamine is present in cereals, green vegetables, liver and peanuts. Lack causes neurasthenia, paraesthesia and anorexia

Vitamin B₂, Plasma (Riboflavine)

RI: 2.6–3.7 µg/100 mL
IND: Poor nutrition, stunted growth
INT: LOW – Malnutrition or malabsorption with cheilosis, glossitis and photophobia
PHYS: Vit. B₂ is found in milk, liver and green vegetables

Vitamin B₃ (Nicotinic Acid)

RI: 0.6 mg/100 mL
IND: Malnutrition
INT: LOW – Pellagra
PHYS: Nicotinic acid is present in whole grain, lean pork and beef, and peanuts. Lack causes lassitude, dermatitis, diarrhoea and glossitis

Vitamin B₁₂, Serum (Cyanocobalamin)

RI: 150–660 pmol/L (200–900 ng/mL)
IND: Anaemia
INT: LOW – Pernicious anaemia (Hb?), gastrectomy, intestinal blind loops, Crohn's disease, sprue, chronic pancreatitis, subacute combined degeneration of the cord, congenital, vegan diet. False low due to folate deficiency, late pregnancy, oral contraceptives, multiple myeloma, megadose vitamin C therapy HIGH – Hepatic disease. False high due to chronic leukaemia, polycythaemia rubra vera, metastatic malignancy
PHYS: Vit. B₁₂ is required for the formation of erythrocytes. Intrinsic factor of stomach required for its absorption from the gut

See also Schilling Test

Vitamin C, Serum (Ascorbic Acid)

RI: 23–86 µmol/L (0.4–1.5 mg/100 mL)
IND: Dietary deficiency
INT: LOW – Scurvy,rickets (ALP,Ca?)
PHYS: Lack of vit. C leads to impaired wound healing, and poor resistance to infections and stress. Plentiful in citrus and berry fruits

Vitamin D, Serum (Hydroxycalciferol)

RI: 35–120 pmol/L
IND: Bone disease
INT: LOW – Rickets (Ca, P?), stunted growth, tetany, osteomalacia, proximal myopathy HIGH – Metastatic calcification with excess intake of calcium or its mobilisation from bone

PHYS: Vit. D is formed by the irradiation of ergosterol in the skin. Low levels may be due to sun deprivation. Recommended dietary allowance 10 µg/day. Fast for 12 hours before test. Collect blood without using tourniquet

See also 25-Hydroxyvitamin D, Blood; Calcium, Serum

Vitamin E, Serum

RI: Adult: 11–46 µmol/L
Child: 7–35µmol/L
IND: Haemolysis, fat malabsorption
INT: LOW – Deficiency due to haemolysis or malabsorption
FALSE NORMAL – Hyperlipidaemia, cholestasis

Vitamin K, Serum (Phytomenadione)

RI: Refer to laboratory
IND: Undiagnosed bleeding disorder
INT: LOW – Malabsorption, cholestasis, small bowel diseases, haemorrhagic disease of newborn, dietary insufficiency, long term antibiotics
PHYS: Lack of vitamin K causes excessive bleeding and bruising. Test not yet routinely available

VLDL

See Very Low Density Lipoprotein Cholesterol, Blood

VMA

See 4-Hydroxy-3-Methoxy Mandelic Acid

von Willebrand Factor, Plasma (vWf) (Ristocetin Cofactor; Collagen Binding Assay, von Willebrand Factor)

RI: Variable
IND: von Willebrand's disease
INT: LOW – von Willebrand's disease
PHYS: ELISA test, measuring qualitative and quantitative abnormalities of von Willebrand factor. Subtypes of disease can be identified by variables within test

vWf

See von Willebrand Factor, Plasma

Waaler-Rose Test

See Rheumatoid Factor, Serum

Wasserman Complement Fixation Test [WR]

RI: Negative
IND: Sexually transmitted disease
INT: POSITIVE – Syphilis (FTA?), yaws
PHYS: Nonspecific screening test for syphilis

See also Rapid Plasma reagin Test, Serum

Water Deprivation Test
See Fluid Deprivation Test

WCC
See White Cell Count, Blood; White Cell Count, Urine

Weil-Felix Reaction (Rickettsial Serology)

RI: Negative (titre < 1:160)
ND: Typhus
INT: POSITIVE – Epidemic typhus, murine typhus, scrub typhus, rocky mountain spotted fever, tick typhus
       NEGATIVE – Q fever, other rickettsiae, normal persons
PHYS: Nonspecific agglutination of Proteus strain by serum of affected patient

White Cell Count, Blood [WCC] (Leucocyte Count)

RI: Neonate 10–30 x 10^9/L (10,000–30,000/mm³)
       Infant 6–20 x 10^9/L (6,000–20,000/mm³)
       Child 5–15 x 10^9/L (5,000–15,000/mm³)
       Adult 4–10 x 10^9/L (4,000–10,000/mm³)
ND: Infection, blood disease
INT: HIGH – Bacterial infection, leukaemias, alcoholic hepatitis, cholecystitis, pregnancy
       LOW – Leukaemia, viraemia (eg. viral hepatitis), autoimmune disease, post splenectomy, elderly
       ABNORMAL FORMS – Bloch-Sulzberger syn., Bloom syn., eosinophilia-myalgia syn., May-Hegglin anomaly, myelodysplastic syn., Sézary syn., leukaemia

See also entries for individual white cell types

White Cell Count, Urine (Addis Count)

RI: < 3000/mL (1–2/HPF) (< 5/mm³)
ND: Renal disease
INT: HIGH – Inflammation of urinary tract (eg. infection, irritation, nephropathy collagen diseases etc.)
       RED CELL CASTS HIGH – Glomerular bleeding
       HYALINE CASTS HIGH – Fever, diuretics, exercise, severe renal disease
       WHITE CELL CASTS HIGH – Pyelonephritis
       GRANULAR CASTS HIGH – Nonspecific renal disease
       WAXY CASTS HIGH – Chronic renal disease
PHYS: White cells are nonspecific signs of renal tract damage. Cell casts localise damage to kidney. Cells counted on a grid under a x40 microscope lens

Vidal Test (Typhoid Antibodies, Blood)

RI: Negative
ND: Typhoid fever
INT: RISING TITRE – Typhoid fever

       POSITIVE – Typhoid vaccination, carrier state
PHYS: False positives and negatives common. Rising titre more significant

WR
See Wasserman Complement Fixation Test

Xylose Absorption Test, Urine

RI: 5–8 g/5 hours
IND: Malabsorption
INT: LOW – Sprue, renal insufficiency, coeliac disease
PHYS: 25 g of xylose is given, and its urinary excretion over 5 hours is measured. Xylose is absorbed in the jejunum. Unreliable test

Zarontin
See Ethosuximide, Serum

Zinc, Serum [Zn]

RI: 12–20 µmol/L (80–140 µg/100 mL)
INT: LOW – Cirrhosis, diarrhoea, malabsorption syn., alcoholism (GGT?), drugs (eg. steroids, diuretics)
       HIGH – May be due to zinc therapy

Zinc, Urine

RI: 8–11 µmol/day
IND: Zinc lack or excess
INT: HIGH – Catabolic states, excess zinc in blood
       LOW – Zinc deficiency, liver disease, poor wound healing
PHYS: Indication of amount of exchangeable zinc in body

Zn
See Zinc

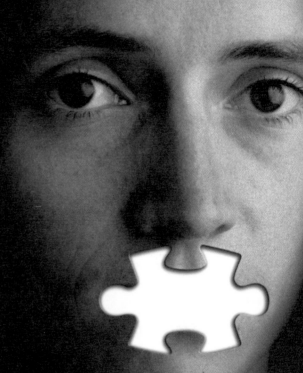

You're trying to piece her life together

She won't swallow it

Indication: Schizophrenia, both as initial therapy and for maintenance.
Legal Category: POM.
Further/Prescribing Information is available from:
Eli Lilly and Company Limited, Dextra Court, Chapel Hill, Basingstoke, Hampshire, RG21 5SY.

Removing the obstacles to care **ZYPREXA** Velota

Orodispersible Tablets, Olanzapir

SECTION FIVE
TREATMENT

THERAPY AND PROGNOSIS

FORMAT

Disease [Abbreviation] (Alternate Name)
THER: A commonly recognised form of therapy
OR other recognised forms of treatment
AND additional therapy normally required
ADD additional types of therapy if above does not prove effective.

1. First step in a therapeutic crescendo or format.
2. Second and subsequent steps in crescendo format are numbered sequentially.

PREC: Precautions that should be observed in the treatment of this disease. For further information on contraindications, precautions, adverse reactions, interactions, use in pregnancy, use in children, dosage and administration, consult a pharmacopoeia such as MIMS or MIMS Annual.

PROG: Prognosis. The expected result of treatment, statistically treated if appropriate.

See also Other Relevant Diseases

Abbreviation
See Disease Name

Alternate name
See Disease Name

Acetaminophen Poisoning
See Paracetamol Poisoning

Acne
THER: Minimise facial oils by regular washing with an unperfumed soap.
AVOID skin abrasives
1. Peeling agents (eg. retinoic acid, benzyl peroxide)
OR adapalene gel
OR isotretinoin cream
OR azaleic acid cream
ADD topical steroid lotions
ADD topical antibiotics (eg. clindamycin erythromycin)
ADD comedo extractor
2. Oral antibiotics (eg. tetracycline, doxycycline minocycline, erythromycin) long-term
3. Antiandrogens – women only (eg. cyproterone acetate, spironolactone)
4. Isotretinoin in severe cystic cases
ADD intralesional triamcinolone
ADD dermabrasion for chronic scarring
PREC: Isotretinoin is teratogenic.
PROG: Often chronic. Scarring may occur if poorly controlled. Cases in adults more resistant to treatment than teenagers.

Acquired Immune Deficiency Syndrome [AIDS]
THER: 1. Prevent contagion by safe sex practices, not sharing needles, testing blood products and taking care in the disposal of sharp instruments.
2. Start combination antiretroviral treatment early choosing from AZT, ddC, interferon, 3TC, saquinavir, indinavir, etc. Treatment regimes are altering frequently.
3. Treat opportunistic infections and complications.
PROG: No cure or vaccine available yet.
Combination therapies appear to slow progress of HIV infection from one stage to the next.
Stages of AIDS are currently categorised thus:
• HIV category 1. A glandular fever-like disease that lasts a few days to weeks with adenitis, fever, rash, malaise, and HIV test is positive.
• HIV category 2. HIV test positive but no symptoms.
• HIV category 3. Generalised lymphadenopathy.
• HIV category 4 and 5 (AIDS). Varied symptoms and signs include fever, weight loss, diarrhoea, nerve and brain disorders, severe infections, lymphadenomas, sarcomas, and other cancers. Very susceptible to all infections.

Acromegaly
THER: Bromocriptine
OR octreotide
OR pituitary deep X-ray therapy
OR hypophysectomy and yttrium implantation.

PREC: Other treatments limited to highly specialised centres.
PROG: Mortality rate twice normal for age and sex. Considerable morbidity due to cardiac disease, diabetes etc.

Actinomycosis
THER: Benzyl penicillin (IV or IM), then long-term orally
ADD surgical drainage and resection of affected areas.
PROG: Good, provided pretreatment tissue damage is not extensive.

Addiction
See Alcoholism; Narcotic Addiction

Addison's Disease
(Adrenocortical Insufficiency)
THER: Hydrocortisone
AND fludrocortisone
Adrenal crisis — Hydrocortisone
PREC: Patient susceptible to intercurrent infections. Significant problems with overuse of steroids.
PROG: Increased incidence of thyroiditis, diabetes, pernicious anaemia etc. Prognosis excellent if properly treated.

Adrenocortical Insufficiency
See Addison's Disease

Agranulocytosis
THER: 1. Withdraw responsible agent (eg. drug).
2. Corticosteroid therapy (controversial).
3. Protect against contact with infection.
4. Aggressively treat any infection.
5. Leucocyte transfusions.
PROG: Mortality rate 10–30%.

AIDS
See Acquired Immune Deficiency Syndrome

Alcoholism
THER: **Acute withdrawal:**
1. Admit to hospital; observe carefully.
2. Chlordiazepoxide
OR diazepam
OR chlomethiazole
3. Maintain fluid, nutrition and electrolytes.
4. Replace vitamin and mineral deficits (eg. vitamin B complex, iron, folic acid).
Maintenance of withdrawal:
1. Goal of total abstinence set.
2. Extensive education, continued counselling and support (eg. Alcoholics Anonymous, social workers).
3. Disulfiram. Interacts with alcohol to produce

vomiting, flushes, headaches, chest pain and fear.
4. Psychotherapy.
PROG: Extremely variable between therapists. Totally dependent on patient motivation.

Aldosteronism
See Hyperaldosteronism

Allergic Conjunctivitis (Atopic Conjunctivitis)
THER: 1. Cold compress to eye.
2. Vasoconstrictor drops (eg. naphazoline, antazoline, adrenaline.
3. Antihistamines orally.
4. Sodium cromoglycate drops – may take up to 30 days to work.
5. Lodaximide and other newer agents topically.
PROG: Very good, but may recur.

Allergic Rhinitis (Hay Fever)
THER: 1. Oral or topical antihistamines.
2. Corticosteroid nasal sprays.
3. Pseudoephedrine.
4. Sodium cromoglycate nasal spray.
5. Specific allergen hyposensitisation.
6. Oral steroids if acutely distressing.
PROG: Seasonally chronic. Satisfactory control.

Allergy
See Anaphylactic Shock; Allergic Rhinitis

Alopecia Areata
THER: 1. Intradermal methylprednisolone acetate OR triamcinolone acetonide.
2. Systemic corticosteroids if progressive.
3. Topical minoxidil OR dithranol
4. Allergen therapy
5. PUVA photochemotherapy
5. Wigs or hair transplantation.
PROG: Only average. Often recurrent or progressive.

Altitude Sickness
(Acute Mountain Sickness)
THER: 1. Descent to lower altitude.
2. Rest.
3. Oxygen supplementation.
4. Avoid alcohol, sedatives.
5. Paracetamol for headache.
6. Dexamethasone.
7. Acetazolamide.
8. Nifedipine for pulmonary oedema.
Prevention:
1. Ascent slowly or in stages (acclimatisation).
2. Avoid strenuous exertion, alcohol.
3. Frequent, small meals.
4. Acetazolamide.
5. Dexamethasone.

PROG: Occurrence and severity depend on elevation, rate of ascent and individual susceptibility. Uncommon below 2500 metres in persons without cardiac or pulmonary disease. Symptoms abate with acclimatisation in 3-7 days.

Alzheimer's Disease
THER: 1. Regular routine in familiar environment.
2. Aid orientation with clocks, calendars, message board, diary, night lights etc.
3. Stimulating simple activities.
4. Adequate time for demonstrating, teaching and socialisation. Avoid rushing any activity.
5. Protect against falls and self-injury.
6. Treat any complicating conditions (eg. Parkinsonism, heart failure, diabetes).
7. Antidepressant medication (eg. nortriptyline, desipramine, doxepin).
8. Psychotropic medication (eg. thioridazine, haloperidol, trifluoperazine).
9. Antipsychotic medication (eg. haloperidol, trifluoperazine).
10. Donepezil or tacrine (should only be prescribed by, or following consultation with, clinicians, who are experienced in the diagnosis and management of Alzheimer's Disease).
PREC: All medications may worsen confusion, and increase risk of falls.
PROG: Incurable, but highly variable rate of progression.

Amenorrhoea, Primary
See Infertility, Female

Amenorrhoea, Secondary
THER: Investigate cause and treat as appropriate. Amenorrhoea due to anxiety or stress may be relieved by short course of norethisterone OR ethinyloestradiol.
PREC: Pregnancy commonest cause. Beware of anorexia nervosa.

See also Infertility, Female

Amoebiasis, Intestinal
THER: **Amoebic dysentery**
Metronidazole orally
ADD surgery in fulminating cases.
Carriers
Diiodohydroxyquin orally for 20 days
OR diloxanide furoate orally for 10 days.
Amoebic liver abscess
Metronidazole
AND dehydroemetine
ADD aspiration of abscess.
PROG: 98% cure with good treatment. Relapses possible. High mortality untreated.

Amyloidosis

THER: No method of promoting fibril resorption. Prevention of fibril precursor protein product only treatment.
Cyclophosphamide
OR chlorambucil
OR other cytotoxic combinations
ADD vitamin C supplements (experimental).

PROG: Systemic amyloidosis mean survival time 12 to 15 months. Reactive systemic amyloidosis survival varies widely depending on underlying cause.

Anaemia

See Aplastic Anaemia; Megaloblastic Anaemia; Iron Deficiency Anaemia; Haemolytic Anaemias, Idiopathic

Anaerobic Infections

THER: 1. Take specimen for culture.
2. Metronidazole AND/OR clindamycin.

Anal Fissure (Fissure-in-Ano)

THER: 1. Warm baths.
2. Fibre supplements to keep stool soft.
3. 0.2% glyceryl trinitrate ointment daily for a month.
4. Botulinum injection into sphincter
5. Surgical sphincterotomy.

PROG: 5% require sphincterotomy eventually, which is very successful. Small proportion develop faecal incontinence after procedure..

Anaphylactic Shock

THER: 1. Adrenaline 1:1000 S.C. 0.3mL – repeat in 1 minute prn.
2. Maintain airway (intubate or tracheostomy), oxygen and establish IV line; elevate legs.
3. Maintain fluid and electrolyte balance intravenously.
4. Diphenhydramine IVI or IMI
OR promethazine IVI or IMI.
5. Hydrocortisone sodium succinate IVI.
6. Observe in hospital for 24 hours.
7. Investigate cause if possible and advise preventive measures

PROG: Good if treated rapidly.

Ancyclostomiasis, Intestinal (Hookworm)

THER: Mebendazole
OR pyrantel pamoate.
ADD iron supplementation

PROG: Good.

See also Cutaneous Larva Migrans

Angina Pectoris

THER: **Acute:**
Glyceryl trinitrate sublingually
OR isosorbide nitrate sublingually
Prophylaxis:
1. Glyceryl trinitrate ointment or patches.
OR isosorbide nitrate orally.
2. Aspirin orally.
3. Beta-blocker
4. Calcium antagonist.
5. Coronary artery surgery or dilatation if fails to respond.

PREC: Do not combine beta-blocker with perhexiline or verapamil.

PROG: Mortality 4% per annum; significant morbidity.

See also Myocardial infarct

Ankle Sprain

See Sprained Ankle

Ankylosing Spondylitis

THER: 1. Physiotherapy and regular exercises.
2. NSAIDs.
3. Analgesics.
4. Local steroid injections.
5. Prednisolone.
6. Radiotherapy.

PREC: Radiotherapy: greatly increased risk of leukaemia.

PROG: Uveitis, glaucoma and pulmonary fibrosis cause significant morbidity. Only a small proportion develop spinal fusion with adequate treatment.

Anorexia Nervosa

THER: 1. Involve family members in problem.
2. Warn patient of long-term problems.
3. Admit to hospital for bed rest and normal feeding until target weight attained.
4. Psychotherapy and conditioning programme.
5. Amitriptyline
OR other tricyclic antidepressants.
6. Modified insulin therapy (controversial).

PREC: Patient rejection of treatment; all measures must be taken to encourage compliance.

PROG: Reasonable long-term; relapses common. Significant psychiatric morbidity.

Anthrax

THER: Benzylpenicillin
OR tetracycline.

PROG: Poor in pulmonary and septicaemic forms. Very good in cutaneous forms.

Anticoagulant (Oral), Overdose

THER: **For overdoses of coumarins and indanediones:**
1. Vitamin K (phytomenadione) IVI slowly.
2. Fresh frozen plasma.

Anxiety

THER: 1. Support and psychotherapy.
2. Benzodiazepines.

3. Tricyclic antidepressants.
4. Buspirone.
5. Beta-blockers.
6. Meprobamate
OR trifluoperazine
OR phenobarbitone.
ROG: Good, depending on cause; often chronic.

phthous Ulcer
ee Mouth Ulcers

plastic Anaemia
HER: 1. Prevent and treat infection by isolation, scrupulous nursing and aggressive antibiotic therapy.
2. Androgens in high doses, eg. oxymetholone, methandienone.
3. Prednisolone
OR methylprednisone reducing over a month (experimental).
4. Transfusion of appropriate cells.
5. Antilymphocytic globulin and bone marrow transplantation in specialist centres.
ROG: Mortality 50% in 6 months, 80% in 2 years; most survivors can live normal, but often shortened, lives.

Apnoea
See Sleep Apnoea

Appetite, Excess
See Obesity

Arrhythmias
See Atrial Flutter/Fibrillation; Cardiac Arrest; Paroxysmal Supraventricular (Atrial) Tachycardia; Paroxysmal Ventricular Tachycardia; Ventricular Tachycardia; Wolff-Parkinson-White Syndrome

Arterial Gas Embolism
See Bends

Arteritis
See Temporal Arteritis

Arthritis
See Ankylosing Spondylitis; Dermatomyositis and Polymyositis; Gout; Lupus Erythematosus, Systemic; Osteoarthritis; Polymyalgia Rheumatica; Rheumatic Fever; Rheumatoid Arthritis; Scleroderma; Septic Arthritis

Asbestosis
THER : 1. No specific treatment.
2. Smoking cessation.
3. Supplemental oxygen if $PaO_2 < 55$.
PREC: Observe for development of lung cancer, mesothelioma.
PROG: Established disease may progress despite withdrawal from exposure but new cases of asbestosis are not being seen. 50% of patients with asbestosis die of lung cancer.

Ascariasis (Roundworms)
THER: Pyrantel pamoate
OR Mebendazole
OR Pyrvinium pamoate.
PROG: Good.

Aseptic Meningitis
See Meningitis, Viral

Aspergillosis
THER: Amphotericin B.
PROG: Poor.

Asteatotic Dermatitis
See Dermatitis

Asthma
THER: **For all asthmatics:**
1. Objective assessment of airway function.
2. Patient education.
3. Written action plan.
4. Avoidance of precipitating factors (allergens, dust, fumes, aspirins , NSAID's, beta-blockers, oesophageal reflux).
5. Avoidance of active/passive smoking.
6. Regular exercise desirable.
7. Nasal steroids if rhinitis also present.
8. Early, aggressive treatment of exacerbations.
Mild, intermittent asthma:
1. Beta-agonist bronchodilator inhaler prn (eg. salbutamol, terbutaline).
2. Sodium cromoglycate for allergen, cold- or exercise-induced asthma pre-exposure.
More frequent asthma:
Inhaled corticosteroids on a regular basis (eg. beclomethasone, budesonide)
AND/OR sodium cromoglycate OR nedocromil
AND bronchodilator inhalers regularly (eg. efomoterol, salmeterol) OR as required (eg. salbutamol, terbutaline)
ADD ipratropium bromide spray
ADD higher doses of inhaled steroids
ADD zafirlukast
ADD theophylline.
Acute asthma:
1. Beta-agonist bronchodilator by nebuliser frequently
AND nebulised ipratropium bromide
AND oral prednisone short-term.
2. Usually continue inhaled steroids.

Status asthmaticus:
1. Hospitalisation.
2. Oxygen
AND aggressive beta-agonist bronchodilator inhalation
AND nebulised ipratropium bromide
ADD methylprednisolone OR hydrocortisone IV
ADD IV salbutamol OR IV aminophylline
ADD mechanical ventilation.
PROG: Rarely fatal; significant morbidity unless well controlled. Adequate prophylaxis should be aimed for, and is usually possible

Astrocytoma

See Intracranial Tumour

Asystole

See Cardiac Arrest

Atherosclerosis

See Claudication

Athetosis

- THER: Levodopa
OR diazepam in high doses
OR other muscle relaxants and sedatives.
PROG: No effective treatment. Levodopa most successful so far. Usually occurs with cerebral palsy.

See also SIGNS SECTION 2.

Athlete's Foot

See Tinea

Atopic Conjunctivitis

See Allergic Conjunctivitis

Atopic Eczema

THER: 1. Avoid irritant clothing (eg. wool) and soaps.
2. Moisturising creams.
3. Antihistamines orally.
4. Hydrocortisone 1.0% cream.
5. Stronger steroid creams if unresponsive, eg. betamethasone, triamcinolone in 0.05% or 0.1% strengths.
6. Tar creams
7. Short-term oral steroids in acute unresponsive cases.
8. PUVA or UVB radiation
9. Oral azathioprine OR cyclosporin A
PROG: Steady improvement with age in children; but only 10% totally cured by time. Usually well controlled by treatment.

Atrial Flutter/Fibrillation

THER: Digoxin

OR Beta-blockers (sotalol)
ADD DC cardioversion if fails to convert.
PROG: Good.

Attention Deficit Hyperactivity Disorder (ADHD

THER: 1. Psychostimulant medication (eg. methylphenidate, dexamphetamine).
2. Tricyclic antidepressants (eg. imipramine).
3. MAOI.
4. Moclobemide.
5. Behaviour modification/social skills training.
6. Sensory integration.
7. Family counselling.
8. Occupational therapy.
9. Diet modification (controversial).
PREC: Psychostimulants may be addictive. Tricyclics contraindicated in cardiovascular disorders. MAOI require strict diet.
PROG: Most cases of ADHD can be controlled provided there is adequate parental commitment.

Back Pain, Non-Specific

THER: 1. Exclude specific cause of pain.
2. Bed rest on firm mattress.
3. Traction, manipulation,
AND hydrotherapy.
4. Paracetamol AND/OR codeine.
5. NSAIDs.
6. Clonazepam OR diazepam.
7. Immobilisation with spinal support by corset or cast.
8. Epidural injection of steroid and local anaesthetic.
9. Tricyclic antidepressants.
10. Chymopapain (chemonucleolysis) injection for disc herniation.
11. Laminectomy OR discectomy where appropriate.
12. Rehabilitation by occupational and physiotherapists.
PREC: Extreme care required with epidural steroids. Exclude significant pathology before traction.
PROG: Very good; recurrence common.

Balanitis

THER: Clean subpreputial space carefully and take culture.
Yeasts present — nystatin cream.
OR miconazole cream
OR clotrimazole cream.
Trichomonads present — metronidazole.
Bacteria present — use appropriate antibiotic.
PROG: Moderate; may require circumcision to prevent recurrences.

Baldness

THER: 1. Determine cause (see SYMPTOMS SECTION 1)
2. Treat specific cause if possible
3. Minoxidil topically or orally

4. Finasteride orally
5. Antiandrogens (women only) (eg.
spironolactone)
6. Hair transplantation AND/OR scalp flap
rotation AND/OR scalp reduction surgery
7. Camouflage (eg. hair thickeners, wigs)

REC: Minoxidil – hypotension (orally), skin irritation.
Finasteride – loss of libido. Spironolactone –
renal and electrolyte problems.

ROG: Hair counts increase about 10% per annum with
minoxidil. Long-term treatment necessary with
all drugs.

d Sores (Pressure Ulcers)

HER: 1. Good nursing care in position to avoid
pressure to sore.
2. Ripple mattress OR water bed OR sheep skin
etc.
3. Careful attention to patient hygiene, nutrition
and general health.
4. Debridement of necrotic tissue.
5. Antiseptic swabs (eg. chlorhexidine,
povidone iodine etc).
6. Dextranomer.
7. Benzoyl peroxide 20% solution.

REC: Dextranomer interacts with other topical
preparations.

ROG: Good with high quality nursing care and good
nutrition.

ed Wetting

ee Enuresis

ell's Palsy

HER: None specific. High dose prednisolone may be
beneficial in acute stage. Nerve stimulation and
facial exercises during recovery.

ROG: 85% spontaneous complete recovery.

ends (Arterial Gas Embolism)

HER: 1. Place diver in 30° head-down position.
2. 100% oxygen or oxygen/carbon dioxide
mixture by face mask.
3. Lignocaine infusion to prevent arrhythmias.
4. Anticoagulants (eg. heparin).
5. Transport to hyperbaric chamber. Avoid air
transport unless aircraft flies below 300m.
6. Recompression in hyperbaric chamber.
7. Carefully monitor fluid and electrolyte
balance and ECG.
8. Slow, calculated decompression. Beware of
relapses.

REC: Do not raise head until recompressed.

ROG: Variable depending on severity.

ipolar Disorder

ee Manic-Depressive Disorder

Bites

See Snake Bite

Blastomycosis

THER: Amphotericin B IVI
OR Ketoconazole (pulmonary disease)
OR itraconazole
AND excision of skin lesions and
bronchopleural fistulae.

PREC: South and North American forms differ slightly;
many experimental treatment programmes.

PROG: Poor with pulmonary involvement; relapses.

Bleach Poisoning

THER: 1. Gastric lavage OR emesis.
2. Sodium thiosulfate orally OR milk OR milk of
magnesia.
3. Calcium gluconate 10% IVI.

PREC: Do not use acid antidotes.

PROG: Dose related; danger of gut perforation.

Blepharitis

THER: 1. Bathe crusts off lids regularly.
2. Tetracycline
OR erythromycin ophthalmic ointment.
3. Tetracycline orally

PROG: Good; often recurs. Chronic.

Blood Disorders

*See Agranulocytosis; Anaemia;Christmas Disease;
Disseminated Intravascular Coagulation; Haemophilia;
Leukaemia, Acute Lymphoblastic; Leukaemia, Acute
Myeloid; Leukaemia, Chronic Lymphoid; Leukaemia,
Chronic Myeloid. Thrombocytopenia; Von Willebrand's
Disease;*

Boils

See Furunculosis, Cutaneous; Impetigo

Brain Tumour

See Intracranial Tumour

Breast Carcinoma

THER: Surgery (radical or simple mastectomy, or
lumpectomy)
AND cytotoxic chemotherapy (eg.
cyclophosphamide, methotrexate, fluorouracil,
etc)
AND/OR radiotherapy
AND/OR tamoxifen (anti-oestrogen)
AND/OR oophorectomy
AND/OR adrenalectomy
AND/OR hypophysectomy (controversial)
AND/OR progestagens.

PROG: Depends on stage of disease. Untreated 18%
survive 5 years. Overall 55% + five year survival
with treatment.

Bronchial Carcinoma
See Lung Carcinoma

Bronchiectasis
THER: 1. Patient education.
2. Smoking cessation essential.
3. Regular exercise important.
4. Postural drainage by patient.
5. Yearly flu vaccine, pneumovax every 6 years.
6. Bronchodilator inhaler.
7. Empiric antibiotic at the first sign of exacerbation (eg. amoxicillin, tetracycline, ciprofloxacin, cefuroxime).
8. Consider intermittent, prolonged prophylactic antibiotic for frequent infections.
9. Referral to specialist.
10. Oxygen if PaO_2 <55.
11. Resectional surgery rarely indicated.
PREC: Complications include: recurrent acute exacerbations, pneumonia, lung abscess, empyema, haemoptysis, cor pulmonale, respiratory failure and rarely, brain abscess, amyloidosis.
PROG: Generally normal life expectancy unless disease severe.

Bronchiolitis
THER: 1. Usually no specific treatment required.
2. If severe:
– hospitalisation
– oxygen if hypoxaemic
– hydration
– bronchodilators
– aerosolised ribavirin.
PREC: Must distinguish from acute asthma.
PROG: Most children recover at home with no specific treatment. Relatively high frequency of respiratory symptoms and asthma later in life.

Bronchitis, Acute
THER: 1. Smoking cessation essential.
2. Symptomatic: rest, paracetamol, adequate hydration.
3. Antibiotic (eg. amoxicillin, erythromycin, cefaclor) only for patients with protracted course, underlying chronic illness.
PREC: Avoid cough suppressants, decongestants.

Bronchitis, Chronic
THER: 1. Patient education.
2. Smoking cessation essential.
3. Regular exercise programme.
4. Adequate hydration.
5. Consider trial of bronchodilator inhaler (eg. salbutamol, ipratropium bromide).
6. Oxygen if PaO_2 <55.
7. For exacerbations:
– empiric antibiotic therapy (eg. amoxicillin, tetracycline, clarithromycin, trimethoprim-sulfamethoxazole, cefuroxime).
– short course of corticosteroids.
PREC: Avoid cough suppressants, mucolytics, sedatives. Yearly flu vaccine, pneumovax eve 6 years.
PROG: High rate of progressive chronic airflow limitation. May lead to respiratory and/or right heart failure.

Bronchopneumonia
See Pneumonia, Bacterial

Brucellosis
THER: Tetracycline
OR doxycycline for 6 weeks
ADD co-trimoxazole
OR streptomycin IMI for 3 weeks in severe case
PREC: Beware of bone, joint, cardiac and meningeal infection. Destroy affected cattle and vaccina cattle contacts.
PHYS: Good; 20% become chronic; rarely fatal.

Bulimia
THER: 1. Tolerant, concerned therapist who can take time to motivate patient.
2. Teach new attitudes about desirable weight
3. Teach new attitudes towards food.
4. Determine precipitating factors, and teach coping techniques and factor avoidance.
5. Counselling to make patient aware of risks associated with disease.
6. Avoid alcohol.
7. Relaxation techniques.
8. Psychotropics and antidepressants in selected patients and in small quantities.
9. Psychoanalysis.
PREC: Psychotropics and antidepressants — risk of suicide, sedation.
PROG: Up to 30% suicide. Various studies show cure rates of 20–40% and similar control rates.

Bunion
THER: 1. Shoe modifications (eg. expanded uppers, metatarsal bar).
2. Felt padding over bunion.
3. Surgical correction of halux valgus and removal of exostosis.
4. Replacement arthroplasty.
PROG: Good.

Burns
THER: 1. Immerse burnt area in cool water immediate for 30 min.
2. Control pain, eg. morphine IMI or IVI.
3. Wash and debride wound, under general anaesthetic if necessary.
4. Nurse under strictly aseptic conditions.
5. Closed treatment (deep burn) — dress burn

with petroleum gauze dressings OR silver sulfadiazine cream OR silver nitrate solution soaked pads. Open treatment (superficial burn) — expose burns to air and allow to dry out under aseptic conditions.
6. Treat any topical or systemic infection aggressively on culture results with appropriate antibiotic.
7. Maintain fluid and electrolyte balance, by IV line in acute stages and large burns. Transfuse whole blood if necessary.
8. Tetanus vaccination.
9. Subsequent dressings and debriding may need to be done under general anaesthesia or IV narcotics.
10. Skin grafts.
PROG: Depends on depth of burn and area covered. Critical over 30%, shock over 15% of surface area burnt.

See also Flash Burns, Eye

Bursitis
THER: 1. Rest and immobilisation of affected joint.
2. Analgesia.
3. Local heat, physiotherapy.
4. NSAIDs.
5. Antibiotics.
6. Local corticosteroid injections into bursa.
PROG: Good.

Calculi
See Ureteric Calculi

Cancer
See Breast Carcinoma; Choriocarcinoma and Invasive Moles; Colonic Carcinoma; Hodgkin's Disease; Intracranial Tumour; Leukaemia; Lung Carcinoma; Myelomatosis

Candidiasis, Oral (Thrush; Moniliasis)
THER: Nystatin drops or cream
ADD ketoconazole
PROG: Very good; may be secondary to inhaled or oral steroids.

Candidiasis, Vaginal (Thrush)
THER: Nystatin vaginal cream or pessaries
OR imidazole vaginal cream or pessaries
AND antifungal creams for male partner
AND nystatin orally in recurrent cases
AND advice on personal and sexual hygiene
ADD ketoconazole OR fluconazole orally in resistant cases
ADD sodium bicarbonate douche.
PREC: Beware of diabetes as cause. Caution with applicators in pregnancy.
PROG: 85% cure on one course of treatment; relapses common.

Carcinoid Syndrome
THER: Surgery to tumour tissue (controversial)
AND/OR 5-fluorouracil intra-arterially
OR cyclophosphamide
AND codeine phosphate
OR methysergide
OR phenclomine for diarrhoea
AND phenoxybenzamine
OR propranolol for flushing
AND isoprenaline
AND/OR prednisone for bronchospasm.
PROG: Poor; 50% survive 3 years from diagnosis.

Carcinoma
See Cancer

Cardiac Arrest
THER: 1. Confirm that arrest has occurred.
2. Insert oropharyngeal airway.
3. Ventilate with bag, mask and 100% oxygen OR mouth to mouth resuscitation at 10/min.
4. Cardiac compression by firm blows to sternum, followed by rhythmic sternal pressure at rate of 70/min.
5. Insert endotracheal tube rapidly when convenient.
6. Blind DC defibrillation with 200–400 joules.
7. Insert IV line and maintain with 5% dextrose. If IV line cannot be inserted, all drugs, except sodium bicarbonate, may be given in diluted form through endotracheal tube.
8. If arrest continues for more than 15 min. infuse 100 mL sodium bicarbonate IV rapidly. Repeat every 15 min.
9. Obtain continuous ECG read-out if possible and proceed further on results:
Asystole:
1. Atropine 0.6 mg IV stat and repeat after one minute.
2. Isoprenaline 0.2 mg IV stat.
3. Adrenaline 1:1000 1 mL IV or intracardiac stat. Repeat if necessary.
4. Calcium gluconate 10%, 10 mL IV.
5. If bradycardia occurs use external pacemaker.
If ventricular fibrillation occurs proceed as follows:
Ventricular Fibrillation:
1. Repeated DC shocks of 200–400 joules.
2. If debrillation fails:
Isoprenaline 0.02 mg IV repeating every minute OR bretylium 5 mg/kg IV to max of 25 mg/kg in divided doses.
3. Calcium gluconate 10%, 10 mL IV.
4. Adrenaline 1:1000 1 mL IV or intracardiac.
5. If sinus rhythm obtained:
Lignocaine 1% 5 mL IV stat.
ADD procainamide 100–800 mg IV if unstable. Continue these at lower dose in IV infusion.
Complete Heart Block:
1. Atropine 0.6–1.2 mg IVI or IMI unless given previously.

2. Isoprenaline 0.2 mg IVI unless given previously.
3. Hydrocortisone 300 mg IV stat.
4. Pacemaker.
PROG: In good centres, 10% survive asystole, 40% survive ventricular fibrillation.

See also Myocardial Infarct

Cardiomyopathy, Hypertrophic

THER: Propranolol
OR disopyramide
ADD diuretics for congestive failure
ADD DC electroversion for serious arrhythmias
ADD Beta-blocker (eg. sotalol) for prevention of atrial arrythmias.
PROG: Guarded; worse with arrhythmias.

Carpal Tunnel Syndrome

THER: 1. Diuretics.
2. NSAIDs.
3. Splint wrist in extension 12 hours a day.
4. Hydrocortisone acetate injection into carpal tunnel.
5. Surgical division of ligaments.
PROG: Good; exclude precipitating cause (eg. pregnancy, hypothyroidism).

Cellulitis

THER: 1. Aspirin for pain and fever.
2. Rest and elevate affected part.
3. Cephalexin orally
OR cefazolin IVI
OR amoxycillin ± clavulanic acid
OR flucloxacillin IVI
PROG: Very good.

Cerebral Abscess

THER: 1. Antibiotic treatment of original focus of infection.
2. Operative drainage or excision of abscess cavity.
3. Irrigation of abscess cavity with antibiotic solution.
4. If patient debilitated, spread of infection may be controlled by intensive treatment with appropriate antibiotic.
PROG: Reasonable if aggressively treated. Fatal untreated.

Cerebral Palsy

THER: 1. Intensive physiotherapy.
2. Control muscle spasm with diazepam or lorazepam
AND/OR dantrolene
AND/OR baclofen
AND/OR clonidine.
3. Surgery to lengthen or cut tendons.
4. Neurosurgery (eg. dorsal rhizotomy).

5. Intrathecal drugs (eg. baclofen).
PROG: No cure. Reasonable control of spasm.

Cerebral Tumour

See Intracranial Tumour

Cerebrovascular Accident

THER: 1. Bed rest, elevate head, IV fluids and sedatior if necessary. Monitor blood pathology and ECG
2. Tube feed and catheterise if comatose
3. Investigate by CT scan OR angiography to exclude clot, pressure, shift.
4. Anticoagulants if appropriate
5. Treat other concurrent conditions.
6. Neurosurgery if appropriate
7. Intensive rehabilitation by speech therapists, occupational therapists, physiotherapists, social workers, ophthalmologists.
8. Domestic care programme.
PREC: Anticoagulants may cause further haemorrhage. Medications may have abnorma effects and side effects, particularly CNS depressants.
PROG: Extremely variable, depending on cause, site, and nature. Delayed initial recovery indicates poorer long-term prognosis.

See also Transient Ischaemic Attack

Cestode Infestation (Tapeworms)

THER: Praziquantel
AND purgative 6 hours after treatment.
PROG: Good provided treated early and followed carefully.

Chancroid

THER: Azithromycin stat.
OR spectinomycin stat.
OR ciprofloxacin stat.
OR enoxacin
OR amoxycillin
OR erythromycin
AND drain fluctuant buboes.
PREC: Higher doses than normal course of treatment often required.
PROG: Responds well to treatment.

Chickenpox (Varicella)

THER: 1. None specific, vaccination available in some countries.
2. Antiseptics and antipruritics, eg. calamine lotion, to lesions.
3. Oral antihistamines for itch.
4. Penicillin
OR erythromycin for significant secondary infection.
5. Acyclovir for immunocompromised host.
PREC: Antihistamines — sedation.
PROG: Good; encephalitis and pneumonia occur rarely.

Infectious from 5 days before rash appears to 6 days after last crop erupts.

Chilblains
HER: 1. Elevation.
2. Gradual warming.
3. Avoid trauma.
4. Treat secondary infection.
5. Topical corticosteroid creams.
6. Vasodilators (eg. nicotinic acid) may prevent recurrences.
PROG: Very good; may recur easily if further cold exposure.

Chlamydia, Venereal
THER: Azithromycin
OR doxycycline
OR erythromycin
AND treat sexual partner(s).
PROG: Very good, provided treatment adequate.

Cholecystitis, Acute
THER: 1. Nil by mouth and intravenous feeding.
2. Pentazocine for analgesia.
3. Atropine OR propantheline parenterally.
4. Gentamicin AND ampicillin IM
OR fluoroquinolones
OR cephalosporins IM
OR clindamycin IM.
5. Cholecystectomy after recovery
OR cholecystostomy if patient deteriorating
OR chenodeoxycholic acid long-term if surgery impractical.
6. Endoscopic sphincterotomy for ductal stones.
7. Extracorporeal shockwave lithotripsy with single or few large stones.
8. Transhepatic infusion of gall bladder by methyl tertiary butyl ether.
PREC: Avoid morphine; causes sphincter of Oddi spasm. Observe closely for perforation or gangrene. Surgery mandatory in recurrent cases.
PROG: Good; surgery curative.

Cholera
THER: 1. Rapid fluid and electrolyte replacement by oral glucose/salt formula (see below)
OR IV infusion.
Use interosseous or peritoneal route in children if necessary. Monitor carefully.
2. Tetracycline
AND/OR co-trimoxazole
AND/OR chloramphenicol
World Health Organisation oral rehydration formula:
To 1 litre boiled water add common salt (NaCl) 3.5g, sodium bicarbonate (NaHCO$_3$)2.5g, potassium chloride 1.5g, and glucose 20g.

PROG: Untreated 35–80% mortality; less than 1% if adequately treated.

Cholesterol, Excess
See Hypercholesterolaemia

Chondrocalcinosis
See Pseudogout

Chorea, Huntington's and Sydenham's
THER: Chlorpromazine
OR tetrabenazine
OR thiopropazate
OR pimozide
OR haloperidol.
PROG: Sydenham's self-limiting with cure after 1–3 months. Huntington's congenital.

Choriocarcinoma and Invasive Moles
THER: 1. Evacuation of mole surgically.
2. Methotrexate OR actinomycin D prophylactically after evacuation.
3. Methotrexate
AND/OR 6-mercaptopurine
OR actinomycin D for acute disease.
4. Chlorambucil
OR diazo-oxonorleucine in resistant cases.
PROG: Choriocarcinoma 40% 5 year survival. Invasive moles 90% 5 year survival.

Christmas Disease
THER: Replacement therapy with factor IX. Otherwise as for Haemophilia.

Chronic Bronchitis
See Bronchitis, Chronic.

Chronic Fatigue Syndrome (Post Viral Fatigue Syndrome; Royal Free Disease: Myalgic Encephalomyelitis; Tapanui Flu; Neuromyasthenia)
THER: No specific therapy available. Psychological/psychiatric support appropriate. Patients should be allowed to try some of the wide variety of purported (but unproven) treatments available, provided they are not potentially harmful.
PROG: Eventual recovery with many relapses and remissions over several years.

See also SYNDROMES SECTION 6.

Ciguatera Poisoning
THER: Supportive and symptomatic treatment only.
Mannitol IV slowly
ADD amitriptyline
AND paracetamol AND/OR indomethacin

AND cyproheptadine
PREC: Ensure adequate hydration before using mannitol. Avoid tropical reef fish in future
PROG: Settles after days to months but may be easily triggered again by much lower doses of toxin.

Cirrhosis, Primary Biliary

THER: 1. Cholestyramine
OR phenobarbitone for itching.
2. Penicillamine
OR azathioprine in selected patients.
3. Spironolactone.
4. Vitamins A, D and K IM.
5. Triglyceride supplements to diet.
6. Surgery (eg portal shunts)
7. Liver transplantation
PREC: Avoid steroids.
PROG: Inevitably progressive at variable rates.

Claudication

THER: 1. Stop smoking.
2. Diet — low cholesterol, low fat.
3. Exercise and physiotherapy to improve collateral circulation.
4. Calcium channel blockers (eg. nifedipine, felodipine).
5. Peripheral vasodilators (eg. isoxsuprine).
6. Oxpentifylline
7. Reconstructive vascular surgery
OR percutaneous transluminal dilation
AND/OR lumbar sympathectomy.
PROG: Useful exercise tolerance can usually be obtained.

Cluster Headache (Migrainous Neuralgia)

THER: **Prophylaxis:**
Methysergide
AND/OR prednisone
AND/OR lithium carbonate
OR propranolol
OR ergotamine
OR indomethacin.
Acute:
Ergotamine sublingually, inhaled or rectally
OR sumatriptan
AND/OR pethidine IMI with prochlorperazine IMI
AND/OR oxygen hyperventilation for 10 min.
PREC: See Migraine.
PROG: Recurrences common; some cases resist treatment.

Coagulation Defects

See Christmas Disease; Disseminated Intravascular Coagulation; Haemophilia; Thrombocytopenia; Thrombosis, Deep Venous; von Willebrand's Disease

Coccidiomycosis

THER: Amphoterecin B
OR ketoconazole

OR itraconazole
ADD resection of lesion
PROG: May resolve spontaneously or disseminate, particularly in patients with AIDS, lymphoma or immunosuppression

Coeliac Disease

THER: 1. Gluten-free diet (eg. avoid wheat, rye, barley)
2. High protein, low fat diet.
3. Vitamin and mineral supplementation (eg. folic acid, vitamin D, iron).
4. Prednisone.
PROG: Good; above average incidence of gut carcinomas and lymphomas.

Cold, Common

See Coryza

Cold Injury

See Frostbite

Colic, Infantile

See Infantile Colic

Cold Sore

See Herpes Simplex

Colitis, Pseudomembranous

See Pseudomembranous Colitis

Colonic Carcinoma

THER: Wide surgical resection of affected area (if possible) with recto-colic anastomosis or colostomy
ADD cytotoxic chemotherapy
ADD radiotherapy.
PROG: Five year survival:
• Duke class A – 95%
• Duke class B – 60%
• Duke class C – 25%
• Duke class D – <1%

Coma

THER: 1. Secure airway and support respiration if necessary.
2. Control shock (see separate entry).
3. Determine circumstances of onset and history from friends, relatives or onlookers (eg. sudden or slow onset, seizure, head injury, vomit, incontinence, etc – see SYMPTOMS SECTION 1).
4. Determine level of coma (eg. responds to commands or only pain, eyes open spontaneously or not at all, confused speech or none etc).
5. Detailed physical examination (eg. papilloedema, pupil reactions, eye movements, hemiplegia, respiratory etc – see SIGNS

SECTION 2).
6. Attempt to make definitive diagnosis of cause (see SYMPTOMS SECTION 1) by specific pathological (eg. B .glucose), radiological (eg. CAT scan) and electro-physiological (eg. EEG investigations).
7. Treat any specific cause found, or support in coma with close monitoring, naso-gastric or parenteral feeding and careful nursing while investigations continue.

PROG: Exclude pseudocoma or hysterical coma. Depends on cause.

Concussion

THER: 1. Exclude increased intracranial pressure by watching for signs of drowsiness, vomiting, increasing headache, unequal pupil size, ocular palsy, nystagmus, confusion, incoherence, paralysis, coma, slow pulse, increased BP.
2. Avoid sedatives, alcohol, aspirin and sedating analgesics. Use paracetamol only.
3. Rest. Avoid physical activity until asymptomatic.
4. Investigate if symptoms persist for 2 weeks, or signs listed in 1. above occur.

PREC: Beware of combinations of multiple mild signs.
PROG: Usually very good. If prior concussion recently, avoid contact sports.

Condylomata Acuminata

THER: 20–50% podophyllum topically; wash off after 8 hours.
ADD surgical removal by liquid nitrogen, cautery or excision.
PREC: Podophyllum — start with lower concentration to avoid burns.
Biopsy lesion before destructive surgery to exclude malignancy.
PROG: Significant risk of recurrence; should have Pap smear 6 monthly.

Congestive Heart Failure
See Heart Failure, Congestive

Conjunctivitis, Bacterial

THER: 1. Compresses to clean off secretions.
2. Broad spectrum antibiotic drops, such as polymyxin/bacitracin.
3. Gentamycin or tobramycin drops.

Conjunctivitis, Purulent

THER: Sulfacetamide drops
OR neomycin/polymyxin drops
OR gentamicin 0.3% ophthalmic drops.
Ointments of above drops may be used at night.
PREC: Check for blocked tear duct in infants and recurrent cases.
PROG: Excellent if treated rapidly. If hyperacute – suspect gonococcal infection.

Conjunctivitis, Viral

THER: 1. Warm compresses to clean secretions.
2. Vasoconstriction drops.
3. Antibacterial drops only if secondarily infected.
PROG: Self-limited process.

Constipation

THER: 1. Exclude specific pathological cause.
2. High fibre, high fluid diet.
3. Fibre supplements and bulking agents.
4. Oral laxatives (eg. bisacodyl, docusate, lactulose, sennosides).
5. Rectal laxatives.
6. Wash out and manual removal if impacted.
PREC: Beware of dependence on therapy.
PROG: Often chronic.

See also SYMPTOMS SECTION 1

Contraception
See Fertility Control

Convulsion (Fit)

THER: **Acute**
1. Diazepam IV
OR lorazepam IV
AND/OR phenytoin IV.
2. Determine cause (see SYMPTOMS SECTION 1) and take appropriate prophylactic measures.
Refractory cases
1. Barbiturate OR midazolam IV.
2. General anaesthesia.
PREC: Beware of aspiration and respiratory arrest.
PROG: Generally good; depends on cause.

See also Epilepsy, Febrile Convulsions; Status Epilepticus

Cor Pulmonale

THER: 1. Oxygen therapy titrated against arterial pO_2 (maximum 30% O_2).
2. Frusemide
ADD spironolactone.
3. Potassium supplements if necessary.
4. Digoxin in selected patients.
5. Venesection if haematocrit very high.
PROG: Five year survival rate 40%. Significant morbidity. Up to 30% mortality within one year of diagnosis.

Coryza (Common Cold)

THER: Aspirin OR paracetamol for fever and pain
AND medicated steam inhalations, eg. menthol
AND maintain adequate fluid intake
ADD antihistamines
AND/OR pseudoephedrine
AND/OR xylometazoline 0.05%
OR phenylephrine nasal drops

AND/OR cough suppressants.

PREC: Antibiotics are contraindicated without evidence of secondary bacterial infection. Nasal drops must not be overused or rebound effect occurs.

PROG: Excellent; may become chronic through winter.

Crabs

See Pediculosis

Cramps, Nocturnal

THER: 1. Adequate evening fluid intake.
2. Biperiden OR quinine sulphate taken in evening as prophylaxis.
3. Massage and heat to affected muscles.
4. Benzodiazepines if severe.

PROG: Prophylaxis usually successful.

Cretinism

See Hypothyroidism

Crohn's Disease (Regional Enteritis)

THER: No satisfactory medical or surgical therapy. Treatments that may be tried include:
— Oral or parenteral steroids in acute stages
— Sulfasalazine or mesalazine in acute stages
— High fibre, low fat diet
— Codeine phosphate for recurrent diarrhoea.
— Metronidazole AND/OR ciprofloxacin for fistulae.
— Azathioprine OR cyclosporin OR methotrexate for unresponsive cases.
— Surgery to affected part of gut.

PREC: Beware of perforation or obstruction.

PROG: 60% relapse after surgery. Significant morbidity. Mortality rate double expected age and sex.

Croup (Laryngotracheobronchitis)

THER: Humidified atmosphere
AND antihistamines for sedation and catarrh
AND aspirin for fever and inflammation
AND inhaled budesonide OR prednisolone orally stat.
ADD oxygen if necessary
ADD dexamethasone if severe stridor or IMI *in extremis*.
ADD nasogastric suction if intubated or tracheostomy

PROG: Good if adequately managed. Regular assessment essential. Mediastinal emphysema and pneumothorax may occur. Disease unusual over 4 years of age.

Cryptococcosis

THER: Amphotericin B
ADD flucytosine in meningitis.

PROG: Poor.

Cushing's Disease

THER: Depends on cause, which should be determined first.
Treatments include:
— Surgery or radiotherapy to adrenal gland or tumour and pituitary irradiation if appropriate
— Metyrapone under plasma cortisol control
— Aminoglutethamide
— Ketoconazole
— Pituitary surgery

PREC: Commonest cause iatrogenic.

PROG: Surgical mortality may be significant without adequate preparation. 50% mortality in five years without treatment. Greatly improved with adequate therapy.

Cutaneous Larva Migrans (Ancylostomiasis)

THER: Thiabendazole
OR freeze spray eruption with ethyl chloride

PROG: Second or third courses often necessary for cure. Freeze spraying less effective.

See also Ancylostomiasis, Intestinal

CVA

See Cerebrovascular Accident

Cyanide Poisoning

THER: 1. Positive pressure respiration with oxygen.
2. Amyl nitrate inhalations every 3 minutes.
3. Cobalt edetate 1.5%, 40 mL IVI slowly; repeat if necessary.
4. Sodium thiosulfate 50% 25 mL IVI.
5. Sodium nitrate 3% 10 mL IVI.
6. Gastric lavage with sodium bicarbonate 2%, and place 300 mL sodium thiosulfate solution 25% in stomach.

PREC: Cobalt edetate — severe side effects, particularly if used when no cyanide in blood.

PROG: Poor; dose related.

Cystic Fibrosis (Fibrocystic Disease)

THER: **General:**
1. Best supervised in specialised CF units.
2. Patient and family education.
3. Nutritional supplementation.
4. Regular exercise.
5. Bronchodilators.
6. Avoid mucolytics, steroids.
7. Forced coughing, postural drainage, chest percussion.
8. Lung transplant (heart-lung or double-lung).
Pulmonary infections:
1. Admit if patient ill.
2. Intensive physiotherapy.
3. Antibiotics based on culture. Start with:
aminoglycoside + antipseudomonal penicillin
OR ceftazidime
OR ciprofloxacin.

4. Trial of suppressive antibiotics if infections frequent.
Malabsorption:
1. Enteric-coated pancreatic enzyme replacement
AND H$_2$ antagonist.
PROG: Incurable. Improving with median survival >25 years.Males sterile. 10% develop diabetes.

Cystinosis

THER: None specific. Correct biochemical abnormalities. Haemodialysis offers some hope. Renal transplants of temporary benefit only.
PROG: Death before puberty unless haemodialysed from early age.

Cystitis

THER: Take urine sample for M/C/S
AND high fluid intake (except with sulphas and nalidixic acid)
AND antibiotics (eg. trimethoprim, cotrimoxazole, amoxycillin ± clavulanic acid, cefaclor, norfloxacin)
ADD urinary alkalinisers
THEN alter antibiotic if necessary when urine culture and sensitivity results available.
PROG: Very good; investigate for cause if recurrent.

Cytomegalovirus (CMV) Infection

THER: Normally mild or subclinical and requires no treatment. In immunodeficient patients, ganciclovir and anti-CMV immunoglobulin are used.
PROG: Excellent, except in pregnancy when congenital deformities may occur in fetus.

Dandruff

THER: 1. Detergent shampoo or hair rinse 3 times a week containing selenium sulfide
OR zinc pyrithione
OR cetrimide.
2. Tar gels (10% coal tar in detergent).
3. Corticosteroid lotions for initial control of very severe cases.
PREC: Severe cases may be confused with psoriasis. Some forms due to fungal infection.
PROG: Often chronic; control reasonable.

Deep Venous Thrombosis

See Thrombosis, Deep Venous

Defibrination Syndrome

See Disseminated Intravascular Coagulation

Dehydration

THER: 1. Electrolyte solution containing approximately sodium 90 mmol/L, potassium 20 mmol/L,

chloride 80 mmol/L, citrate 10 mmol/L and glucose 2% in water by mouth or a nasogastric drip.
2. Intravenous OR intraperitoneal infusion of 0.45% saline in 2.5% dextrose with added potassium chloride if dehydration due to diarrhoea.
3. Carefully monitor fluid and electrolyte balance.
PREC: Electrolyte balance from dehydration due to burns, diabetic ketoacidosis, diarrhoea and water deprivation will vary dramatically and may alter choice of rehydration fluid.

See also Cholera

Delirium Tremens

See Alcoholism

Dementia

THER: 1. Exclude secondary cause of dementia.
2. Treat associated physical disease.
3. Treat psychological symptoms with phenothiazines
OR benzodiazepines
OR chloral hydrate.
4. Analgesia where appropriate.
5. Social worker/occupational therapist.
PREC: Medications should be kept to minimal dosages to avoid sedation and further confusion.
PROG: Poor unless cause treatable; slowly progressive.

Dengue Fever

THER: 1. Bed rest and cool sponging
2. Intravenous replacement of fluid and electrolytes
3. Paracetamol AND/OR codeine for pain
4. Diazepam for agitation
5. Blood transfusion for coagulopathies
PREC: Salicylates and NSAID are contraindicated
PROG: Recovery in a few weeks normal unless haemorrhagic fever occurs when death is possible

Dental Infections

THER: Benzylpenicillin IMI (severe cases)
AND amoxycillin ± clavulanic acid
AND/OR metronidazole
OR erythromycin
AND analgesics
AND hot saline mouth washes
AND soft diet.
PROG: Treatment is a for acute situation. Specific cause should be sought and treated by a dentist.

Depression

THER: 1. Emotional support

ADD benzodiazepine (eg. diazepam) for short-term relief of stress.
2. Tricyclic antidepressant
OR moclobemide
OR SSRI (eg. fluoxetine, fluvoxamine, paroxetine, sertraline).
OR nefazodone
OR venlafaxine
3. Buspirone.
4. MAOI.
5. Major or minor tranquillisers.
6. Electroconvulsive therapy.
7. Psychotherapy.

PREC: MAOI — severe reaction with certain foods and drugs, eg. cheese, red wine, beans, liver; other tyramines, tricyclic antidepressants; amphetamines.

PROG: Generally good. Often recurrent. Very disruptive to family. Beware of potential for suicide.

See also Postnatal Depression

Dermatitis Herpetiformis

THER: Dapsone
OR sulfapyridine
AND gluten-free diet.

PROG: Drugs do not cure, only control and help skin lesions and not those in gut. Gluten-free diet life-long necessary. May be associated with thyroid disorders, pernicious anaemia, lymphoma and diabetes.

Dermatitis, Most Forms of, Dry (Xerotic and Asteatotic Dermatitis)

THER: 1. Avoid irritant clothing, chapping, sweating.
2. Avoid soaps and other allergens.
3. Moisturising creams.
4. 10% urea preparations.
5. Hydrocortisone 1.0% cream or ointment.
6. Oral antihistamines for pruritus.
7. Oral antibiotics for severe infections.
8. Stronger steroid creams or ointments.
9. Oral prednisone short-term.

PROG: Cure rare, control normally adequate. Often recurrent, or may subside spontaneously.

See also Atopic Eczema; Perioral Dermatitis; Rash; Seborrhoeic Dermatitis

Dermatomyositis and Polymyositis

THER: Prednisone
ADD methotrexate
OR azathioprine
OR cyclophosphamide
AND physiotherapy.

PROG: Poor; 30% of patients have intercurrent carcinoma.

Diabetes Insipidus

THER: 1. Increase water intake.

2. Thiazide diuretics (act paradoxically to reduce urine flow in nephrogenic form).
3. Vasopressin in oil IMI short-term.
4. Desmopressin intranasally.

PROG: Cannot be cured. May be very well controlled. Nephrogenic form more severe, particularly in infants.

Diabetes Mellitus

THER: 1. Education of patient.
2. Diet (reduce rapidly absorbed carbohydrates, animal and dairy fat; increase polyunsaturated fats and fibre).
3. Exercise and weight reduction programme.
4. Type 2 only – Oral hypoglycaemics singly or combined, eg. sulfonylureas if thin (chlorpropamide, glipizide, tolbutamide, glibenclamide), biguanides if obese (metformin, phenformin).
5. Type 2 only – acarbose
6. Insulin in one to three daily injections of one or more of the different types, eg. soluble (peak 4h, duration 8h), isophane (peak 10h, duration 24h), protamine zinc* (peak 16h, duration 36h), lente zinc suspension (peak 8h, duration 24h), semilente zinc suspension (peak 4h, duration 12h), biphasic (peak 2h, duration 24h).
7. Clofibrate.

PREC: *Protamine zinc insulin cannot be mixed with other insulins. Only soluble insulin can be given IVI.
Clofibrate increases half-life of tolbutamide and chlorpropamide.

PROG: Good with adequate control.

See also Hyperinsulinism, Hypoglycaemia

Diabetic Ketoacidosis

THER: 1. Establish diagnosis and severity by appropriate laboratory investigations.
2. Nasogastric tube if unconscious.
3. Oxygen.
4. Fluid replacement with isotonic saline to correct electrolyte imbalance and shock.
5. Soluble insulin by intravenous infusion.
6. Potassium supplements.
7. Bicarbonate if pH low (<7).
8. IM insulin once stabilised.
9. Antibiotics to prevent secondary infection.
10. Heparin to prevent thrombosis in elderly, unconscious or hyperosmolar patients.

PREC: Fluid and electrolyte balance critical; monitor all relevant biochemical levels constantly.

PROG: Generally good with adequate treatment.

Diarrhoea

See Cholera; Enteritis, Viral; Salmonellosis, Intestinal; Typhoid.
See also SYMPTOMS SECTION 1.

Diphtheria

THER: 1. Diphtheria antitoxin IVI after skin testing for

sensitivity.
2. Penicillin OR erythromycin in high doses.
3. Prednisolone for severe cases, eg. laryngeal inflammation.
4. Treat shock and arrhythmias of myocarditis as appropriate.
5. Intubation OR tracheostomy for laryngeal obstruction.
REC: Isolate patient and carriers. Nursing and medical attendants should have been previously vaccinated.
ROG: Mortality 10–30%; higher with myocarditis. Vaccine available.

Disseminated Intravascular Coagulation [DIC] (Defibrination Syndrome)
THER: 1. Restore fluid and electrolyte balance IV.
2. Oxygen.
3. Heparin IVI.
4. Fresh frozen plasma platelet concentrates for haemorrhagic states OR fibrinogen IVI.
5. Aprotinin if fibrinolysis proven by laboratory tests.
6. Treat underlying cause, eg. remove dead fetus, antibiotics for sepsis, malignancy, liver disease etc.
REC: Anticoagulant therapy requires close monitoring.
ROG: Mortality rate 50%; lower in obstetrics.

Diverticulitis, Colonic
THER: 1. High fibre diet.
2. Fibre supplements.
3. Tetracycline OR penicillin orally in acute attacks.
4. Antispasmodics.
5. Laxatives when necessary, eg. vegetable oil OR paraffin.
6. Surgery for perforation or fistula.
ROG: Good response to treatment.

Donavanosis
See Granuloma Inguinale

Drowning
HER: 1. Cardiopulmonary resuscitation (CPR) at site (ie. external cardiac massage and mouth to mouth resuscitation).
2. Prevent hypothermia by warm coverings.
3. Transport to hospital while maintaining CPR.
4. Intubate, oxygen, positive pressure ventilation with paralysis if moribund or in hypertonic coma.
5. Correct metabolic acidosis with sodium bicarbonate IVI.
6. Frusemide OR mannitol to produce mild dehydration.
7. Corticosteroids parenterally.
8. Maintain in intensive care unit.

PREC: Prevent hypo or hyperthermia. Intensive resuscitation protocols are still controversial and protocols may vary between centres.
PROG: Depends almost entirely on period of immersion and effectiveness of initial CPR.

Drug Addiction
See Narcotic Addiction

Duodenal Ulcer
See Peptic Ulcer

Dysentery
See Cholera; Enteritis, Bacterial; Salmonellosis, Intestinal; Shigellosis

Dysmenorrhoea
THER: 1. Paracetamol, aspirin, codeine.
2. Combined oestrogen/progestogen pills (oral contraceptive)
OR dydrogesterone
OR mefenamic acid
OR other NSAIDs
OR nifedipine
OR belladonna ergotamine/phenobarbitone combinations
OR dicyclomine
ADD uterine curettage in chronic cases
ADD hysterectomy if severely disabling.
PREC: Exclude pathological causes (see SYMPTOMS SECTION 1).

Ear Disease
See Furunculosis, Otic; Glue Ear; Mastoiditis; Meniere's Disease; Otitis Externa; Otitis Media

Echinococcus
See Hydatid Disease

Eclampsia
THER: Diazepam
OR chlormethiazole
AND maintain airway, fluid and electrolyte balance
OR hydralazine
ADD epidural block
AND deliver child as rapidly as possible
ADD diazoxide postpartum.
PREC: Beware of patient trauma, disseminated intravascular coagulation and postpartum haemorrhage. Neonate may be sedated and require respiratory assistance. Dosage of hydralazine and diazoxide should be monitored carefully.
PROG: Good for both mother and child if carefully treated and monitored.

Eczema
See Atopic Eczema

Ejaculation, Premature
THER: 1. Investigate causes (eg. stress, guilt).
          2. Counselling. Emphasise lack of pathology.
          3. Obtain cooperation of partner.
          4. "Squeeze" technique on penis.
          5. Psychotherapy.
PROG: Success rates as high as 98% claimed.

Ejaculation, Retrograde
THER: 1. Investigate to exclude cause (eg. diabetes).
          2. Explanation and reassurance.
          If fertility desired:
          1. Imipramine OR phenylephrine OR
          pseudophedrine OR brompheniramine OR
          cyproheptadine.
          2. Urological surgery.
          3. Sperm retrieval and artificial insemination.
PROG: Using all above techniques, provided sperm are
          being produced in the testes, successful
          pregnancy in a partner is usually possible.

Elephantiasis
See Filariasis

Embolism, Pulmonary
See Pulmonary Embolism

Emphysema
THER: 1. Patient education.
          2. Smoking cessation essential.
          3. Regular exercise programme (esp. walking).
          4. Energy conservation, control of breathing
          pursed-lip breathing instruction.
          5. Consider trial of bronchodilator (eg.
          salbutamol, ipratropium bromide).
          6. Oxygen if pO_2 <55.
          7. Lung transplantation if age <60, limited life
          expectancy and otherwise reasonably fit.
PREC: Avoid oral steroids.
          Yearly flu vaccine and pneumovax every 6
          years.
PROG: Highly variable depending on FEV_1.
          Development of acute respiratory failure is an
          ominous sign.

Encephalitis, Acute Viral
THER: 1. Acyclovir IV if *Herpes simplex* suspected.
          2. Corticosteroids (controversial).
          3. Control convulsions (see separate entry).
          4. Reduce cerebral oedema (eg. mannitol IV).
          5. Oxygen and maintain airway.
PROG: Mortality 40–90%. Significant residual
          morbidity. Often follows mumps, measles or
          chickenpox.

Encephalitis, Japanese
See Japanese Encephalitis

Endocarditis, Bacterial
THER: 1. Take several blood specimens for culture
          2. Benzylpenicillin IV
          AND gentamicin IV
          OR vancomycin IVI
          AND cloxacillin IVI
          3. Alter antibiotic if necessary when culture
          results available
          THEN after antibiotic if necessary when culture
          results available.
PREC: Adequate dosage and length of treatment
          essential.
PROG: Significant morbidity and mortality 60% of
          prosthetic valve infections fatal.

Endometriosis
THER: Combined oestrogen/progestogen (oral
          contraceptive) constantly for 12 months
          OR norethisterone for 12 months
          OR danazol for 6 months
          OR GnRH (eg. buserelin, nafarelin)
          ADD surgery.
PROG: 80% cure rate (ie. pregnancy or loss of
          symptoms)

Enteric Fever
See Salmonellosis, Intestinal

Enteritis Bacterial
THER: 1. Take faeces sample for M/C/S.
          2. Treat dehydration (see separate entry).
          3. Restrict fats in diet.
          4. Use antibiotics in severe systemic infections
          only.
          5. Change antibiotic if necessary when culture
          results available.

See also Cholera; Salmonellosis, Intestinal; Shigellosis

Enteritis, Regional
See Crohn's Disease

Enteritis, Viral
THER: 1. Correct fluid loss with oral glucose, salt and
          water (see WHO rehydration formula under
          Cholera entry). Avoid plain water and non-
          breast milk.
          2. Avoid antibiotics and antidiarrhoeals.
          3. Correct fluid loss intravenously if signs of
          dehydration (normal saline 20 mL/kg/hr)
          OR 1/3 normal saline with 3% dextrose 150 mL/
          kg/d).
          4. Correct electrolyte imbalances.
          5. Introduce solids and dairy products gradually
PREC: Antidiarrhoeals may give temporary relief, but

prolong disease. Post-infection milk intolerance may necessitate lactose free formula in infants.
PROG: Very good unless poorly managed or late presentation.

See also Dehydration
See also Diarrhoea in SYMPTOMS SECTION 1

Enterobiasis (Threadworm, Pinworm)

THER: Careful personal hygiene
Pyrantel pamoate
OR mebendazole
OR pyrvinium pamoate
AND treat all members of family.
PROG: Good.

Enuresis (Bed Wetting)

THER: 1. Exclude pathological cause by urine M/C/S.
2. Positive parental support and encouragement.
3. Reward system, eg. star chart.
4. Restrict evening fluids.
5. Lift child out of bed to toilet at parents' bed time.
6. Bell alarm that is activated by wetting (5 years of age +).
7. Imipramine (school children and adults).
8. Desmopressin in difficult cases.
PROG: 80% cure by one of above methods within 3 months.

Epididymo-Orchitis

THER: 1. Support scrotum with bandages or jockstrap; ice packs to scrotum
2. erythromycin
OR tetracycline
OR doxycycline
OR fluoroquinolone
OR co-trimoxazole
3. Aspirin OR paracetamol
4. Surgical drainage of abscess.
PROG: Very good; testicular torsion must be excluded.

Epiglottitis

THER: Cefotaxime IV
OR ceftriaxone IV
AND dexamethasone
ADD oxygen if distressed
ADD intubation OR tracheostomy *in extremis.*
PREC: Significant side effects with dexamethasone.
PROG: Good provided adequate airway maintained.

Epilepsy, Absence (Petit Mal)

THER: Valproate
OR ethosuximide
OR clonazepam
OR acetazolamide.
PROG: Easily controlled; remits in adult life.

Epilepsy, Tonic-clonic (Grand Mal)

THER: **Acute:**
See Status Epilepticus; Convulsions.
Prophylaxis:
Generalised seizure:
1. Valproate.
2. Carbamazepine OR gabapentin OR lamotrigine OR phenytoin OR vigabatrin.
3. Phenobarbitone.
4. Surgery in strictly selected cases.
Partial seizure:
1. Carbamazepine.
2. Gabapentin OR lamotrigine OR phenytoin OR vigabatrin.
3. Phenobarbitone
PREC: Measure serum concentrations of drugs regularly.
PROG: Trial of gradual drug withdrawal after 2 years. If recurrence, lifelong treatment probably necessary. Total remission of seizures on treatment occurs in 30–50% of patients.

Erysipelas

THER: 1. Topical antibiotics (eg. fusidic acid, tetracycline, neomycin, miconazole)
AND aspirin OR paracetamol
2. Oral antibiotics (eg. cephalexin, dicloxacillin, erythromycin, flucloxacillin)
3. IV antibiotics (eg. flucloxacillin)
PROG: Very good.

Erythema Multiforme Minor

THER: 1. Bed rest,
2. Soothing dressings to lesions
3. Eliminate precipitants.
4. Corticosteroids OR acyclovir if persistent/recurrent.
PROG: Small percentage progress to Stevens-Johnson syndrome. Usually settles in 2–6 weeks.

Erythema Nodosum

THER: 1. Eliminate or treat cause, eg. toxins, infection, inflammatory bowel disease.
2. Rest in bed.
3. Potassium iodide solution.
4. Corticosteroids orally if persistent.
PROG: Depends on cause; usually settles in 4–8 weeks.

Eye Disease

See Allergic Conjunctivitis; Blepharitis; Conjunctivitis; Flash Burns, Eye; Glaucoma; Keratitis; Stye

Familial Mediterranean Fever

THER: Colchicine prophylaxis
PREC: Diarrhoea as side effect
PROG: 25% develop amyloidosis. Symptom control successful in 85%

Fanconi's Syndrome, Idiopathic

THER: 1. Replace vitamin D losses.
2. Maintain electrolyte balance carefully.
3. Monitor and control blood pH.
PROG: Good if carefully controlled; no cure.

See also Cystinosis

Febrile Convulsions

THER: **Acute:**
Diazepam, OR lorazepam IM, IV or rectally
AND maintain adequate airway
AND cool sponging or bath
AND paracetamol
AND nurse in cool conditions, eg. fan
AND treat cause of fever
ADD admit to hospital for further investigation if first attack.
Prophylaxis:
1. Control fever with paracetamol and sponging.
2. Treat infections aggressively.
3. Phenobarbitone
OR sodium valproate.
PREC: Beware of aspiration pneumonia.
PROG: Initial seizure under 1 year of age gives 50% chance of recurrence, over 3 years 15%. Does not usually predispose to epilepsy.

Fertility Control (Contraception)

THER: **Pre-conceptive:**
1. Coitus interruptus (f/r: 15–25%).
OR Fertility awareness (rhythm method) using dates, cervical mucus detection and basal body temperature recordings (f/r: 2–25%).
OR Spermicidal creams or foams (f/r: 5–20%).
OR Vaginal diaphragm with spermicide (f/r: 2–20%).
OR Condom (penile sheath) with spermicide (f/r: 2–10%).
OR Intrauterine device (f/r: 1–5%).
OR Progestagen only oral contraceptive pill (f/r: 1–2%).
OR Combined oestrogen and progestagen oral contraceptive (monophasic or multiphasic) (f/r: 0.5–2.0%).
OR Depot medroxyprogesterone acetate injection (f/r: 0.25%).
OR Vasectomy or tubal ligation (f/r: 0.1%).
Post-conceptive:
Two tablets of medium to high potency combined oestrogen and progestagen oral contraceptive within 72 hours of sex. Repeat 12 hours later (f/r: 4%).
AND Metoclopramide to prevent vomiting medication
OR Five norethisterone 0.35 mg tablets daily for five days, starting within 72 hours of sex.
OR Five ethinyl oestradiol 1 mg tablets daily for five days.
OR Insert intrauterine device within five days of sex.
OR Abortefacients eg. mifepristone [RU486].

OR Abortion by curretage and/or suction.
PREC: The patient's personal religious, ethical and moral beliefs, and any relevant legislation, must be carefully considered by the physician when prescribing any form of contraception.
Combined oral contraceptive: increased risk of cardiovascular complications in smokers especially if aged over 35; contraindicated in ischaemic heart disease, thrombosis, cerebral haemorrhage, severe migraine, liver disease, breast cancer; contraceptive effectiveness reduced by rifampicin, most anticonvulsants and antibiotics.
Intrauterine device: increased risk of pelvic infection and ectopic pregnancy; may cause dysmenorrhoea; may be expelled.
High-dose post-contraceptive oral contraceptive: risk of nausea, vomiting.
High-dose ethinyl oestradiol: significant risk of nausea, vomiting, embolism.
Abortion: risk of pelvic infection, haemorrhage, perforation, psychological problems.

Fibrocystic Disease

See Cystic Fibrosis

Filariasis (Elephantiasis)

THER: Diethylcarbamazine
AND prednisone
ALTERNATING with suramin IVI weekly
ADD antibiotics for abscesses and ulcer.
PREC: Hypersensitivity reactions occur due to death of microfilariae.
PROG: Deformity of elephantiasis reversible by surgery only; otherwise good.

Fissure-in-Ano

See Anal Fissure

Fit

See Convulsion; Epilepsy; Febrile Convulsions

Flash Burns, Eye (From Welding, Ultraviolet Light etc)

THER: 1. Topical anaesthetic drops once only.
2. Homatropine drops
3. Analgesics.
4. Antibiotic eye ointment.
5. Firm eye padding.
6. Ensure protective eye wear used in future.
PREC: Topical anaesthetics: eye damage may occur with continued use.
PROG: Heals within 48 hours unless foreign body present.

Folliculitis

THER: 1. Oral flucloxacillin OR erythromycin OR cepalexin.

2. Intranasal antibiotics to eliminate reservoir
3. Antiseptic soaps and shampoo.
4. Prolonged antibiotics (eg. cepalexin, dicloxacillin, minocycline, cotrimoxazole) for recurrent attacks
5. Firm eye padding.
ROG: Responds rapidly to antibiotics, but recurrences common

___

Frostbite

THER: 1. Rewarm rapidly by immersion in 42°C water.
2. Elevate affected part.
3. Analgesia.
4. Antibiotics only if secondary infection present.
5. Ensure tetanus prophylaxis.
6. Surgical debridement at a later stage.
REC: Avoid thawing and refreezing. Do not debride early, but wait until dead tissue dried and mummified unless gangrene occurs.
PROG: If only erythema and blistering occur — good.
If skin loss — partial loss of function.
If gangrene — amputation.

___

Frozen Shoulder

THER: 1. Exercises.
2. Heat.
3. Physiotherapy.
4. Corticosteroid injections.
5. Manipulation under anaesthetic.
6. Systemic steroids.
PREC: Manipulation may cause capsular or bony damage.
PROG: Often chronic; control reasonable.

___

Fungal Infection

See Aspergillosis; Blastomycosis; Candidiasis, Oral; Candidiasis, Vaginal; Cryptococcosis; Histoplasmosis; Onychomycosis; Pityriasis Versicolor; Tinea

___

Furunculosis, Cutaneous (Boils)

THER: 1. Exclude systemic cause (eg. diabetes).
2. Check personal hygiene.
3. Swab culture from lesions and nose in recurrent cases.
4. Oral antibiotics (eg. clindamycin, minomycin, sodium fusidate, erythromycin, rifampicin)
5. Antiseptic soap and nasal mupirocin to prevent recurrence.
PROG: Good; often recurrent. Abscess formation possible.

___

Furunculosis, Otic

THER: 1. Careful ear cleansing.
2. Adequate analgesia eg. narcotics initially, then codeine and aspirin.
3. Gentamicin ointment wick.
4. Erythromycin
OR cloxacillin.

PROG: Good; often recurrent. Cerebral or bone disease possible.

___

Gall Bladder

Se Cholecystitis, Acute

___

Gangrene, Gas

See Gas Gangrene

___

Gas Embolism

See Bends

___

Gas Gangrene (*Clostridium welchii* Infection)

THER: 1. Polyvalent gas gangrene antitoxin.
2. Penicillin IM OR IV.
3. Surgical debridement of infected area. Amputation may be necessary well above infected area.
4. Hyperbaric oxygen in specialised centre.
5. Maintain fluid and electrolyte balance.
PREC: Careful nursing to prevent inoculation of staff with *Clostridium welchii*, particularly during surgery.
PROG: 95% +mortality without treatment. Only average chance of survival with treatment.

___

Gastric Ulcer

See Peptic Ulcer

___

Gastritis

THER: 1. Diet; clear fluids only initially.
2. Treat cause if known (eg. alcohol excess, smoking, stress, other irritants).
3. Antacids (eg. aluminium and/or magnesium hydroxide, simethicone, oxethazaine).
4. H_2-blockers (eg. cimetidine, ranitidine, famotidine).
OR proton pump inhibitors (eg. lansoprazole, omeprazole, pantoprazole)
OR misoprostol
OR sucralfate.
5. Antibiotics if bacterial infection present.
PROG: Depends on cause; may progress to peptic ulcer. Generally good.

___

Gastroenteritis

See Enteritis Bacterial; Enteritis, Viral

___

Gastro-oesophageal Reflux

See Reflux Oesophagitis

___

Genital Herpes

See Herpes, Genital

___

Genital Warts

See Warts, Ano-Genital

___

Giant Cell Arteritis
See Temporal Arteritis

Giardiasis, Intestinal
THER: Metronidazole
PROG: Very good.

Glandular Fever
See Infectious Mononucleosis

Glaucoma
THER: **Acute Narrow Angle:**
1. Pilocarpine drops.
2. 20% mannitol IV OR glycerol 50% solution orally.
3. Acetazolamide IV and orally.
4. Corticosteroids orally or IVI if poor response.
5. Laser surgery once pressure normalised.
Open Angle:
1. Topical beta-blocker eye drops
ADD pilocarpine drops
ADD epinephrine or dipivefrin drops
ADD oral acetazolamide.
2. Laser trabeculoplasty.
3. Filtering surgery, if indicated.
PREC: Avoid pupil dilation and cycloplegics in narrow angle glaucoma.
PROG: Very good with correct and rapid treatment.

Glioma
See Intracranial Tumour

Globus
See Oesophageal Spasm

Glomerulonephritis, Acute
THER: 1. Eradicate causative or coexistent β-haemolytic streptococcal infection with penicillin.
2. Cyclophosphamide when appropriate.
3. Correct any nephrotic syndrome with steroids if necessary.
4. Low protein, high carbohydrate, low sodium diet.
5. Renal dialysis.
6. Control electrolyte and fluid balance.
7. Frusemide in high doses for oedema.
PREC: Perform regular blood smears with cyclophosphamide.
PROG: 90% cure; 5% chronic; 5% mortality.

See also Nephrotic Syndrome

Glomerulonephritis, Latent
THER: 1. Treat acute attacks as above.
2. High fluid, moderate protein, high carbohydate diet.
3. Avoid strenuous exercise.

4. Packed cell transfusion for severe anaemia.
PROG: Eventual death from uraemia common, but often after 20–30 years.

Glue Ear (Middle Ear Effusion)
THER: 1. Observe progress of condition for weeks or months
2. Prolonged course of amoxycillin
3. Teach valsalva manoeuvre. Assist with autoinflation devices
4. Oral steroids (controversial)
5. Insert tympanoplasty tubes (grommets)
6. Adenoidectomy
PREC: Hearing loss possible if inadequately treated. Avoid underwater swimming with grommets *in situ.*
PROG: Good with appropriate treatment

See also Nephrotic Syndrome

Goitre
See Hyperthyroidism; Hypothyroidism

Gonorrhoea
THER: Ceftriaxone with Lignocaine IMI
OR ciprofloxacin orally
OR amoxycillin 3 g orally WITH probenecid (only if strain known to be penicillin sensitive)
OR spectinomycin IMI for resistant strains
OR cefixime orally
OR other appropriate antibiotic after culture
AND doxycycline orally
AND treat sexual partner(s).
PREC: Exclude other concurrent forms of VD, eg. syphilis. Notifiable disease in most countries.
PROG: Good. Beware of resistant strains. Follow-up carefully.

Gout
THER: **Acute:**
NSAIDs
AND/OR colchicine
ADD corticotrophin gel IMI.
Prophylaxis:
Allopurinol
AND/OR colchicine
OR probenecid
OR sulfinpyrazone WITH colchicine
AND avoid excess purines (eg. liver, shellfish) and alcohol in diet
AND reduce weight gradually if obese.
PROG: Excellent on correct treatment and with good compliance.

See also Hyperuricaemia

Granuloma Annulare
THER: 1. Confirm diagnosis by biopsy.
2. Exclude diabetes mellitus.
3. Intralesional steroids

OR strong topical steroids AND retinoids.
4. Cryotherapy
5. Systemic treatment (eg. dapsone OR oral steroids OR chloroquine OR oxpentifylline OR retinoids OR cyclosporin OR chlorambucil OR nicotinamide).
6. PUVA
PROG: No ideal treatment exists, but many different treatments have been successful in different cases. Spontaneous regression possible over years.

Granuloma Inguinale (Donavanosis)

THER: Tetracycline orally
OR doxycycline orally
OR sulphadiazine orally
OR erythromycin orally
OR norfloxacin orally.
REC: Follow-up long-term to detect any cancer.
PROG: Recurrence common. Neoplastic change possible. Stenosis or gross swelling of urethra, anus and vagina possible.

Graves' Disease
See Hyperthyroidism

Guillain-Barré Syndrome

THER: 1. Hospitalise and monitor lung function.
2. Treat respiratory failure with tracheostomy, intubation and artificial respiration if necessary.
3. Intragastric OR intravenous feeding.
4. Plasmapheresis OR IV immunoglobulin.
5. Physiotherapy (eg. splints, walking aids).
6. Psychological support.
REC: Respiratory paralysis may develop rapidly.
PROG: 20% have permanent residual paralysis.

See also SYNDROMES SECTION 6

Haemochromatosis, Idiopathic

THER: 1. Screen all blood relatives for iron accumulation and treat early.
2. Venesection of 500 mL blood at regular intervals to keep Hb below 110 g/L and serum iron normal.
3. Desferrioxamine IMI or subcutaneous infusion.
REC: Desferrioxamine very painful injection.
PROG: Good provided treated before major organ damage occurs. Life-long treatment required.

Haemolytic Anaemias, Idiopathic

THER: 1. Transfusion of carefully matched blood if acute.
2. Prednisone for 2–4 weeks.
3. Exclude any treatable cause, eg. leukaemia, lymphoma, drugs, diabetes.
4. Splenectomy.
5. Immunosuppressive drugs, eg. 6-

mercaptopurine, azathioprine.
PROG: Depends on cause; significant mortality.

Haemophilia

THER: **Acute:**
1. Rest area affected by bleed.
2. Transfusion of cryoprecipitate/factor VIII.
3. Surgical drainage or aspiration of haematoma or joint if necessary.
4. Maintain high fluid intake/urine output.
Chronic:
1. Treat joint arthritis with naproxen OR sulindac
ADD corticosteroids if needed.
2. Physiotherapy, eg. swimming.
3. Protection and support of patient.
4. Analgesics (non-salicylate).
PROG: Severe morbidity; significant mortality. Life expectancy markedly reduced.

Haemorrhagic Fever
See Lassa Fever; Dengue Fever

Haemorrhoids (Piles)

THER: 1. Avoid constipation and straining at stool.
2. Bulky diet, eg. bran.
3. Glycerin or other soothing suppositories and creams.
4. Steroid/antiseptic/antibiotic combination creams AND/OR suppositories.
5. Injection sclerotherapy of small piles.
6. Rubber band ligation of large 2nd degree piles.
7. Surgical evacuation of thrombosed external pile.
8. Alternative therapies of 2nd degree piles include cryotherapy, sphincterotomy and anal dilation.
9. Haemorrhoidectomy.
PREC: Beware of carcinoma development in chronic pile.
PROG: Recurrences common; control good.

Hair Loss
See Alopecia Areata; Baldness

Hallux Valgus
See Bunion

Hartnup Disease

THER: Nicotinamide AND high protein diet.
PROG: Mental retardation and neurological problems in 25%, otherwise good outlook.

Hay Fever
See Allergic Rhinitis

Headache, Non-specific

THER: 1. Paracetamol
AND/OR codeine
ADD NSAIDs
ADD massage, physiotherapy, relaxation
therapy, acupuncture.
2. Investigate to determine cause of headache
(eg. migraine, tension, cluster, meningitis,
sinusitis, etc – see SYMPTOMS SECTION 1).
PROG: Depends on cause.

*See also Cluster Headache; Meningitis, Bacterial (Septic);
Meningitis, Viral (Aseptic); Migraine; Otitis Media;
Sinusitis; Tension Headache; Trigeminal Neuralgia*

Head Injury

See Concussion

Heart Attack

See Myocardial Infarct

Heartburn

See Reflux Oesophagitis

Heart Disease

*See Angina Pectoris; Atrial Flutter/Fibrillation; Cardiac
Arrest; Cardiomyopathy, Hypertrophic; Cor Pulmonale;
Endocarditis, Bacterial; Hypertension, Essential;
Myocardial Infarct; Myocarditis; Pericarditis, Acute;
Rheumatic Fever; Ventricular Tachycardia*

Heart Failure, Congestive (CCF)

THER: 1. Rest sitting up with oxygen if needed.
2. ACE inhibitor.
3. Diuretics for pulmonary and peripheral
oedema.
4. Restrict salt in diet.
5. Correct potassium depletion.
6. Digoxin.
7. Anticoagulants if bed-fast.
8. Isosorbide nitrate sublingually.
PREC: Careful monitoring of anticoagulants
necessary.
PROG: Generally good in short-term. Greatly increased
long-term morbidity and mortality rate.

Helminthiasis

*See Ancylostomiasis, Intestinal; Ascariasis; Cestode
Infestation; Enterobiasis; Hydatid Disease;
Strongyloidiasis; Trichuriasis*

Hepatic Abscess

THER: 1. Identify specific causative agent and treat
according to bacteriology report.
2. Gentamicin AND clindamycin
AND/OR metronidazole may be used while
awaiting results.
3. Surgical drainage
PROG: Significant mortality unless treated early.

Hepatic Carcinoma

THER: Surgical resection if possible
AND/OR chemotherapy.
PROG: Very poor.

Hepatitis, Acute Viral (Hepatitis A, B, C, D and E)

THER: No specific treatment available for any form.
Supportive measures include:
• Total rest until completely recovered.
• Low protein, high carbohydrate diet.
• Control vomiting.
• Monitor prothrombin time.
• Stop all medication if possible.
• Barrier nursing.
• Paracetamol for analgesia. Avoid aspirin and
NSAIDs.
• Cholestyramine for pruritus.
• Avoid alcohol until 3 months after recovery.
• Interferon AND/OR ribavarin may be useful in
Hepatitis B and C.
• Liver transplantation in fulminant viral
hepatitis.
Vaccination available against Hepatitis A and B.
Human immunoglobulin prophylactic against
other forms.
PREC: No evidence that corticosteroids are beneficial.
PROG: *Hepatitis A:* Recovery within 2 months normal.
Mortality 0.15%.
Hepatitis B: 10–20% chronic infection. 15% of
chronic eventually fatal. Fulminant in 1%. Risk
of hepatoma increased 200 times.
Hepatitis C: 50% develop chronic infection, 20%
develop cirrhosis. Fulminant in 1%. Some
increase in risk of malignancy.
Hepatitis D: Chronic infection in more than 50%
Sometimes fulminant. Probable increase in risk
of malignancy.
Hepatitis E: Self-limiting and very rarely chronic
Fulminant form rare, except during pregnancy
when fulminant form occurs in 20%. Risk of
malignancy unknown.

Herpes, Genital

THER: 1. Exclude syphilis, gonorrhoea,
trichomoniasis. Take swabs for viral culture.
2. Aciclovir or valaciclovir.
3. Topical anaesthetic creams (eg. lignocaine).
4. Idoxuridine/dimethylsulfoxide lotions for
chronic lesions.
5. Antibiotics for concurrent secondary infection
PROG: Recurrent attacks, that may resolve
spontaneously. Regular Pap smears are
recommended.

Herpes Simplex (Cold Sore)

THER: 1. Idoxuridine paint or ointment in first 24 hours
2. Drying agents (eg. ether, povidone-iodine).

3. Acyclovir topical
   OR oral (not recommended routinely for "cold sores".)
4. High lysine diet prophylaxis (eg. potatoes, milk) (controversial).
   Treat secondary infections with topical antibiotics.
PROG: Spontaneous resolution, recurrences common.

Herpes Zoster
See Chickenpox; Shingles

Hiatus Hernia
See Reflux Oesophagitis

Hiccoughs (Hiccups)
THER: **For brief episodes:**
   Breath holding, rebreathing air in paper bag, swallowing ice water, sudden fright, pulling out tongue, sneezing etc.
   For chronic episodes:
   1. Exclude organic cause (see SYMPTOMS SECTION 1).
   2. Chlorpromazine orally or IVI.
   3. Metoclopramide IVI every 4 hours.
   4. Quinidine sulfate OR phenytoin OR valproic acid.
   5. Psychotherapy OR hypnosis OR acupuncture.
   6. General anaesthetic.
   7. Phrenic nerve block.
   8. Very rarely — phrenic nerve transection.
PREC: Phrenic nerve block and transection — impaired pulmonary function.

Hirsutism
THER: Spironolactone long-term
   AND/OR cyproterone acetate
   AND/OR hydrogen peroxide bleaching of hairs
   ADD surgical depilation.
PREC: Exclude any ovarian, adrenal or pituitary pathology.
PROG: Reasonable after 6 months use.

Histoplasmosis
THER: Amphotericin B
   AND bed rest until recovered
   ADD resection of cavitated lung
   ADD sulfadiazine if no response.
   For pulmonary disease:
   ketoconazole
   OR itraconazole
PROG: Good if primary and localised, poor if generalised.

HIV
See AIDS

Hives
See Urticaria

Hodgkin's Disease (Malignant Lymphoma)
THER: 1. Staging biopsy of lymphoid tissue.
   2. Radiotherapy.
   3. Chemotherapy with 2 or more drugs.
PROG: Five year survival rates – Stage 1, 85%; stage 2, 75%; stage 3, 50%; stage 4A, 35%; stage 4B, 20%.

Hookworm
See Ancylostomiasis, Intestinal

Huntington's Chorea
See Chorea, Huntington's and Sydenham's

Hydatid Disease (Echinococcus)
THER: 1. Mebendazole OR albendazole.
   2. Operative removal of cyst or organ involved.
PREC   Drugs must be taken very long-term. Essential to avoid spillage of cyst contents during surgery.
PROG: Depends on cyst site: good in spleen, poor in brain and lungs.

Hydatidiform Mole
See Choriocarcinoma and Invasive Moles

Hyperactivity
See Overactivity, Paediatric

Hyperaldosteronism
THER: Sugical removal of adrenocortical adenoma
   AND/OR spironolactone
   OR amiloride.
PROG: Good, unless kidney damage prior to therapy.

Hypercholesterolaemia
THER: Low cholesterol diet to reduce blood cholesterol levels:
   —If overweight, reduce total fat and carbohydrate intake, and increase exercise, to lose weight.
   —Increase intake of wholegrain cereals, fruit and vegetables.
   —Avoid offal (brains, liver), prawns, squid (calamari), octopus.
   —Limit eggs to two per week.
   —Avoid full cream milk, cheese, ice cream, pizza.
   —Limit dairy products to skimmed milk, low fat yoghurt and cottage cheese.
   —Use polyunsaturated margarine instead of butter.
   —Select lean cuts of red meat.

—Avoid sausage, rissoles, bacon, salami, hamburger.
—Remove skin from chicken.
—Eat fish in preference to other flesh.
—Avoid fried food (eg. chips, potato crisps, fried fish or chicken).
ADD hypolipidaemic drugs if response inadequate (see Hyperlipidaemia entry).

PROG: Long-term high levels of blood cholesterol can lead to premature atherosclerosis, myocardial infarct and cerebral ischaemia.

Hyperemesis Gravidarum
See Morning Sickness

Hyperhidrosis
See Sweating, Excess

Hyperinsulinism
THER: Glucose enriched diet
AND/OR diazoxide
AND/OR pancreatectomy
ADD glucose IVI when acute.
PROG: Good with adequate therapy. Brain damage may occur in infants before diagnosis.

Hyperlipidaemia
THER: 1. Deal with secondary factors (eg. diabetes, alcoholism, hypothyroidism, renal or liver disease, oral contraceptives, etc).
2. Reduce bodyweight to desirable limits.
3. Treat aggressively those with bad family history, diabetics, obese, smokers, hypertensives, those with coronary artery disease, low level of high density lipoprotein. Treat mildly the elderly, premenopausal women, those with short-life expectancy from other disease.
Elevated LDL-Cholesterol:
1. Low cholesterol, polyunsaturated fat diet.
2. Statin AND/OR resin.
Elevated Triglycerides and/or low HDL-Cholesterol:
1. Low fat diet.
2. Fibrate or nicotinic acid.
Low HDL-Cholesterol and/or elevated Triglycerides:
1. Low fat diet.
2. Nicotinic acid or fibrate.
PROG: Control leads to lessening of coronary artery disease and associate risks. Patient compliance a large factor.

Hyperparathyroidism, Primary
THER: Surgical removal of abnormal parathyroids OR medical treatment
1. High fluid intake.
2. Urinary acidification.
3. (Female) oral oestrogens

AND/OR progestogens.
4. Vitamin D supplements.
5. Diuretics for hypercalcaemia.
6. Oral phosphate and calcitonin.
PREC: Significant side-effects with calcitonin.
PROG: Satisfactory with good management. Renal and bone disease may occur. Hypertension common.

Hyperprolactinaemia
THER: 1. Exclude drug or hypothyroid induced cause of disease.
2. Bromocriptine.
2. Surgery AND/OR radiotherapy to pituitary gland.
PROG: Good.

Hypertension, Essential
THER: 1. Withdraw exacerbating drugs, (eg. oral contraceptives).
2. Stop smoking, reduce alcohol, reduce salt intake, reduce weight if obese, check cholesterol.
3. Reduce stress and anxiety. Relaxation techniques.
4. Drug treatment:

Hypertension and	Use first	Use Second
Cardiac failure	A	D
Peripheral vascular disease	C,D	A
Ischaemic heart disease	B	C
Renal disease	B,C	D
L. ventricular diastolic failure	A	B,C
Bradycardia	A	D
Tachycardia	B	C
Conduction disease	A	D,C
Hyperlipidaemia	A,C	
Diabetes	A,C	
Asthma	A,C	D
Constipation	A,B	
Depression	A,C	D
Impotence	A,C	
Venous hypertension	A,D	B
Raynaud's phenomenon	C	A,D
Gout	A,C	

A=ACE inhibitor   B=β-blocker
C= Calcium antagonist   D=Diuretic
5. Other drugs (eg. methyldopa, alpha-blockers).
6. In resistant cases try minoxidil OR hydralazine OR clonidine.
7. *In extremis* use diazoxide IVI.
8. For phaeochromocytoma use phentolamine.
PREC: Potassium supplements or amiloride may be needed with diuretics. Avoid thiazide diuretics in diabetes and gout. Avoid beta-blockers in asthma, heart failure, diabetes and peripheral vascular disease. Avoid calcium antagonists in heart failure.
PROG: Greatly increased cardiovascular and cerebral morbidity and mortality without treatment. Normal life expectancy if well controlled.

yperthyroidism (Thyrotoxicosis)

HER: Anti-thyroid drugs, eg. carbimazole,
       propylthiouracil
       AND/OR propranolol
       AND/OR surgery (partial thyroidectomy)
       AND/OR radioactive iodine (I^{131}).
ROG: Some morbidity, negligible mortality. May
       progress to Graves' disease.

ypertrophic Cardiomyopathy

ee Cardiomyopathy, Hypertrophic

yperuricaemia

HER: 1. Maintain adequate hydration.
       2. Reduce excess weight.
       3. Reduce intakes of purines (eg. offal,
          shellfish).
       4. Alkalinise urine (eg. sodium bicarbonate).
       5. Reduce alcohol intake.
       6. Allopurinol OR probenecid
          OR sulfinpyrazone.
       7. Colchicine short term to reduce very high
          urate levels.
REC: See GOUT entry.
ROG: Risk of gout and/or renal damage if not
       adequately controlled.

ee also Gout

ypoglycaemia

HER: 1. Oral glucose drink or tablets.
       2. Glucose 10% 20 mL IVI stat.
       3. Glucagon IMI stat.
       4. Treat precipitating factor.
ROG: Recovery within minute usual. Brain damage
       with prolonged hypoglycaemia.

ee also Diabetes Mellitus; Hyperinsulinism

ypoparathyroidism

HER: Vitamin D
       OR dihydrotachysterol
       OR a-hydroxycholecalciferol.
ROG: Satisfactory with good management; significant
       morbidity; very low mortality.

ypopituitarism (Simmonds' Disease; heehan's Postpartum Necrosis)

HER: 1. Individually tailored hormone augmentation
       therapy depending on assay levels. Hormones
       that may be replaced are ACTH (by
       dexamethasone or hydrocortisone); TSH (by
       thyroxine); growth hormone in children;
       oestrogens, clomiphene, LH, testosterone and
       FSH to maintain sexual function.
       2. Surgery, radiotherapy, cryosurgery or yttrium
       implantation for treatment of primary pituitary
       tumour.
       3. Bromocriptine for lactation and amenorrhoea.

PROG: Depends on cause, age and areas of pituitary
       affected. Good compliance essential.

Hypotension, Postural

THER: 1. Avoid sudden postural changes.
       2. Treat underlying diseases, see SIGNS
          SECTION 2. Check for drug and other
          iatrogenic causes (eg. diuretics, alpha-
          blockers, tricyclic antidepressants,
          methyldopa).
       3. Promote exercise and physical fitness.
       4. Elastic stockings.
       5. High sodium diet.
       6. Fludrocortisone.
       7. Phenylephrine and dihydroergotamine.
       8. Drugs being used experimentally and acting
          idiosyncratically include: caffeine,
          indomethacin, metoclopramide, propranolol.
       9. Vasopressin.
       10. Sympathomimetics eg. ephedrine,
           amphetamines, methylphenidate). ADD MAOIs
           with caution (eg. tranylcypromine*).
PREC: *Interaction between sympathomimetics and
       tranylcypromine potentially dangerous.
PROG: Control difficult and poor in many patients.

Hypothermia

Ther: 1. Cardiopulmonary resuscitation (CPR).
       2. Establish airway, Administer warm humidified
          oxygen
       3. Prevent further heat loss (eg. warm blankets).
       4. Admit to intensive care and determine cause
          of low temperature
       5. Monitor rectal temperature, ECG, fluid and
          electrolyte balance closely
       6. Rewarm – immerse in 40°C water bath, use
          heating pads, blow hot air into bag surrounding
          patient etc.
       7. Warm and humidify inspired gases.
       8. Treat cardiac arrhythmias.
PREC: Do not cease resuscitation efforts until warmed
       above 32°C. Cardiac arrhythmias cannot be
       effectively treated below 30°C. Treat thin males
       and children first when large numbers involved.
       Warm infants slowly.
PROG: Better than many physicians expect. Depends
       on temperature and duration of exposure.

See also SIGNS SECTION 2.

Hypothyroidism (Myxoedema; Cretinism)

THER: 1. L-thyroxine.
       2. Monitor thyroid function regularly.
PREC: Caution in use with angina or cardiac failure.
PROG: Very good in adult; significant mental
       retardation in children even with therapy.

Ichthyosis

THER: 1. Add oils and surfactant to bath.
       2. Emollients (eg. glycerin in cream base,

lanolin, paraffin).
3. Lactic acid creams.
4. Compound tincture of benzene.
5. Antiseptic soaps to reduce chance of infection.
6. Oral antibiotics for skin infections.
7. Isotretinoin.
8. Acetretin.
PREC: Isotretinoin is teratogenic.
PROG: Depends on cause and form. Usually chronic with poor to moderate control.

Impetigo
THER: 1. Antiseptic cleansing of skin and remove crusts.
2. Topical mupirocin
OR fusidic acid cream
OR bacitracin
OR polysporin.
3. Cloxacillin
OR erythromycin
OR cephalexin
OR amoxicillin ± clavulanic acid.
PREC: Treat underlying skin disease if present (eg. dermatitis).
PROG: Very good; contagious.

Impotence
THER: 1. Investigate cause thoroughly, see INVESTIGATIONS SECTION 3.
2. Depending on cause, treatments may include one or more of the following:
—Psychotherapy for functional disorders
—Androgen supplementation for hormone deficiency
—Bromocriptine for hyperprolactinaemia
—Sildenafil
—Intrapenile injections of Prostaglandin E_1 AND/OR papaverine
—Vacuum penile pump
—Inflatable penile prostheses
—Ligation of penile veins.
PREC: Sildenafil – interacts with nitrates. Papaverine - prolonged painful erection.
PROG: Varies dramatically between centres and depends on cause.

Incontinence, Urinary, Female
THER: 1. Reduce weight if obese.
2. Reduce caffeine (coffee, tea, colas) and alcohol intake.
3. Cease potentially aggravating drugs (eg. prazosin, labetolol, diuretics, anticholinergics, tricyclic antidepressants, antihistamines, lithium etc).
4. Pelvic floor exercises taught by a physiotherapist.
5. Systemic or topical oestrogen replacement therapy if post-menopausal.
6. Oxybutynin
OR imipramine
OR propantheline
OR pseudoephedrine

7. Surgical correction of uterine or vaginal prolapse
8. Supra-pubic urethral suspension or similar operation.
9. Artificial urethral device.
PROG: Good control usually achieved.

Infantile Colic (3 Month Colic)
THER: 1. Alter feeding technique and types of food (alter mother's diet if breastfeeding)
2. Use white noise (eg. vacuum cleaner) near crying baby
3. Rock or move baby regularly
4. Gentle abdominal massage
5. Chloral hydrate
6. Sedating antihistamines
PREC: Do not use chloral hydrate for a prolonged period
PROG: Self limiting condition after 6 to 12 weeks

Infant, Premature
See Labour, Premature

Infarct, Cerebral
See Stroke

Infarct, Myocardial
See Myocardial Infarct

Infectious Mononucleosis (Glandular Fever)
THER: No specific treatment, supportive measures only. Antibiotics only used if intercurrent bacterial infection present.
PREC: Rash with penicillin.
PROG: Good. Recovery slow over 2–8 weeks.

Infertility, Female
THER: Carefully investigate cause (see INVESTIGATIONS SECTION 3):
Anatomical blockage or abnormality — surgery.
Hypothyroid — thyroxine.
Hypoprolactinaemia — bromocriptine.
Anovulatory — clomiphene AND/OR gonadotrophin.
PREC: Exclude male partner as cause.
PROG: 12–15% of females infertile, half can be helped by therapy.

Infertility, Male
THER: Carefully investigate cause (see INVESTIGATIONS SECTION 3):
Anorchia and Klinefelter's syndrome — testosterone.
Cryptorchidism, obstructive azoospermia and varicocele — surgery.
Hypogonadism — HCG and FSH.
Hypospermatogenesis — clomiphene (experimental).

REC: Involve female partner.
ROG: Depends on cause; generally poor.

Influenza

THER: 1. Zanamivir if within 36 hours of onset
      2. Paracetamol
      AND/OR NSAIDs for fever and arthralgia
      AND tepid sponging and bathing for fevers
      AND adequate fluid intake
      ADD decongestants
      ADD antihistamines for rhinitis and catarrh
      Vaccination available.
      Amantadine for prophylaxis.
PREC: Antibiotics contraindicated unless significant risk of secondary bacterial infection.
PROG: Good except in elderly and debilitated.

Insecticide Poisoning

See Organophosphate Poisoning

Insect Sting

See Anaphylactic Shock

Insomnia

THER: 1. Explanation and reassurance.
      2. Exclude and treat causes, eg. coffee, drugs, anxiety, depression.
      3. Nitrazepam
      OR temazepam
      OR flurazepam
      OR zopiclone
      OR choral hydrate
      OR dichloralphenazone.
      4. Tricyclic antidepressants.
PREC: Barbiturates contraindicated due to danger of dependency.
PROG: Good if used appropriately. Danger of dependence with all drugs.

Intertrigo

THER: 1. Keep skin surfaces apart.
      2. If candidiasis present use miconazole, econazole, clotrimazole, terbinafine, naftifine, ketoconazole or nystatin lotion.
      If infection present use mupirocin/fusidic acid.
      3. Hydrocortisone 1% cream.
PROG: Often recurrent unless skin kept dry. Powders help.

Intestinal Salmonellosis

See Salmonellosis, Intestinal

Intracranial Tumour

THER: 1. Diagnose specifically, the type of tumour present by biopsy AND/OR surgical excision of as much tumour as possible.
      2. Radiotherapy (pinealomas, medulloblastomas, craniopharyngioma)

AND/OR chemotherapy (pineal germinomas)
AND/OR immunotherapy (disseminated intracerebral neoplasms) as appropriate to tumour type.
3. Headaches treated by simple analgesics; opiates other than codeine are contraindicated.
4. Control cerebral oedema with intermittent use of dexamethasone.
5. Ventriculo-atrial or ventriculo-peritoneal shunt for obstructive hydrocephalus.
6. Aspiration of recurrent cysts through burr holes.
7. Epilepsy controlling medication when appropriate (see separate Epilepsy entry).
8. Antiemetics.
9. Tricyclic antidepressants and psychotropic drugs useful for control of symptoms in some patients.
PROG: Results vary between centres.
      Reasonable expectations would be:
      Astrocytoma — 5yr. survival 50%.
      Medulloblastoma — 1yr. survival 50%.
      Glioblastoma — 1yr. survival 20%.
      Ependymoma — 5yr. survival 35%.
      Meningioma — 10yr. survival 90%.
      Schwannoma — 10yr. survival 95%.
      Craniopharyngioma — 5yr. survival 90% + endocrine dysfunction.
      Pituitary adenoma — 5yr. survival 85%.

Iritis (Anterior Uveitis)

THER: 1. Identify associated conditions such as rheumatoid arthritis, ankylosing spondylitis and sarcoidosis and treat it appropriately if present.
      2. If no contraindication: topical steroid drops and mydriatics.
PREC: Extreme care in use of topical steroids necessary, as may allow secondary infection, corneal thinning, cataract and glaucoma.
      Treatment required to prevent secondary glaucoma.
PROG: Spontaneous resolution in 4–6 weeks; 40% recur.

Iron Deficiency Anaemia

THER: 1. Determine and correct cause of iron deficit, eg. poor diet, gut bleed, pregnancy, menorrhagia.
      2. Ferrous gluconate or sulfate
      OR parenteral iron IMI.
      3. Folic acid.
      4. Blood transfusion if acute.
PROG: Depends on cause.

Iron Overload

See Haemochromatosis, Idiopathic; Iron Poisoning, Acute

Iron Poisoning, Acute

THER: 1. Desferrioxamine IMI.
      2. Desferrioxamine IV infusion.
      3. Lavage stomach.

4. Desferrioxamine in water in stomach.
5. Fluid replacement.
PROG: Good if treated early.

Irritable Bowel Syndrome (Spastic Colon)

THER: 1. High fibre, low fat diet.
2. Bulking agents, high fluid intake, senna. AND/OR lactulose for constipation.
3. Antispasmodics OR pinaverium bromide.
4. Diphenoxylate OR codeine OR loperamide for diarrhoea.
5. Dopamine antagonists for bloating and flatus (eg. domperidone, metoclopramide).
6. Anxiolytics eg. benzodiazepines.
7. Tricyclic antidepressants.
PROG: Control reasonable, often chronic. Exclude other bowel pathology.

Ischaemic Heart Disease

See Angina Pectoris

Jaundice

See Hepatitis, Acute Viral. See also SYMPTOMS SECTION 1

Jet Lag

THER: 1. Jet lag does not occur on long North-South flights (eg. London to Cape Town, Sydney to Tokyo).
2. Break journey with long East-West or West-East flights. If only one stop-over possible, make that on the East-West leg (eg. London to Sydney) as jet lag is worse when travelling against time.
3. Select departure and arrival times to give lowest possible time coefficient (see table).
4. Adjust to new time zone as soon as possible after departure from home (eg. sleep and eat at destination times rather than local times).
5. Drink adequate non-alcoholic fluids to avoid dehydration on aircraft.
6. Mild hypnotics to regulate sleep pattern, eg. temazepam.
7. Melantoin (experimental prophylaxis).
PREC: Hypnotics — give trial prior to journey to judge effects.
PROG: Modified international Civil Aviation Organisation formula for estimating recovery time after arrival:

$$\text{Rest time in hours} = \left(\frac{\text{Travel time in hours}}{2} + \text{Time zones in excess of 4} + \text{Departure time coefficient} + \text{Arrival time coefficient}\right) \times 2.4$$

1 time zone = 1 hour difference in time

Time period	0800-1200	1200-1800	1800-2200	2200-0100	0100-0800
Departure time coefficient	0	1	3	4	3
Arrival time coefficient	4	2	0	1	3

eg. Rest time in hours $\left(\frac{16}{2} + 3 + 1 + 2\right) \times 2 = 28\,\text{hrs}$

The example after the equation allows for a16 hour trip crossing 7 time zones (7 hours time difference), leaving at 5pm and arriving at 1pm local time

Keratitis

THER: **Herpes Simplex:**
1. Trifluorothymidine eye drops every 2 hours, nine times daily.
2. Cycloplegics.
3. Arrange ophthalmological consultation.
Other viral keratitis:
1. Self-limiting condition.
2. Topical astringents or lubricants.
3. Antibiotic drops if secondarily infected.
Fungal keratitis:
1. Swab eye for culture and sensitivity.
2. Obtain ophthalmological consultation, as fungal keratitis is extremely rare and difficult to treat.
PREC: Avoid corticosteroid eye drops.
PROG: Slow healing can be expected. Subsequent scarring possible but uncommon.

Kidney Disease

See Cystinosis; Cystitis; Enuresis; Fanconi's Syndrome, Idiopathic; Glomerulonephritis; Glomerulonephritis, Acute; Nephrotic Syndrome; Pyelonephritis; Renal Failure, Chronic; Ureteric Calculi

Labour, Premature

THER: **Ruptured Membranes Only:**
1. >32 weeks – transport to adequate neonatal facility and deliver. Dexamethazone if <34 weeks.
2. <32 weeks – dexamethasone if >27 weeks.
—salbutamol, ritodrine or terbutaline until >32 weeks.
—prophylactic antibiotics
—deliver immediately if infection supervenes.
Ruptured Membranes and Contractions:
As above, but do not persist with salbutamol etc, unless <28 weeks.
Contractions Only:
1. >34 weeks – deliver.
2. <34 weeks – dexamethasone
—salbutamol, ritodrine or terbutaline until 34 weeks, then deliver.
—do not use steroids if <27 weeks.
PREC: Dexamethasone reduces incidence of hyaline membrane disease.
PROG: Birth weight:
<500g — survival 10%.
500–750g — 50%.
750–1000g — 66%.
1000–1500g — 90%.
Figures vary widely between centres.

Lactation Suppression

THER: 1. Prevent nipple stimulation.

2. Diuretics.
3. Bromocriptine.
4. Oral contraceptives.
PREC: Oestrogens should not be used because of the
        increased risk of thromboembolism.

Larva Migrans
See Cutaneous Larva Migrans

Laryngotracheobronchitis
See Croup

Lead Poisoning, Acute
THER: 1. Gastric lavage with 1% sodium sulphate
        solution, leaving some in stomach.
        2. Calcium disodium edetate IV.
        3. Dimercaprol IM AND mannitol IV
        OR dexamethasone IV for encephalopathy.
PROG: Good. Renal damage in chronic cases.

Legionnaire's Disease
THER: Erythromycin orally or IVI
        ADD rifampicin orally.
PROG: 12% mortality with Legionella pneumonia;
        occasional pulmonary, neurological and mental
        sequelae.

Leg Ulcers
See Venous Leg Ulcer

Leptospirosis
THER: Penicillin IMI daily for a week. Only effective
        early in illness. Higher doses may be necessary
        OR tetracycline
        OR erythromycin
        ADD renal dialysis in late stages.
PROG: Good except with renal involvement.

Leukaemia, Acute Lymphoblastic
THER: **Acute:**
        Prednisolone orally daily
        AND vincristine
        AND allopurinol to prevent hyperuricaemia
        AND high fluid intake
        ADD packed cell transfusions for anaemia
        ADD L-asparaginase OR daunorubicin
        OR doxorubicin OR other cytotoxics.
        Continuing:
        Many different drug schedules varying in
        complexity, but usually containing several drugs
        on a rotating routine, eg. mercaptopurine,
        methotrexate etc. Continued for 2–3 years.
        Relapse:
        As for acute stage PLUS bone marrow
        transplantation
        AND/OR radiotherapy
        AND/OR intrathecal methotrexate.

PREC: Immunosuppressive and cytotoxic drugs – bone
        marrow depression, intercurrent infections,
        neutropenia, neurological deterioration,
        alopecia.
PROG: Extremely viable. 90% initial remission, 40%+
        cure rate; 5–10% develop meningeal leukaemia.

Leukaemia, Acute Myeloid
THER: 1. Intensive combination cytotoxic drug therapy,
        eg. anthracycline, cytarabine.
        2. Intrathecal cytarabine or methotrexate.
        3. Red cell, granulocyte and platelet
        transfusions as indicated.
        4. Active prevention and treatment of infection.
        These may be fatal. Reverse barrier nursing
        essential.
        5. Immunotherapy.
        6. Bone marrow transplants
PROG: 20% 3 year survival, 50% 12 month survival.

Leukaemia, Chronic Lymphoid
THER: 1. Chlorambucil OR cyclophosphamide in short
        courses.
        2. Prednisolone.
        3. Radiotherapy.
        4. Prophylactic antibiotics.
        5. Blood transfusions as indicated.
        6. Human immunoglobulin IMI (controversial).
PROG: Slow progression of disease to death almost
        inevitable. Treatment does not usually affect
        course, but may reduce lymphoid mass and
        help symptoms. Occurs only in elderly.

Leukaemia, Chronic Myeloid
THER: 1. Busulfan AND thioguanine
        OR hydroxyurea.
        2. Radiotherapy of specific organs.
        3. Splenectomy (controversial).
        4. Vincristine and prednisolone in patients with
        lymphoid blastic transformation.
PREC: Neutropenia and infection common.
PROG: Median survival 3.5 years.

Lice
See Pediculosis

Lichen Planus
THER: 1. Topical corticosteroids eg.
        fluocinomide/halcinonide.
        2. Psoralens plus long-wave untraviolet light
        (PUVA).
        3. Oral prednisone
        4. Tretinoin AND/OR corticosteroid cream
        under occlusion.
        5. Intralesional corticosteroids
        6. Oral Isotretinoin OR acetretin.
        7. Dapsone OR griseofulvin OR antimalarials.
        8. Oral cyclosporin A
PREC: Oral isotretinoin amd acetretin teratogenic.

PROG: Usually a benign self-limiting disease. May persist for months or years. Neoplastic degeneration of oral lesions known.

Listeriosis

THER: Amoxycillin OR penicillin
ADD gentamicin.
PROG: Good in adults and older children. Poor in infants and with meningo-encephalitis. Transmitted by contaminated food (eg. soft cheeses, raw meat) particularly from mother to infant at birth, and the immunocompromised.

Liver Disease

See Cholecystitis, Acute; Cirrhosis, Primary Biliary; Hepatic Carcinoma; Hepatitis Abscess; Hepatitis, Acute Viral

Lung Carcinoma

THER: Surgical resection and radiotherapy
AND/OR cytotoxic chemotherapy for oat-cell forms, eg. methotrexate, vincristine, cyclophosphamide, etc
AND/OR immunotherapy (controversial).
PROG: 40% 1 year survival, 15% 5 year survival. Worse with oat-cell carcinomas.

Lung Diseases

See Asthma; Asbestosis; Bronchitis Pneumothorax; Bronchiolitis; Bronchiectasis; Lung Carcinoma; Pulmonary Abscess; Pulmonary Embolism; Respiratory Distress Syndrome, Infantile; Tuberculosis

Lupus Erythematosus, Systemic [SLE]

THER: 1. Emotional support.
2. Avoid sun exposure.
3. Prednisone OR NSAIDs
ADD chloroquine OR mepacrine
ADD immunosuppressive agents (eg. azathioprine, cyclophosphamide, chlorambucil)
ADD warfarin for abnormal clotting
ADD danazol for thrombocytopenia.
PREC: Avoid salicylates. Eye checks regularly while using antimalarials.
PROG: Significant morbidity, 97% 5 year survival.

Lyme Disease

THER: Penicillins
OR ceftriaxone IVI
OR tetracyclines.
PROG: Good if treated early. Chronic arthritis may occur if left untreated. Caused by tick transmitted spirochaetae.

Lymphoedema

THER: 1. Elevation of affected limb when at rest.
2. Intensive prolonged massage in direction of lymphatic drainage. Control proximal lymphoedema before treating more distal areas.
3. Skin care to prevent infection and improve skin tone.
4. Compression bandages and/or stockings.
5. Regular prolonged exercise.
6. Sequential pumps and compression devices.
7. Benzopyrones.
8. Surgery in carefully selected patients with specific small areas involved.
PROG: With combination of therapies most patients will obtain at least 50% reduction in affected limb circumference.

Lymphogranuloma Venereum

THER: Doxycycline OR minocycline OR erythromycin OR sulphadiazine
AND analgesics
AND drain fluctuant buboes
ADD sulfadiazine for bacterial complications
ADD anorectal surgery if required.
PREC: Lymphatic blockage may cause gross disfigurement of external genitalia.
PROG: Good if treatment prompt, delayed treatment leads to scarring and difficulty in eradicating *Chlamydia trachomatis* infection. Higher incidence of rectal carcinoma.

Lymphoma

See Hodgkin's Disease

Malaria

THER: **Prophylaxis:**
Start prophylaxis 2 weeks before entering area and continue for 4 weeks after leaving.
Most Tropical Areas:
— Chloroquine weekly
SE Asia, India, S America, SW Pacific.
High risk:
— Doxycycline
OR chloroquine
AND pyrimethamine
OR mefloquine
Low risk:
— Chloroquine AND proguanil
OR sulfadoxine with dapsone
AND pyrimethamine
(Risk factors higher with longer stay, wet season, staying outside cities, etc).
Treatment:
SEVERE MALARIA
Quinidine dihydrochloride IVI
AND maintain correct fluid and electrolyte balance.
UNCOMPLICATED MALARIA
Plasmodium malariae, vivax and ovale:
– Chloroquine orally OR IMI
P. falciparum:
– Quinine sulfate orally
AND pyrimethamine/sulfadoxine orally

OR doxycycline orally
LIVE INFECTIONS
Primaquine after blood infection eliminated
PREC: Dosage schedules complex. Refer to
manufacturer's literature. Higher dosages and
prolonged therapy may be required in resistant
cases. IV quinine use requires expert advice as
doses may be toxic.
PROG: Good if treated early; relapses may occur.

Mallory-Weiss Syndrome

THER: 1. Urgent intravenous replacement of fluids with
plasma expander and blood when available.
2. Balloon tamponade in emergency.
3. Gastroscopy to control bleeding once patient
stabilised.
4. Gastric lavage by nasogastric tube.
5. Antacids AND cimetidine OR ranitidine.
6. Surgical gastrotomy if bleeding persists.
PROG: Exsanguination from massive blood loss
possible in acute situation. Good prognosis
once bleeding controlled.

Manic-Depressive Disorders (Bipolar Disorder)

THER: 1. Tricyclic antidepressants
OR other antidepressant medication (see
separate entry).
2. Haloperidol
OR other antipsychotic medication.
3. Electroconvulsive therapy.
4. Lithium OR valproate OR carbamazepine for
long-term maintenance. Check plasma levels
regularly (see PATHOLOGY SECTION 4).
PROG: Good with adequate compliance. Cyclical and
episodic.

Mastalgia

THER: Diuretics (premenstrual mastalgia)
OR bromocriptine (severe cases)
OR progestogens (premenstrual tension and
dysmenorrhoea)
OR danazol (cystic breast disease)
OR pyridoxine.
PROG: Control reasonable; often recurrent.

Mastitis, Puerperal

THER: 1. Antipyretics AND analgesics.
2. Flucloxacillin
OR cephalexin
OR erythromycin
ADD flucloxacillin IV.
3. Drain breast by breast pump regularly.
4. Incise and drain abscesses.
PROG: Good.

Mastoiditis

THER: 1. Obtain pus for culture if possible.
2. Amoxycillin OR flucloxacillin IMI or IVI

3. Surgical drainage of mastoid.
4. Alter antibiotic on culture result.
5. Long-term antibiotic treatment often necessary.
PROG: Generally satisfactory, often chronic.

Measles (Morbilli)

THER: None specific. Penicillin or erythromycin for
secondary bacterial complications. Vaccination
available.
PROG: Good. Pneumonia, otitis media and encephalitis
may occur. Infectious from onset of prodromal
symptoms until 4 days after start of rash.

Megaloblastic Anaemia

See Pernicious Anaemia

Melanoma

THER: 1. Wide excision of primary lesion.
2. Surgical removal of draining lymph nodes.
3. Immunotherapy with allogenic or autologous
vaccines (experimental).
PROG: Five year survival depends on tumour thickness.
<0.75mm – 99%
0.75 to 2.5mm – 85%
2.5 to 4.0mm – 70%
>4.0mm – 44%
Disseminated melanoma – 6%

Melioidosis

THER: Ceftazidime IMI
OR ticarcillin IMI
OR tetracycline IMI
OR kanamycin IMI
ADD chloramphenicol IMI OR orally
ADD surgery for localised lung lesions.
PROG: 6 to 12 months treatment necessary. 50%
mortality with septicaemia.

Menière's Disease (Menière's Syndrome)

THER: 1. Stop smoking.
2. Stop caffeine (eg. coffee, tea, colas).
2. Avoid alcohol.
4. Low sodium, high potassium diet.
5. Medications:
Amitriptyline
AND/OR diphenhydrinate
AND/OR betahistine*
OR antihistamines* orally or IM
OR prochlorperazine
AND/OR meclizine
AND/OR atropine sulfate IM
AND/OR diuretics
AND/OR oxpentifyline
6. Tinnitus masker
7. Endolymph surgery.
PREC: *Betahistine, antihistamines and
prochlorperazine interact adversely.
PROG: Poorly controlled, significant morbidity.
Spontaneous recovery common.

Meningioma

See Intracranial Tumour

Meningitis, Bacterial (Septic Meningitis)

THER: 1. CSF and/or blood culture.
2. **Neonate:**
Cefotaxime AND penicillin
OR aminoglycoside AND ampicillin.
Child:
Ampicillin
AND chloramphenicol
OR cefotaxime or ceftriaxone IM or IV.
Adult:
Ampicillin 400mg/kg AND chloramphenicol
100mg/kg per day OR cefotaxime or ceftriaxone
IM or IV.
3. Change to specific antibiotic when culture
results available.
4. Anticonvulsants if fitting.
5. Prednisone (controversial).
PROG: Mortality rate 5–30%, higher with children and
pneumococcal meningitis.

See also Meningococcal Infections

Meningitis, Viral (Aseptic Meningitis)

THER: 1. Exclude bacterial form by lumbar puncture
and CSF microscopy and culture.
2. No specific therapy, symptomatic and
supportive treatment only.
PROG: Very good.

Meningococcal Infections

THER: **Treatment:**
Penicillin G IV in large doses
OR ceftriaxone
OR chloramphenicol
AND maintain fluid and electrolyte balance.
Prophylaxis:
Vaccination
OR oral rifampicin
OR ceftriaxone.
PROG: Infection most common in children under five
years of age. Incubation period 3–4 days.
Vaccination takes some weeks to be effective.
98% mortality within 48 hours without
antibiotics, <10% mortality with appropriate
antibiotic treatment. Neurological sequelae now
rare.

Menopause

THER: Nil, unless symptoms distressing then:
conjugated oestrogens cyclically orally
OR oestradiol patches
OR oestradiol implants
OR oestriol cyclically
AND norethisterone acetate for last 5–7 days of
cycle
ADD diuretics for oedema
ADD antidepressants if necessary

ADD clonidine for flushing.
PREC: Long-term use of oestrogens may lead to higher
incidence of endometrial carcinoma, this
problem usually overcome by addition of
progestogen at end of cycle.
PROG: Symptoms may be difficult to control.

Menorrhagia

THER: Norethisterone days 15–25 of cycle
OR oestrogen/progestogen combination pills
(oral contraceptives) cyclically.
OR tranexamic acid during menstruation.

See also Dysmenorrhoea

Menstrual Disorders

*See Dysmenorrhoea; Endometriosis; Fertility Control;
Infertility, Female; Menopause; Menorrhagia*

Mercury Poisoning, Acute (Heavy Metal Poisoning)

THER: 1. Copious egg whites and milk.
2. Gastric lavage.
3. D-penicillamine OR dimercaprol.
4. Fluid replacement.
5. Haemodialysis.
PROG: Good in acute, severe morbidity in chronic.
Mean lethal dose $HgCl_2$ 70mg.

Mesothelioma

See Asbestosis

Migraine

THER: **Acute:**
1. Rest in dark room.
2. Aspirin in high doses OR paracetamol
OR naproxen in high doses.
3. Sumatriptan OR naratriptan OR zolmitriptan.
4. Prochlorperazine
OR metoclopramide
OR chlorpromazine parenterally, rectally or IMI
with additional fluids.
5. Ergotamine tartrate orally.
6. Diazepam IM or orally.
7. IV-dihydroergotamine.
8. Pentazocine OR pethidine IM in moderate
doses, infrequently, for intractable cases.
9. Demerol sparingly.
Prophylaxis:
1. Avoid precipitants, eg. stress, foods, drugs.
2. Methysergide
OR clonidine
OR pizotifen
OR bellergal
OR beta-blocker (eg. propranolol)
OR calcium channel blocker (eg. verapamil)
OR phenelzine and other MAOIs
OR tricyclic (eg. amitryptyline)
OR NSAID (eg. naproxen).

PREC: Do not give ergotamine or sumatriptan within 12 hours of each other. Sumatriptan — care with heart disease. Narcotics — beware of dependency; addicts often use migraine as excuse to obtain supply.

PROG: Frequency and severity tend to decrease with age. Onset unusual over 40 years. Spontaneous remissions common. Prophylaxis often successful.

Migrainous Neuralgia
See Cluster Headache

Mole, Invasive Uterine
See Choriocarcinoma and Invasive Moles

Molluscum Contagiosum
THER: Leave lesions to settle spontaneously OR incison, curettage or diathermy of lesions AND cantharidin solution.

PROG: Spontaneous resolution after 3–18 months; mildly infectious.

Moniliasis
See Candidiasis, Vaginal and Oral ; Tinea

Mononucleosis
See Infectious Mononucleosis

Morbilli
See Measles

Morning After' Pill
See Fertility Control

Morning Sickness (Hyperemesis Gravidarum)
THER: 1. Dietary advice — frequent dry meals.
2. Concentrated carbohydrate solution (eg. emetrol).
3. Pyridoxine hydrochloride
OR meclozine
OR promethazine
OR doxylamine succinate and pyridoxine hydrochloride
ADD acupuncture (controversial)
ADD IV fluids and hospitalisation for hyperemesis gravidarum.

PROG: Nausea occurs in 80% of pregnancies. Only 20% persist beyond 14 weeks. Only 1% develop hyperemesis gravidarum.

Motor Neurone Disease
THER: No cure possible. Management of specific symptoms using physiotherapists, dietitians, speech therapists, psychologists, occupational therapists and nurses as well as doctors. Tricyclic antidepressants for depression. Oxygen therapy for hypoxia from poor respiratory muscle function. Fluid diet to cope with dehydration and dysphagia. Nasogastric tube may be required. Anticholinergics to reduce dribbling and salivation. Careful posturing and physiotherapy to avoid food or mucus aspiration. Baclofen AND/OR diazepam for spasticity. Communication aids for dysarthria (eg computers). Surgery of selected patients (eg tracheostomy, gastrostomy).

PROG: Slowly progressive with remissions and relapses. Death due to respiratory problems or suicide. Complicated by dehydration and malnutrition.

Mountain Sickness
See Altitude Sickness

Mouth Ulcers (Aphthous Ulcers)
THER: 1. Stop smoking.
2. Check for causes, eg dentures, Diabetes, drugs (eg. tetracycline), Crohn's disease, pernicious anaemia, iron deficit.
3. Benzocaine and other local anaesthetic lotions, pastes and lozenges.
4. Carboxymethylcellulose paste.
5. Triamcinolone 0.1% or other steroid pastes or pellets.
6. Antiseptic mouthwashes (eg chlorhexidine, hydrogen peroxide, povidone-iodine).
7. Antifungal lozenges or paints.
8. Tetracycline mouth rinse.
9. Prednisone tablets orally.

PROG: Often recurrent, but attacks self-limiting.

Multiple Myeloma
See Myelomatosis

Multiple Sclerosis
THER: **Acute:**
Prednisone orally
OR methylprednisolone pulse therapy
OR interferon beta 1b.
Chronic:
Diazepam OR baclofen for spasms
AND treat intercurrent infections aggressively
AND carbamazepine for neuralgia
AND avoid temperature changes
AND have adequate rest periods
AND physiotherapy
AND appropriate sphincter management
AND informed counselling

PREC: Doubtful claims of efficacy for many drugs.

PROG: Unpredictable course with variable remission periods. Average survival after diagnosis 25–35 years. Significant morbidity.

Mumps

THER: None specific, supportive and symptomatic measures only. Vaccine available.
PROG: Good. Orchitis occurs in 25% of adult males. Meningitis, pancreatitis, oophoritis may occur. Infectious from 3 days before paratoid swelling starts to 7 days after.

Myalgic Encephalomyelitis

See Chronic Fatigue Syndrome

Myasthenia Gravis

THER: Neostigmine orally or IMI
AND/OR ephedrine sulphate
ADD intermittent positive pressure respiration if acute; tracheostomy may be needed
AND maintain fluid and electrolyte balance
OR steroid therapy (selected cases)
ADD azathioprine
ADD thymectomy by surgery or radiation.
PREC: Beware of drug side-effects mimicking myasthenia gravis, eg neostigmine overdose.
PROG: Spontaneous remissions and relapses. Sudden death from myasthenic crisis possible.

Mycoplasma Pneumonia

THER: 1. Take sputum for culture to confirm diagnosis before starting antibiotics.
2. Erythromycin
OR tetracyclines.
3. Bronchodilators.
4. Chest physiotherapy.
PREC: Beware of specific antibiotic sensitivities. Disease may cause haemolytic anaemia.
PROG: Good with correct treatment. Often responsible for chronic lung infections in young adults.

Mycoses

See Aspergillosis; Candidiasis; Cryptococcosis

Myelofibrosis

THER: Symptomatic treatment only:
1. Folic acid AND/OR pyridoxine for anaemia.
2. Oxymetholone for severe anaemia.
3. Myelosuppressive therapy in selected patients.
4. Splenectomy in selected patients.
5. Blood transfusion *in extremis*.
PREC: Splenectomy — thrombocytopenia. Acute 'blastic' crisis may occur due to thrombocytopenia and haemolytic anaemia. Beware of haemorrhages and secondary infection.
PROG: Average survival 3 years from diagnosis.

Myelomatosis (Multiple Myeloma)

THER: 1. Variable combinations of one or more cytotoxic drugs, eg vincristine, melphalan, cyclophosphamide, prednisone.
2. Irradiation of specific areas.
3. Decompression operations.
4. Physiotherapy.
5. High fluid intake AND mannitol in selected patients.
6. Transfusion for anaemia if severe.
7. Analgesia.
PROG: Five-year survival 20%, 18-month survival 50%.

Myocardial Infarct

THER: **On suspected diagnosis:**
1. Glyceryl trinitrate sublingual tablet OR spray.
2. Insert intravenous line.
3. Morphine IMI or IVI.
4. Prochlorperazine OR metoclopramide IVI to prevent vomiting.
5. Oxygen.
6. Soluble aspirin sublingually if conscious
7. Atropine IVI for bradycardia and shock.
8. Lignocaine IVI for ventricular arrhythmias provided pulse rate above 50/min.
9. Frusemide IVI for left heart failure or hypertension provided systolic pressure above 90mmHg.
On diagnosis and hospital admission:
1. Monitor all functions in intensive care. Take blood for cardiac enzymes.
2. Oxygen.
3. Atropine IVI for bradycardia
ADD pacemaker if persistent.
4. Verapamil IVI slowly for paroxysmal atrial tachycardia. Digoxin if needed, provided no heart block present for atrial flutter/fibrillation.
5. Lignocaine IVI stat then as IV infusion for ventricular ectopics and tachycardia.
6. Electrical cardioversion immediately for ventricular fibrillation* or atrial fibrillation with haemodynamic compromise.
7. Dopamine IVI for hypotension.
8. Thrombolytic (eg. streptokinase), early.
9. Pacemaker for second degree or severe heart block.
Continuing hospital management:
1. Strict bed rest 24–48 hours; gradually mobilise to full activity over 5–7 days.
2. Light diet and mild laxative.
3. Heparinisation in selected patients to prevent pulmonary emboli and after thrombolysis consider a β-blocker as long-term prophylaxis.
4. Diazepam for anxiety.
5. Test cardiac enzymes daily x 3 days.
6. Discharge at 6–8 days if no complications.
After discharge:
1. Reduce risk factors.
2. Exercise test.
3. Maintain beta-blocker compliance by regular visits.
4. Aspirin in low doses long-term.
5. Keep blood cholesterol level within normal limits.

PROG: 40% fatal in one hour, 15% fatal in next 2 days. Higher rates over 75 years, with left ventricular failure, large Q waves, large enzyme release, persistent tachycardia, cardiomegaly, prolonged hypotension.

See also Cardiac Arrest

Myocarditis

THER: **Bacterial:**
Penicillin IVI or other suitable antibiotic as selected by blood culture.
Viral or Toxic:
1. Bed rest.
2. Diuretics as required.
3. Antiarrhythmic drugs as required.
4. Steroid therapy if deteriorating (not proven).
5. Pacemaker if necessary.

PROG: Bacterial — good. Other — significant morbidity and mortality.

Myxoedema
See Hypothyroidism

Nail Infection
See Onychogryphosis; Onychomycosis; Paronychia

Narcolepsy

THER: Amphetamines in slowly increasing doses AND/OR tricyclic and antidepressants.
PREC: Care must be taken to prevent danger to self or others (eg. car driving).
PROG: Variable. Control often difficult. No cure.

Narcotic Addiction

THER: 1. Detoxification in hospital, under close outpatient supervision or in specialised unit. Screen for hepatitis B and C, and AIDS. Correct malnutrition and intercurrent illnesses.
2. Methadone programme. Dosage slowly decreased.
3. Extensive counselling by trained professionals who are available for crisis situations.
4. Self-help groups.
PREC: Methadone — urinalysis advisable to monitor compliance, care in use with asthmatics and in pregnancy.
PROG: Extremely variable depending on motivation of patient and devotion of therapist.

Narcotic Poisoning
THER: Naloxone IVI; repeat if necessary.
PREC: Beware of withdrawal symptoms. Respiratory depression likely.
PROG: Good.

Nausea
See Vomiting
See also SYMPTOMS SECTION 1

Needle Stick Injury

THER: 1. Wash area immediately and thoroughly while expressing blood through puncture wound
2. Immerse wound in antiseptic solution (eg. povidone-iodine)
3. baseline testing for hepatitis B and C, HIV.
4. Hepatitis B vaccine if not vaccinated
5. Consider administration of zidovudine or other anti-HIV medication
6. With consent, test suspect individual initially in contact with needle for hepatitis B and C, and HIV
7. Repeat testing for hepatitis B and C, and HIV after 3 and 6 months
PREC: Negative results of testing in suspect individual do not exclude disease in early stage. Practice safe sex until follow-up test negative
PROG: Risk of developing HIV 1:250, hepatitis B 1:2 and hepatitis C 1:20 in a needle stick injury from a patient with these diseases

Nematode Infestation
See Toxocariasis

Neoplasm
See Cancer

Nephrotic Syndrome
THER: 1. Strict, prolonged bed rest.
2. High calorie, moderate protein, low sodium diet.
3. Frusemide
OR ethacrynic acid
AND spironolactone
OR amiloride.
4. Salt-free albumin infusions.
5. Maintain electrolyte balance.
PROG: Depends on cause. Membranous nephropathy has worst prognosis at 75% five-year survival if not dialysed.

Neuralgia
See Trigeminal Neuralgia

Neurosis
See Obsessive Compulsive Neurosis

Non-Specific Urethritis [NSU] (Non-Gonoccocal Urethritis [NGU])

THER: Azithromycin
OR minocycline
OR doxycycline

AND treat sexual partner(s).
PREC: Exclude other forms of venereal disease.
PROG: 85% cure; relapses common.

NSU

See Non-Specific Urethritis

Obesity

THER: 1. Diet. Restrict intake to 4200 kJ/d under maintenance level. 1 kg fat contains 37,800 kJ.
2. Exercise. Increase slowly to significant levels. 420kJ consumed by 20 min. walking, 17 min. tennis, swimming 400 m in 9 min., cycling @ 20 kph for 9 min, running @ 16 kph for 5 min.
3. Anorectic drugs to suppress appetite, eg. fenfluramine, mazindol, diethylpropion
4. Dexfenfluramine
5. Behaviour or group therapy.
6. Fasting under medical supervision with fluid, protein, vitamin and mineral supplements.
7. Jaw wiring (controversial).
8. Surgery — gastric stapling, vagotomy, jejuno-ileostomy, gastric banding (controversial).
9. Acupuncture (controversial).
PREC: Surgery — significant morbidity.
PROG: Mortality rate doubles with body/mass index over 35 kg/m^2.

Obsessive Compulsive Neurosis

THER: 1. Close liaison with supportive doctor.
2. Clomipramine long-term and in high doses that are reached by slow increases.
OR other tricyclic antidepressants
OR SSRI (eg. paroxetine, fluoxetine, fluvoxamine)
OR MAOIs.
3. Psychotherapy.
4. Behavioural therapy. Rituals should not be supported by family members or therapist.
PREC: MAOIs — dangerous reactions with certain foods and drugs.
PROG: Poor; long-term therapy usually required.

Oesophageal Spasm

THER: 1. Exclude cardiac or pulmonary disease.
2. Glyceryl trinitrate OR isosorbide dinitrate sublingually for acute attacks.
3. Hyoscine butylbromide
OR benzodiazepines for prophylaxis.
4. Cardiomyotomy if uncontrolled.
PREC: Glyceryl trinitrate and isosorbide dinitrate — headache, flushing.
PROG: Depends on cause.

Oesophagitis

See Reflux Oesophagitis

Onychogryphosis

THER: Careful clipping. Special gloves.

2. Griseofulvin orally
OR terbinafine orally
OR fluconazole orally
AND ticonazole lotion
PREC: Cholestatic jaundice may occur with all but griseofulvin. Medication must be given longterm
PROG: Complete resolution in only 30% after 12 months treatment.

Onychomycosis

THER: Amorolfine topically
OR terbinafine orally
OR itraconazole orally.
PROG: Good. Longterm treatment required

Oral Contraceptives

See Fertility Control

Orchitis

See Epididymo-Orchitis

Orf

THER: None specific. Antibiotics for secondary infections of lesions.
PROG: Excellent.

Organophosphate Poisoning (Insecticides)

THER: 1. Pralidoxime IVI slowly, repeat in one hour.
2. Atropine IVI stat, then every 10 minutes as necessary. Large doses may be required.
3. Artificial respiration.
PREC: Atropine — increases intraocular pressure.
PROG: Dose related.

Osteoarthritis

THER: 1. Structured activity programme and physiotherapy.
2. Analgesics, eg. aspirin OR paracetamol
AND/OR dextropropoxyphene
AND/OR codeine.
3. NSAIDs.
4. Intra-articular steroid injections.
5. Psychotherapeutic drugs (eg. tricyclics)
6. Surgery, particularly for hip.
PREC: See under Rheumatoid Arthritis.
PROG: No mortality, significant morbidity. Usually slowly progressive despite therapy.

Osteomalacia and Rickets

THER: 1. Calciferol orally or IMI.
2. Ultraviolet light.
3. Vitamin D supplements.
4. Phosphate supplements.
PROG: Good, but often very slow to control.

Osteomyelitis

THER: 1. Blood and needle taps of bone sent for culture

(*S. aureus* common cause).
2. Flucloxacillin OR cefotaxime IV.
3. Switch to appropriate antibiotic after culture result received (eg. cephalosporins, benzylpenicillin).
4. Surgical drainage of affected parts.
5. Immobilisation of affected parts.

PROG: Very good with proper treatment. Poor without treatment.

Osteoporosis

THER: 1. Exercise programme.
2. Analgesics, eg. paracetamol
AND/OR aspirin
AND/OR codeine.
3. Female — cyclical oestrogen therapy.
Male — testosterone enanthate.
4. Disodium etidronate OR alendronate sodium OR salcatonin
5. Effervescent calcium
OR other calcium compounds (eg. calcium gluconate)
AND/OR calcium fortified dairy products.
6. Vitamin D (calciferol).
7. Sodium fluoride.
8. Calcitonin.
9. Raloxifene (post-menopausal women)
10. Nandrolone IM every 2 to 4 weeks.
11. Thiazide diuretic (controversial).

PROG: Successful treatment prevents progression of disease. Existing bone damage cannot be corrected.

Otitis Externa

THER: 1. Thoroughly clean external canal.
2. Antibiotic/corticosteroid otic drops.
3. Antibiotic/corticosteroid otic wick.
4. Oral steroids short-term for acute swelling.
5. Promethazine or other antihistamines for itch.
6. Oral antibiotics for middle ear spread.
7. 5% acetic acid in 50% alcohol drops as prophylaxis after swimming.

PREC: Beware of infection in diabetics.
PROG: Good, but may become recurrent.

Otitis Media

THER: Amoxycillin ± clavulanic acid
OR doxycycline
OR cefaclor
AND adequate oral analgesia (eg. aspirin and codeine) and aural analgesia (eg. lignocaine or benzocaine drops)
ADD nasal decongestants, eg. oxymetazoline or xylometazoline drops
ADD myringotomy if progressive.

PROG: May progress to mastoiditis, labyrinthitis, or meningitis if inadequately treated. 'Glue ear' (serous otitis media) may result from inadequate resolution.

See also Glue Ear

Overactivity, Paediatric (Hyperactivity)

THER: 1. Exclude pathological cause in child or parents.
2. Exclude misbehaviour and impulsivity.
3. Parent and teacher counselling.
4. Behaviour modification by psychologist.
5. Psychotherapy by psychiatrist.
6. Methylphenidate.
7. Haloperidol.

PREC: No substantive evidence to support use of specific diets.
PROG: Good in long-term.

Paget's Disease of Bone

THER: Analgesics, eg. aspirin OR paracetamol
AND/OR codeine
AND/OR biphosphonate drugs
OR calcitonin
OR pamidronate IV
OR glucagon
OR mithramycin
OR actinomycin.

PROG: Severe morbidity with bone and cardiac complications. Life expectancy significantly reduced.

Pain, Severe, Terminal Disease

THER: 1. Identify individual areas, types and causes of pain.
2. Arrange adequate social and psychological support.
3. Physiotherapy, eg. transcutaneous electrical nerve stimulation, massage, manipulation, heat.
4. Allow conscious patient to manage own analgesic requirements.
5. Aspirin AND/OR paracetamol.
6. Dextropropoxyphene and paracetamol.
7. NSAIDs.
8. Codeine.
9. Narcotics (eg. morphine, pethidine) orally, rectally, IM or IV.
10. Benzodiazepines AND/OR tricyclic antidepressants.
11. Radiotherapy for bone pain:
12. Carbamezapine OR clonazepam for neuralgia.
13. Baclofen for muscle spasm.
14. Elevate and strap oedematous limbs.
15. Prednisone OR dexamethasone.
16. Intrathecal narcotics or anaesthetics.
17. Surgical nerve destruction.

PROG: Adequate pain control should be available for all patients with terminal disease.

PAN

See Polyarteritis Nodosa

Pancreatitis, Acute

THER: 1. Relieve shock with intravenous fluids (avoid

sodium overload), calcium gluconate IVI and insulin for hyperglycaemia.
2. Plasma or blood transfusion.
3. Relieve pain with pethidine IMI.
4. Nasogastric suction.
5. Oxygen and parenteral frusemide for respiratory distress; ventilation may be necessary.
6. Antibiotics for intercurrent sepsis.
7. Surgery in carefully selected patients with fulminating pancreatitis (pancreatectomy), gall stone pancreatitis and pancreatic pseudocyst.
8. Diet — low fat, no alcohol, high protein, vitamin supplements.

PREC: Beware of delayed pulmonary oedema, renal failure, abscess formation.

PROG: Mortality 20% overall; higher with elderly, hypotension, oliguria, uraemia, hypoxia, disseminated intravascular coagulation.

Panhypopituitarism

See Hypopituitarism

Panic Attacks

THER: **Prevention:**
beta-blockers (eg. propranolol)
AND/OR alprazolam
AND/OR imipramine
AND/OR phenelzine
AND psychotherapy
OR behavioural therapy.
Treatment:
Paroxetine
OR benzodiazepines (eg. diazepam, oxazepam)
AND supportive therapy.

Paracetamol Poisoning

THER: 1. Take blood for S. paracetamol levels.
2. Gastric lavage if within 4 hours of ingestion.
3. N-acetylcysteine IVI AND methionine orally as soon as possible, and within 15 hours of poisoning.
4. Assess liver function regularly.

PREC: N-acetylcysteine — anaphylactoid reactions in 5%.

PROG: Significant liver damage (up to 10% of cases admitted to hospital) and death possible (up to 2% of cases admitted to hospital) with high-dose paracetamol poisoning (eg. in excess of 150–250 mg/kg). Urgent treatment essential.

Paralysis Agitans

See Parkinson's Disease

Parathyroid Disease

See Hyperparathyroidism; Hypoparathyroidism

Parkinson's Disease

THER: Selegiline
OR levodopa/carbidopa
OR levodopa/benserazide
AND bromocriptine
OR pergolide
OR benztropine
OR trihexyphenidyl
OR amantadine.
ADD benzhexol
OR biperiden
OR orphenadrine
OR procyclidine
OR tolcapone
ADD apomorphine IM for severe episodes
All patients:
Physiotherapy
Consider neurosurgery in selected patients.
Experimental procedures include pallidotomy, stimulators, transplants and neurotrophic factors.

PREC: All drugs act synergistically. Use controlled release preparations (CR) when possible.

PROG: Slowly progressive. Depression common. Amelioration usually adequate. Environmental aetiology probable.

Paronychia, Acute (Infection of Periungal Tissue)

THER: 1. Oral antibiotics (eg. cephalexin).
2. Topical fusidic acid cream.

PROG: Good. May be recurrent if treatment not complete or nails allowed to become wet.

Paronychia, Chronic (Infection of Periungal Tissue)

THER: 1. Keep nail dry and clean by use of cotton lined gloves if necessary. Avoid detergent exposure.
2. Drying agents to nail (eg. chloroform, Betadine, surgical spirit).
3. Miconazole to nail if yeast present.
4. Ketoconazole orally for yeast.
5. Wedge resection of nail and bed for recurrent infections and ingrown nail.

PROG: Good. May be recurrent if treatment not complete or nails allowed to become wet.

Paroxysmal Atrial Supraventricular Tachycardia [PAT]

THER: **Acute:**
Verapamil IV slowly
ADD cardioversion by DC shock.
Prophylaxis:
Verapamil
OR metoprolol
OR sotalol
OR propanolol
OR digoxin.

PROG: Very good.

Paroxysmal Ventricular Tachycardia

THER: Lignocaine IVI stat
ADD cardioversion by DC shock
THEN propranolol
OR amiodarone.
PREC: Avoid digoxin.
PROG: Depends on cause, often accompanies
myocardial infarct.

Pediculosis (Lice, Crabs)

THER: Topical lindane
OR permethrin
OR maldison
OR 1% gamma benzene hexachloride
AND fine comb affected hair
AND treat other family members and sexual
partner(s).
PREC: Gamma benzene hexachloride — avoid eyes
and mucous membranes.
PROG: Good.

Pelvic Inflammatory Disease and Salpingitis

THER: Doxycycline orally
AND metronidazole
OR tinidazole orally
AND analgesia with hypnotics and narcotics if
necessary
ADD ciprofloxacin orally
ADD cefotaxime IV
ADD surgical drainage of abscess
ADD hysterectomy if intractable.
PHYS: Often chronic. Infertility may ensue. Significant
morbidity.

See also INVESTIGATIONS SECTION 3

Pemphigoid, Bullous

THER: Prednisone orally
ADD azathioprine
OR methotrexate
OR cyclophosphamide.
PREC: Disease may recur if dose of steroids reduced
too rapidly.
PROG: Maintenance therapy often required.

Pemphigus, Vulgaris

THER: Prednisone orally
ADD azathioprine
OR methotrexate
OR cyclophosphamide.
PREC: Disease may recur if dose of steroids reduced
too rapidly.
PROG: Maintenance therapy often required.

Peptic Ulcer

THER: 1. Stop smoking. Restrict alcohol, salicylates
and NSAIDs.
2. Antacid liquids or tablets in high doses, eg.
magnesium trisilicate, aluminium hydroxide.

3. H_2-receptor antagonists (eg. famotidine,
nizatidine, ranitidine)
OR misoprostol
OR colloidal bismuth
OR sucralfate
OR carbenoxolone.
4. Proton pump inhibitors (eg. lansoprazole,
omeprazine, pantoprazole).
5. Triple therapy for *Helicobacter pylori* infection
(eg. colloidal bismuth, tetracycline and
metronidazole
OR proton pump inhibitor, amoxycillin and
clarithromycin).
6. Surgery (eg. vagotomy, antrectomy,
pyloroplasty, gastro-jejunostomy).
7. Acute bleeding ulcer treated by
hospitalisation, transfusion, sedation,
parenteral cimetidine
OR ranitidine.
8. Surgery if unresponsive or recurrent despite
conservative treatment.
PREC: Nausea common with triple therapy. Exclude
malignancy, particularly with gastric ulcer.
PROG: Good; relapses common.

Pericarditis, Acute

THER: 1. Treat underlying condition, eg. myocardial
infarct, rheumatic fever, viraemia, TB,
septicaemia.
2. Analgesia if viral or idiopathic, then aspirin.
3. Hydrocortisone.
4. Surgical pericardial paracentesis if effusion
with tamponade.
PREC: Beware of long-term steroid use. Great skill and
care required for paracentesis.
PROG: Depends on cause. Viral and bacterial forms
have good prognosis.

Perioral Dermatitis

THER: 1. Moisturisers
2. Oral antibiotics (eg. tetracycline, doxycycline,
erythromycin)
3. Hydrocortisone 1% cream
PREC: Avoid fluorinated steroid creams. Avoid
tetracyclines in pregnancy
PROG: Recurrences common

See also Rosacea

Peripheral Vascular Disease

See Claudication

Pernicious Anaemia
(Megaloblastic Anaemia)

THER: 1. Vitamin B_{12}/hydroxycobalamin IMI twice
weekly initially, then every 1–3 months.
2. Folic acid after B_{12} levels stable.
3. Diuretics and digitalis for cardiac failure.
4. Iron supplements if needed.
PROG: Very good. Symptomatic recovery in 2–3 days,

haematological recovery in 4–6 weeks.
Continuous therapy required.

Pertussis (Whooping Cough)

THER: Erythromycin
AND symptomatic management (eg. paracetamol)
ADD gammaglobulin IMI in infants
ADD oxygen if paroxysms severe
ADD sedatives, (eg. phenobarbitone,
diazepam, promethazine) in small doses if
distressed or convulsing.
PREC: Antibiotics only useful prophylactically and are
not curative.
PROG: Mortality 0.5–1%, significant morbidity from
cerebral hypoxia and bronchiectasis.
Vaccination available.

Phaeochromocytoma

THER: Surgery.
Pre- and post-operative care difficult.
Pre-Op: Phenoxybenzamine or labetalol.
Post-Op: Noradrenaline and cortisone
ADD propranolol or labetalol for arrhythmias.
PREC: Hypertensive crises may occur. Several
tumours may be present.
PROG: Significant operative mortality. Post-operative
prognosis excellent. Medical management
alone difficult and life expectancy without
surgery is limited.

Pharyngitis, Bacterial

THER: Phenoxymethylpenicillin
OR amoxycillin ± clavulanic acid
OR erythromycin
OR other appropriate antibiotics
AND rest with adequate fluid intake
AND analgesia, eg. aspirin OR paracetamol
AND soothing gargles
ADD tonsillectomy and adenoidectomy if chronic.
PREC: Watch for quinsy or other abscess formation.
PROG: Excellent.

Phenylketonuria

THER: Low phenylalanine diet commenced within one
month of birth until 8+ years of age.
PROG: Good if detected early by Guthrie or similar test.
More common in Irish or Scots, rare in Blacks.
Infants not treated early suffer severe brain
damage.

Phobias

THER: 1. Behaviour therapy.
2. Anxiolytics (eg. benzodiazepines).
3. Beta-blockers to control physical symptoms.
PROG: Reasonable in most. Occasionally disabling.

PID

See Pelvic Inflammatory Disease

Pigmentation Defects

See Vitiligo

Piles

See Haemorrhoids

Pimples

See Acne

Pinworm

See Enterobiasis

Pityriasis Rosea

THER: None
OR oral antihistamines for irritation
AND/OR hydrocortisone cream.
ADD UVB phototherapy
PROG: Self-limiting disease. Clears in 6–10 weeks.
Recurs in 20%.

Pityriasis Versicolor (Tinea Versicolor)

THER: Selenium sulphide lotion
OR sodium thiosulfate 20% solution
OR clotrimazole cream or lotion
OR miconazole cream or lotion
OR ketoconazole cream
OR terbinafine cream
OR benzoic acid ointment.
ADD ketoconazole orally
ADD intraconazole orally
PROG: Good short-term, relapses very common.

Pneumoconiosis

See Asbestosis; Silicosis

Pneumonia, Bacterial

THER: 1. Obtain sputum or aspirate for culture.
2. **Community based treatment:**
Roxithromycin
OR erythromycin
OR amoxycillin ± clavulanic acid
OR doxycycline
OR cefaclor
Hospital based treatment:
Ceftriaxone IV
OR cefotaxime IV
OR flucloxacillin IM
OR gentamicin IM
3. Paracetamol OR aspirin for discomfort.
4. Linctus codeine or similar for cough.
5. Switch to appropriate antibiotic when culture
result available.
6. Physiotherapy for segmental drainage.
7. Oxygen if distressed or cyanotic.
8. Treat intercurrent cardiac failure.
9. Delirium in severe cases treated with diazepam.

10. Maintain nutrition and fluid and electrolyte balance.
11. Vaccination against pneumococcal pneumonia available for highly vulnerable patients.

PREC: Beware of empyema, endocarditis, pericarditis and pleural effusion.

PROG: Recovery expected except in debilitated, elderly or neonates where small mortality rate occurs.

Pneumothorax

THER: **Small with mild symptoms:**
Observation only.
Larger with symptoms:
Small-calibre intercostal tube with flutter valve OR large-calibre intercostal tube with underwater seal or under suction.
Recurrent pneumothoraces:
1. Oversewing of apical subpleural blebs.
2. Pleurodesis with talc poudrage or apical pleurectomy.

PROG: Recurrence rate after 1st episode, 20%; after 2nd episode, 60%; after 3rd episode, >85%.

Poisoning

See Anticoagulant, Overdose; Bleach Poisoning; Cyanide Poisoning; Iron Poisoning, Acute; Lead Poisoning; Mercury Poisoning; Narcotic Poisoning; Organophosphate Poisoning; Paracetamol Poisoning; Snake, Spider or Scorpion Bite

Poliomyelitis

THER: No specific cure.
Symptomatic management of mild cases. Paralytic forms require fluid and electrolyte management, adequate nutrition, orthopaedic care, artificial respiration. Oral vaccine available.

PROG: Mortality 5–10%. Severe morbidity.

Polyarteritis Nodosa [PAN]

THER: Prednisone
ADD immunosuppressive agents (eg. cyclophosphamide, azathioprine) if progressive
AND antibiotics for chest and other infections
AND hypotensive agents for hypertension.

PROG: 30% mortality in first few weeks, 50% five-year survival overall. Spontaneous remissions may occur.

Polycystic Ovarian Syndrome

See Stein-Leventhal Syndrome in SYNDROMES SECTION 6

Polycythaemia (Rubra) Vera

THER: 1. Repeated venesection to lower packed cell volume below 50%.
2. Dextran IV weekly for high platelet count.
3. Radioactive phosphorus IV.

4. Myelosuppressive drugs, eg. busulfan, chlorambucil, melphalan.

PREC: Leukaemia and gout may be induced. Extreme care necessary with all surgery due to increased bleeding tendency.

PROG: Average survival time 13 years with good treatment.

Polymyalgia Rheumatica

THER: 1. Prednisolone reducing slowly.
2. Analgesics, eg. aspirin, paracetamol.
3. NSAIDs.
4. Calcium supplements in women.

PREC: See under rheumatoid arthritis.

PROG: Significant morbidity, often lasting 12–36 months.

Polymyositis

See Dermatomyositis and Polymyositis

Porphyria, Acute

THER: 1. Identify and remove precipitants, eg. barbiturates and other drugs, alcohol.
2. Maintain fluid and electrolyte balance.
3. Maintain high calorie diet with IV laevulose if necessary.
4. Chlorpromazine
OR metoclopramide for nausea.
5. Diazepam
OR sodium valproate for convulsions.
6. Aspirin
OR paracetamol
AND/OR dihydrocodeine for pain.
7. Propranolol for tachycardia and hypertension; may also help acute attack in high doses.
8. Physiotherapy.
9. Haematin IV for acute attack.
10. Splenectomy.

PREC: Avoid barbiturates and alcohol. May mimic many acute abdominal conditions. Rebound effect after laevulose.

PROG: Mortality 25% during acute attack. Significant cardiovascular morbidity. Life expectancy reasonable after surviving acute attack.

Porphyria Cutanea Tarda

THER: 1. Avoid precipitating factors, (eg. drugs, alcohol).
2. Venesection of 500 mL/2 weeks until urinary uroporphyrin normal.
3. Avoid sunlight, use sunscreen creams.
4. Hydrochloroquine (can cause hepatic disease).

PROG: Reasonable. Remissions common.

Post-Herpetic Neuralgia

THER: 1. Prevent complications of shingles by using aciclovir, valaciclovir or high-dose steroids early in course of disease.

2. Simple analgesics (eg. paracetamol)
AND/OR capsaicin cream
AND/OR tricyclic antidepressants
AND/OR phenothiazines
AND/OR carbamazepine
AND/OR phenytoin.
3. Heat, physiotherapy, acupuncture, TENS.
PROG: Treatment very difficult and often unsuccessful.

See also Shingles

Postnatal Depression

THER: 1. Explanation and reassurance to patient and spouse.
2. Arrange home nursing and housekeeping support.
3. Allow mother time alone from infant.
4. Tricyclic antidepressant drug, while allowing breast feeding to continue.
5. Beware of suicidal or infanticidal thoughts. Admit to hospital if necessary.
PREC: Underdosage of tricyclics most common therapeutic error.
PROG: Self-limiting, but may be prolonged.

Post-Viral Syndrome

See Chronic Fatigue Syndrome

Pre-Eclampsia

THER: 1. Limit all physical activity.
2. Diazepam
OR chlomethiazole.
3. Diazoxide.
4. Frusemide.
PROG: Very good, should not proceed to eclampsia.

See also Eclampsia

Pregnancy

See Eclampsia; Fertility Control; Infertility, Female; Labour, Premature; Morning sickness; Pre-Eclampsia;

Premature Ejaculation

See Ejaculation, premature

Premature Labour

See Labour, Premature

Premenstrual Syndrome/Tension [PMS/T]

THER: 1. Exclude specific gynaecological or systemic disease.
2. Oral contraceptives
OR progestogens (eg. dydrogesterone, norethisterone)
AND/OR diuretic
AND/OR pyridoxine
AND/OR mefenamic acid
OR indomethacin.

3. Bromocriptine
OR danazol.
PROG: Control reasonable. Often chronic. Symptoms may decrease after pregnancy.

Pressure Ulcers

See Bed Sores

Priapism

THER: 1. Pseudoephedrine 120 mg orally.
2. Walk around briskly.
3. Empty bladder.
4. Hot packs to penis and perineum.
5. Repeat pseudoephedrine after two hours.
6. alpha-blocker (eg. prazosin).
7. Needle aspiration of penis.
8. Surgical drainage of penis.
PREC: Ejaculation does not ease priapism
PROG: Treatment should start if erection persists for two hours. Success is common by point 4. Priapism beyond 12 hours may cause permanent penile damage.

See also SYMPTOMS SECTION 1

Prostatic Carcinoma

THER: Depends on staging of disease. Treatment protocols include prostatectomy with excision of seminal vesicles and lymph nodes, radiotherapy, irradiation of bone metastases, orchidectomy, oestrogen therapy (now controversial), cytotoxic drugs, luteinising hormone releasing hormone analogues and antiandrogen therapy.
PROG: Judged by serial measurement of serum acid phosphatase, prostate specific antigen and alkaline phosphatase. Overall 70% 5-year survival.

Prostatitis

THER: Trimethoprim
OR norfloxacin
OR amoxycillin
OR ciprofloxacin
AND high fluid intake
AND analgesics
ADD gentamicin IV
ADD prostatic massage in chronic cases
ADD surgery (significant problems involved).
PROG: Acute cases settle well after two weeks. Chronic cases difficult to cure and require prolonged treatment.

Prostatomegaly

THER: 1. Prazosin
OR finasteride
OR terazosin
OR alfuzosin.
2. Transurethral resection.
3. Prostatectomy.

REC: Hypotension with prazosin. Acute urinary
        retention may require suprapubic
        catheterisation.
PROG: 60%+ controlled medically, but long-term
        treatment may be required. Surgical mortality
        <1%, morbidity 15%.

Pruritus Ani
THER: 1. Avoid scratching at all cost.
        2. Exclude iatrogenic causes (eg. antibiotics,
        other drugs) and systemic disease (eg.
        diabetes, worms, carcinoma).
        3. Treat local infections (eg. thrush).
        4. High fibre diet to avoid constipation.
        5. Avoid moisture, nylon underwear and other
        irritants.
        6. Wash anus with water after defaecation and
        dry carefully.
        7. Avoid spicy foods and red wine.
        8. Ice pack.
        9. Hydrocortisone creams.
        10. Sitz baths (eg. silver nitrate, potassium
        permanganate).
        11. Surgical correction of anal lesions (eg. piles,
        fissure).
REC: Avoid long-term use of fluorinated topical
        corticosteroids.
PROG: Benign, but often chronic and recurrent.

Pseudogout (Chondrocalcinosis; Calcium Pyrophosphate Crystal Deposition Disease)
THER: 1. Analgesics, eg. aspirin
        OR paracetamol
        AND/OR codeine
        OR pentazocine.
        2. Indomethacin
        OR other NSAIDs.
        3. Intra-articular corticosteroids.
        4. Joint fluid aspiration.
PROG: Chronic, no prophylaxis available.

Pseudomembranous Colitis
THER: 1. Stop all antibiotics.
        2. Maintain fluid and electrolyte balance,
        including plasma and whole blood if needed.
        3. Corticosteroids for shock.
        4. Vancomycin
        OR metronidazole
        OR bacitracin.
        5. Colectomy if chronic.
PROG: Clindamycin induced form common and often
        responds better than other forms. Mortality rate
        25–70% overall.

Psittacosis
THER: Tetracycline for one month
        ADD oxygen as required.
REC: Tetracycline only effective if started early.
        Myocarditis and secondary bacterial infections
        may occur.

PROG: Often chronic, rarely fatal.

Psoriasis
THER: 1. Topical steroid creams eg. betamethasone
        valerate.
        2. Dithranol ointment on alternate days; weaker
        and less frequently on sensitive areas, stronger
        and more often on thick patches ± UVB.
        3. Calcipotriol ointment.
        4. Coal tar dressings daily for thick patches, with
        or without salicylic acid ointment ± UVB.
        5. Cyclosporin emulsion.
        6. PUVA (psoralen + ultraviolet light).
        7. Acetretin orally.
        8. Intralesional triamcinolone injections.
        9. Oral corticosteroids (controversial).
        10. Methotrexate
        OR cyclosporin for severe disabling cases.
PREC: Acetretin is teratogenic. Dithranol – burning,
        sensitisation, avoid face. PUVA – avoid
        sunlight; cataracts, pruritus, blisters, squamous
        cell carcinomas, basal cell carcinomas,
        melanoma may occur; premature skin ageing.
PROG: Cure rare, morbidity moderate to mild,
        prolonged remissions may occur, arthritis can
        develop. Disease may be aggravated by lithium,
        beta-blockers, indomethacin and antimalarials.

Pulmonary Abscess
THER: 1. Aggressive chest physiotherapy.
        2. Bronchodilator sprays, eg. salbutamol,
        terbutaline.
        3. Sputum or bronchoscopy sample for
        culture.
        4. Benzylpenicillin IMI AND metronidazole.
        5. Alter antibiotics if necessary when culture
        results available.
        6. Surgical drainage of abscess.
PREC: Beware of empyema, haemorrhage, metastatic
        emboli, bronchiectasis, amyloidosis.
PROG: Good.

Pulmonary Embolism [PE]
THER: 1. Heparin IV bolus + infusion.
        2. Oxygen.
        3. Narcotics if severe pain.
        4. Thrombolytic therapy with streptokinase,
        t-PA, urokinase if massive acute PE and no
        contraindications.
        5. Oral anticoagulation for at least 3 months.
PREC: Under-dosing with heparin to be avoided.
        Thromboprophylaxis for all high risk patients.
PROG: Generally very good. Small proportion of
        patients do not lyse their emboli and develop
        chronic pulmonary hypertension.

Pulmonary Fibrosis (Fibrosing Alveolitis)
THER: 1. Exclude reversible causes (eg. drugs,
        organic dusts, mouldy hay).
        2. Establish specific cause and disease activity.

3. Smoking cessation.
4. Regular exercise.
5. Observation without treatment for many patients (because of poor response and major toxicity of the anti-inflammatory agents)
OR trial of prednisone
OR cyclophosphamide
AND/OR penicillamine.
6. Oxygen supplementation if pO_2 <55.
7. Referral to a specialist.
8. Single-lung transplant.

PROG: Variable but often poor with 50% 5-year survival. Only 20% have even a small objective response to steroids.

Pulmonary Hypertension

THER: 1. Referral to specialist.
2. Seek causative and contributing factors.
3. Avoid strenuous exertion, pregnancy.
4. Oxygen if hypoxaemic.
5. Anticoagulation if no contraindications.
6. Vasodilators if acute benefit has been demonstrated.
7. Surgical options:
– valve replacement for mitral stenosis
– repair of atrial septal defect
– thromboendarterectomy if chronic large vessel emboli
– lung or heart-lung transplantation.

PREC: Vasodilator use requires extreme caution
PROG: Primary pulmonary hypertension three year survival 50%.

Pyelonephritis

THER: 1. Take midstream urine for M/C/S.
2. High fluid intake.
3. Amoxycillin ± clavulanic acid
OR trimethoprim
OR co-trimoxazole
4. Urinary alkalinisers
5. Gentamicin IM
6. Alter antibiotic if necessary when urine culture result available.

PROG: Very good. Investigate any possible cause by IVP.

Q Fever

THER: Tetracycline
OR ciprofloxacin
AND symptomatic treatment.
PROG: Good long-term.

Quinsy

THER: 1. Penicillin in high doses IM or orally
OR erythromycin IM or orally.
2. Aspirin and gargles.
3. Surgical drainage of abscess.
4. Tonsillectomy after stabilisation.
PROG: Good.

Rabies

THER: 1. Heavily sedate,(eg. promethazine, diazepam)
2. Use major analgesics, eg. morphia, heroin.
3. Intensive care monitoring.
Post-exposure with HRIG and vaccine essential before symptoms appear.
PROG: Mortality rate 99% within 2–3 days if not vaccinated.

Rash

See Acne; Alopecia Areata; Atopic Eczema; Dandruff; Dermatitis ; Dermatomyositis and Polymyositis; Herpes Simplex; Molluscum Contagiosum; Perioral Dermatitis; Pityriasis Versicolor; Psoriasis; Scabies; Scarlet Fever; Scleroderma; Seborrhoeic Dermatitis; Shingles; Tinea; Urticaria; Vitiligo

Raynaud's Phenomenon

THER: 1. Gloves and thick socks.
2. Stop smoking.
3. Alcohol in regular low doses useful.
4. Vasodilator drugs, (eg. tolazoline, prazosin) of temporary use in some cases.
5. Topical glyceryl trinitrate, nifedipine, long-acting oral nitrates, methyldopa, reserpine and griseofulvin, have all been used experimentally with varying degrees of success.
6. Acupuncture (controversial).
7. Sympathectomy in severe cases.
PROG: Some morbidity, no mortality.

Rectal Carcinoma

THER: Abdominoperineal or anterior resection of rectum
ADD radiotherapy
ADD chemotherapy, eg. 5-fluorouracil, mitomycin-C.
PROG: Five-year survival 40% post-operative, 5% inoperable at diagnosis. Significant operative mortality.

Reflux Oesophagitis (Heartburn)

THER: 1. Reduce weight if obese and stop smoking.
2. Raise head of bed, avoid stooping, avoid nocturnal food and drink, eat small meals.
3. Antacids, eg. aluminium or magnesium compounds.
4. Oxethazaine compounds.
5. Alginate compounds.
6. Metoclopramide.
7. H_2-blockers, eg. ranitidine, nizatidine.
8. Cisapride.
9. Omeprazole.
10. Antacid nasogastric drip.
11. Surgery; selective vagotomy or hiatus hernia repair.
PREC: May mimic cardiac disease. Peptic ulceration of oesophagus possible.
PROG: Good, often chronic.

Regional Enteritis
See Crohn's Disease

Reiter Syndrome
THER: 1. Rest.
      2. Analgesics, (eg. paracetamol)
      3. NSAIDs.
      4. Tetracycline for urethritis.
      5. Symptomatic treatment for mouth lesions and conjunctivitis.
PROG: Attacks last from a few days to months. Arthritis may become chronic.

Renal Calculi
See Ureteric Calculi

Renal Failure, Acute
THER: 1. Treat cause of failure (eg. blocked ureters, transfusion reaction, heavy metals etc.)
      2. Correct fluid and electrolyte imbalances.
      3. 20% mannitol IV (controversial).
      4. Frusemide IM or IV.
      5. Calcium gluconate IV for hyperkalaemia.
      6. Sodium bicarbonate IV for acidosis.
      7. Low protein, low sodium, low potassium diet.
      8. Glucose OR parenteral hyperalimentation.
      9. Haemodialysis OR peritoneal dialysis.
      10. Restrict fluids in oliguric stage, free fluids in diuretic stage.
PREC: Beware of anaemia, infections, congestive cardiac failure, convulsions.
PROG: Depends on cause. Some mortality, seldom residual morbidity.

Renal Failure, Chronic
THER: 1. Control blood pressure and cardiac failure.
      2. Control fluid and electrolyte balance.
      3. Control calcium and phosphate levels with phosphate binders, calcium supplements and vitamin D.
      4. Low protein diet.
      5. Avoid drug toxicity.
      6. Treat infections carefully.
      7. Treat anaemia.
      8. Haemodialysis.
      9. Renal transplantation.
PROG: Satisfactory if cause of renal failure can be found and controlled, and if patient complies carefully with correct management.

Repetitive Strain Injury [RSI]
THER: 1. Exclude pathological cause for pain. Treat tendinitis, tenosynovitis, carpal tunnel syndrome, etc as appropriate.
      2. Rest. Splint if necessary.
      3. Occupational therapy and work practice management.
      4. Physiotherapy (eg. interferential therapy, ultrasound, hot/cold packs).
      5. NSAIDs.
      6. Psychological assessment.
PROG: As diagnosis is controversial, no definitive prognostic studies available. Some cases become chronic.

See also Occupational Overuse Syndrome in SYNDROMES SECTION 6

Respiratory Distress Syndrome, Infantile
THER: 1. Oxygen to give arterial pO_2 of 50-90mm Hg (6.7-12 kPa).
      2. Mechanical ventilation if acidotic.
      3. Maintain caloric and fluid intake, prevent sepsis and hypothermia, check for coagulopathies and anaemia.
      4. May be prevented by antenatal corticosteroids to mother.
PREC: Retrolental fibroplasia with prolonged high arterial pO_2.
PROG: Recovery or death within 3 days.

Retrograde Ejaculation
See Ejaculation, retrograde

Reye Syndrome
THER: 1. 10% glucose 1.2 L/m^2/d IVI.
      2. Positive pressure respiration and oxygen.
      3. Correct biochemical and electrolyte imbalances.
      4. Mannitol IVI for cerebral oedema.
PROG: Mortality rate 40%.

Rheumatic Fever
THER: 1. Bed rest; joint immobilisation if arthritis bad.
      2. Penicillin.
      3. Soluble aspirin for fever and arthritis.
      4. Digitalis and diuretics for cardiac failure.
      5. Aspiration of pericardial effusions.
      6. Prednisolone for some severe cardiac complications.
PREC: Salicylates - may precipitate heart failure.
PROG: 60% develop valvular disease. Antibiotic prophylaxis gives good long-term outlook.

Rheumatoid Arthritis
THER: 1. Aspirin
      OR paracetamol
      OR dextropropoxyphene
      AND/OR codeine.
      2. NSAIDs.
      3. Disease modifying antirheumatic drugs (eg. auranofin OR methotrexate OR sulfasalazine OR hydroxychloroquine OR leflunomide OR aurothiomalate IMI OR cyclosporin)
      4. Prednisolone OR ACTH depot injections short-term.
      5. Intra-articular steroids infrequently.
      6. Synovectomy.

7. Tricyclic antidepressants adjunctively.
PROG: Significant morbidity. Majority adequately controlled, minority progress to severe disablement.

See also Still's Disease

Rhinitis, Acute

THER: 1. Oxymetazoline
OR xylometazoline nasal drops.
2. Steam vaporiser.
3. Decongestants.
4. Pseudoephedrine.
5. Antihistamines, oral or topical.
6. Anticholinergics topically.
7. Nasal corticosteroids.
8. Antibiotics, orally, for secondary infection.
PREC: Nasal drops - rebound congestion if overused.
PROG: Good, often recurrent.

See also Allergic Rhinitis

Rickets
See Osteomalacia and Rickets

Rickettsioses

THER: Tetracycline
OR chloramphenicol
OR doxycycline
ADD parenteral rehydration
ADD oxygen.
PROG: Good. Vaccinations available for some forms.

See also Typhus, All Forms

Ringworm
See Tinea

Rosacea

THER: 1. Avoid alcohol, environmental extremes, hot drinks, spicy foods and aggravating medications.
2. Use sunscreen regularly
3. Topical metronidazole gel
OR topical 1% sulphur
4. Oral antibiotics (eg. tetracycline, doxycycline, minocycline, erythromycin) long-term
5. Hydrocortisone 1% cream.
6. Oral metronidazole
7. Topical isotretinoin
8. Surgical shaving or laser of rhinophyma.
PREC: Avoid potent topical steroids.
PROG: Good over several months. May need chronic therapy.

Roseola Infantum

THER: No specific treatment. Paracetamol.
No vaccine available.
PROG: Excellent. Incubation period 2 weeks.

Rotavirus Infection
See Enteritis, Viral

Roundworms
See Ascariasis

Royal Free Disease
See Chronic Fatigue Syndrome

Rubella (German Measles)

THER: None specific, symptomatic only.
Vaccination available.
PROG: Very good, may cause fetal abnormalities in early pregnancy. Incubation period 14-21 days.

Salmonellosis, Intestinal

THER: 1. IV infusion to correct fluid and electrolyte losses.
2. Diphenoxylate
OR codeine phosphate.
PREC: Only use antibiotics if essential as may prolong carrier state.
PROG: Good if correctly managed.

Salpingitis
See Pelvic Inflammatory Disease and Salpingitis

Sarcoidosis

THER: 1. Usually no treatment required.
2. Oral prednisone in intermediate doses for:
– significant respiratory symptoms
– pulmonary function impairment
– involvement of heart, CNS, hypercalcaemia
– disabling systemic symptoms.
3. Nonsteroidal anti-inflammatory agent for joint symptoms.
4. Topical or oral steroids for eye involvement.
5. Chloroquine for severe skin disease.
6. Referral to a specialist.
PROG: Generally very good. Majority resolve spontaneously. Fewer than 10% with radiological parenchymal involvement become disabled and fewer than 5% die of the disease.

See also Löfgren's Syndrome in SYNDROMES SECTION 6

Scabies

THER: 1. Permethrin or lindane 8–12 hour topical exposure.
2. Treat all family members.
3. Oral antihistamines for itch.
4. Antibiotics for secondary infection.
5. Betamethasone valerate for dermatitic areas
6. 10% sulphur cream OR crotamiton cream for resistant cases

7. Oral ivermectin for Norwegian scabies
PREC: Skin irritation; protect eyes and mouth
PROG: Good

Scarlet Fever

THER: Benzylpenicillin IM
OR phenoxymethylpenicillin
OR erythromycin.
PREC: Diarrhoea from antibiotics.
PROG: Good with treatment.

Schizophrenia

THER: **Acute:**
For control and sedation:
Haloperidol 10-20 mg IV or IM every 2 hours
OR chlorpromazine orally
OR thioridazine orally
ADD diazepam IM or IV for agitation
For control without sedation:
Haloperidol orally at night only
OR trifluoperazine orally.
OR olanzapine
OR risperidone
Chronic:
Oral antipsychotics (eg. clozapine, haloperidol,
olanzapine, risperidone, thioridazine,
trifluoperazine)
OR fluphenazine IM monthly for poor
compliance
AND psychotherapy in selected patients
AND environmental manipulation
ADD behavioural therapy.
PREC: Dystonic reactions to therapy possible – give
benztropine IV or IM
PROG: Reasonable control in most cases.
Relapses common. No specific cure.

Scleroderma (Systemic Sclerosis)

THER: No specific therapy but treat symptomatically
with following support:
– Physiotherapy regularly.
– Avoid cold.
– ACE inhibitor for hypertension.
– Antibiotics for chest and other infections.
– D-penicillamine for severe skin and deep
organ involvement.
– Calcium channel blocker for Raynaud's
phenomenon and pulmonary hypertension.
– H_2 receptor antagonist
AND/OR omeprazole
AND/OR cisapride forgastro-oesophageal
reflux.
PROG: Five year survival 50% overall. Poorer
prognosis with major organ involvement.

Scoliosis

THER: **Adolescent, Growth Not Complete**
< 20° – observe
20-30° – brace if progressive
> 30° – brace and/or surgery

Adult, Growth Complete
< 45° – no treatment practical
> 45° – surgery
PREC: Careful observation and family cooperation essential
PROG: Good if detected early.

Seborrhoeic Dermatitis

THER: SKIN
1. Hydrocortisone 1% cream
2. Ketaconazole cream
3. Miconazole cream
4. 1% sulphur with 1% salicylic acid
5. Fluorinated steroid cream
SCALP
1. Anti-inflammatory shampoo (eg. selenium
sulphide, zinc pyrithione)
2. Antifungal shampoo (eg. ketaconazole)
3. Keratolytic shampoo (eg. tar, salicylic acid)
4. Fluorinated steroid lotion
5. Sulphur creams applied overnight
EYELASHES
1. Dilute zinc pyrithione shampoo
2. Hydrocortisone 1% cream
PREC: Beware of prolonged use of steroid creams,
particularly near eyes
PROG: Relapses common. Maintenance therapy
necessary

Septicaemia

THER: 1. Take blood for culture.
2. Penicillin IM or IV
OR penicillin derivatives
OR clindamycin IM or IV
OR gentamicin IM or IV
OR cephalosporin IM or IV.
3. Treat source of infection (eg. lance abscess).
4. Modify antibiotics according to culture result.
5. Monitor WCC. Neutropenia indicates poorer
prognosis.
PREC: Medical emergency if shock present and IV
antibiotics necessary.
PROG: Mortality over 10% with severe neutropenia.

Septic Arthritis

THER: 1. Remove pus by repeated joint aspirations or
open drainage. Send pus for culture.
2. Flucloxacillin IV OR cephalosporin IV.
3. Alter antibiotic if necessary on culture result.
4. Splint joint, local heat, elevation.
5. Appropriate analgesia.
6. Mobilise early, but carefully.
PROG: 100% normal function if treated early.

Septic Meningitis

See Meningitis, Bacterial

Septic Shock

THER: 1. Ensure adequate ventilation and use oxygen
if necessary.

2. Take blood for culture while establishing an intravenous line.

3. Monitor all basic functions carefully (eg. blood pressure, pulse, temperature, respiration, urinary output, fluid intake, central venous pressure, etc).

4. Obtain specimens from all possible sites of infection (eg. urine, faeces, throat swab, sputum, CSF, skin sores etc) for gram stain and culture.

5. Initiate broad-spectrum antibiotic treatment. (eg. gentamicin AND flucloxacillin). Change antibiotic if necessary when results of cultures known.

6. Investigate other possible sources of infection by chest X-ray, ECG, haemoglobin, full blood count, platelet count, ESR, prothrombin time, plasma electrolytes, blood glucose, liver function tests, etc.

7. Surgically drain any source of infection.

8. Hyperbaric oxygen for gas gangrene.

9. Folic acid and B group vitamin supplements.

PREC: Beware of acidosis, acute renal failure, coagulopathies and hypoxia.

PROG: Overall mortality 50%, but varies greatly depending on source of infection. Necrosis.

Sheehan's Postpartum Pituitary Necrosis

See Hypopituitarism

Shigellosis (Bacillary Dysentery)

THER: 1. Replace fluid and electrolyte loss orally (see Cholera entry) AND/OR intravenously.

2. Faeces M/C/S before using antibiotics.

3. Reverse barrier nurse and dispose of stools appropriately until diarrhoea ceases and faeces M/C/S clear.

4. Co-trimoxazole OR ciprofloxacin OR oxytetracycline.

5. Diphenoxylate OR codeine phosphate.

6. Identify contacts, test faeces, and treat carriers.

PREC: Do not prolong antibiotic therapy as resistant strains may result. Use antidiarrhoeals sparingly.

PROG: Very good.

Shingles (*Herpes zoster*)

THER: 1. Analgesics, eg. aspirin AND/OR codeine OR pentazocine.

2. Aciclovir or valaciclovir orally in high doses and in early stages.

3. Sedatives, eg. diazepam OR barbiturates.

4. Idoxuridine/dimethylsulphoxide lotions

5. Prednisone.

6. Soothing topical applications, eg. calamine lotion OR spray-on plastic skin.

7. Antibiotics for secondary infection OR silver sulphadiazine cream.

8. Capsaicin cream for post-herpetic neuralgia.

PROG: Settles spontaneously in 2-6 weeks. Complications include persistent neuralgia and blindness from ocular involvement.

See also Post-Herpetic Neuralgia

Shin Splints

See Tibial Stress Syndrome in SYNDROMES SECTION 6

Shock

See Anaphylactic Shock; Cardiac Arrest; Hypotension, Postural; Septic Shock

See also Hypotension in SIGNS SECTION 2

Sick Building Syndrome

THER: 1. Improve ventilation. Ensure pollution not entering air intakes.

2. Ban smoking.

3. Seal vinyl, insulation panels, etc to prevent vaporisation.

4. Increase air flow near printers, photocopiers and other machinery.

5. Clean air conditioning filters and water tanks regularly.

6. Reduce humidity in air conditioned buildings to 50%.

7. Reduce partitioning to improve airflow.

8. Clear air conditioning ducts.

PROG: Extensive renovations may be required for success.

See also SYNDROMES SECTION 6

Sickle Cell Disease

THER: **General:**

1. Treat intercurrent infections aggressively and immunise against pneumococcal infections.

2. Transfuse to raise Hb to 140/gL + with any infection, leg ulcer, pre-operatively or other physical stress.

3. Leg ulcers treated by elevation and debridement.

Acute Crisis:

1. Maintain adequate hydration.

2. Appropriate analgesia.

3. Blood transfusion mandatory.

4. Treat any identifiable infection, or give prophylactic antibiotics.

PREC: Very susceptible to infection, dehydration and shock.

PROG: Variable. Death in childhood from cerebral haemorrhage or shock common. Uraemia common in later life.

Silicosis

THER: Non effective.

PREC: 1. Industrial dust control.
2. Worker removal if early features.
Complications:
1. Mycobacterial infection.
2. Respiratory failure.
PROG: Very good for simple silicosis but those with progressive massive fibrosis are disabled.

Simmonds' Disease
See Hypopituitarism

Sinusitis
THER: Amoxycillin ± clavulanic acid
OR cefaclor
OR doxycycline
OR erythromycin
ADD metronidazole
ADD antihistamines
AND/OR pseudoephedrine.
PROG: Good.

Sjögren's Syndrome
THER: No specific therapy. Supportive and symptomatic measures include mouthwashes and artificial tears. Treat concurrent arthritis.
PROG: Normal lifespan, significant morbidity.

See also Rheumatoid Arthritis

Sleep Apnoea
THER: 1. Establish correct diagnosis.
2. Aggressive weight reduction if obese.
3. Avoid alcohol, sedatives, narcotics.
4. Treat hypothyroidism if present.
5. Referral to specialist.
6. Upper airway surgery if anatomical abnormality.
7. Nasal CPAP the mainstay.
8. Tracheostomy if severe and CPAP not tolerated.
PREC: **Complications:**
Daytime hypersomnolence, personality change, intellectual deterioration, right heart failure, hypertension, motor vehicle accidents, arrhythmias.
PROG: Excellent with compliance to treatment.

See also Snoring

Snake Bite
THER: 1. Apply firm bandage over site of bite and wind firmly along full length of limb above bite.
2. Immobilise affected part.
3. Transport calmly and efficiently to nearest medical facility without exciting patient.
4. Observe vital signs.
5. If evidence of systemic spread of venom, give specific antivenom IV slowly if snake identified OR polyvalent antivenom if snake unknown and patient deteriorating.

6. Antihistamines IM AND/OR adrenaline subcutaneously for vaccine reaction or patient deterioration.
7. Maintain fluid and electrolyte balance.
8. Heparin if disseminated intravascular coagulation present*.
9. Diazepam IMI for anxiety.
10. Digoxin for tachycardia and cardiac failure.
11. Frusemide for renal or cardiac failure.
12. Haemodialysis OR peritoneal dialysis in extremis.
13. Tetanus prophylaxis.
PREC: Beware of anaphylaxis from antivenom *Some venoms may increase bleeding tendency.
PROG: Depends on snake, site of bite, amount of venom and hospital access; generally good.

Snoring
THER: 1. Weight loss if obese.
2. Avoid alcohol, sedatives, smoking.
3. Nasal steroids if rhinitis present.
4. Sleep in lateral position.
PROG: Excellent if patient compliant.

See also Sleep Apnoea

Spastic
See Cerebral Palsy

Spastic Colon
See Irritable Bowel Syndrome

Sprained Ankle
THER: 1. Cold compress in acute stage.
2. Strapping to support ankle.
3. Rest and elevate ankle.
4. NSAIDs to reduce pain and swelling.
5. Physiotherapy after joint stable to rehabilitate.
6. Surgery for severe injury.
PROG: Good, provided mobilisation is not too early.

Status Epilepticus
THER: 1. Insert IV line and secure firmly.
2. IV diazepam
OR IV lorazepam
AND phenytoin.
3. Glucose 50% and thiamine IV ± naloxone.
4. General anaesthesia and ventilation if intractable. Barbiturate or midazole drip.
PROG: Rapid control desired, investigation and treatment of cause essential.

See Convulsion; Epilepsy

Still's Disease (Juvenile Rheumatoid Arthritis)
THER: 1. Aspirin OR indomethacin.
2. Sodium aurothiomalate (gold) IMI.

3. Corticosteroids OR ACTH only when necessary eg. prednisolone on alternate days.

PROG: 50% complete remissions; others chronic with carditis, amyloidosis and iridocyclitis.

See also Rheumatoid Arthritis

Sting, Insect
See Anaphylactic Shock

Stomach Carcinoma
THER: Surgery in selected cases only. Palliative surgery and chemotherapy in others. Symptomatic treatment only in most.
PROG: Five year survival rate 12%.

Stomatitis
See Mouth Ulcers

Stone, Ureteric
See Ureteric Calculi

Stretch Marks
See Striae

Striae (Stretch Marks)
THER: 1. Exclude pathological cause (see SYMPTOMS SECTION 1)
2. Tretinoin topically
PREC: Tretinoin is teratogenic
PROG: Some improvement with treatment and time.

Stroke
See Cerebrovascular Accident

Strongyloidiasis
THER: Thiabendazole
PREC: Significant gastrointestinal side effects
PROG: Autoinfection may lead to very high parasite laod. Treatment usually effective

Stye, Eyelid
THER: 1. Remove lash in stye if possible.
2. Hot compresses, 20 minutes, four times daily.
3. Topical and systemic antibiotics not effective, as infection is localised and devoid of blood supply.
PROG: Good.

Subacute Bacterial Endocarditis [SBE]
See Endocarditis, Bacterial

Sweating, Excess
THER: Aluminium hexahydrate solution topically AND/OR probanthine orally
ADD autonomic nerve resection
ADD iontophoresis
ADD resection of axillary sweat glands.

See also SYMPTOMS SECTION 1

Sydenham's Chorea
See Chorea, Huntington's and Sydenham's

Syphilis
THER: Procaine penicillin IMI daily for 10-14 days
OR benzathine penicillin compound twice weekly for 4 doses
OR doxycycline for 2 weeks
OR erythromycin for 2 weeks
AND treat sexual partner(s).
PREC: Follow-up to ensure cure. Notifiable disease. Jarisch-Herxheimer reaction to massive spirochaete destruction can be modified by steroids.
PROG: Without treatment 60% remain latent with no serious effects, 40% progress to tertiary stage and serious cardiovascular or neurological sequelae. Treatment arrests further progression in most cases, but will not reverse pathological damage.

Systemic Lupus Erythematosus [SLE]
See Lupus Erythematosus, Systemic

Systemic Sclerosis
See Scleroderma

Tachycardia
See Flutter/Fibrillation; Paroxysmal Supraventricular Tachycardia; Paroxysmal Ventricular Tachycardia; Wolff-Parkinson-White Syndrome
See also SIGNS SECTION 2

Tapeworms (Taeniasis)
See Cestode Infestation

Temporal Arteritis (Giant Cell Arteritis, Cranial Arteritis)
THER: 1. Prednisone – treatment may be protracted.
2. Monitor ESR to determine subsequent prednisone dose.
PROG: Significant risk of blindness if inadequately treated.

Tendinitis
THER: 1. Rest. Sling if appropriate. Ice.

2. NSAIDs.
3. Corticosteroid AND local anaesthetic infiltration around tendon.
4. Physiotherapy (eg. ultrasound).
5. Surgery.
REC: NSAIDs – gut irritation. Corticosteroids should not be used excessively.
PROG: Good. Occasionally chronic.

Tension Headache
THER: 1. Remove cause of anxiety if possible.
2. Relaxation exercises and therapy.
3. Aspirin
OR paracetamol.
4. Diazepam
OR lorazepam
OR ibuprofen
OR other minor tranquillizers.
ADD NSAIDs.
5. Analgesic/sedative combinations (eg. paracetamol with codeine and doxylamine succinate).
REC: Sedation and dependence on tranquillizers.
PROG: Good, often recurrent.

Testicle, Undescended
See Undescended Testicle

Testicular Cancer
THER: 1. Measure S.HCG and alpha-fetoprotein (see PATHOLOGY SECTION 4) to assist in diagnosis, staging and prognosis.
2. Inguinal orchiectomy.
3. Radiotherapy to seminomas only.
4. Chemotherapy (eg. bleomycin, cisplatin, etoposide) for all types of testicular cancer.
5. Follow progress by regular measurement of tumour markers.
PROG: Overall 90% 10yr. survival.
Nearly 100% cure of seminomas.

Tetanus
THER: 1. Debride responsible wound.
2. IVI antitetanus serus stat.
3. Intrathecal antitetanus serum AND betamethasone.
4. Diazepam in high doses IMI or IVI OR phenobarbitone and chlorpromazine IMI.
5. Quiet, dark environment.
6. Tracheostomy performed early.
7. Intermittent positive pressure respiration after curarisation.
8. Control fluid and electrolyte balance.
9. Tachycardia and hypertension controlled by propranolol.
10. Bladder catheterisation if curarised.
11. Heparinise in long-term cases.
12. Vaccination available as prophylaxis.
PROG: Neonatal mortality 80%, general mortality

20-90% depending on spasm frequency and incubation period.

Thalassaemia beta Major
THER: 1. Repeated red blood cell transfusions.
2. Desferrioxamine subcutaneously regularly for iron overload (not proven).
3. Ascorbic and folic acid supplements (limited benefit).
4. Splenectomy if needed.
5. Treat infections aggressively.
6. Genetic counselling. Major form requires gene from both parents.
PROG: No cure, haemosiderosis main problem, life span 15-30 years.

Thalassaemia beta Minor
THER: Nil required, genetic counselling advisable.
PROG: No sequelae.

Threadworm
See Enterobiasis

Three Month Colic
See Infantile Colic

Thrombocytopenia
THER: 1. Remove precipitating factor(eg. drug).
2. Corticosteroids in high doses for short period (eg. prednisolone).
3. Prevent trauma or stress likely to cause haemorrhage.
4. Platelet transfusions.
5. Splenectomy if chronic.
PROG: Good. Morbidity due to cerebrovascular accident and other internal haemorrhages.

Thrombosis, Deep Venous [DVT]
THER: **General prophylaxis:**
1. Eliminate stasis in calf by pressure stockings, elevation, physiotherapy
2. Anticoagulants (eg. low dose heparin subcutaneously OR warfarin OR aspirin)
Surgical prophylaxis:
1. Essential for all high risk patients.
2. Early ambulation (but this alone is not sufficient for all but the lowest risk patients).
3. For general surgery, bed rest: low dose heparin.
– For neurosurgery, intracranial bleeding: compression stockings, intermittent pneumatic compression.
– For hip or knee surgery: warfarin, low molecular weight heparin, adjusted dose heparin.
Acute Treatment:
1. Heparin IV bolus + infusion aiming for APTT 2–2.5 times control.

2. Bed rest 24 hours, then mobilise.
3. Start warfarin same day.
4. Overlap warfarin with heparin until INR 2–3 for 2 consecutive days.
5. Continue warfarin (INR 2–3) at least 3 months.
6. Consider thrombolytic therapy for young patient with extensive DVT and no contraindications.
7. Prescription-type support stockings if significant leg swelling still present more than several weeks later.
8. Surgery in extensive and embolising cases

PREC: Daily prothrombin time, INR, platelets while on heparin. Avoid aspirin, NSAIDs. Warfarin contraindicated in pregnancy.

PROG: Pulmonary embolism is commonly associated with proximal DVT. Incidence of postphlebitic leg swelling and discomfort occurs in at least 50% of patients eventually.

See also Pulmonary Embolism

Thrush
See Candidiasis

Thyroiditis, De Quervain's Subacute
THER: Salicylates
ADD propranolol for thyrotoxicosis
ADD prednisolone for severe forms.
PROG: Self-limiting with complete recovery in most cases.

Thyroiditis, Hashimoto's
THER: 1. Determine degree of thyroid activity.
2. If hypothyroid use thyroxine. If hyperthyroid use neomercazole.
3. Suppress any subsequent goitre with thyroxine.
PROG: Usually permanent. May be transient after pregnancy.

Thyrotoxicosis
See Hyperthyroidism

TIA
See Transient Ischaemic Attack

Tic Doloureux
See Trigeminal Neuralgia

Tietze Syndrome
THER: Analgesics
AND NSAIDs
ADD corticosteroid infiltration of affected cartilage.
PROG: Good.

Tinea (*T. cruris; T. barbae; T. corporis; T. capitis; T. pedis*)
THER: 1. Topical hygiene important.
2. Tolnaftate cream for minor skin infection
3. Imidazole creams (eg. miconazole, clotrimazole, econazole).
4. Terbinafine topically or orally for widespread skin infection
5. Griseofulvin OR ketoconazole orally for severe scalp infection
PREC: Care with griseofulvin and ketoconazole.
PROG: Good; recurrences common.

See also Aspergillosis; Candidiasis, Vaginal; Onychomycosis; Pityriasis Versicolor

Tinea Versicolor
See Pityriasis Versicolor

Tinnitus
See Hypertension, Essential; Menière's Disease
See also SYMPTOMS SECTION 1

Tonsillitis
THER: Phenoxymethylpenicillin
OR amoxycillin ± clavulanic acid
OR erythromycin
AND aspirin for fever and pain
AND anaesthetic/antiseptic mouth gargles
ADD benzylpenicillin or other injectable penicillin as initiating treatment in severe cases.
PREC: Beware of quinsy.
PROG: Good.

Toxocariasis
THER: Diethylcarbamazine
OR thiabendazole
ADD oral corticosteroids for ophthalmic oedema and inflammation.
PROG: Partial or total blindness possible with ophthalmic involvement. Often present undiagnosed in latent form.

Toxoplasmosis
THER: No treatment required unless severe, persistent, pregnant or immunologically suppressed.
Pyrimethamine
AND folinic acid (calcium folate)
AND sulphadiazine for 3-6 weeks
OR spiramycin for 2 weeks
ADD corticosteroids for ocular disease.
PROG: Very good. Rarely causes fetal deformities and mental retardation at any stage during pregnancy.

Transient Ischaemic Attack [TIA]
THER: 1. Determine cause of TIA (eg. atheroma,

cardiac) by neurological assessment, risk factors, CAT scan, Doppler, echocardiography,angiography.
2. If acute, admit to hospital. If resolved, may assess as out-patient
3. Anticoagulate with aspirin OR warfarin.
4. Surgery to isolated cardiac or carotid lesions.

PREC: Do not use aspirin and anticoagulants together.
PROG: Risk of stroke after TIA increased five-fold. Treatment can reduce this risk.

Tremor, Essential

THER: 1. Exclude pathological cause of tremor (see SYMPTOMS SECTION 1).
2. Propranolol OR other Beta-blockers.
PROG: Variable. Side effects of medication may be less tolerable than tremor. Some patients fail to respond to any treatment.

Trichomoniasis, Vaginal

THER: Metronidazole for 1 week
OR tinidazole
OR clindamycin
AND treat male partner
ADD clotrimazole pessaries.
PREC: Beware of intercurrent VD.
PROG: 90% cure with single course of treatment.

Trichuriasis (Whipworm Infestation)

THER: Mebendazole
PROG: Very safe and effective treatment.

Trigeminal Neuralgia (Tic Doloureux)

THER: Carbamazepine
OR phenytoin
OR clonazepam
AND appropriate short-term analgesia (eg. pentazocine, pethidine)
ADD baclofen
ADD surgery in intractable cases.
PROG: Rare under 50 years, more common in females. May be secondary to tumours or multiple sclerosis. Usually well controlled.

Tuberculosis, Meningeal

THER: Pyrazinamide
AND isoniazid
AND pyridoxine
AND rifampicin
AND streptomycin
ADD prednisolone
PROG: 80% recovery, but often residual CNS lesions.

Tuberculosis, Pulmonary [TB]

THER: Isoniazid
AND/OR rifampicin
AND/OR streptomycin
AND/OR ethambutol

AND/OR pyrazinamide.
Usually 3 or more of the above drugs are used for three months, then 2 drugs for a further six months.
PROG: 90+% cure rate, relapses often due to poor compliance.

Tumour
See Cancer

Typhoid

THER: **Acute:**
Chloramphenicol
OR co-trimoxazole
OR ampicillin
AND maintain fluid and electrolyte balance orally (see Cholera entry) or IV
AND high calorie, low residue diet
ADD hydrocortisone IVI in extremis
ADD transfusions for haemorrhage
ADD surgery for gut perforation.
Chronic Carrier:
Ampicillin
OR ciprofloxacin long-term.
May persist in gall bladder despite treatment.
PREC: Beware of sudden shock from haemorrhage or perforation.
PROG: Mortality rate 2% with good treatment. Poor prognosis with gut perforation. Oral and injectable vaccination available.

Typhus, All Forms

THER: **Prophylaxis:**
Doxycycline 200 mg per week
Treatment:
Tetracycline
OR chloramphenicol
OR doxycycline.
PROG: Generally good. Circulatory, renal or hepatic collapse possible. Vaccine no longer available.

Ulcer
See Bed Sores; Mouth Ulcers; Peptic Ulcer, Venous Leg Ulcer

Ulcerative Colitis

THER: 1. Regular sigmoidoscopy to exclude carcinoma.
2. High fibre diet.
3. Iron supplements for secondary anaemia.
4. Antidiarrhoeal agents (eg. loperamide)
5. Prophylaxis with aminosalicylic acid derivatives (eg. sulphasalazine, olsalazine, mesalazine
OR azathioprine
OR sodium cromoglycate.
6. Corticosteroids orally AND/OR rectally AND/OR IM.
7. Metronidazole AND/OR ciprofloxacin.

8. Maintain fluid and electrolyte balance in acute attacks.
9. Colectomy with ileostomy.

PROG: 5% acute attack mortality. Recurrent attacks common. Significant morbity. 75% ten year survival rate.

Undescended Testicle

THER: Gonadotrophic releasing hormone by subcutaneous injection (controversial) AND/OR surgical placement of testicle in scrotum if medical treatment fails, or testicle outside line of descent.
PREC: Retractile testes require no treatment.
PROG: Very good if treatment undertaken before two years of age. Infertility and seminoma likely if delayed beyond puberty.

Uraemia

THER: 1. Treat specific cause(s) eg. drugs.
2. Adequate diet.
3. Haemodialysis.
4. Renal transplant.
PROG: Death without adequate therapy inevitable. Convulsions and CNS damage may occur. Significant morbidity with long-term management. Transplants moderately successful.

See also Renal Failure

Ureteric Calculi

THER: 1. High fluid intake.
2. Morphine IM
OR pethidine IM WITH prochlorperazine.
3. NSAIDs.
4. Atropine subcutaneously for spasm.
5. Treat intercurrent urinary infection.
6. Collect all urine to check for stone to analyse.
7. Surgery or lithotripsy for chronic, symptomatic or obstructive stones.
PREC: Beware of narcotic addition.
PROG: Very good.

Urethritis, Non-Specific

See Non-Specific Urethritis

Urinary Infection

See Cystitis; Pyelonephritis

URTI (Upper Respiratory Tract Infection)

See Coryza; Influenza; Pharyngitis, Bacterial; Quinsy; Tonsillitis

Urticaria (Hives)

THER: **Acute:**
1. Remove cause of reaction if known.
2. Adrenaline SCI if severe.

3. Antihistamines IM THEN orally.
4. Oxygen and airway support *in extremis*.
5. Topical soothing treatments (eg. calamine lotion, menthol, phenol etc).
6. Corticosteroids orally OR IM OR IV if airway compromised.
Chronic:
Long-term oral antihistamines
AND topical soothing lotions or creams
ADD tricyclic antidepressants
PROG: Good, relapses possible. Beware of angio-oedema of respiratory tract.

See also Anaphylactic Shock

Uveitis, Anterior

See Iritis

Vaginitis, Bacterial

THER: Triple sulphur cream
AND amoxycillin
OR tetracycline
OR erythromycin
AND metronidazole OR nystatin.
PROG: Good; often recurrent, particularly in pregnant, debilitated or sexually promiscuous women.

See also Candidiasis; Trichomoniais, Vaginal

Varicella

See Chickenpox; Shingles

Varicose Ulcer

See Venous Leg Ulcer

Varicose Veins

THER: **Due to long and short saphenous incompetence:**
– Surgery (eg. stripping, "nick and pick", valve slings).
– Selected sclerotherapy of remaining veins.
Due to perforator incompetence, spider veins
– Injection sclerotherapy (sodium tetradecyl sulphate) with compression.
PREC: Inject only one leg at a time with patient lying and leg elevated. Avoid injecting arteries - this can cause peripheral gangrene - intra-arterial heparin and dextran may save situation. Compression bandages for at least 6 weeks with patient remaining as mobile as possible. Sclerosant may cause allergy, anaphylaxis, skin ulcers and skin staining.
PROG: Reasonable improvement in most patients. Recurrence always possible.

VD (Venereal Disease)

See Gonorrhoea; Non-Specific Urethritis; Syphilis; Trichomoniasis, Vaginal; Warts, Ano-Genital

enereal Warts
ee Warts, Ano -Genital

enomous Bite
ee Snake Bite

enous Leg Ulcer (Varicose Ulcer)
HER: 1. Strong elastic stockings or bandages
         AND mobilisation.
       2. Saline/paraffin or other bland dressings.
       3. Chlorhexidine solution for infected ulcers.
       4. Amoxycillin
         OR co-trimoxazole orally for cellulitis.
       5. Dextranomer
         OR fibrinolysin ointment
         OR Duoderm.
       6. Elevation of leg, bed rest, careful nursing.
       7. Skin grafting.
       8. Vein ligation
         AND/OR stripping.
REC: Fibrinolysin – pain in clean ulcer.
       Dextranomer– treat infection before use;
       contra-indicated in deep ulcers. Avoid topical
       antibiotics.
ROG: Often chronic. Slow improvement with careful
       treatment. Healing usually possible.

enous Thrombosis
ee Thrombosis, Deep Venous

entricular Arrhythmia
ee Atrial Flutter/Fibrillation; Cardiac Arrest; Paroxysmal
upraventricular (Atrial) Tachycardia; Paroxysmal
entricular Tachycardia; Ventricular Tachycardia;
Volff-Parkinson-White Syndrome

entricular Failure
ee Cardiac Failure, Congestive

entricular Fibrillation
ee Cardiac Arrest

entricular Tachycardia
HER: 1. Lignocaine IVI stat.
       2. DC cardioversion.
       3. IV infusion of lignocaine OR procainamide
         AFTER successful cardioversion.
       4. Quinidine, cease if tachycardia persists after
         2 g given.
       5. Procainamide
         OR disopyramide.
       6. Propranolol as prophylaxis
         OR IVI slowly and repeated *in extremis*.
       7. Procainamide
         OR phenytoin may be given IVI under ECG

control *in extremis*.
PREC: Digitalis normally contraindicated.
PROG: Very high mortality rate if progresses to
       fibrillation.

Vertigo
See Menière's Disease
See also SYMPTOMS SECTION 1

Vincent's Angina (Trench Mouth)
THER: Penicillin
       OR erythromycin
       AND/OR metronidazole
       AND sodium bicarbonate solution gargles.
PROG: Good; highly infectious.

Viral Infections
THER: None specific except in Herpes and influenza
       (see separate entry). Symptomatic treatment
       only available.
       Soluble aspirin
       OR paracetamol for pain, fever and
       inflammation.
       Vidarabine may be used in some severe cases
       eg. herpes.
       Human gammaglobulin IMI may prevent or
       mitigate infection in some cases. Vaccinations
       often available eg. influenza, mumps, measles
       etc.
PREC: Beware of fulminating cases with severe
       specific organ damage.
PROG: Generally good with prolonged rest.

See also Chickenpox; Coryza; Hepatitis; Infectious
Mononucleosis; Influenza; Measles; Mumps; Shingles

Visceral Larva Migrans
See Toxocariasis

Vitiligo
THER: 1. Protect from sun.
       2. Methoxsalen and UVA light
         OR trioxysalen and UVA light.
       3. Cosmetics and dyes.
       4. Melanocyte autotransplantation.
PROG: Poor, less than 15% respond satisfactorily.

Vomiting
THER: 1. Determine pathological cause (see
         SYMPTOMS SECTION 1) and treat specifically
         if possible.
       2. Concentrated carbohydrate solution
         (Emetrol).
       3. Prochlorperazine
         OR metoclopramide
         OR chlorpromazine orally OR IM OR IV.
       4. Maintain fluid and electrolyte balance.

5. Hyoscine patches for prophylaxis (motion sickness).
PREC: Beware of vomiting associated with early pregnancy.
PROG: Depends on cause.

von Willebrand's Disease

THER: 1. Rest affected area.
2. Transfusion of cryoprecipitate OR fresh frozen plasma.
3. Local pressure on bleeding point with thrombin soaked Gelfoam. Treatment normally only required after trauma during surgery or pregnancy.
PROG: Fatal bleeding occurs occasionally; generally a normal life span with moderate morbidity.

See also Haemophilia

Warts, Ano-Genital

THER: Imiquimod cream
OR cautery
OR laser coagulation
OR freeze with liquid nitrogen
OR paint with acid preparations (eg. podophyllum, trichloroacetic acid)
AND/OR surgical excision of warts.
ADD topical fluorouracil
AND examine and treat sexual partners
AND regular follow up (eg. Pap smear, colposcopy).
PREC: Wide margin around obvious wart should be treated to prevent recurrence. Do not use imiquimod in pregnancy or lactation.
PROG: Cervical lesions may be linked to dysplasia and cervical cancer. Often recurrent, but usually settle after adequate treatment.

Warts, Skin

THER: 1. Most warts will resolve spontaneously with time, but may be many years and may spread initially.
2. Topical acid preparations (eg. podophyllim 15–50% paint, salicylic acid 10-25% ointment, formaldehyde1.5%, formalin 3–6% soaks)
3. Cryotherapy (CO_2 or N_2)
4. 5-fluorouracil 5% with salicylic acid OR diathermy/cautery OR excision (rarely)
5. Inject bleomycin under resistant warts
6. Cimetidine (experimental) or retinoids orally
7. Immunotherapy with dinitrochlorobenzene or diphencyprone.
PREC: Protect surrounding normal skin from acid ointments by use of vaseline. Cautery and cryotherapy may cause scarring.
PROG: Good long-term.

Wegener's Granulomatosis

THER: Prednisolone

ADD cyclophosphamide OR azathioprine.
PROG: Mortality 10% per annum in good centres.

Wernicke's Encephalopathy (Wernicke-Korsakoff Syndrome)

THER: 1. Stop alcohol intake.
2. Thiamine IV or IM initially, orally later.
3. Good diet.
4. Follow up to prevent recurrence of alcoholism and/or malnutrition.
PREC: Do not use IV glucose in acute stage.
PROG: Neurological symptoms normally settle rapidly, but psychoses may remain. Significant mortality in acute stage.

See also SYNDROMES SECTION 6

Whiplash

THER: 1. X-ray to exclude further pathology.
2. NSAIDs.
3. Analgesics.
4. Mild tranquillizers (eg. low dose diazepam).
5. Neck collar.
6. Physiotherapy after acute stage.
7. Depot steroid injection of trigger sites.
8. Tricyclic antidepressants in chronic cases.
9. Surgery in small number of selected cases.
PROG: Of those still complaining of symptoms after one month, 45% persist for more than 2 years.

Whipworm Infestation

See Trichuriasis

Whooping Cough

See Pertussis

Wilson's Disease

THER: Penicillamine A
OR trientine (triethylenetetramine dihydrochloride) life-long
AND pyridoxine
AND zinc supplements
ADD prednisone for adverse reactions to drugs
ADD liver transplantation *in extremis*.
PROG: Often irreparable liver damage present by time of diagnosis. If adequately controlled at an early stage, life expectancy reasonable but rarely normal.

Wolff-Parkinson-White Syndrome [WPW]

THER: **Acute:**
1. Vagal stimulation.
2. Verapamil
OR propranolol stat slowly
OR procainamide IV
OR DC cardioversion.
Prophylaxis of atrial ectopics:

Propranolol
OR other beta-blockers.
Prophylaxis of ventricular ectopics:
Disopyramide
OR quinidine
OR procainamide
ADD pacemaker
ADD surgical division of aberrant pathway.
REC: Do not use disopyramide, quinidine or
         procainamide concurrently. Avoid digoxin.
ROG: Sudden death may occur, but rare. Adequate
         control normal.

ee also SYNDROMES SECTION 6

Worms

ee Ancylostomiasis, Intestinal; Ascariasis; Cestode
festation; Enterobiasis; Hydatid Disease;
rongyloidiasis; Trichuriasis

---

erotic Dermatitis
ee Dermatitis

---

ollinger-Ellison Syndrome
HER: Total gastrectomy
         AND gastrinoma excision
         OR H_2 antagonist (eg. cimetidine, ranitidine)
         OR Proton pump inhibitors (eg lansoprazole,
         omeprazole, pantoprazole).
         AND antacids as required.
REC: Surgical treatment preferable in long-term.
ROG: Good.

ee also SYNDROMES SECTION 6

SECTION SIX
SYNDROMES

THEIR SYMPTOMS, DIAGNOSIS, TREATMENT AND COMPLICATIONS
PREFACE

Syndromes seem to be multiplying exponentially in modern medicine. Some are just a passing fad, or have only local significance; others, though, become diagnostic classics, and are handed down with the combinations of the original describers' surnames (the etymology of which can be quite fascinating at times), or Latin/Greek hybrids that are designed to paralyse even the most articulate tongue.

Unfortunately, remembering the details about this multitude of syndromes is fast becoming an impossible task for the busy clinician. This section, and the syndromes under the appropriate symptoms in SECTION 1, should overcome that problem by directing the doctor's thoughts towards an appropriate, although sometimes unusual, diagnosis. Bizarre collections of presenting symptoms may suddenly resolve themselves into one of the less common, but previously recognised syndromes. Not every described syndrome can possibly be described in any tome shorter than a thousand pages, but this section should cover the majority of those encountered by most physicians.

Syndrome: A concurrence of several symptoms in a disease.

Oxford English Dictionary

FORMAT

Syndrome Name [Abbreviation] (Alternate Name)

DES: Description. Characteristic symptoms and signs of the syndrome. (Symptoms and signs that are not always present are shown in brackets.)

TEST: Pathological, radiological, electrophysiological and other appropriate tests used in the diagnosis, with the expected result of the test in a patient with the syndrome shown in (brackets). See also INVESTIGATIONS SECTIONS 3 and PATHOLOGY SECTION 4.

TRT: Treatment. The available treatments for the syndrome, if any.

COMM: Comment. Further discussions on the epidemiology and complications of the syndrome.

See also Other Relevant Syndromes

Abbreviation
See Disease Name

Alternate name
See Disease Name

NB: See list of symtoms, organs etc. In SIGNS SECTION 1 to make the diagnosis of a syndrome

Abetalipoproteinaemia
See Bassen-Kornzweig Syndrome

Accelerated Conduction Syndrome
See Wolff-Parkinson-White Syndrome

Acquired Immune Deficiency Syndrome (AIDS)
DES: **Group I HIV+ (Acute Infection)**
Fever, malaise, arthropathy, sore throat, myalgia, nausea, vomiting, headache, diarrhoea, transient rash and adenitis, (convulsions, photophobia, coma).
Group II HIV+ (Asymptomatic)
No symptoms.
Group III HIV+ (Persistent Lymphadenopathy)
Generalised lymphadenopathy.
Group IV AIDS-Related Complex
Diarrhoea, fever, weight loss, sweats, skin infections (eg. tinea, shingles, warts, folliculitis).
Group IV AIDS
Dyspnoea, cough, fatigue rashes, vomiting, headaches, lung infections (eg. *Pneumocystis carinii* pneumonia), Kaposi's sarcoma, intracranial lesions, coma, death.
TEST: See INVESTIGATIONS SECTION 3.
TRT: See TREATMENT SECTION 5.
COMM: Transmitted by blood products and semen. Occurs mainly in homosexuals and IV drug abusers. May remain latent in Group II for years. No cure or vaccine available yet. Mortality close to 100%

Acrocephalopolysyndactyly
See Carpenter Syndrome

Acrocephalosyndactyly of Apert
See Apert Syndrome

Acute Brain Syndrome (Acute Confusional Syndrome)
DES: Elderly, psychotic, clouding of consciousness, disorientation, impaired thought processes, poor short-term memory, illusions, misinterpretations, hallucinations (visual, tactile, auditory, olfactory), anxiety, fear, restlessness, apathy.
TEST: Psychiatric assessment.
TRT: Careful nursing, haloperidol. Other sedatives may aggravate confusion.
COMM: Abrupt onset. Common in suddenly hospitalised elderly patients. May settle spontaneously with time.

Acute Febrile Neutrophilic Dermatosis
See Sweet Syndrome

Adams-Stokes Syndrome
See Stokes-Adams Syndrome

Adrenocortical Hyperfunction
See Cushing Syndrome

Adrenogenital Syndrome, Adult Women
DES: Amenorrhoea, acne, rough skin, hirsutism, bromhidrosis, voice deepening, breast atrophy, increased musculature.
TEST: U.17-ketosteroids (H), dexamethasone suppression test (AB), S.testosterone (H), CT scan for adrenal tumour, ultrasound for ovarian tumour.
TRT: Depends on cause of excess androgen. Surgery for tumours, prednisone in other cases.
COMM: Many different causes and sub-forms of syndrome. Pituitary, ovarian, placental and thymic forms.

See also Stein-Leventhal Syndrome

Adrenogenital Syndrome, Child (Congenital Adrenal Hyperplasia
DES: Masculinsation of female, premature virilisation in male; hypocorticalism; (hypertension).
TEST: S.ACTH (H), P.androgens (H), U.pregnanetriol (H), U.17-ketosteroids (H).
TRT: Glucocorticoids or mineralocorticoids long-term.
COMM: Due to enzymatic error of metabolism involved in cortisol synthesis.

Adult Respiratory Distress Syndrome
See Respiratory Distress Syndrome, Adult

Afferent Loop Syndrome
DES: Postprandial abdominal pain relieved by vomiting, malabsorption, steatorrhoea, (pernicious anaemia).
TEST: Ba meal (AB), faecal fat (H).
TRT: Tetracycline or lincomycin, surgical resection of afferent loop.
COMM: Only occurs after Bilroth II gastrectomy or gastrojejunostomy, and is caused by stasis and distension in the bowel afferent loop.

AIDS
See Acquired Immune Deficiency Syndrome

Alagille Syndrome
DES: Peripheral pulmonary artery stenosis, biliary hypoplasia with variable hepatic impairment, deep set eyes, prominent forehead, mental retardation.
TEST: Chromosomal analysis.
TRT: Surgical correction of arterial and biliary abnormalities.
COMM: Congenital condition localised to chromosome 20p11.2.

Albright Syndrome (Fibrous Dysplasia; McCune-Albright Syndrome)

DES: Precocious puberty, polyostotic fibrous
        dysplasia, (hyperthyroidism, acromegaly).
TEST: Skeletal X-ray (AB), S.ALP (H),
        U.hydroxyproline (H).
TRT: Surgical correciton of deformities, steroids
        (variable results).
COMM: Usually occurs in young females.

Alport Syndrome

DES: Deafness, progressive glomerulonephritis,
        haematuria (otitis media, renal failure,
        cataracts).
TEST: U.Hb (+), renal function tests (AB).
TRT: Nil. Disease recurs in transplanted kidneys.
COMM: Autosomal recessive disorder of boys.

Amnestic Syndrome

DES: Memory disturbance, alcoholism, thiamine
        deficit.
TEST: LFT (AB), S.thiamine (L).
TRT: Treat alcoholism.
COMM: Sudden onset, amnesia chronic.

Amsterdam Dwarf

See de Lange Syndrome

Anaphylactoid Purpura

See Henoch-Schoenlein Syndrome

Andersen's Syndrome (Type IV Glycogen Storage Disease)

DES: Hepatosplenomegaly, glycogen storage
        disease caused by lack of a liver
        transglucosidase that is inevitably fatal in
        childhood.
TEST: Liver biopsy.
TRT: Nil available.

Angelman Syndrome (Happy Puppet Syndrome)

DES: Severe mental retardation, mute, ataxic gait,
        intractable seizures, inappropriate laughter,
        microcephaly, facial dysmorphia.
TEST: Chromosome analysis.
TRT: Nil.
COMM: Sporadic occurrence 1:25,000. Due to
        chromosome 15 damage.

Anterior Chest Wall Syndrome

See Tietze Syndrome

Anterior Compartment Syndrome

DES: Pain in anterolateral muscular compartment of
        the lower part of the leg, worse with exercise,

        (weak foot dorsiflexion).
TRT: Rest, NSAIDs, physiotherapy, surgical
        decompression (rarely).
COMM: Due to increasing pressure in the rigid
        compartment between tibia, fibula, deep fascia
        and interosseous membrane. Caused by
        exercise stress (eg. long distance running).

Anterior Impingement Syndrome (Footballer's Ankle)

DES: Chronic ankle pain worse with running or
        descending stairs, ankle stiffness, pain on ankle
        dorsiflexion.
TEST: X-ray ankle (+ exostoses on upper surface of
        talus and lower end of tibia at ankle joint
        margin).
TRT: Rest, NSAIDs, surgical removal of osteophyte.
COMM: Caused by repeated forced dorsiflexion on the
        ankle, as in kicking.

Antiphospholipid Syndrome

DES: Arterial and venous thromboses, recurrent
        miscarriage, thrombocytopenia, livedo
        reticularis, valvular heart disease, Coombs'
        positive autoimmune haemolytic anaemia,
        chorea, dementia.
TEST: Antiphospholipid antibodies (+), Hb (L), lupus
        anticoagulant antibody (+).
TRT: Anticoagulants.
COMM: Aetiology includes drugs (eg. phenothiazine,
        phenytoin, hydralazine, procainamide) and
        infections (eg. TB, syphilis, malaria, mumps,
        rubella, parvovirus). Caused by lack of
        circulatory blood coagulation inhibitors.

Apert Syndrome (Acrocephalosyndactyly of Apert)

DES: Frontal bossing, exophthalmos, hypoplastic
        maxillae, syndactyly.
TRT: Surgical opening of cranial sutures.
COMM: Autosomal dominant inheritance

See also Carpenter Syndrome

Asherman Syndrome

DES: Amenorrhoea and infertility after uterine
        curettage for postpartum haemorrhage.
COMM: Due to over vigorous curettage of uterus to
        control severe bleeding with subsequent
        adhesion of uterine walls and failure of
        endometrium to redevelop.

Asperger Syndrome

DES: Inappropriate social interaction, lack of
        empathy, abnormal speech pattern, paucity of
        facial expression, unusual preoccupations,
        poor communication skills, mental retardation,
        poor coordination, (poor posture, poor
        imagination, poor ability to specifically
        memorise data, hypo- or hyper sensitive to

sensations, violent).
TEST: Psychiatric and psychological assessment.
TRT: Managed by psychologists, social workers, occupational therapists and psychiatrists.
COMM: Developmental disorder. More common in males. No cure, but normal life expectancy.

Auriculotemporal Syndrome
See Frey Syndrome

Azorean Disease
See Machado-Joseph Syndrome

Bard-Pic Syndrome
DES: Progressive jaundice associated with carcinoma of the head of pancreas, cachexia.

Barlow Syndrome
DES: Mitral valve prolapse (arrhythmias, syncope, transient ischaemic attacks).
TEST: Echocardiography (AB), auscultation (late systolic click).
TRT: Reassurance if asymptomatic. Beta-blockers for mildly affected. Surgical repair if severe. Antibiotic cover to prevent endocarditis.
COMM: May be genetic.

Barrett Syndrome
DES: Chronic reflux eosophagitis, distal oesophageal ulceration, oesophageal stricture.
TEST: Delicate reticular mucosal pattern on double contrast barium meal, characteristic progressive columnar metaplasia of distal oesophagus.
COMM: Acquired premalignant condition.

Bartter Syndrome
DES: Child or young adult, short stature, polydipsia, polyuria, enuresis, nocturia, muscle weakness (tetany, cramps, salt craving, vomiting, constipation).
TEST: Metabolic alkalosis (+), S.potassium (L), U.potassium (H), P.renin (H), P.aldosterone (N or H), Chvostek's sign (+) and Trousseau's sign (+) (see SIGNS SECTION 2).
TRT: Indomethacin to inhibit prostaglandin activity, potassium supplements.
COMM: Recessive disorder giving the metabolic effects of hyperaldosteronism without hypertension. Caused by failure of kidney to conserve potassium. Rare. Females > males.

Basal Cell Carcinoma Naevus Syndrome
See Gorlin-Goltz Syndrome

Bassen-Kornzweig Syndrome (Abetalipoproteinaemia)
DES: Fat malabsorption, low body weight,

acanthocytosis, retinitis pigmentosa, ataxia, growth retardation.
TEST: P.cholesterol (L), P.triglycerides (VL).
TRT: Fat restricted diet, medium chain triglyceride supplements.
COMM: Due to inability to synthesise chylomicrons and very low density lipoproteins. Poor prognosis.

Beal Syndrome (Contractural Arachnodactyly)
DES: Long slim arms and legs, long fingers and toes, multiple joint contractures particularly the knees, calf muscle hypoplasia, crumpled ears, (progressive kyphoscoliosis in 50%, mitral valve prolapse, cardiac septal defects, aortic hypoplasia).
TEST: Nil.
TRT: Symptomatic, cardiac surgery.
COMM: Uncommon. Autosomal dominant inheritance. Joint contractures improve spontaneously. Differentiate from Marfan syndrome.

Beckwith-Wiedemann Syndrome
DES: Exomphalos, macroglossia, visceral enlargment, hypoglycaemia.
TRT> Parenteral nutrition, protection of visceral sac from trauma and infection, surgical closure at a later time.
COMM: Often normal developmental outcome. May be familial.

Behcet Syndrome
DES: Recurrent oral and genital ulcers, uveitis, arthritis, cerebral abnormalities (eg. convulsions, palsies, mental disturbances, encephalitis), (erythema nodosum, thrombophlebitis, skin ulcers, vasculitis, blindness).
TEST: WCC (H), ESR (H).
TRT: Corticosteroids, immunosuppressants.
COMM: Seriously disabling and sometimes fatal. Chronic course with spontaneous temporary remissions.

See also Reiter Syndrome

Bell's Palsy
DES: Paralysis of muscles on one side of face.
TEST: Nil.
TRT: Reassurance, physiotherapy, protect eye and face, prednisone.
COMM: Complete recovery usual in 2-10 weeks. If partial recovery occurs, this will be unresponsive to treatment. May be triggered by trauma or exposure.

Benign Lymphoepithelial Lesion
See Mikulicz Syndrome

Bernard-Soulier Syndrome
DES: Prolonged bleeding time, purpura, petechiae on dependent areas, mucocutaneous bleeding.

EST: Bleeding time (H), coagulation screen (AB, see PATHOLOGY SECTION 4), clotting factors (N).
OMM: Due to poor platelet adhesion from a platelet membrane defect. Aggravated by aspirin. Autosomal recessive inheritance. Similar to Glanzmann syn.

ackfan-Diamond Syndrome (Erythrogenesis nperfecta)

ES: Progressive anaemia (abnormal tryptophan metabolism, Turner syndrome appearance with normal karyotype).
EST: RCC (VL), Hb (L), B.WCC (N), B.reticulocytes (L), platelets (H), U. erythropoietin (H).
RT: Blood transfusion, steroids intermittently.
OMM: Very rare neonatal disorder.

lock-Sulzberger Syndrome (Incontinentia igmenti)

ES: Neonate, linear grouped vesicles on skin, eosinophilia, vesicles become warty then subside to leave pigmented streaks, (usually female, CNS lesions, dental lesions, eye abnormalities).
RT: Nil.
OMM: Causes abortion of male. Present at birth.

loom Syndrome

ES: Small at birth, photosensitive skin, malar hypoplasia, Jewish, leukaemia and other malignant disease (facial telangiectasia).
EST: S.IgA (L), S.IgM (L), lymphoreticular abnormalities.
RT: Nil.
OMM: Extremely rare. Death in adolescence common. Heterozygous carriers prone to malignant disease.

lue Diaper Syndrome

ES: Mental retardation, hypercalcaemia, nephrocalcinosis.
OMM: Due to defect in tryptophan absorption. Degraded to indoles which are excreted and react with napkin starch to produce a blue stain.

lue Rubber Bleb Naevus Syndrome

ES: Multiple blue tinged rubbery blebs in skin, small bowel haemangiomas, (haemangiomas of liver, spleen, brain).
EST: Faecal occult blood (+), blood Hb (L), S.Fe (L).
RT: Resection of gut sometimes helps, iron orally or parenterally, transfusion.
OMM: Chronic condition with poor prognosis.

oerhaave Syndrome

ES: Spontaneous rupture of oesophagus.
RT: Surgical repair.
OMM: May be fatal. Often follows gluttony.

Bonnet Syndrome
See Charles Bonnet Syndrome

Brachial Amyotrophy
See Parsnich-Turner Syndrome

Brachioradialis Pruritis
See Itchy Upper Arm Syndrome

Brachmann-de Lange Syndrome
See de Lange Syndrome

Brain Syndrome, Organic

DES: Emotional disturbances (eg. anxiety, depression), cognitive impairment (eg. memory disorders, disorientation, poor logic, inappropriate sensations), behavioural changes (eg. exhibitionism, aggression), pathological causes (eg. alcohol, drugs, neoplasm, infection, metabolic or endocrine disorders, collagen diseases, epilepsy, etc).
TEST: Extensive investigation of CNS to elicit cause.
TRT: Treat cause, supportive environment, thioridazine, counselling and behavioural therapy.
COMM: Chronic unless reversed early. Always secondary to an organic cause.

Briquet Syndrome (Somatisation Disorder)

DES: Multiple, unexplained, recurrent symptoms with no physical basis.
TEST: All normal.
TRT: Psychiatric counselling. Intractable.
COMM: Form of hysteria. Family history common.

Brown Syndrome

DES: Unilateral eye movement disorder. Limited eye elevation in adduction, normal eye elevation in abduction, (downshoot in adduction, hypotropia in primary position, anomalous head tilt with chin up and ipsilateral head tilt).
TEST: Clinical diagnosis
TRT: Superior oblique tenotomy. Steroids may assist in inflammatory causes
COMM: Usually congenital, but may be acquired due to trauma, surgery, infection or autoimmune inflammation

Brown-Séquard Syndrome

DES: Hemisection of spinal cord causing ipsilateral spastic paralysis and loss of proprioception, contralateral loss of pain and temperature sense, lower motor neurone signs immediately below lesion, light touch preserved bilaterally.
TRT: Treatment of cause if possible.
COMM: May be due to trauma, transverse myelitis,

vascular lesions, tumours or lateral compression. Complete syndrome uncommon.

Brugada Syndrome (laitai)

DES: Sudden onset of ventricular fibrillation followed by collapse and death in 30%. May be cause of undiagnosed sudden death.
TEST: ECG (R bundal branch block with ST elevation in V1 to V3), all physical and ultrasound cardiac tests normal.
TRT: Implanted cardioverter-defribrillator, quinidine.
COMM: Congenital electrocardiographic abnormality more common in males (90%) and those with southeast Asian origins (1:2500).

Bruton Syndrome

DES: Congenital agammaglobulinaemia, leukaemia, lymphomas.
TEST: S.IgG (V), WCC (AB).
TRT: Human γ globulin injections. Treat leukaemia and lymphoma.
COMM: Immune deficiency syndrome.

Budd-Chiari Syndrome

DES: Hepatomegaly, splenomegaly, abdominal pain, ascites, portal hypertension (upper intestinal bleeds).
Test: Ultrasound scan (AB), liver biopsy (+), radionuclide liver scan (+).
TRT: Liver transplant.
COMM: Due to hepatic vein thrombosis secondary to clotting diseases or local tumours. Usually fatal within 2 years.

Burning Vulva Syndrome (Vulvodynia)

DES: Exquisite tenderness of vulval vestibule, infective and dermatological causes excluded.
TEST: Vaginal and vulval swabs (—), STD screen (—), herpes virology (—).
TRT: Loose clothing, reduce washing, reduce irritation of area including sexual activity until healed.
COMM: Diagnosis of exclusion.

Capgras Syndrome (L'illusion de Sosies')

DES: Psychotic delusion that a near relative has been replaced by a double or impersonator, (paranoid schizophrenia).
TEST: EEG (temporal dysrhythmia).
TRT: Nil specific. Try chlorpromazine, trifluoperazine or fluphenazine.
COMM: Rare. May be transient in the elderly.

Carcinoid Syndrome

DES: Facial flushing, oedema of head and neck, abdominal cramps, diarrhoea, asthma, cardiac valve lesions, hepatomegaly, telangiectasia, (hypotension, pulmonary oedema).
TEST: U.5HIAA (H), adrenaline provocation test (+).
TRT: Surgical resection of argentaffinoma, cytotoxic drugs, prednisone in emergency situation and long-term in some cases, cimetidine for flushing, diphenoxylate and atropine for diarrhoea.
COMM: Tumours may arise in ileum, stomach or bronchi.

Carney's Complex

DES: Atrial myxoma, spotty mucocutaneous pigmentation, (cutaneous myxomas, endocrine tumours [eg. Cushing syndrome], dominant inheritance).
TEST: Histology of cutaneous myxomas (AB), echocardiography (AB).
TRT: Surgical removal of cardiac and endocrine myxomas.
COMM: Rare. Metachronous postsurgical tumours may occur.

Carotid Sinus Syndrome

DES: Episodic hypotension, vertigo, syncope, (bradycardia)
TEST: Carotid massage causes brief asystole and hypotension
TRT: Pacemaker
COMM: Exaggerated baroceptor response in the caroti body. Do not perform test in patients with caroti bruit or recent cerebrovascular accident or myocardial infarct

Carotidynia Syndrome

DES: Discomfort to intense pain in and behind angle of jaw that radiates across face and temple, tender carotid artery and bulb, stiff neck muscles, neck oedema, (rhinorrhoea, Horner syndrome, hoarseness).
TEST: WCC, ESR, S.ANA, skull X-ray to exclude temporal arteritis, dental abscess and temporomandibular joint pain.
TRT: Pizotifen, propranolol.
COMM: Migraine-like vascular reaction.

Carpal Tunnel Syndrome

DES: Hand pain (usually in median nerve area and may radiate up arm), impaired median nerve sensation in hand, muscular weakness of hand
TEST: EMG.
TRT: Splinting, NSAIDs, diuretics, surgical relief of carpal tunnel compression.
COMM: Due to compression of median and other nerve in carpal tunnel of wrist. May be associated with rheumatoid arthritis, connective tissue disorders, diabetes and hypocalcaemia.

Carpenter Syndrome (Acrocephalopolysyndactyly)

DES: Peculiar facies, skull deformity, finger

brachysyndactyly, toe syndactyly, obesity,
mental retardation, hypogenitalism.
RT: Plastic surgery for deformities
COMM: Due to premature closure of coronal sutures.
Autosomal recessive inheritance.

See also Apert Syndrome

Catatonic Syndrome
DES: Increased muscular tone at rest that is
abolished during movement, sudden impulsive
movements and excitement.
EST: Exclude pathological or toxic cause.
RT: Hospitalisation, haloperidol or fluphenazine or
thiothixene, psychotherapy, behavioural and
social therapy.
COMM: Usually associated with schizophrenia, but may
be due to neoplasms, encephalopathies, CNS
haemorrhage, drugs, toxins and metabolic
disorders.

Causalgia
See Complex Regional Pain Syndrome Type Two

Cerebrohepatorenal Syndrome
See Zellweger Syndrome

Cervical Rib Syndrome (Naffziger Syndrome, Scalenus Anticus Syndrome, Thoracic Outlet Obstruction Syndrome)
DES: Pain and paraesthesia in arm and hand in
distribution of ulnar nerve, muscular weakness
of small hand muscles, altered sensation in
forearm and hand, (cold blue hands, reduced
pulsation of radial and ulnar arteries, Horner
syndrome).
EST: Adson's test (+), X-ray (cervical rib present).
RT: Rest, traction, surgical excision of rib.
COMM: Slowly progressive, intermittent course.

Charcot Joints
DES: Painless swelling of weight bearing joint with
hypermobility and loss of joint contour. Joint
surface disintegrates.
EST: X-ray (AB), FTA (+), RPR (+).
RT: Orthopaedic support or surgery.
COMM: Usually secondary to syphilis but may occur in
syringomyelia.

See also SIGNS SECTION 2

CHARGE Syndrome
DES: Coloboma of iris-retina, congenital heart
disease, choanal atresia, retarded growth and
development, genital hypoplasia, ear
abnormalities and deafness (oesophageal
atresia, facial palsy, renal abnormalities,
structural brain defects, cleft lip and palate,
endocrine defects).

TRT: Feeding gastrostomy, heart surgery,
symptomatic.
COMM: Name is an acronym for major clinical features.
Often die soon after birth, but if survive first year,
prognosis reasonable. Result of an embryonic
neural crest defect.

Charles Bonnet Syndrome
DES: Vivid, elaborate and recurrent visual
hallucinations in elderly patients with ocular
disorders, affective reactions (olfactory
hallucinations).
TRT: Psychological counselling and support,
psychiatric therapy.
COMM: Often found in widows deprived of any company
or outside contact.

Chediak-Higashi Syndrome
DES: Recurrent skin infections, partial albinism
(hepatosplenomegaly, respiratory, infections,
pancytopenia).
TEST: B.leukocytes (giant inclusion lysosomes), B.T
cell lymphocyte CD16(L).
TRT: Steroids. Bone marrow transplants. Vitamin C.
COMM: Autosomal recessive disease.

Chiari-Frommel Syndrome
DES: Abnormal secondary amenorrhoea after
cessation of breast feeding following
confinement, continued lactation.
TEST: Prolactin Assay (H or N), pituitary tomography
or CT scan.
TRT: Surgery for pituitary tumour.
COMM: May be due to prolactin secreting pituitary
tumour.

Chinese Restaurant Syndrome
DES: Facial pressure, headache, nausea, chest pain,
burning sensation of head and upper trunk.
TRT: Symptomatic. Settles spontaneously after 12 to
48 hours.
COMM: Caused by overuse of sodium glutamate.
Aggravated by alcohol.

Chorda Tympani Syndrome
DES: Submental sweating after eating
TEST: Surgical section of chorda tympani

Chronic Fatigue Syndrome (Myalgic Encephalomyelitis)
DES: The diagnosis of this condition can only be
confirmed if both major criteria are met, plus six
symptoms and two signs from the minor criteria.
Major criteria:
— New persistent or relapsing, debilitating
fatigue severe enough to reduce or impair
average daily activity below 50% of premorbid
activity of a period of more than 6 months

— Exclusion of all other causes by thorough clinical evaluation and haematological and biochemical investigations

Minor criteria — Symptoms:
— Generalised fatigue lasting more than 24 hours following levels of exertion that would have been easily tolerated previously
— Generalised headache
— Mild fever <38.6°C
— Unexplained general muscle weakness
— Myalgia
— Migratory arthralgia without signs
— Sore throat
— Painful cervical or axillary lymph nodes
— One or more of the following neuropsychological problems (photophobia, forgetfulness, irritability, confusion, poor concentration, depression, transient visual disturbances, difficulty thinking)
— Insomnia or hypersomnia
— Rapid onset over hours or days of major criteria

Minor criteria – Signs documented by a physician on at least two occasions at least a month apart
— Mild fever <38.6°C
— Nonexudative pharyngitis
— Palpable or tender cervical or axillary lymphadenopathy

TEST: FBC, ESR, C-RP, LFT, S. creatinine, TFT and other tests considered justified by the physician to exclude any other cause of the symptoms.

TRT: Symptomatic, supportive.

COMM: More common in young females. May follow a viral infection. Tends to run a relapsing course for one to four years or more before settling spontaneously. Prognosis poor if the patient has a social or psychological reason for remaining ill. May be severely debilitating.

Churg-Strauss Syndrome

DES: Asthma, systemic vasculitis involving two or more extrapulmonary organs, blood eosinophilia, (peripheral neuropathy, cardiac disease, pulmonary infiltrates, pulmonary haemorrhage, diarrhoea, rash, glomerulonephritis).

TEST: B.eosinophils (H), S.ANCA (+), tissue biopsy eosinophils (H), tissue biopsy (AB).

TRT: Prednisone, cyclophosphamide, azathioprine.

COMM: Long-term follow up essential.

Circulatory Shock
See Shock Syndrome

Clérambault Syndrome
See de Clérambault Syndrome

Climacteric Syndrome
See Menopausal Syndrome

Cockayne Syndrome

DES: Mental retardation, dwarfism, optic atrophy, neural deafness, hypersensitivity to sunlight, cataracts, retinal pigmentary degeneration, (cerebellar defects, peripheral neuropathy)

TEST: Skin biopsy shows defective fibroblast DNA

TRT: None available

COMM: Rare. Autosomal recessive inheritance.

Coffin-Lowry Syndrome

DES: Prominent lips, coarse facial features, tapering fingers, antimongoloid eye slant, mental retardation, kyphosis and scoliosis.

TEST: Nil specific.

TRT: Nil.

COMM: X-linked recessive inheritance.

Coffin-Siris Syndrome

DES: Hypoplastic toenails, generalised hirsutism at birth, mental retardation, coarse facial features, sparse hair in later life.

COMM: Autosomal recessive inheritance .

Cogan Syndrome

DES: Interstitial keratitis, tinnitus, vertigo, deafness, (fever, lymphadenopathy, arthralgia, abdominal pain, splenomegaly, melaena, cardiac abnormalities eg. aortic valve disease).

TEST: ESR (H), WCC (H), B.eosinophils (H).

TRT: Corticosteroids, cyclophosphamide.

COMM: Rapid onset in young adults. Rare. Variable self-limiting course.

Collet-Sicard Syndrome
See Sicard Syndrome

Complex Regional Pain Syndrome Type One
See Reflex Sympathetic Dystrophy Syndrome

Complex Regional Pain Syndrome Type Two (Causalgia)

DES: Sudden onset of limb pain in the tissue supplied by the affected nerve, limb dysfunction, oedema, sudomotor abnormalities, vasomotor abnormalities, abnormal sweating

TEST: None diagnostic.

TRT: Physiotherapy, systemic steroids, calcium channel blockers, NSAID

COMM: Regional pain syndrome that develops after injury to a peripheral nerve

Congenital Adrenal Hyperplasia
See Adrenogenital Syndrome, Child

Conn Syndrome

DES: Primary aldosteronism due to an aldosterone

secreting adenoma. Symptoms include hypertension, muscular weakness, hyporeflexia, paraesthesiae, arrhythmias, tetany.
EST: S.sodium (H), S.potassium (L), ECG (AB).
RT: Surgical excision of adenoma in adrenal gland. Spironolactone.
OMM: Fatal without treatment.

onradi-Hunermann Syndrome
ES: Ventricular septal defect, patent ductus arteriosus, asymmetric limb shortness, large skin pores, (early punctate mineralisation)
RT: Cardiac Surgery

onrad Syndrome
ES: Cataract, limb contractures, deafness, retardation, stippled ephiphyses on X-ray.
RT: Surgery for cataract and limb contractures.
OMM: Congenital.

ontractural Arachnodactyly
ee Beal Syndrome

ori's Syndrome (Type III Glycogen Storage isease)
ES: Mild glycogen storage disease, hepatomegaly, growth retardation, diarrhoea, peripheral myopathy, cirrhosis, cardiomyopathy, late onset.
EST: B.lactate (H), glucagon stimulation test (AB).
RT: High glucose diet, liver transplant.
OMM: Caused by lack of amylo-1-6-glucosidase.

osten Syndrome
ES: Ear pain and discomfort, temporal headache, tinnitus, impaired hearing, dental malocclusion.
EST: X-rays of temporomandibular joint with mouth open and closed (AB).
RT: Dental or surgical correction of malocclusion.
OMM: Due to abnormal stress on temporomandibular joint and muscles used in mastication.

ostochondral Syndrome
ee Tietze Syndrome

ot Death
ee Sudden Infant Death Syndrome

owden Disease
ee Multiple Hamartoma Syndrome

REST Syndrome
ES: Calcinosis, Raynaud's phenomenon, oesophageal pathology, sclerodactyly, telangiectasia.

TEST: B.centromere autoantibodies (+).
COMM: Subform of scleroderma. Name an acronym for symptoms. Good prognosis.

Creutzfeldt-Jakob Syndrome
DES: Myoclonic jerks, seizures, dementia, aphasia, paralysis, visual disturbances, primitive reflexes.
TEST: EEG (AB).
TRT: Nil.
COMM: Rapidly progressive to death within 12 months. May be caused by a prion infection.

Cri-du-Chat Syndrome
DES: Mental retardation, ocular hypertelorism, microcephaly, round face, low set ears, cat-like cry ("cri du chat") as newborn.
TEST: Chromosome studies (deletion of short arm of fifth chromosome).
TRT: Nil.
COMM: Cat cry disappears with age.

Crigler-Najjar Syndrome
DES: Severe nonhaemorrhagic jaundice of neonate, kernicterus.
TEST: S.unconjugated bilirubin (VH).
TRT: Phenobarbitone helps some types.
COMM: Due to glucuronyl transferase deficiency.
See also Gilbert Syndrome

Crocodile Tears Syndrome
DES: Tears pour from affected eye with eating, occurs after recovery from Bells' palsy.
TRT: Surgical division of tympanic nerve division conveying glossopharyngeal salivary fibres.
COMM: Possibly due to regenerating salivary branches of the facial nerve being misdirected to the lacrimal gland during recovery from Bell's palsy.

Cronkhite Syndrome
DES: Abnormal pigmentation of fingers, hands, palms and soles.
See also Cronkhite-Canada Syndrome

Cronkhite-Canada Syndrome
DES: Abnormal pigmentation of fingers, hands, palms and soles, mucosal thickening in the stomach, small bowel and colon to form non-cancerous polyp-like lumps
TEST: Gastroscopy and colonoscopy
COMM: Intestinal haemorrhage may cause anaemia.

Crouzon Syndrome
DES: Craniofacial dysostosis, exophthalmos, divergent squint, optic atrophy.
TEST: Skull X-ray (AB).

TRT: Major facial surgery.
COMM: Familial.

CRST Syndrome
See CREST Syndrome

Cubital Tunnel Syndrome
DES: Sensory loss in the fifth finger and half the fourth
        finger, wasting and weakness of ulnar supplied
        intrinsic muscles and flexor digitorum
        profundus, frequently bilateral.
TRT: Operative release of ulnar nerve trapped under
        flexor carpi ulnaris aponeurosis 3 cm distal to
        medial epicondyle of elbow.
COMM: Due to ulnar nerve entrapment. No history of
        trauma necessary.

Cushing Syndrome (Adrenocortical Hyperfunction)
DES: Central obesity (moon face, buffalo hump,
        abdominal protuberance), purple striae,
        psychosis, plethoric, oligomenorrhoea or
        impotence, weakness, headache, backache,
        hypertension, acne, chloasma.
TEST: Blood pressure (H), X-ray (osteoporosis), IVP
        (nephrolithiasis, adrenal enlargement), CT scan
        (adrenal enlargement), adrenal angiography
        (adrenal enlargement), ECG (short P-R
        interval), S.17-hydroxy steroids (H),
        S.potassium (L), S.chloride (L), B.eosinophils
        (L), dexamethasone suppression test (+),
        ACTH stimulation test (+), P.ACTH (VH), U.free
        cortisol (H), B.WCC (L).
TRT: Surgical removal of adrenal tumour with
        cortisone cover, irradiation of pituitary,
        hypophysectomy, correction of iatrogenic
        causes.
COMM: Usually due to pituitary or adrenal disease. May
        be due to ACTH secretion by other neoplasms
        (eg. oat cell carcinoma of lung), or steroid
        therapy.

Cutis Hyperelastica
See Ehlers-Danlos Syndrome

Cystic Duct Syndrome
DES: Cystic duct obstruction by fibrosis or adhesion,
        pain on gall bladder stimulation, normal gall
        bladder.
TEST: IV cholangiogram ('golf-ball' gall bladder after
        stimulation, no gall stones).
TRT: Cholecystectomy.
COMM: Mimics cholelithiasis.

DaCosta Syndrome (Effort Syndrome)
DES: Chronic palpitations resistant to psychiatric
        care; triggered by anxiety, exercise or stress;
        wide pulse pressure.

TEST: ECG (AB).
TRT: Beta-blockers.
COMM: Functional state with no underlying pathology.

Dandy Syndrome
DES: Total bilateral loss of vestibular function,
        horizon bounces up and down as patient walks
        (loss of foveation), vertigo

Dandy-Walker Syndrome
DES: Craniomegaly, vomiting, irritability, poor head
        control, cleft palate, nystagmus,
        (hydrocephalus, wide ataxic gait, headaches,
        polycystic kidneys, abnormal lumbar vertebrae,
        subnormal mentality, delayed motor
        development)
TEST: X-ray & CT skull (AB)
TRT: Surgery to cerebellum and upper spinal canal,
        CSF shunt
COMM: Failure of the midline portion of the cerebellum
        to develop

---

de Clerambault Syndrome (Erotomania)
DES: Monomania, fixed delusional conviction that
        another is in love with them despite minimal
        contact, majority are female, may persecute
        victim, who is often a doctor.
TRT: Psychoanalysis, phenothiazines,
        clomipramine.
COMM: Poor prognosis. Treatment extremely difficult
        and often unsuccessful. Certification
        occasionally necessary.

Defibrination Syndrome
DES: Bleeding excessively from mucous membranes
        and skin, ecchymoses, melaena, epistaxis.
TEST: Clot formation (poor), B.platelets (L),
        prothrombin time (H), B.fibrinogen (L), Hb (L),
        APTT (VH), thrombin time (H), bleeding time
        (H).
TRT: Treat underlying disorder (eg. sepsis, shock),
        heparin may control pathological clotting and
        bleeding, fresh blood transfusions, blood
        cryoprecipitate.
COMM: Diffuse, pathological intravascular coagulation
        secondary to sepsis, shock or childbirth. Fibrin
        levels depleted causing secondary bleeding.
        Prognosis serious.

Déjerine-Roussy Syndrome (Thalamic pain Syndrome)
DES: Excruciating, unrelenting pain involving the
        entire one side of the body
TEST: MRI or CT (AB)
TRT: Neurosurgery to ablate thalamus
COMM: Caused by stroke or head injury involving
        posterolateral thalamus.

See also Lateral Medullary Syndrome

e Lange Syndrome (Brachmann-de Lange yndrome, Amsterdam Dwarf)

ES: Microcephaly, severe mental retardation, bushy eyebrows that meet in centre, low birth weight and failure to thrive, low hairline, hirsute, (skeletal malformations).
RT: Nil.
OMM: Congenital. Rarely survive beyond 10 years.

e Toni-Fanconi-Debré Syndrome

ES: Osteomalacia, aminoaciduria, phosphaturia, glycosuria, renal tubular acidosis.
EST: U.glucose (H), U.phosphate (H), U.pH (L), U.amino acids (H), S.potassium (L), S.phosphate (L).
RT: Correct cation deficits, vitamin D and calcium supplements.
OMM: Defect of renal tubular function.

Demons-Meigs Syndrome

See Meigs Syndrome

Denervation Syndrome

DES: Gas bloat syndrome (see separate entry), diarrhoea, gastric dilation, retention of gastric contents, recent oesophageal surgery.
TEST: Gastroscopy.
TRT: Diet, pyloroplasty.
COMM: Due to vagal nerve damage during operative mobilisation of the oesophagus.

Devic Syndrome (Neuromyelitis Optica)

DES: Acute bilateral optic neuritis (total or partial vision loss), transverse myelitis (paraplegia), (multiple sclerosis).
TEST: CSF WCC (H), CSF protein (H)
TRT: Immunosuppressive drugs
COMM: Course similar to that of MS

DiGeorge Syndrome (Thymic Hypoplasia)

DES: Neonatal tetany, hypertelorism, recurrent severe infections, hypocalcaemia.
TEST: S.Ig (N), antibody response (L), S.Ca (L), B.lymphocytes (L), B.T-cells (absent), lymph node biopsy (AB).
TRT: Thymic tissue transplantation.
COMM: Due to embryogenic failure of the thymus and parathyroid glands.

See also Good Syndrome; Nezelof Syndrome

Diencephalic Syndrome

DES: Cachexia, pallor, vomiting, (nystagmus, optic atrophy, tremor, sweats, hypoglycaemia, polyuria).
Usually male child.
COMM: Poor prognosis. Due to anterior hypothalamic tumour.

Diogenes Syndrome

DES: Recluse, live in filth and squalor, male >> female, (substance abuse, mental subnormality)
TEST: Exclude organic cause of mental disorder
TRT: Treat psychoses, dementia
COMM: More a symptom of underlying problem than a syndrom in itself.

Down Syndrome (Trisomy 21, Mongolism)

DES: Mental retardation, flattened facial features, dwarfism, low-set ears, heavily fissured protruding tongue, spotty depigmentation of iris, broad hands with single transverse crease, (congenital heart lesions, lenticular opacities).
TEST: Chromosomal studies (trisomy 21).
TRT: Nil. Social support of parents and patient.
COMM: More common in older mothers. Rare familial form. Higher than average mortality rate.

Dressler Syndrome

DES: After myocardial infarct, pericarditis, pericardial friction rub, fever, (pneumonitis).
TEST: B.myocardial autoantibodies (+). Cardiac enzymes and other biochemical criteria used to differentiate syndrome from new infarct of myocardium, cardiac failure or pulmonary embolism.
TRT: Spontaneous resolution accelerated by indomethacin or corticosteroids.
COMM: Hypersensitivity reaction.

Dry Eye Syndrome

DES: Significantly reduced tear production, dry scratchy irritated eye (xerophthalmia).
TEST: Schirmer tear test (+).
TRT: Artificial tear drops or ointment. Surgical blockage of tear duct to prevent tear drainage.
COMM: Common.

Duane Syndrome

DES: Congenital absence fo 6th nerve resulting in deficient horizontal eye movement.
TRT: Surgery if strabismus severe.
COMM: Rare. Visual acuity normal.

Dubin-Johnson Syndrome

DES: Asymptomatic neonatal jaundice, gall bladder not seen on oral cholecystogram.
TEST: S.conjugated bilirubin (VH), BSP excretion (L), darkly pigmented liver on biopsy.
TRT: Nil necessary.
COMM: Good prognosis.

Dubowitz Syndrome

DES: Intrauterine growth retardation, ptosis, micrognathia, sparse hair, short stature, mild mental retardation, eczema.
COMM: Autosomal recessive inheritance.

Ductus Arteriosus
See Eisenmenger Syndrome ; Patent Ductus Arteriosus

Dumping Syndrome (Postgastrectomy Syndrome)
DES: Sweating, tachycardia, pallor, epigastric discomfort, nausea, weakness, abdominal cramps, (syncope, vomiting, diarrhoea). All symptoms occur within 20 minutes of eating in a patient who has had a partial gastrectomy.
TEST: S.glucose (N), glucose tolerance test (late hypoglycaemia), ECG (non-specific AB).
TRT: Frequent small meals with low carbohydrate content. No fluids with meal. Sedatives and anticholinergics.
COMM: Occurs in 10% of postgastrectomy patients.

Dysautonomia
See Riley-Day Syndrome

Dyscontrol Syndrome, Episodic
See Episodic Dyscontrol Syndrome

Dysplastic Naevus Syndrome
DES: Naevus <10mm diameter, irregular pigmentation, irregular colouration, poorly defined edge, irregular border, greater than 40 moles on body, usually on trunk.
TEST: Histology.
TRT: Excision of some, observation of all moles.
COMM: Often progress to malignant melanomas.

Dystrophia Adiposgenitalis
See Fröhlich Syndrome

Eaton-Lambert Syndrome (Myasthenic Syndrome)
DES: Presynaptic disorder characterised by impaired release of acetylcholine from nerve endings, (bronchial carcinoma).
TRT: Immunosuppressive drugs.
COMM: Autoimmune aetiology similar to myasthenia gravis.

Ebstein Anomaly
DES: Tricuspid valve dysplasia and displacement into the right ventricle, tricuspid valve regurgitation, impaired right ventricular function, right to left atrial shunt, (cyanosis, paroxysmal atrial tachycardia, Wolff-Parkinson-White syndrome)
TEST: Echocardiography
TRT: Propranolol, valve replacement surgery, transection of abnormal conduction tracts
COMM: Congenital

Edwards' Syndrome (Trisomy 18)
DES: Micrognathia, cardiac malformations, rocker-bottom feet.
TRT: Nil.
COMM: Congenital.

Effort Syndrome
See Da Costa Syndrome

Ehlers-Danlos Syndrome (Cutis Hyperelastica)
DES: Hyperextensible joints, skin fragility, skin hyperelasticity, knee and elbow scarring and pseudotumours.
TRT: Nil.
COMM: Eight clinically and genetically different variants

Eisenmenger Syndrome
DES: Patent ductus arteriosus with bidirectional or right to left flow, pulmonary hypertension, machinery murmur.
TEST: ECG (N or L ventricular hypertrophy), cardiac catheterisation (AB).
TRT: Surgery, indomethacin sometimes successful.
COMM: Due to failure of ductus arteriosus to close and obliterative changes to pulmonary arterioles.

See also Patent Ductus Arteriosus

Ellis-van Creveld Syndrome
DES: Polydactyly, excess oral frenula, small nails, short arms and legs, small chest, atrial septal defect, ventricular septal defect.
TEST: Nil.
TRT: Surgical repair of defects.
COMM: Autosomal recessive inheritance.

Ekbom Syndrome
See Restless legs Syndrome

Eosinophilia-Myalgia Syndrome (EMS)
DES: Marked eosinophilia, severe myalgia, cough, dyspnoea, arthralgia, peripheral oedema, thick skin, rashes, neuritis.
TEST: B.eosinophils (VH), S.transaminases (H), WCC (H).
TRT: Nil other than stopping L-tryptophan ingestion.
COMM: Triggered by ingestion of high dose L-tryptophan. Mortality 1%.

Episodic Dyscontrol Syndrome
DES: Physical abuse of family, severe episodic intoxication, impulsive sexual misconduct, irresponsible social behaviour.
TEST: EEG (AB or N), exclude CNS tumour or lesion.
TRT: Avoid alcohol, phenytoin and/or thioridazine, legal restraints.

COMM: Not related to recognised mental disorders (eg. schizophrenia).

Erb-Duchenne Palsy

DES: Neonate flaccid paralysis of shoulder girdle muscles, (sensory loss over deltoid muscle, diaphragmatic palsy).
TEST: Arm hangs in 'porter's tip' position (see Waiter's Hand)
TRT: Rest arm with shoulder abducted, arm prone and elbow flexed. Strap to infant's pillow.
COMM: Usually due to excess traction on head during delivery, and trauma to 5th cervical nerve.

See also Parsnich-Turner Syndrome

Erotomania

See De Clérambault Syndrome

Erythema Infectiosum

See Slapped Cheek Syndrome

Erythrogenesis Imperfecta

See Blackfan-Diamond Syndrome

Fallot's Pentalogy

DES: Atrial septal defect, pulmonary artery stenosis, dextroposition of aorta, right ventricular hypertrophy, ventricular septal defect.

See also Fallot's Tetralogy

Fallot's Tetralogy

DES: Pulmonary artery stenosis, ventricular septal defect, dextroposition of aorta, right ventricular hypertrophy, (cyanosis on exertion, retarded physique, dyspnoea relieved by squatting, finger clubbing).
TEST: Chest X-ray (clear lung fields, abnormal heart shadow), ECG (AB), angiocardiography (AB), cardiac catheterisation (AB), heart sounds (harsh systolic murmur and thrill at left sternal border), echocardiography (AB).
TRT: Surgical correction of defects.
COMM: Most common congenital heart disease. Operative mortality 3%. Small chance of survival to adult life without surgery.

See also Fallot's Pentalogy; Fallot's Trilogy

Fallot's Trilogy

DES: Pulmonary artery stenosis, atrial septal defect, right ventricular hypertrophy.

See also Fallot's Tetralogy

Fanconi Syndrome

See De Toni-Fanconi-Debré Syndrome

Felty Syndrome

DES: Febrile migratory polyarthritis, splenomegaly, leucopenia, (hyperpigmentation, leg ulcers, lymphadenopathy, hepatomegaly). Usually associated with advanced rheumatoid disease.
TEST: Rheumatoid factor (VH), B.LE cells (H), B.antinuclear antibodies (VH), Hb (L), B.leukocytes (L), B.neutrophils (VL), B.platelets (L or N).
TRT: Splenectomy, symptomatic treatment of arthritis.

Fetal Alcohol Syndrome

DES: Intrauterine growth retardation, mid-face hypoplasia, hirsute, small fingernails, short palpebral fissures, mild mental retardation, (microcephaly, hypotonia, hyperactive, poor coordination, micrognathia).
TRT: Nil.
COMM: Due to excess alcohol intake (>80 g per day) by pregnant mother. Incidence 1:1000.

Fibrositis Syndrome (Fibromyalgia Syndrome)

DES: Trunk and/or limb pain with multiple variable tender points, stiffness, exhaustion, aggravated by cold, eased by heat.
TRT: Salicylates, NSAIDs, benzodiazepines, amitriptyline.
COMM: Often precipitated by sleep disturbances.

Fibrous Dysplasia

See Albright Syndrome

Fitz-Hugh-Curtis Syndrome

DES: Perihepatitis secondary to salpingitis. Abdominal pain worse lying down and turning, vaginal discharge, vulval itch, dysuria.
TEST: Peritoneal fluid (+ for Chlamydia).
TRT: Tetracycline for patient and partner(s).

Floppy Baby Syndrome

DES: Partial widespread muscular paralysis in an infant.
TEST: Faecal botulism test (+). False negative very common.
TRT: Supportive.
COMM: Babies fed honey contaminated with dust containing Clostridium botulinum are affected by the toxin produced by this bacteria. Rarely fatal. Self-limiting.

Floppy Eyelid Syndrome

DES: Obesity, slack rubbery tarsal plate, papillary conjunctivitis, lax canthal tendons, spontaneous eversion of upper eyelid during sleep (corneal ulceration).
TRT: Weight loss, tape eyelid at night, surgical correction.

Focal Dermal Hypoplasia
See Goltz Syndrome

Foetal Alcohol Syndrome
See Fetal Alcohol Syndrome

Fong Syndrome
See Nail-Patella Syndrome

Fragile X Syndrome
DES: Mental subnormality, hyperactivity, autism, epilepsy, large infant, large jaw, ears and forehead, myopia, enlarged testes, single palmar crease, flat feet, (fourth heart sound, cleft palate, lax joints, nystagmus). More common and severe in males, normal females may be carriers.
TEST: Cytogenetics (variable AB), chorionic villus biopsy (95% reliable at 15 weeks pregnant). Carriers may be normal.
TRT: Appropriate support servcies, thioridazine or methylphenidate for hyperactivity. Family genetic counselling.
COMM: Common cause of mental retardation (1 in 2000 men, 25% of all mentally retarded males).

France's Triad
DES: Asthma, aspirin sensitivity, allergic rhinitis (nasal polyposis).

Freeman-Sheldon Syndrome (Whistling Face Syndrome)
DES: Talipes, club hands, pursed lips, difficulty opening mouth, facial grimace, normal mentality.
TRT: Plastic and orthopaedic surgery
COMM: Autosomal dominant.

Frey Syndrome (Auriculo-Temporal Syndrome)
DES: Sweating and vasodilation in the distribution of the auriculo-temporal nerve when eating.
TRT: Surgery.
COMM: Due to disturbance between the sympathetic and parasympathetic nerves. May follow infection or surgery to the parotid gland.

Fröhlich Syndrome (Dystrophia Adiposogenitalis)
DES: Puberty or later onset, loss of libido and sexual function, thin skin that wrinkles prematurely, scanty body hair, fine scalp hair, obesity of buttocks, genitals and thighs, lethargy.
TEST: Exclude pituitary tumour.
TRT: Hormone supplements.
COMM: Rare.

Fuchs Syndrome (Fuchs Uveitis, Heterochromic Cyclitis)
DES: Chronic non-granulomatous anterior uveitis, different coloured irises, blurred vision, slow onset, unilateral, young adult or child, (secondary cataract, glaucoma)
TEST: Abnormal gonioscopy
TRT: None available
COMM: Regular checks for glaucoma or cataract formation

Gaisböck Syndrome (Stress Erythrocytosis)
DES: Polycythaemia, hypertension, smoker, plethora (middle-aged, overweight, white male, alcohol abuse)
TEST: B.erythrocytes (H), plasma volume (L), PCV (H)
TRT: None necessary
COMM: No splenic enlargement. May be familial

Gardner Syndrome
DES: Adenomatosis coli, mandibular osteomas, sebaceous cysts, soft tissue tumours, (melaena).
TEST: Faecal occult blood (+ or –), Ba enema (AB), colonoscopy (AB), S.CEA (+ or –).
TRT: Surgical.
COMM: Genetic problem. Significant risk of large bowel cancer.

Gas Bloat Syndrome
DES: Postprandial abdominal distension, inability to vomit or belch.
TEST: Gastroscopy or barium meal.
TRT: Operative release of cardiac sphincter.
COMM: Supercontinence of the cardiac sphincter after a Nissen fundoplication. Aggravated by air swallowing.

Gastrinoma
See Zollinger-Ellison Syndrome

Gay Bowel Syndrome
DES: Infective enterocolitis, diarrhoea, tenesmus, homosexual male.
TEST: Faeces M/C/S (+).
TRT: Appropriate antibiotic.
COMM: Due to anal or oral sex. May be due to many different bacteria (eg. Shigella, Salmonella), viruses (eg. herpes), chlamydia or protozoa.

Geniculate Herpes
See Ramsay Hunt Syndrome

Gerstmann Syndrome
DES: Total agnosia, agraphia, unable to calculate, unable to recognise own body parts, unable to distinguish left from right
COMM: Caused by lesions of the dominant parietal lobe

erstmann-Straussler-Scheinker Syndrome

ES: Onset in mid-life, clumsiness, unsteadiness,
      incoordination, abnormal gait, (ataxia,
      dysarthria, deafness, blindness)
RT: Nil available
OMM: Hereditary spino-cerebellar degeneration
      caused by a prion

ianotti-Crosti Syndrome

ES: Multiple papular dull red spots develop on thighs,
      buttocks, arms and face over 3-4 days, spots
      become purple espedcially on the legs due to
      capillary leakage, mild fever, mild itch, axillary
      and groin lymphadenopahy, hepatomegaly
EST: Viral serology (AB), LFT (AB)
RT: Mild steroid cream for itch.
OMM: Affects children from 6 months to 12 years. Skin
      response to viral infection (eg. Hepatitis B,
      Epstein Barr virus, Coxsackie viruses, Echo
      viruses, respiratory syncitial virus). Rash fades
      in 2-8 weeks with mild scaling. Recurrence
      unlikely but possible

ilbert Syndrome

ES: Benign asymptomatic hereditary jaundice, dark
      complexion.
EST: S.bilirubin (H, VH with 24 hour fast),
      S. unconjugated bilirubin (H).
RT: Nil usually necessary. Phenobarbitone or
      aminopyrine induce synthesis of microsomal
      enzymes in liver to relieve jaundice.
OMM: Due to glucuronyl transferase deficiency.
      Autosomal dominant trait.

illes de la Tourette's Syndrome

ES: Onset in childhood, seizures, involuntary
      movements, uncontrollable involuntary
      vocalisations.
RT: Dopamine antagonists, haloperidol.
COMM: Rare.

See also Crigler-Najjar Syndrome

illespie Syndrome

DES: Aniridia (lack of iris), mental retardation,
      cerebellar ataxia
EST: Non specific
RT: None available
COMM: recessively inherited

See also Miller Syndrome

lanzmann Syndrome

DES: Prolonged bleeding time, recurrent episodes of
      severe mucosal haemorrhage.
EST: Bleeding time (H).
RT: Whole blood or platelet transfusion.
COMM: Defect in platelet membrane structure.
      Autosomal recessive inheritance. Similar to
      Bernard-Soulier syn.

Glycogen Storage Diseases

See Andersen Syndrom; Cori Syndrome; Hers
Syndrome; McArdle Syndrome; Pompe Syndrome; von
Gierke Syndrome

Goltz Syndrome (Focal Dermal Hypoplasia)

DES: Scar-like areas of skin atrophy on scalp, thighs
      and iliac crests, (hypotrichosis, nail
      abnormalities).
TRT: Nil available.
COMM: Due to partial or complete dermal absence in
      affected areas.

Good Syndrome

DES: Thymic hypoplasia, hypothyroidism.
COMM: Very rare.

See also DiGeorge Syndrome; Nezelof Syndrome

Goodpasture Syndrome

DES: Recurrent haemoptysis, dyspnoea, anaemia,
      cough, pulmonary haemosiderosis,
      glomerulonephritis, (renal failure).
TEST: Hb (L), S.Fe (L), lung or renal biopsy (AB),
      B.glomerular basement membrane
      autoantibodies (+).
TRT: Prednisone, cyclophosphamide,
      plasmaphoresis, haemodialysis, nephrectomy
      and renal transplantation.
COMM: Poor prognosis. Immunological mechanism.

Gorlin-Goltz Syndrome (Basal Cell Carcinoma Naevus Syndrome

DES: Multiple naevoid basal cell carcinomas,
      intracranial calcification, vertebral and rib
      abnormalities, multiple odontogenic
      keratocysts of the mandible, palm pitting, onset
      in childhood (macrocephaly, epidermal cysts,
      spina bifida occulta, pectus excavatum, cardiac
      fibroma, cleft lip, polydactyly).
TEST: Radiology of jaw, vertebrae and ribs (AB).
TRT: Excision of mandibular cysts and basal cell
      carcinomas.
COMM: Recurrence of mandibular cysts after excision is
      common. Inherited.

Gradenigo Syndrome (Petrositis)

DES: Headache, diplopia, facial pain, middle ear
      infection.
TRT: Antibiotics, mastoidectomy.
COMM: Due to infection of petrous bone apex involving
      sixth cranial nerve.

Grey Baby Syndrome

DES: Chloramphenicol use, cardiovascular collapse.
COMM: Fatal chloramphenicol toxicity due to liver
      impairment and failure to eliminate drug.

Growing Pains
See Limb Pain Syndrome

Guillain-Barré Syndrome
DES: Polyneuritis, progressive symmetrical weakening of limbs or face, hand and foot paraesthesia, back pain, dysarthria, dysphagia, flaccid respiratory paralysis.
TEST: CFS (AB), CSF protein (H), depressed or absent reflexes.
TRT: Symptomatic, respiratory support, corticosteroids controversial.
COMM: Progressive symptoms with peak disability at one month. May follow a viral infection or vaccination. Spontaneous recovery in 80%. Rarely may progress to death.

Guyton's Canal Syndrome
DES: Sensory loss in the fifth finger and half the fourth finger, wasting and weakness of ulnar supplied intrinsic muscles of the hand.
TRT: NSAIDs, operative release of ulnar nerve at wrist.
COMM: Due to ulnar nerve entrapment at wrist.

Haemolytic Uraemic Syndrome
DES: Haematuria, proteinuria, anaemia, thrombocytopenia, (acute renal insufficiency, vomiting, diarrhoea).
TEST: Renal biopsy (AB), U.blood (+), U.protein (+), platelets (L), Hb (L), FBC (AB), S.creatinine (H), S.urea (H).
TRT: Transfusion, conservative management of renal failure.
COMM: Due to renal microangiopathy and reduced glomerular filtration rate with associated haemolytic anaemia. Familial and acquired forms. May follow gut infections or occur with pregnancy. Mortality rate 30%.

Hajdu-Cheney Syndrome
DES: Child, lax joints, premature tooth loss, small unusually shaped facies, micrognathia, unusual eye and eyebrow shape, slow growth, excess body hair, generalised weakness and pain, (finger abnormalities)
TRT: Nil
COMM: Autosomal dominant inheritance

Hallermann-Streiff Syndrome
DES: Cataracts, facial and dental anomalies, hypotrichosis, dwarfism.
TRT: Surgical correction of deformities and cataract.
COMM: Congenital.

Hamman-Rich Syndrome (Idiopathic diffuse Interstitial Fibrosis)
DES: Diffuse progressive interstitial fibrosis of lungs with severe respiratory embarrassment.

TEST: Chest X-ray (diffuse reticulation).
TRT: Nil effective.
COMM: Usually fatal. May follow acute pneumonia

Hand-Schueller-Christian Syndrome (Histiocytosis X)
DES: Diabetes insipidus, exophthalmos, skull bone absorption, otitis externa, (skin rashes, gingivitis)
TEST: Skull X-ray (map like areas of decreased density), chest X-ray (mottled or honeycomb lung), skin biopsy (foam cells), bone marrow biopsy (foam cells or N).
TRT: Treat diabetes insipidus, deep X-ray to bone lesions, chemotherapy (eg. vinblastine, prednisone, cyclophosphamide).
COMM: Usually occurs in children. Non-familial.

Happy Puppet Syndrome
See Angelman Syndrome

Harlequin Syndrome
DES: Severe khthyosis, disordered keratinisation, distorted features.
TRT: Moisturising cream in large quantities.
COMM: Most die *in utero*. Long-term survival rare. Congenital.

Heerfordt Syndrome (Uveoparotid Syndrome)
DES: Salivary adenitis, uni or bilateral facial paralysis (Bell's palsy), uveitis, sarcoidosis
COMM: Self-limiting benign lymphoepithelial lesion

Heiner Syndrome
DES: Cows' milk allergy, chronic pulmonary disease, anaemia, eosinophilia
TEST: FBC (AB), Hb (L)
TRT: Avoid cows' milk. Treat pulmonary symptoms

HELLP Syndrome
DES: Haemolysis, elevated liver enzyme activity, low platelet count, pregnant woman, (hypertension, pre-eclampsia, abdominal pain).
TEST: LFTs (AB), FBC (haemolysis, low platelets).
TRT: Early confinement if possible.
COMM: Name is an acronym for characteristic blood picture.

Henoch-Schoenlein Syndrome (Anaphylactoid Purpura)
DES: Purpura, generalised vasculitis, (abdominal pain, intestinal bleeding, haemoptysis, haematuria, arthralgia).
TEST: Coagulation screen (N).
TRT: Steroids. Usually self-limiting.
COMM: Acquired immunological disorder.

See also SIGNS SECTION 2: Henoch-Schoenlein Purpura

Hers Syndrome

DES: Hepatomegaly, variable hypoglycaemia
TEST: B.lipids (N or H)
TRT: Dietary
COMM: Mildest of the glycogen storage diseases
        caused by hepatic phosphorylase deficiency.
        Rare and often undiagnosed until late
        childhood. Autosomal recessive

Histiocytosis X

See Hand-Schueller-Christian Syndrome

HIV-Associated Lipodystrophy Syndrome

See lipodystrophy Syndrome

Holmes-Adie Syndrome

DES: Pupil asymmetry, poor light pupillary light
        response, sluggish accommodation, absent
        tendon reflexes, (female more common).
TRT: Nil.
COMM: Benign condition.

Horner Syndrome

DES: Ipsilateral miosis, ptosis, enophthalmos,
        reduced sweating.
TEST: Nil.
TRT: Treat underlying cause.
COMM: Due to compression of sympathetic outflow
        pathways from pneumothorax, brain stem
        lesion, basilar artery insufficiency, lung
        carcinoma, syringomyelia, etc.

See also Pancoast Syndrome

Hunter Syndrome (Mucopolysaccharoidosis II)

DES: Stiff joints, grotesque facies,
        hepatosplenomegaly, cardiac anomalies, mild
        mental retardation, (deafness).
TEST: B.leukocytes (AB), bone marrow (AB), lumbar
        X-ray (N), 'gargoyle cells' in connective tissue,
        U.heparitin sulfate (H).
TRT: Nil.
COMM: Congenital mucopolysaccharoidosis, milder
        than Hurler's syndrome. Reasonable life
        expectancy.

See also Sanfilippo Syndrome

Hurler Syndrome (Mucopolysaccharoidosis I)

DES: Dwarfism, gross facies, stiff joints, lumbar
        gibbus, mental retardation, cardiac disorders,
        corneal clouding, hepatosplenomegaly, (claw
        hand).
TEST: B.leukocytes (AB), bone marrow (AB), lumbar
        X-ray (AB), 'gargoyle cells' in connective tissue,
        U.heparitin sulfate (H).
TRT: Nil.

COMM: Congenital mucopolysaccharoidosis. Usually
        fatal in childhood.

See also Hunter Syndrome; Sanfilippo Syndrome

Hyaline Membrane Disease

See Respiratory Distress Syndrome, Infant

Hyperkinetic Syndrome

DES: Early onset of developmental problems,
        overactivity, poor motor co-ordination, learning
        disorders, antisocial behaviour.
TEST: EEG.
TRT: Behaviour modification techniques,
        methylphenidate, dexamphetamine, special
        education programmes, environmental
        modification.
COMM: A form of minimal brain dysfunction.

Hypermobility Syndrome

DES: Passive dorsiflexion of little fingers beyond 90°
        (1 point each side), passive apposition of the
        thumb to the front of the forearm (1 point each
        side), hyperextension of knees beyond 10° (1
        point each side), hyperextension of elbows
        beyond 10° (1 point each side), resting palms
        easily on floor when bending from waist with
        knees straight (1 point). Diagnosis positive if
        score of 6 or more. Joint pain intermittently,
        swelling of joints, tenderness of joints, ease of
        joint dislocation.
TRT: Joint protection, physiotherapy, supports,
        splints, exercise programme, counselling,
        NSAIDs, analgesics, local anaesthetic and
        steroid injections.
COMM: Disability from recurrent spains or dislocations.
        Osteoarthritis may develop.

Hypoplastic Left Heart Syndrome

DES: Neonate, rapid onset heart failure, weak
        peripheral pulses, cyanosis.
TEST: Cardiac catheterisation (mitral and/or aortic
        atresia with patent ductus arteriosus).
TRT: Nil satisfactory.
COMM: Death within days of birth usual.

Ichabod Syndrome

DES: Syndrome of imminent death from any chronic
        cause. The characteristic signs may be useful in
        prognostication.
        Immobility —<20% patients weightbear within
        two days death.
        Confusion and coma — 40% become comatose
        and 30% confused in the two days before death.
        Homeostatic failure — Failure of temperature
        regulation, blood pressure control and
        peripheral circulation common in last two days
        before death.
        Anorexia — Very common in final week before
        death.

Blood — Haematological changes of imminent death include rising bilirubin, low serum albumin, low haemoglobin, high serum calcium, rising liver enzymes.
Observation — Occasional (rather than regular) observation of facial appearance shows marked deterioration in personality features.
Dypsnoea — 30% become dyspnoeaic in last two days. Cheyne-Stokes respiration very common in last few hours.
COMM: As well as being an acronym for the signs of impending death, the syndrome name was derived from the Old Testament daughter-in-law of Eli who, before dying in childbirth, named her son Ichabod, which translates as "the glory has departed".

Idiopathic Diffuse Interstitial Fibrosis
See Hamman-Rich Syndrome

Idiopathic Lymphadenopathy Syndrome
DES: Homosexual, generalised chronic lymphadenopathy, (immunodeficiency).
TEST: Human T leukaemia virus antibody type III (+).
COMM: Closely related to AIDS and may be a prodromal state.

Idiopathic Renal Acidosis
See Lightwood Syndrome

Idiot Savant Syndrome
See Savant Syndrome

Iliolumbar Syndrome
DES: Sciatica, pain and tenderness of posterior portion of one or both iliac crests, lateral bending away from involved side worsens pain.
TRT: Injection of local anaesthetic and depot steroid into iliac crest at insertion of iliolumbar ligament.
COMM: Caused by damage to the iliolumbar ligament from lifting and twisting movements.

Illiotibial Band Friction Syndrome
DES: Long distance runner, lateral knee pain in distal part of illiotibial band, pain on compression of lateral femoral epicondyle, (crepitus over lateral femoral epicondyle).
TRT: Rest, NSAIDs, physiotherapy.
COMM: Caused by running on sloped surface (eg. beach, road shoulder).

Impingement Syndromes
See Anterior Impingement Syndrome; Posterior Impingement Syndrome; Shoulder Impingement Syndrome

Incontinentia Pigmenti
See Bloch-Sulzberger Syndrome

Insulin Resistance Syndrome
See Reaven Syndrome

Intermediate Coronary Syndrome (Unstable Angina)
DES: Anginal pain of variable character, severity, duration, radiation, timing and causation from one attack to another or even during attacks.
TEST: ECG (AB).
TRT: Rest, nitrates and beta-blockers, or verapamil or nifedipine. Should be stabilised in hospital.
COMM: Intermediate stage between angina and myocardial infarct, to which they may progress. Mortality 15% per annum.

Irritable Bowel Syndrome
DES: Abdominal pain, constipation and/or diarrhoea, dyspepsia, mucous stools, anxiety or depression.
TEST: Sigmoidoscopy and barium enema show colonic hypermotility, blood and faecal studies normal.
TRT: Diet (eg. high fibre), psychotherapy, gut antispasmodics, sedatives, vegetable mucilages.
COMM: May be secondary to stress or low fibre diet.

Irukandji Syndrome
DES: Jellyfish sting, acute pulmonary oedema, acute respiratory failure, severe generalised pain, tachycardia, profuse sweating, shaking, systemic hypertension.
TRT: Intravenous narcotics in high doses, phentolamine IVI, diuretics, nitrates, intermittent positive pressure ventilation via endotracheal tube.
COMM: May be due to massive catecholamine release.

Itchy Upper Arm Syndrome (Brachioradialis Pruritus)
DES: Chronic sun damage to skin, intense itching and burning on extensor surface of arm, no apparent rash, worse in summer.
TEST: Skin biopsy (mast cell infiltration).
TRT: Potent topical corticosteroids. Generally resistant to treatment.
COMM: Due to constant subcutaneous histamine release by mast cells.

Jaccoud Syndrome
DES: Repeated attacks of rheumatic fever or lupus synovitis resulting in rheumatoid-like changes to hands and feet. Ulnar deviation and subluxation at metacarpophalangeal joints and metatarsophalangeal joints, pain free, no oedema, normal movement, signs of rheumatic heart disease.

TEST: ESR (N), rheumatoid factor (–), anti-DNA
antibody (–).
TRT: Nil specific.

Jamaican Neuritis
See Strachan Syndrome

Jervell-Lange-Nielsen Syndrome
DES: Deafness, syncopal attacks.
TEST: ECG (prolonged Q-T interval).
COMM: Autosomal recessive. Sudden death possible.

Job-Buckley Syndrome (Hyper-IgE Syndrome)
DES: Recurrent staphylococcal infections of the skin
or lungs, elevated IgE, osteopenia with
recurrent fractures, (coarse facial features, red
hair, fair skin, allergies)
TEST: S.IgE (H), B and T cell (L), B.eosinophils (H)
TRT: Long-term prophylactic antibiotics
COMM: May be autosomal dominant inheritance

Johanson-Blizzard Syndrome
DES: Aplastic ala nasi, anal atresia, aplasia cutis
congenita, deaf, mild mental retardation, failure
to thrive.
TRT: Nil.
COMM: Autosomal recessive inheritance.

Johansson-Sinding-Larsen Syndrome
DES: Knee pain in adolescents caused by disruption
to the lower pole of the patella at the tendon
attachment resulting in ossicle formation.
TEST: X-ray (AB in some cases).
TRT: Reset, splint if severe.
COMM: Good prognosis.

Joseph Syndrome
See Machado-Joseph Syndrome

Kallmann Syndrome
DES: Prepubertal hypogonadism, anosmia, familial,
long arms and legs, male, female body shape.
TEST: S.testosterone (VL).
TRT: Hormone replacement therapy.
COMM: Due to hormonal dysfunction of the
hypothalamus.

Kartagener Syndrome
DES: Dextrocardia, bronchiectasis, sinusitis,
(transposition of viscera).
TEST: X-ray chest (AB), barium meal (AB).
TRT: Surgical correction of defects if required.
Antibiotic and symptomatic treatment of lung
and sinus problems.
COMM: Hereditary.

Kawasaki Syndrome (Mucocutaneous Lymph Node Syndrome)
DES: Infant, high fever, stomatitis, polymorphous
rash, conjunctivitis, cervical adenitis, redness
and swelling of hands and feet followed by
desquamation, lethargy, vasculitis, (diarrhoea,
coronary aneurysm in 15-35%, death in 1-3%).
TEST: U.albumin (H), ESR (H), CSF WCC (H),
B.polymorphs (H), platelets (H late),
echocardiography (AB), B.culture (N).
TRT: Aspirin reduces fever and complication rate.
Unresponsive to antibiotics. Aggravated by
steroids.
COMM: Cause uncertain, but may be a bacterial
infection.

Kleine-Levin Syndrome
DES: Recurrent periods of severe excessive
sleepiness, increased appetite, mood
disturbances, sexual hyperactivity,
disorientation, hallucinations, memory loss,
may be asymptomatic for months between
attacks,more common in men, onset 12 to 20
years.
TEST: CSF WCC (H or N).
TRT: Stimulants.
COMM: Aetiology unknown. Self-limiting by fourth decade.

Klinefelter Syndrome
DES: Delayed puberty, hypoplastic testes and penis,
infertile, tall and slim, (gynaecomastia, mental
retardation, emotional disturbances).
TEST: Buccal smear (Barr body present),
chromosomal screen (XXY, XXXY or XXXXY).
TRT: Testosterone.
COMM: Common chromosomal disorder.

Klippel-Feil Syndrome
DES: Short neck, limited head movement, congenital,
(webbed neck).
TEST: Cervical radiology (fusion of 2 or more cervical
vertebrae).
TRT: Cosmetic surgery.
COMM: Non-familial.

Klippel-Trenaunay Syndrome
DES: Vascular malformation on the limbs, port wine
stain, local overgrowth of soft tissue, (local
overgrowth of bone, arteriovenous
malformations).
TRT: Surgery, compression bandages.

Klumpke's Palsy
DES: Hand held limply at wrist in neonate.
TRT: Wrist splinted in neutral position.
COMM: Due to lower brachial plexus damage during a
traction delivery.

See also Erb-Duchenne Palsy

Köebner Phenomenon

DES: Psoriasis or lichen planus developing at sites of skin trauma. Often linear pattern.
TRT: As for psoriasis or lichen planus.

Korsakoff Syndrome

See Wernicke-Korsakoff Syndrome

Kugelberg-Welander Syndrome

DES: Muscular weakness of shoulder girdle and pelvis, (abnormal gait, hypertrophic calves, tongue weakness).
TEST: S.CK (H), EMG (AB), nerve conduction studies (AB), muscle biopsy (AB).
TRT: Nil.
COMM: Muscle end plate abnormality that is slowly progressive. Normal life-span. Familial. Extensor plantar response, negative knee jerks.

Laitai

See Brugada Syndrome

Landau-Kleffner Syndrome

DES: Motor seizures, acquired receptive and expressive aphasia, behavioural disorders, onset 4 to 9 years of age
TRT: Anticonvulsants, speech therapy
COMM: 50% recovery. Poor prognosis with early onset

Landry-Guillain-Barré Syndrome

See Guillain-Barré Syndrome

Lange Syndrome

See de Lange Syndrome

Langer-Giedion Syndrome

DES: Sparse hair, bulbous nose, mild microcephaly, multiple exostoses.
TEST: Chromosomal analysis.
TRT: Plastic surgery.
COMM: Congenital condition localised to chromosome 8q24–>24.13.

Lateral Medullary Syndrome

DES: Excruciating, unrelenting pain involving one side of the body and the opposite side of the face
TEST: MRI or CT (AB)
TRT: Neurosurgery to ablate affected area
COMM: Caused by stroke or head injury involving lateral medulla

See also Déjerine-Roussy Syndrome

Laurence-Moon-Biedl Syndrome

DES: Retinitis pigmentosa, obesity, mental retardation, polydactyly, hypogenitalism.
TEST: Ophthalmoscopy (AB).
TRT: Nil.
COMM: Night blindness usual. Hereditary.

Leigh Syndrome (Subacute necrotising encephalomyelopathy)

DES: Onset from infancy to 6 years. Progressive development of vomiting, weight loss, weakness, seizures, dementia, vision loss, nystagmus, irregular respiration, stupor, death.
TEST: None specific.
TRT: Thiamine used experimentally. May remit temporarily.
COMM: Autosomal recessive inheritance. Possible due to an inborn error of thiamine metabolism.

Lennox-Gastaut Syndrome

DES: Multiple variable form seizures, mental retardation, drop attacks, status epilepticus.
TEST: EEG (slow-spike and wave discharges and slow background rhythms).
TRT: Combination of sodium valproate, lamotrigine and clobazam. Surgical corpus callosotomy in resistant cases.
COMM: Control of seizures usually very difficult.

Leopard Syndrome

DES: Multiple lentigines, hyperpigmentation, pulmonary stenosis, ECG abnormalities, cardiomyopathy, hypertelorism, (sensorineural deafness).
TEST: ECG (specific abnormality).
COMM: Dominant genetic inheritance.

Leriche Syndrome

DES: Calf claudication with walking, erectile failure, cold feet, femoral pulses absent or weak, aortic bruit, (thigh and buttock claudication).
TEST: Aortography (AB), Doppler flow studies (AB).
TRT: Surgery (graft, thromboendarterectomy and/or sympathectomy).
COMM: Due to atherosclerotic occlusion of distal aorta and iliac arteries. Postoperative prognosis good.

Leschke Syndrome

DES: Brown pigment spots on skin, asthenia, hyperglycaemia

Lesch-Nyhan Syndrome

DES: Mental deficit, gout, self-mutilation, choreoathetosis.
TEST: S.uric acid (VH), U.uric acid (H).
TRT: Symptomatic.
COMM: X-linked recessive error of metabolism.

Letterer-Siwe Syndrome
DES: Infant under 2 years, fever, wasting, pruritic papular rash, hepatosplenomegaly, lymphadenopathy.
TEST: Hb (L), WCC (L), chest X-ray (AB with infiltrates).
TRT: Chemotherapy, radiotherapy. Natural regression possible in Stage 1.
COMM: A Histiocytosis X disease. Staging determined by biopsy. Prognosis very good in Stage 1. Stage 2, 25% mortality. Stage 3, 66% mortality.

Liddle Syndrome
DES: Hypoaldosteronism, hypertension, hypokalaemia, alkalosis.
TEST: S.potassium (L).
TRT: Triamterene.
COMM: Rare. Inherited. Renal disease with preservation of sodium to the detriment of potassium.

Lightwood Syndrome (Idiopathic Renal Acidosis)
DES: Weight loss, vomiting, constipation, child.
TEST: U.pH (H), B.pH (L), renal biopsy (renal tubular calcification).

L'Illusion de Sosies
See Capgras Syndrome

Limb Girdle Syndrome
DES: Weak anterior neck flexor muscles, weak upper limb girdle muscles (eg. serratus anterior, supraspinatus, deltoid, biceps, triceps, brachioradialis), weak lower limb girdle muscles (eg. iliopsoas, gluteals).
TEST: EMG (AB), muscle biopsy (AB), S.CK (H or N).
TRT: Physiotherapy.
COMM: Relatively common cause of muscle weakness. Often progressive.

Limb Pain Syndrome (Growing Pains)
DES: Non-articular aching limb pains, bilateral, often nocturnal, affect both sexes in children from 6 to 14 years of age, worse in legs, intermittent, restless legs.
TEST: Exclude other limb pain pathology (see SYMPTOMS SECTION 1).
TRT: Reassurance, minor analgesics, massage, heat. Settles spontaneously.
COMM: May affect up to 33% of children. Familial.

Lipodystrophy Syndrome (HIV-Associated Lipodystrophy Syndrome)
DES: Excessive fat deposition over upper thoracic vertebrae (buffalo hump), circumferentially around neck, in breasts (both sexes) and in central abdomen. Loss of fat from proximal limbs and cheeks
TEST: S.cholesterol (H), S.triglycerides (H), C-peptide (H), B.glucose (H), GTT (AB), HIV antibodies (+)
TRT: Cease causative medicaiton, but this may result in worsening of HIV/AIDS
COMM: Adverse effect of protease inhibitor drugs used to treat HIV/AIDS. 80% of patients affected within 18 months, but only 10% severely affected.

Lip-Pit Syndrome
DES: Small bilateral pits on lower lip, cleft palate and/or cleft lip.
TRT: Plastic surgical correction.
COMM: Autosomal dominant syndrome with 50% penetration to siblings and offspring

Lissencephaly Syndrome
DES: Seizures, hypotonia, jaundice, corneal opacity, wrinkled forehead skin.
TRT: Nil.
COMM: Autosomal recessive inheritance. Early death normal.

Locked-in Syndrome
DES: Total paralysis of limbs and lower cranial nerves, normal consciousness
COMM: Due to infarct or damage to ventral pons, multiple sclerosis or pontine tumours. Able to communicate only by eye blinks. Poor prognosis

Loeffler Syndrome (PIE Syndrome)
DES: Pulmonary infiltrates with eosinophilia (PIE), wheeze, cough, fever.
TEST: Lung biopsy (AB), B.eosinophils (H).
TRT: Treat underlying cause which may be drugs, allergen, toxocara, microfilaria.
COMM: Asthmatics prone to this syndrome.

Löfgren Syndrome
DES: Erythema nodosum, bilateral hilar adenopathy on chest X-ray, sarcoidosis.
TEST: Chest X-ray (AB), tissue histology (AB).
TRT: NSAIDs control leg and skin symptoms.
COMM: 80% chance of spontaneous recovery.

Loose Anagen Syndrome
DES: Cild, telogen effluvium, loose wispy hair, fair colour, normal hair growth
TEST: Hair pulls easily from scalp without pain
COMM: Good prognosis. Improves with age and gentle hair care

Louis-Bar Syndrome
DES: Telangiectasia of conjunctivae, face and flexor

areas, mental retardation, recurrent infections of lungs and ears, cerebellar ataxia, (athetosis, nystagmus, malignancies).

TEST: S.IgA (VL), S.IgE (VL), S.alpha-fetoprotein (H).
TRT: Nil.
COMM: Death in teenage years usual. Due to cerebellar and spinal cord degeneration.

Lowe Syndrome

DES: Mental retardation, cataracts, corneal clouding, epicanthal folds, buphthalmos, (rickets, Fanconi syndrome).
TEST: U.amino acids (H), U.phosphate (H), U.pH (L).
TRT: Nil.
COMM: X-linked recessive error of metabolism.

Lown-Ganong-Levine Syndrome

DES: Atrial arrhythmia, characteristic ECG.
TEST: ECG (AB).
TRT: Vagal stimulation, procainamide, quinidine, verapamil, beta-blockers, DC cardioversion.
COMM: Preexcitation of ventricles by impulse bypassing the AV node through the James accessory tract.

Lyell Syndrome

See Scalded Skin Syndrome

Machado-Joseph Syndrome (Azorean Disease)

DES: Spasticity, rigidity, ataxia, dysarthria, limb weakness, fixed facies, (tremor, ophthalmoplegia, uncontrolled eye movement)
TRT: Levodopa and baclofen for rigidity and spasticity
COMM: Progressive degeneration of the spinocerebellum. Autosomal dominant. First discovered in the Azores Is.

Mallory-Weiss Syndrome

DES: Forceful vomiting, haematemesis.
TEST: Endoscopy (cardio-oesophageal tear).
TRT: Conservative unless prolonged, then balloon pressure to bleeding point, or surgery.
COMM: Tear in cardio-oesophagel mucosa caused by severe vomiting.

Marfan Syndrome

DES: Arachnodactyly, anomalous skeletal proportions, extra long tubular bones, kyphoscoliosis, joint hyperextensibility, genu recurvatum, lens dislocation, aortic regurgitation and dilation, mitral valve prolapse, (endocarditis, myopia, detached retina).
TEST: Specific chromosomal analysis (AB), skeletal X-ray (AB), echocardiography (AB).
TRT: Surgical correction of heart defects, propranolol, reserpine, physiotherapy.

COMM: Generalised inherited disorder of connective tissue. Mean survival 32 years. Cardiac complications often severe.

Marinesco-Sjögren Syndrome

DES: Onset in childhood with progressive cerebellar atrophy, ataxia, cataracts, multiple skeletal abnormalities, mental retardation, hypogonadism
TRT: Non available
COMM: Unknown enzymatic defect. Rare

Maroteaux-Lamy Syndrome

DES: Bone dysplasia, cardiac lesions, corneal clouding, deafness, short trunk, short neck, retarded growth, waddling gait, genu valgum, pes planus.
TEST: Specific enzyme tests (AB), chorionic villi sampling antenatally (AB).
TRT: Marrow transplantation (controversial).
COMM: Mucopolysaccharoidosis that accumulates dermatan sulfate. Survival beyond 40 years unusual.

Mauriac Syndrome

DES: Reduced stature, obese, hepatomegaly, diabetic
TRT: Correct diet, insulin dose modification.
COMM: Iatrogenic. Due to high dose, once daily, short-acting insulin injections.

May-Hegglin Anamoly

DES: Inflammatory leucocyte dysfunction, thrombocytopenia, large platelets.
TEST: Blood smear (AB).

McArdle Syndrome (Type V Glycogen Storage Disease)

DES: Progressive muscle weakness, muscle cramps myopathy.
TEST: Muscle histology (AB), specific enzyme assay (AB).
TRT: High protein diet, subcutaneous injections of glucagon.
COMM: Muscle phosphorylase enzyme deficiency.

McCune-Albright Syndrome

See Albright Syndrome

Meckel Syndrome

DES: Polydactyly, encephalocoele, cleft lip and palate, cystic dysplastic kidneys, (eye defects, hepatic fibrosis).
TRT: Chorionic villus sampling (+).
COMM: Autosomal recessive inheritance. Early death.

Meigs Syndrome (Demons-Meigs Syndrome)

DES: Ascites, hydrothorax, ovarian fibroma.

TEST: Sex hormone levels (AB).
TRT: Surgical removal of ovarian fibroma.

MEN Syndrome
See Multiple Endocrine Neoplasia Syndrome Type 2; Werner Syndrome

Mendelson Syndrome
DES: Bronchospasm and chemical pneumonitis associated with general anaesthesia or coma.
TRT: Intubation, oxygen, bronchodilators, hydrocortisone, antibiotics, maintenance of acid-base balance, artificial ventilation.
COMM: Due to aspiration of gastric acid.

Menière Syndrome (Menière's Disease)
DES: Vertigo, tinnitus, progressive deafness, (elderly, difficult concentration, depression).
TEST: Nil specific.
TRT: See TREATMENT SECTION 5.

Menopausal Syndrome
DES: Menstrual irregularities, hot flushes, depression, weight gain, 45-55 years old, (libido changes, breast discomfort).
TEST: Vaginal smear (atrophic), S.FSH (H), U.FSH (H), S.LH (H), X-ray (osteoporosis).
TRT: Oestrogen supplements, psychological support, vaginal oestrogens, calcium supplements, symptomatic management.
COMM: Most require no treatment, rarely psychoses develop. Control reasonable with treatment.

Mikulicz Syndrome (Benign Lymphoepithelial Lesion)
DES: Enlargement of salivary glands (parotid, submandibular), enlargement of lacrimal glands, (TB, sarcoidosis, syphilis, recurrent parotitis, actinomycosis, mucous gland atrophy in nose, larynx and vagina, keratoconjunctivitis sicca).
TEST: B.gamma-globulin (H), specific antibodies (+), biopsy histology (AB).
TRT: Conservative unless specific gland painful when surgical excision possible.
COMM: Benign. Common in Scandinavia.

Milkman Syndrome
DES: Multiple, bilateral, symmetrical pseudofractures on X-ray, osteomalacia.
TEST: X-ray (AB), S.calcium (L or N), S.ALP (H).
TRT: Vitamin D in high doses.
COMM: Adult version of rickets.

Miller Syndrome
DES: Inherited aniridia (lack of iris), Wilm's tumour, genito-urinary anomalies, mental retardation

TEST: Chromosome studies (deletion of short arm of chromosome 11)
TRT: None available
See also Gillespie Syndrome

Miller-Dieker Syndrome
DES: Lissencephaly, abnormal facies, mental retardation, growth retardation, low birth weight.
TEST: Specific chromosomal analysis (AB), CT scan (fewer brain gyri).
COMM: Congenital condition localised to chromosome 17. Prenatal diagnosis possible.

Mirrizzi Syndrome
DES: Impacted stone at the neck of the gall bladder causes inflammation that involves the common bile duct and results in biliary obstruction, (fistula of stone from gall bladder to common bile duct).
TEST: LFT (AB), ultrasound of gall bladder (AB).
TRT: Cholecystectomy.
COMM: Uncommon.

Moebius Syndrome
DES: Ptosis, ophthalmoplegia, fixed facies, drooling, dysphagia, normal intelligence, unable to close eyes, dysarthria, uni- or bilateral.
TRT: Plastic surgery.
COMM: Due to aplasia of cranial nerves VI and VII.

Mongolism
See Down Syndrome

Morquio Syndrome
DES: Severe progressive bone dysplasia, cardiac lesions, cataracts, deafness, short neck, short trunk, retarded growth, pes planus, genu valgum.
TEST: Specific enzyme tests (AB).
TRT: Nil necessary.
COMM: Normal life-span expected. Mucopolysaccharoidosis that accumulates keratin sulfate.

Morton Syndrome
DES: Congenital or acquired shortening of the first metatarsal, adduction deformity of first metatarsal, hypermobility of first tarso-metatarsal joint.
TRT: Surgery to correct deformity if severe.
COMM: May cause nerve entrapment and foot pain.

Mucocutaneous Lymph Node Syndrome
See Kawasaki Syndrome

Mucopolysaccharoidoses
See Hunter Syndrome; Hurler Syndrome; Sanfilippo Syndrome

Multiple Endocrine Neoplasia Syndrome Type 1 (MEN1)
See Werner Syndrome

Multiple Endocrine Neoplasia Syndrome Type 2 (MEN2)
DES: MEN2A – medullary thyroid carcinoma, phaeochromocytoma (50%), hyperparathyroidism (15%)
MEN2B – medullary thyroid carcinoma, phaechromocytoma, multiple mucosal neuromas, Marfan syndrome, intestinal ganglioneuromas
TEST: Specific gene testing
TRT: Thyroidectomy (prophylactically if inherited trait detected)
COMM: Autosomal dominant inheritance. Incidence 1:25,000

Multiple Hamartoma Syndrome (Cowden Disease)
DES: Multiple benign stomach hamartomas
TEST: Gastroscopy
TRT: Gastroscopic diathermy or gastric resection
COMM: Familial. May bleed extensively

Munchausen Syndrome
DES: Falsification of symptoms and signs by elaborate means in order to obtain attention, surgery, investigations and medication. Present repeatedly to different hospitals.
TRT: Psychiatric counselling. Further surgery must be avoided.
COMM: Extreme form of attention seeking. May go to great lengths to simulate emergency situations requiring urgent surgery.

See also Polle Syndrome; SHAFT Syndrome

Myalgic Encephalomyelitis
See Chronic Fatigue Syndrome

Myasthenic Syndrome
See Eaton-Lambert Syndrome

Myelodysplastic Syndrome
DES: Refractory anaemia, abnormal white cell morphology, abnormal marrow cell morphology, excess blast cells, malaise, tiredness, frequent infections, abnormal bleeding.
TEST: WCC (AB), Hb (L), marrow biopsy (AB).
TRT: Antibiotics, blood transfusions, platelet concentrate transfusions, bone marrow transplantation. Specific treatment if leukaemia develops.
COMM: May be forerunner to acute leukaemia.

Myofascial Pain Syndrome
DES: Severe muscle spasm (mainly neck, back, chest, shoulders) triggered by touch or use, deep ache and burn in affected muscles, (osteoarthritis neck and back)
TRT: Physiotherapy, NSAIDs, muscle relaxants
COMM: Due to overuse (eg. typing) or poor posture. Fibrocytis a complication

Naffziger Syndrome
See Cervical Rib Syndrome

Nail-Patella Syndrome (Fong Syndrome)
DES: Gross nail defects, small or absent patellae, iliac horns, elbow joint abnormalities, (renal failure).
TEST: U.protein (++).
COMM: Autosomal dominant disorder.

Nelson Syndrome
DES: Skin and tongue pigmentation, pituitary enlargement, postadrenalectomy, (visual field abnormalities).
TEST: Skull X-ray (AB), P.cortisol (L).
TRT: Hormone replacement.
COMM: Usually follows bilateral adrenalectomy for Cushing syndrome.

Nephrotic Syndrome
DES: Gross oedema, ascites, hydrothorax, skin striae, (hypertension).
TEST: U.protein (VH), U.casts (H), U.erythrocytes (+), Hb (L), B.cholesterol (H), P.protein (L), P.albumin (VL), S.gamma-globulin (L or N), renal biopsy (AB).
TRT: Nil specific. Treat underlying cause (eg. chronic infection, excise tumour, stop causative drug) and secondary infections or complications. Restrict sodium. Prednisone used in some cases.
COMM: Many different subtypes and causes. May be associated with collagen or autoimmune disease. More benign in children.

Neu-Lexova Syndrome
DES: Absent eyelids, hypoplastic nose, micrognathia, collodion skin, peripheral oedema, multiple contractures, mental retardation.
COMM: Inheritance is autosomal recessive.

Nuroleptic Malignant Syndrome
DES: Major tranquilliser use, hyperpyrexia, muscular rigidity, tremor, autonomic dysfunction, diaphoresis, confusion, impaired consciousness, (rhabdomyolysis, death in 20%).
TEST: S.CK (H), B.leucocytes (H), LFT (AB).
TRT: Cease neuroleptic medication, symptomatic support, trial medications include l-dopa, bromocriptine, amantadine and dantrolene.
COMM: May occur early or late in use of major

tranquillisers and at normal serum levels. Drugs implicated include phenothiazines, butyrophones, thioxanthines and loxapine. Early treatment improves morbidity and mortality. Rare under 200 cases reported.

See also Serotonin Syndrome

Nezelof Syndrome (Thymic Dysplasia)

DES: Infant, diarrhoea, severe infections, failure to thrive, fever, rashes, thrush.
TEST: S.Ig (N), B.lymphocytes (VL), thymic biopsy (Hassall's corpuscles absent).
TRT: Bone marrow transplant.
COMM: Due to defective colonisation of thymus by medullary stem cells.

See also DiGeorge Syndrome; Good Syndrome

Noonan Syndrome

DES: Short stature, webbed neck, shield chest, pulmonary stenosis, antimongoloid eye slant, ptosis, depressed nasal bridge, low set ears, broad nose tip, affects both sexes equally, (40% mental retardation).
TEST: Chromosomes (N).
TRT: Surgical correction of cardiac anomalies, plastic surgery.
COMM: Appearance of Turner syndrome, but with normal gonadal function.

Occupational Overuse Syndrome (Repetitive Strain Injury)

DES: Arm pain, hand pain, pain burning in nature, may be triggered by movement, (muscle weakness).
TEST: Nil specific.
TRT: Rest, NSAIDs, paracetamol, tricyclic antidepressants, improved posture, physiotherapy.
COMM: May be due to poor posture when typing or using computer terminal for prolonged periods and nerve root compression in neck.

Organic Brain Syndrome
See Brain Syndrome, Organic

Organic Personality Syndrome

DES: Personality change, emotional ability, loss of impulse control, (social inappropriateness, lack of concern about action consequences).
TEST: Nil.
TRT: Thioridazine, behavioural therapy, social support.
COMM: Various underlying causes. May be chronic or transient after frontal lobe trauma.

Orofacial Pain Syndrome

DES: Dull constant ache in muslces of jaw,

tenderness, difficulty opening mouth, (bruxism).
TRT: Physiotherapy, NSAIDs
COMM: Due to muscle spasm. Dental problems may be implicated

Oto-Palato-Digital Syndrome

DES: Conductive deafness, pugilistic facies, hypertelorism, syndactyly, cleft palate.
TRT: Surgical correction of deformities.
COMM: Recessive X-linked trait.

Overactivity Syndrome
See Hyperkinetic Syndrome

Painful Arc Syndrome (Supraspinatus Syndrome)

DES: Pain during mid-range movement of the shoulder joint in abduction, no pain at upper and lower parts of movement range.
TEST: Radiology (N or greater tuberosity fracture or calcified supraspinatus tendon).
TRT: Syndrome may be due to several causes, which may be treated differently:
         GREATER TUBEROSITY TRAUMA — mobilising exercises and physiotherapy once any fracture stable.
         SUPRASPINUS TENDONITIS OR STRAIN, SUBACHROMIAL BURSITIS — interferential and short-wave therapy by physiotherapist, mobilising exercises.
         SUPRASPINATUS CALCIFICATION — as above, or in acute cases, excision of deposit from tendon
         CHRONIC CASES — excision of acromial process.
COMM: Due to nipping of tissue between tuberosity of humerus and the under surface of the acromion or coraco-acromial ligament.

See also Rotator Cuff Syndrome

Painful Bruising Syndrome

DES: Young woman, paraesthesiae of limbs and trunk followed by crops of bruises, (may follow emotional or physical stress).
TEST: All haematological and coagulation tests normal.
TRT: Nil. Self-limited.

Painless Thyroiditis Syndrome

DES: Postpartum female, transient episodes of hypothyroidism and hyperthyroidism, firm goitre.
TEST: Microsomal antibodies (+), thyroid uptake iodine[131] (L).
TRT: Propranolol or thyroxine replacement therapy as necessary.
COMM: More common in North America and Japan. Some progress to permanent hypothyroidism.

Pancoast Syndrome

DES: Shoulder, arm and chest wall pain, ipsilateral Horner syndrome, bronchogenic carcinoma of lung apex.
TEST: Chest X-ray (AB), sputum cytology (+), biopsy (AB).
TRT: Surgery, radiation therapy and chemotherapy for carcinoma.
COMM: Poor survival rate, as spread usual by the time this syndrome presents.

Papillon-Le Fevre Syndrome

DES: Child, mobile anterior teeth, gingival recession, widely spaced teeth.
TEST: Diagnosed by physical examination.
TRT: Impeccable dental hygiene.
COMM: May result in premature loss of teeth.

Parinaud Syndrome (Pretectal Syndrome)

DES: Loss of voluntary upward gaze, loss of pupillary light reflex, retention of miosis with close vision, nystagmus retractorius (retraction of globe on attempted upward vision), (accommodative spasm, ptosis, loss of voluntary downward gaze, papilloedema, third nerve palsy).
TRT: Treat underlying cause.
COMM: Due to pinealoma, glioma, pretectal trauma or cerebrovascular lesions.

Parkinsonism

DES: Tremor maximal at rest, fixed facies, generalised rigidity, shuffling festinating gait, motor weakness, over 50 years old.
TEST: Nil.
TRT: Propranolol, levodopa, amantadine, diphenhydramine, trihexylphenidyl, physiotherapy, psychological support, neurosurgery.
COMM: No specific cause in most cases. Slowly progressive.

Parsnich-Turner Syndrome (Brachial Amyotrophy)

DES: Irregular disturbances of motor and sensory nerves to the arm, muscle wasting, paraesthesia
TEST: Electrophysiological tests (AB)
TRT: None specific. Physio may help retain function
COMM: Very rare brachial plexus disturbance of unknown aetiology that may follow trauma, surgery or childbirth. Usually settles gradually over several years

Patau Syndrome (Trisomy 13-15)

DES: Polydactyly, cardiac malformations, cleft lip and palate, microphthalmia, cerebral malformation.
TRT: Nil.
COMM: Congenital. Rare.

Patello-Femoral Pain Syndrome

DES: Pain in anterior part of knee behind or around patella, dull ache with sharp exacerbations, aggravated by climbing or descending stairs or slopes, no crepitus present.
TEST: Pain on patella compression, pain eased by medial deflection of patella during movement and worsened by lateral deflection.
TRT: Physiotherapy, strapping, rest, NSAIDs.
COMM: Common. Chondromalacia patellae will usually cause crepitus.

Patent Ductus Arteriosus

DES: Ductus arteriosus with left to right flow, machinery murmur, cardiac thrill, (left ventricular hypertrophy and failure).
TEST: ECG (N or L ventricular hypertrophy), cardiac catheterisation (AB).
TRT: Indomethacin in neonate, surgery.
COMM: Congenital failure of duct to close. Good prognosis.

See also Eisenmenger Syndrome

Paterson-Brown-Kelly Syndrome

See Plummer-Vinson Syndrome

Pendred Syndrome

DES: Deaf from birth, goitre from puberty.
TEST: TFT (N).
TRT: Thyroxine for goitre.
COMM: Autosomal recessive.

Perineal Descent Syndrome

DES: Slack pelvic floor muscles causing constipation, straining at stool, incontinence of urine.
TEST: Radiological defaecogram (AB).
TRT: Surgical.
COMM: Caused by old age, difficult labour or chronic constipation. Due to excessive descent of pelvic floor during defaecation.

Petrositis

See Gradenigo Syndrome

Peutz-Jegher Syndrome

DES: Pigmented buccal mucosa, lips and fingers, hamartomatous (haematomatous) polyps of gastrointestinal tract.
TEST: Endoscopy (AB).
TRT: Nil.
COMM: Benign condition. Complications include gut obstruction and bleeding.

Pickwickian Syndrome

DES: Hypoxia, obesity, somnolence, cyanosis, hypoventilation, hypercapnia, respiratory acidosis, right ventricular hypertension, cardiac

failure, pulmonary hypertension, polycythaemia.
TEST: B.pO$_2$ (L), B.pCO$_2$ (H), S.bicarbonate (H),
          respiratory function tests (AB), chest X-ray
          (pulmonary oedema, right heart enlarged).
TRT: Weight loss, progesterone, tracheostomy *in
          extremis.*
COMM: Due to gross obesity.

PIE Syndrome
See Loeffler's Syndrome

Pierre-Robin Syndrome
DES: Cleft palate, micrognathos.
TRT: Craniofacial surgery. Maintenance of airway
          and feeding prior to surgery often difficult.

Piriformis Syndrome
DES: Sciatica caused by compression of the sciatic
          nerve at the sciatic notch by spasm of the
          piriformis muscle, secondary to trauma, hip
          osteoarthritis, strain or sprain. Persistent
          external rotation of hip when supine. More
          common in females.
TEST: Pain and weakness on resisted
          abduction/external rotation of hip.
TRT: Injection of local anaesthetic/corticosteroid
          combination into belly of piriformis muscle via
          sciatic notch, or division of piriformis muscle.

Plica Syndrome
See Synovial Plica Syndrome

Plummer-Vinson Syndrome (Paterson-Brown-Kelly Syndrome)
DES: Dysphagia, oesophageal web, splenomegaly,
          iron deficit anaemia, glossitis, nail spooning,
          premenopausal female, (thin lips, beak shaped
          mouth).
TEST: Ba swallow (AB), oesophagoscopy (AB), Hb (L),
          B.smear (microcythemia).
TRT: Bouginage with oesophageal dilators, iron
          supplements, good diet.
COMM: Often precancerous.

Poikiloderma, Congenital
See Rothmund-Thomson Syndrome

Polle Syndrome
DES: Obscure forms of child abuse, apparently caring
          parents, over consultation with doctors and
          hospitals, demands for extensive investigation
          of child, emotionally stressed child, deliberate
          falsification of symptoms or test by parent.
TRT: Psychotherapy, family counselling.
COMM: Has been described as 'Munchausen syndrome
          by proxy'.

Polycystic Ovarian Syndrome
See Stein-Leventhal Syndrome

Polyglandular Autoimmune Syndromes
DES: TYPE 1 – Child, mucocutaneous candidiasis,
          hypoparathyroidism, adrenal insufficiency,
          (hypogonadism, alopecia, hypothyroidism)
          TYPE 2 – Adult, adrenal insufficiency,
          autoimmune thyroid disease, insulin dependent
          diabetes mellitus, (hypogonadism, myasthenia
          gravis, vitiligo)
          TYPE 3 – Adult, autoimmune thyroid disease
          and insulin dependent diabetes mellitus, or
          adrenal insufficiency and Hashimoto's
          thyroiditis
TEST: Depending on form abnormal results may occur
          with TSH, S.thyroxine, LH, FSH, B.glucose,
          S.Ca, S.phosphorus
TRT: Manage individual hormone deficiencies and
          thyroid disease.
COMM: Type 1 autosomal recessive, types 2 and 3
          autosomal dominant inheritance. Potentially
          fatal

Pompe Syndrome
DES: Hypotonia, mental retardation, hepatomegaly,
          cardiomegaly, abnormal ECG, cardiac failure.
TEST: Specific lysosomal enzyme assay (AB).
TRT: Nil available.
COMM: Death by two years of age normal. Lysosomal
          storage disease caused by acid-glucosidase
          enzyme deficiency.

Posner-Schlossman Syndrome (Glaucomatocyclitic crisis)
DES: Recurrent unilateral acute open-angle
          glaucoma, anterior uveitis, young adult
TEST: Intraocular pressure high
TRT: Steroid eye drops, standard glaucoma
          treatments

Posterior Facet Syndrome
DES: Pain in lower back that is referred to the leg
          caused by chronic synovial inflammation,
          degenerative disease and instability of the
          posterior facet joints of the lumbar vertebrae.
          (Degenerative disc disease, spinal stenosis.)
TEST: Greatest pain with lateral bending of spine when
          spine extended.
TRT: Physiotherapy, manipulation, injection of local
          anaesthetic/corticosteroid combination into
          facet joints, surgical fusion.

Posterior Impingement Syndrome
DES: Posterior ankle pain caused by impingement of
          the posterior talar process on the posterior
          aspect of the tibia, tender at back of ankle.
TEST: Ankle X-ray (+ enlarged posterior tubercle of
          talus or os trigonum present), passive plantar

fixation of ankle causes pain.
TRT: Rest, physiotherapy, NSAIDs, surgery.
COMM: Common in footballers, ballet dancers, gymnasts and others who forcibly plantar flex their ankles.

Postgastrectomy Syndrome
See Dumping Syndrome

Postphlebitic Syndrome
DES: Stasis dermatitis, distal leg ulcers, oedema of legs, varicose veins, post-deep vein thrombosis.
TEST: Venography (AB).
TRT: Bed rest, elevation, support stockings, treat dermatitis and ulceration, surgical removal of varicosities.
COMM: Due to destruction of deep venous valves by thrombophlebitis, and subsequent increase in superficial vein pressure.

Post-Polio Syndrome
DES: Unusual fatigue, arthralgia, myalgia, muscle weakness, onset decades after initial polio infection, (reduced respiratory reserve)
TEST: Nil
TRT: Symptomatic
COMM: May be due to overuse of polio-weakened muscles and excess strain on poorly supported joints.

Post-Traumatic Cerebral Syndrome
DES: Vertigo, headache, asthenia, poor memory, poor concentration, (personality change).
TEST: Cerebral CT scan (N or cortical atrophy and ventricular dilatation).
TRT: Symptomatic.
COMM: Slow recovery normal. Occurs after head injury, sometimes of a minor nature. Aggravated by changes in temperature or posture, alcohol or exercise.

Post-Traumatic Stress Syndrome
DES: Patients must have at least one symptom from each of the following categories for the diagnosis to be confirmed.
General:
— Symptom duration >1 month
— Significant distress or functional incapacity
Traumatic experience:
— Threatening or traumatic event
— Period of provoked fear, helplessness or horror
Re-experiencing phenomena:
— Intrusive recollections
— Nightmares
— Flashbacks as if the event was recurring
— Psychological distress on exposure to cues
— Physiological effects on exposure to cues

Avoidance behaviour:
— Avoid thoughts, feelings or conversations
— Avoid places, people or activities
— Selective amnesia
— Reduced interest
— Detachment from others
— Foreshortened future
— Abnormal affect
Hyperarousal:
— Insomnia
— Irritability or anger
— Poor concentration
— Increased vigilance
— Increased startle response
TRT: Psychiatric or psychological debriefing immediately after event, resume normal work and activities as soon as possible, continued appropriate counselling, alprazolam, tricyclic antidepressants.
COMM: Delayed onset form (with symptoms starting more than six months after incident) may occur. Normal duration three to six months, but may become chronic.

Postassium Wastage Syndrome
DES: Polyuria, muscle weakness, hypokalaemia, metabolic alkalosis, dilute urine.
TEST: U.potassium (VH), S.potassium (L), S.bicarbonate (H), U.SG (VL).
TRT: Correct potassium deficit, treat underlying cause.
COMM: May be due to Fanconi syndrome, aldosteronism and hyperadrenocorticism, chronic renal insufficiency, idiopathic causes.

Potter Syndrome
DES: Renal agenesis, hypoplastic lungs, small jaw, low set ears, loose upper lip, exaggerated epicanthic folds, wide set eyes, contractures, neonate. Risk of recurrence in subsequent pregnancy 1:40.
TRT: Nil.
COMM: Associated with oligohydramnios. No urine passed and death within hours of birth.

Prader-Willi Syndrome
DES: Low birth weight, hypotonia, compulsive eating and obesity, small genitalia, more common in males, (mental retardation, diabetes, small hands and feet).
TEST: Specific chromosomal analysis (AB).
TRT: Nil.
COMM: Hypothalamic disorder caused by chromosome 15 deletion. Not inherited.

Premenstrual Tension Syndrome
DES: Mastalgia, nausea, headache, bowel habit changes, personality changes, oedema, (anxiety, insomnia, poor concentration, depression, appetite changes, vomiting, acne, palpitations). All symptoms ease after

menstruation.

TEST: S.prolactin (N or H). No specific test.

TRT: Psychological support, diuretics, oral contraceptives, symptomatic treatment, mild sedatives, premenstrual progestogens, mild psychotropics, NSAIDs.

COMM: Self-limiting. Usually worse soon after puberty and just before menopause.

Pretectal Syndrome

See Parinaud Syndrome

Progressive Supranuclear Palsy

See Steele-Richardson-Olszewski Syndrome

Pronator Syndrome

DES: Pain and tenderness in proximal forearm, paraesthesia in thumb, paraesthesia in second and third fingers and half fourth finger, weakness of flexor pollicis longus and adductor pollicis brevis.

TRT: Surgical release of median nerve entrapment.

COMM: Due to median nerve entrapment in proximal forearm.

Proteus Syndrome

DES: Severe facial and body disfigurement caused by abnormal, unequal bone growth in face, arms, legs and hands; bony growths on skull causing a great increase in skull circumference; wrinkled subcutaneous bumps on feet, face and hands.

COMM: Rare. Believed to be the cause of John Merrick's 'Elephant Man' deformity.

Prune Belly Syndrome

DES: Potter syndrome, abdominal muscle deficiency, mega-ureter, megacystis, undescended testes, abdominal distension.

TEST: Radiological investigations (AB).

TRT: Nil available.

COMM: Rare. Occurs in 20% of infants with Potter syndrome. Inevitably fatal. Risk of recurrence in subsequent pregnancies <1%.

Pseudo-Cushing Syndrome

DES: Hypercorticalism secondary to alcoholism. Other details as for Cushing syndrome.

Pseudoexfoliation Syndrome

DES: White granular deposits on iris margin and lens, glaucoma, transillumination defects of iris, poor dilation of pupil, corneal pigmentation, more common in females and elderly.

TEST: Slit lamp examination of eye.

TRT: Topical beta-blockers, miotics, argon laser trabeculoplasty, antimetabolites, filtration surgery.

COMM: 33% bilateral.

Punch Drunk Syndrome (Dementia Pugilistica)

DES: Progressive encephalopathy causing cortical, extrapyramidal and cerebellar dysfunction most commonly in boxers. Unsteady gait, tremors, onset delayed years after trauma.

TEST: EEG, CT scan.

COMM: Caused by central cortical and ventricular atrophy.

Ramsay Hunt Syndrome (Geniculate Herpes)

DES: Severe earache, vertigo, herpetic eruption of tympanic membrane, external auditory canal, palate and face, malaise.

TRT: Aciclovir or other antiviral as soon as rash appears, steroids in high doses, analgesics, treat secondary infections.

COMM: Herpes zoster infection of geniculate ganglion. May involve nerves IX, X, V and VI also.

Raynaud's Phenomenon

DES: Pallor, cyanosis and oedema of fingers due to cold, rubor, pain and paraesthesia occur during rewarming, may progress to diminished sensation, chronic pain, fat atrophy and skin ulcers, 90% in women 15–45 years old.

TEST: Nil specific. Exclude precipitating disease by CBC, S.protein, LE cells, B.ANA, etc.

TRT: Keep hands warm, systemic vasodilators, topical nitroglyceryl trinitrate.

COMM: Raynaud's phenomenon differs from Raynaud's disease in that it is usually unilateral, not progressive, but may have more severe local effects on one or two fingers. May be secondary to thoracic outlet syndromes, carpal tunnel syndrome, SLE and other autoimmune diseases. Usually benign.

Reactive Arthritis

See Reiter Syndrome

Reaven Syndrome (Syndrome X, Insulin Resistance Syndrome)

DES: Family history of diabetes, hypertension, dyslipidaemia or obesity; increased body mass index and central obesity; glucose intolerance; hyperinsulinaemia; resistance to insulin stimulated glucose uptake; increased plasma very low density lipoprotein; decreased plasma high density lipoprotein, hypertension.

TEST: S.insulin (H), S.HDL (L), S.VLDL (H).

TRT: Weight loss, low fat diet, stop smoking, increase exercise, manage hypertension, hypolipidaemics.

COMM: Significantly increased risk of stroke, coronary artery disease and myocardial infarct. May affect up to 30% of population in western societies.

Red Man Syndrome

DES: IV vancomycin infusion, erythema, pruritus, urticaria of face, neck and torso, (hypotension, fever, cardiac arrest).

TRT: Reduce rate of IV vancomycin infusion to below 500 g/hr. Resolves spontaneously in majority. Antihistamines if required.

COMM: Usually mild and transient. Occurs in up to 80% of patients receiving IV vancomycin.

Reflex Sympathetic Dystrophy Syndrome (Complex Regional Pain Syndrome Type One)

DES: Prolonged exaggerated burning pain associated with minor trauma, onset immediate or delayed after minor trauma, hot dry limb initially, cold clammy cyanosed limb later.

TEST: Nil.

TRT: Analgesia, physiotherapy, sympathetic nerve blockade, psychotropics.

COMM: Stimulation of the sensory afferent nerves by sympathetic efferent nerves and sensitisation of spinal cord neurons leads to a self perpetuating closed cycle.

Refsum Syndrome

DES: Distal, symmetrical, sensorimotor, genetic polyneuropathy of childhood affecting legs more than arms.

TEST: Nerve biopsy (onion bulb hypertrophy).

TRT: Nil.

COMM: Rare. Due to inability to oxidise phytic acid and its subsequent tissue accumulation.

Reiter Syndrome (Reactive Arthritis)

DES: Conjunctivitis, nonspecific urethritis, arthritis, mucocutaneous lesions (eg. balanitis, stomatitis, punctate skin sores), (uveitis, fever, carditis).

TEST: B.HLA-B27 (+), ESR (H), joint X-ray (AB with recurrent disease).

TRT: Symptomatic, indomethacin.

COMM: Cause unknown, Self-limiting, but recurrences may occur. Usually in young men.

See also Behçet Syndrome

Rendu-Osler-Weber Syndrome

DES: Hereditary haemorrhagic telangiectasia, haemorrhagic lesions on tongue and throughout gastrointestinal tract, severe anaemia, arteriovenous fistulaes.

TEST: Faecal blood (+).

COMM: Autosomal dominant trait.

Repetitive Strain Injury

See Occupational Overuse Syndrome

Respiratory Distress Syndrome, Adult

DES: Posttraumatic, anxiety, dyspnoea, tachypnoea, pulmonary oedema, hypoxia, (cyanosis).

TEST: Chest X-ray (diffuse infiltration or consolidation), $B.pO_2$ (L), S.pH (N or H).

TRT: Oxygen, positive pressure ventilation, maintain fluid balance, diuretics, eradicate infection, control haemorrhage.

COMM: Only occurs in association with severe shock or trauma.

Respiratory Distress Syndrome, Infant (Hyaline Membrane Disease)

DES: Neonate (often pre-term), progressive respiratory difficulty, chest retraction, expiratory grunt, cyanosis, rapid respiration, 'frog' posture.

TEST: Chest X-ray (AB), $B.pO_2$ (L) $B.pCo_2$ (H), BpH (L).

TRT: Corticosteroids to mother before delivery of pre-term infant reduces risk, electrolyte management, oxygen, ventilatory assistance.

COMM: Usually occurs within a few hours of birth. Mortality 20–50%.

Restless Legs Syndrome (Wittmaack-Ekbom Syndrome)

DES: Unpleasant creeping sensation in legs giving the almost irresistable desire to move the legs while at rest.

TRT: Avoid stimulants (eg. coffee, tea, cola), clonazepam, biperiden,oxazepam, diazepam, levodopa and benserazide. Eased by walking.

COMM: More common in women. Exacerbated by pregnancy, warmth and antimotion sickness medications. Exclude anaemia, iron deficiency and diabetes as causes.

Rett Syndrome

DES: Female, normal development to 12-18 months of age then developmental regression, reduced head and body growth, ataxia, episodic hyperventilation, seizures, autism, subnormal mentality, constipation, repetitive 'hand-washing' movements, (sudden cardiovascular death).

TEST: Nil specific. Clinical diagnosis. ECG (prolonged QT interval indicates heart risk)

TRT: Symptomatic. Anticonvulsants. Physiotherapy.

COMM: 1:10,000 female births. Genetic aetiology. Annual mortality 1%

Reye Syndrome

DES: Vomiting, seizures, encephalopathy, tachypnoea and hepatic failure following a viral illness, (mental confusion).

TEST: B.glucose (L), S.transaminase (H), B.ammonia (H), prothrombin time (H), liver biopsy (AB), LFT (AB).

TRT: Nil specific. Mechanical ventilation, control cerebral oedema.

COMM: Mortality 30%. Chronic neurological lesions in a further 30%+. Pathogenesis unknown, but may be associated with aspirin use in children.

Incidence 2-4:1,000,000 children in United Kingdom.

Richner-Hanhart Syndrome (Tyrosinaemia Type II)

DES: Tyrosinaemia causing eye, skin and CNS lesions, eg. photophobia, corneal ulceration, blepharospasm, keratoderma, mental retardation, seizures.
TEST: B.tyrosine (VH).
TRT: Protein restricted diet with exclusion of phenylalanine and tyrosine.
COMM: Due to deficiency of hepatic soluble tyrosine aminotransferase. Autosomal recessive inheritance. Symptoms resolve with treatment.

Rieger Syndrome

DES: Iris dysgenesis, small teeth, oligodontia.
TRT: Nil.
COMM: Autosomal dominant inheritance.

Riley-Day Syndrome (Dysautonomia)

DES: Jewish, lack of lacrimation, excessive sweating, poor temperature control, intermittent fever, variable hypertension and hypotension, corneal anaesthesia, high pain tolerance, (asymptomatic fractures, poor coordination, dysphagia, dysarthria, emotionally labile).
TEST: Tendon reflexes (absent), chest X-ray (patchy infiltrates), U..4-hydroxy-3 methoxy Imandelic acid (H), skin reaction to histamine (absent).
TRT: Nil.
COMM: Familial.

Romano-Ward Syndrome

DES: Elongation of the QT interval on an ECG, sudden collapse due to ventricular arrhythmias, (sudden death from ventricular fibrillation)
TEST: ECG (AB)
TRT: Beta-blockers
COMM: Autosomal dominant inheritance.

Rotator Cuff Syndrome

DES: Tear or rupture of tendons of supraspinatus, infraspinatus and teres minor around the shoulder joint due to ageing.
TEST: Pain with forced forward elevation of humerus against acromion, tenderness over greater tuberosity, painful arc of abduction, pain on resisted abduction
TRT: Rest, NSAIDs, injection of local anaesthetic/corticosteroid combinations, physiotherapy, surgery.

Rothmund-Thomson Syndrome (Congenital Poikiloderma)

DES: Reticulate erythema, skin pigmentation, skin atrophy, telangiectasia, short stature,

hypogonadism, solar sensitivity.
TRT: Nil available.

Rotor Syndrome

DES: Asymptomatic and hereditary neonatal jaundice.
TEST: Oral cholecystogram (N), liver biopsy (no pigment), B.conjugated bilirubin (VH), BSP excretion (L).
TRT: Nil necessary.
COMM: Excellent prognosis.

See also Dubin-Johnson Syndrome

Roussy-Levy Syndrome

DES: Ataxia, kyphoscoliosis, wasting of hands and legs, hypotonia.
TEST: Tendon reflexes (absent).
TRT: Nil available.
COMM: Autosomal dominant. Slowly progressive.

Rubenstein-Taybi Syndrome

DES: Hypoplastic maxilla, broad thumbs and toes, slanted palpebral fissures, patent ductus arteriosus, other cardiac malformations, (mild to moderate subnormal mentality).
COMM: May be hereditary.

Russell-Silver Syndrome

DES: Dwarfism, gestational ages small, 78% significant asymmetry from hemihypertrophy which tends to correct itself with growth, 34% precocious puberty, café-au-lait spots, (incurved and short fifth digit, downturning of mouth, triangular face, syndatyly of toes, mental retardation, renal anomalies, hypospadias).
TRT: Nil.
COMM: Due to retardation of epiphyseal development. Sporadic autosomal dominance within family. Growth and appearance improve in adolescence. 10% develop Wilms' tumour.

Sandifer Syndrome

DES: Paroxysmal neck flexion and muscle stiffening in an infant resembling dystonic posture, but caused by reflux oesophagitis.
TEST: Trial of therapy, Ba swallow.
TRT: Antacids, cisapride, H_2 receptor antagonists.
COMM: May be confused with epileptic seizure.

Sanfilippo Syndrome (Mucopolysaccharidosis III)

DES: Severe mental retardation starting at age 5+, hypertrichosis, gross facies, hepatosplenomegaly.
TEST: U.heparin-N-sulfate (VH).
TRT: Nil available.
COMM: Congenital mucopolysaccharidosis with mild somatic symptoms and late onset.

Savant Syndrome (Idiot Savant Syndrome)

DES: Generally subnormal, but extraordinary talent in one narrow field (eg. music, mathematics).

COMM: Cause unknown, but may be due to antenatal or birth trauma that allows one area of the brain to develop at the expense of others.

Scalded Skin Syndrome (Ritter's Disease, Toxic Epidermal Necrolysis, Lyell Syndrome)

DES: Infant, exfoliative dermatitis commencing on face and genitals and spreading across body.

TEST: Culture swabs from nose, eyes, throat and umbilicus.

TRT: Penicillin or erythromycin.

COMM: Staphylococcal skin infection that spreads from nose, eyes, mouth or umbilicus.

Scalenus Anticus Syndrome

See Cervical Rib Syndrome

Scapulocostal Syndrome

DES: Pain in neck radiating from posterior cervical region to occiput, medial border of scapula and ulnar side of forearm; tender insertion of levator muscle into vertebral border of scapula, (shoulder girdle stiffness, tender trapezius muscle).

TEST: Nil.

TRT: Posture correction, exercise, local anaesthetic infiltration.

COMM: May be due to fatigue associated with chronic faulty posture.

Scheie Syndrome

DES: Recurrent respiratory infections, hepatosplenomegaly, kyphosis, cardiac murmurs, cataracts, slow growth, starts at one to two years of age and progresses to death by ten years.

TEST: Specific enzyme tests (AB).

TRT: Nil effective.

COMM: Mucopolysaccharidosis closely related to Hurler syndrome.

Schmidt Syndrome

DES: Primary thyroid insufficiency, primary adrenal insufficiency.

COMM: Very rare autoimmune disorder.

Seckel Syndrome

DES: Intrauterine growth retardation, low set ears, hip and elbow dislocation, mental retardation, beaked nose.

TRT: Nil.

COMM: Autosomal recessive inheritance.

Serotonin Syndrome

DES: Agitation, vomiting, tremor, myoclonus, vertigo, incoordination, tachycardia, hyper-reflexia, nystagmus, (fever, flush, diarrhoea)

TRT: Stop all antidepressant medication, cyproheptadine, diazepam

COMM: Caused by interaction between different serotonergic antidepressants after inadequate washout periods, or interaciton between antidepressants and other drugs (eg: pethidine, pseudoephedrine, dextromethorphan)

See also Neuroleptic Malignant Syndrome

Sézary Syndrome

DES: Chronic pruritic erythroderma, alopecia, mononuclear infiltration of dermis, lymphadenopathy, abnormal blood lymphocytes.

TEST: Skin biopsy (AB), B.smear (abnormal T lymphocytes).

TRT: Low grade irradiation of lesions, cytotoxic chemotherapy.

COMM: Variant of mycosis fungoides.

SHAFT Syndrome

DES: Sad, hostile, anxious, frustrated, tenacious patient who praises a doctor excessively to obtain unnecessary surgery, then has worsening of imagined symptoms after surgery for which the doctor is blamed.

TRT: Psychotherapy. Avoid surgery unless very strong nonsubjective clinical grounds for intervention.

COMM: Name is an acronym from major personality characteristics.Neurosis. Variation of Munchausen syndrome.

Sheehan Syndrome

DES: Postpartum pituitary necrosis, uterine haemorrhage postpartum, failure of lactation, amenorrhoea, (hypotension).

TEST: S.Thyroxine (L), basal metabolic rate (L), U.17-ketosteroids (L), U.gonadotrophins (VL), B.ACTH (L), Hb (L), WCC (L), B.glucose (L).

TRT: Oral replacement therapy of hormones (eg. thyroxine, cortisone, cyclic oestrogens).

COMM: Varied progressive symptoms of pituitary insufficiency. Due to thrombosis of pituitary circulation during parturition.

Shin Splints

See Tibial Stress Syndrome

Shock Syndrome (Circulatory Shock)

DES: Pallor, hypotension, sensory alteration, rapid weak pulse, clammy skin, oliguria, thirst, dyspnoea, anxiety.

TEST: Determine cause of shock eg. haemorrhage (internal or external), burns, diarrhoea, peritonitis, myocardial infarct, cardiac arrhythmia, pericardial disease, pulmonary embolus, septicaemia, drugs, etc.

RT: Specific to cause. General measures include:
        lie patient supine with legs elevated slightly,
        oxygen, maintain body warmth, intravenous
        fluids, analgesics, ventilatory support.
COMM: Three main subclassifications, hypovolaemic
        shock, cardiogenic shock and vascular shock.
        Correct diagnosis most important step.

Short Bowel Syndrome

DES: Steatorrhoea, pernicious anaemia,
        osteomalacia, hyperoxaluria, secondary to
        bowel resection.
TEST: Faecal fat (H).
RT: Loperimide, codeine, diphenoxylate, vitamin
        B_{12}, folic acid, diet.
COMM: Usually due to extensive bowel resection for
        Crohn's disease or similar.

Shoulder Impingement Syndrome

DES: Painful arc of shoulder movement between 60
        and 120° of abduction
TEST: Local anaesthetic injected into subacromial
        space relieves pain (+)
TRT: Rest, NSAIDs, corticosteroid injections,
        physiotherapy, surgery

Shoulder-Hand Syndrome

DES: Variable painful disorders of hand and shoulder
        of one arm, scapulo-humeral periarthritis,
        Sudeck's atrophy of hand and wrist, (middle
        aged, diabetes).
TEST: X-ray (N).
TRT: Analgesics, passive exercise, steroid injections
        and operative manipulation for shoulder.
        Physiotherapy, trifluoperazine, analgesics,
        prednisone and sympathectomy for hand.
COMM: Prognosis poor if treatment delayed.

Shprintzen Syndrome

See Velocardiofacial Syndrome

Shy-Drager Syndrome

DES: Idiopathic orthostatic hypotension, reduced
        sweating, slight tremor, dysarthria, rigidity,
        ataxia, erectile failure, vertigo, diplegia,
        incontinence.
TEST: MRI brain (AB).
TRT: Care in postural changes, elastic stockings,
        girdle, fluorocortisone, ephedrine sulfate.
COMM: Progressive to death in 5-7 years.

Sicard Syndrome (Collet-Sicard Syndrome)

DES: Paralysis of intrinsic laryngeal, tongue,
        pharyngeal, palatal, sternomastoid and
        trapezius muscles on one side due to a lesion of
        cranial nerves 9, 10, 11 and 12.

Sicca Syndrome

DES: Swelling of salivary and lacrimal glands, dry
        mouth, dry eyes, dry vagina, dry throat.
COMM: Self-limiting benign lymphoepithelial lesion.
        May be part of Sjögren Syndrome, a drug
        reaction or graft versus host disease.

See also Mikulicz Syndrome

Sick Building Syndrome

DES: Nasal, eye and mucous membrane irritation,
        lethargy, dry skin, headache, prolonged time in
        air conditioned building.
TRT: Increase fresh air circulation within building.
COMM: Energy efficient buildings have minimal fresh air
        circulation and allow organic solvents, fungal
        spores and other contaminants to recirculate in
        increasing concentrations.

Sick Sinus Syndrome (Sinus Bradycardia)

DES: Variable heart rate from brief standstill to
        marked tachycardia or atrial fibrillation, atrial
        control of arrhythmias on ECG, syncope.
TEST: Continuous ECG monitoring (AB), cardiac
        enzymes (N).
TRT: Pacemaker and antiarrhythmic drugs.
COMM: Due to sinus node or conduction anomalies.

SIDS Syndrome

See Sudden Infant Death Syndrome

Sjögren Syndrome

DES: Dry eyes, mouth, nose, larynx, vagina and skin,
        rheumatoid arthritis, (pancreatitis).
TEST: Hb (L), B.eosinophils (H), B.HLA-DR3 (+), WCC
        (L), S.rheumatoid factor (+), S.gamma-
        globulins (H), S.FANA (H), S.extractable
        nuclear antibodies (H).
TRT: Symptomatic only. Artificial tears, oral hygiene,
        NSAIDs.
COMM: Syndrome causes many varied symptoms
        arising from mucous membrane dryness.
        Autoimmune disease. May be associated with
        renal tubular acidosis.

Sjögren-Larrson Syndrome

DES: Widespread ichthyosis, spastic diplegia.
COMM: Autosomal recessive trait.

Slapped Cheek Syndrome (Erythema Infectiosum)

DES: Child, erythematous raised rash over cheeks,
        circumoral pallor, mild fever and malaise prior to
        rash, (symmetrical pruritic maculopapular rash
        on extensor surfaces, palms, soles and
        buttocks).
TEST: Specific IgM antibody (RT).

TRT: Paracetamol. Self limiting, with resolution in 10 to 12 days.
COMM: Cause by human parvovirus B19.

Sleep Apnoea Syndrome

DES: More than 30 periods of transient apnoea during full night's sleep, snoring, daytime sleepiness, personality change, irritability, restless sleep, obesity, (pulmonary hypertension, sexual dysfunction, nocturnal enuresis, intellectual impairment, cor pulmonale, cardiac arrhythmias, polycythaemia, sudden death).
TEST: Sleep laboratory studies (AB), B.pO$_2$ (L).
TRT: Weight loss, avoid alcohol and sedatives, continuous positive pressure air supply via face mask, protriptyline, palatal surgery.

Slipping Rib Syndrome

DES: Unattached rib cartilage (usually 10th) overrides the rib above causing pain.
TEST: Chest X-ray (AB).
TRT: Reassurance, corticosteroid/local anaesthetic injections, surgery.

Sly Syndrome

DES: Recurrent respiratory infections, hepatosplenomegaly, kyphosis, cardiac murmurs, cataracts, slow growth, starts at 1-2 years of age and progresses to death by 10 years.
TEST: Specific enzyme tests (AB).
TRT: Nil effective.
COMM: Mucopolysaccharidosis caused by deficiency in beta-glucuronidase that is closely related to Hurler syndrome.

Smith-Lemli-Opitz Syndrome

DES: Ptosis, narrow forehead, mental retardation, hypospadias, anteverted nostrils, syndactyly of toes.
TRT: Surgical correction of deformities.
COMM: Autosomal recessive inheritance.

Smith-Magenis Syndrome

DES: Brachycephaly, mid-face hypoplasia, prognathism, hoarse voice.
TEST: Specific chromosomal analysis (AB).
TRT: Nil.
COMM: Congenital condition localised to chromosome 17p11.2.

Snapping Scapula Syndrome

DES: Snapping noise with shoulder abduction, pain along medial border of scapula, (generalised hypermobility)
TEST: X-ray scapula (bony spur)
TRT: Rest, steroid injection, surgery
COMM: Due to trauma

Sneddon Syndrome

DES: Livedo reticularis (maroon to red, netlike or starburst skin pattern), hypertension, TIA, cerebral ischaemia
TEST: Skin biopsy (AB), antiphospholipid antibodies (+or–)
TRT: Antihypertensives, aspirin or heparin
COMM: Rare and potentially life threatening due to high incidence of myocardial and cerebral infarcts

Somatisation Disorder
See Briquet Syndrome

Soto Syndrome

DES: Development delay as a child, frontal bone bossing, antimongoloid eye slant, accelerated childhood growth, normal adult stature.
TEST: EEG (AB), CT Scan (dilated cerebral ventricles).
COMM: Inherited dominant trait.

Stagardt Syndrome

DES: Deteriorating vision, adolescent, loss of foveal reflex, foveal atrophy.
TEST: Eye fundus examination (AB), fluorescein angiogram (AB).
TRT: Nil.
COMM: Autosomal recessive inheritance. Slowly progressive.

Steele-Richardson-Olszewski Syndrome (Progressive Supranuclear Palsy)

DES: Axial rigidity with extension, dementia, paralysis of downward gaze, upper motor neurone lesion signs, falls backwards easily, elderly, dysphagia.
TRT: Methysergide, benzhexol, l-dopa. Physiotherapy, occupational and speech therapy.
COMM: Aetiology unknown. Male:female = 2:1. Often confused with parkinsonism.

Stein-Leventhal Syndrome (Polycystic Ovarian Syndrome)

DES: Secondary amenorrhoea, infertility, bilateral polycystic ovaries, 15 to 30 year old female, hirsutism, obesity.
TEST: U.17-ketosteroids (H), P.testosterone (H), U.FSH (N).
TRT: Clomiphene, wedge resection of ovaries.
COMM: May be due to defective metabolism of sex steroids.

Stevens-Johnson Syndrome

DES: Erythema multiforme, purulent conjunctivitis (corneal ulcers and perforation), fever, stomatitis, vesicles in nose, vagina, urethra and anal canal.

EST: ESR (H). Nil specific.
RT: Intensive corticosteroid therapy, remove cause of erythema multiforme.
COMM: May be triggered by drugs or infection.

Stewart-Morgagni-Morel Syndrome

DES: Acromegaly, hyperostosis frontalis.
COMM: Hypothalamic-pituitary disorder resulting in excess and androgen production.

Stewart-Treves Syndrome

DES: Angiosarcoma on a lymphoedematous limb, elderly.
EST: Histopathology (+).
RT: Wide excision.
COMM: Lymphoedema often follows mastectomy. Relentlessly aggressive tumour. Poor prognosis.

Sticky Platelet Syndrome

DES: Excess stickness of platelets, migraines, strokes in young patients.
EST: Platelet agglutination rate (VH).
RT: Aspirin, dipyridamole.

Stiff-man Syndrome

DES: Idiopathic tonic muscle rigidity.
EST: EMG (tonic contraction), X-ray (stress fractures and subluxations).
RT: Diazepam, suxamethonium, peripheral nerve block.
COMM: Rare. Most sufferers have rigid limbs with severely painful muscle cramps.

Stokes-Adams Syndrome

DES: Syncope, convulsive movements, bradycardia or transient asystole, reactive hyperaemia on recovery from attack.
EST: ECG (AB).
RT: Eliminate causative drugs, pacemaker, IV atropine.
COMM: May be associated with heart block secondary to myocardial infarction.

Strachan Syndrome (Jamaican Neuritis)

DES: Amblyopia, painful neuropathy, orogenital dermatitis, corneal ulcers, (peripheral sensory loss, ataxia, muscle weakness, spasticity, blindness)
EST: S.vitamin B (L).
RT: Good diet, vitamin B supplements
COMM: Probably due to lack of vitamin B. Worse in alcoholics and smokers

Sturge-Weber Syndrome

DES: Facial port wine stain, convulsions, haemiplegia, mental retardation, buphthalmos,

(glaucoma, retinal detachment, homonymous (haemianopia).
TEST: Skull X-ray (vascular calcifications), EEG (AB).
TRT: Control convulsions, plastic surgery, ophthalmic surgery.
COMM: Congenital.

Subacute Necrotising Encephalomyopathy
See Leigh Syndrome

Subclavian Steal Syndrome

DES: Arm claudication, cerebral symptoms.
TEST: Angiography (AB)
TRT: Nil unless severe, and then surgical arterial bypass.
COMM: Due to occlusion of left subclavian A. or innominate artery. Arm supplied by collateral flow from vertebral artery, resulting in both arm and cerebral ischaemia. Associated with thoracic outlet syndromes.

Sudden Infant Death Syndrome [SIDS]

DES: Infant found dead in cot with no apparent cause of death on examination or autopsy.
TRT: Careful management of parents' guilt and grief.
COMM: More common in lower socio-economic classes. Many theories on causation, but none proven. Prone sleeping is a risk factor. Less common with breast fed infants.

SUNCT Syndrome

DES: Severe headaches that are Shortlasting (seconds to minutes), Unilateral and neuralgiform with associated Conjunctival injection and tear production, occur regularly or spasmodically.
TRT: Sumatriptan, ergotamine, nasal capsaicin, pure oxygen inhalation.
COMM: Name is an acronym of major symptoms. Variant of cluster headaches.

Superior Vena Caval Syndrome

DES: Brawny oedema and flushing of head and neck, dilated neck and arm veins.
TEST: Venography (blocked superior vena cava).
TRT: IV cyclophosphamide, IV ethacrynic acid, mediastinal irradiation.
COMM: Invariably secondary to bronchogenic carcinoma or other mediastinal neoplasms that cause blocking of the superior vena cava. Treatment urgent or cardiac failure occurs. Neoplasms usually inoperable by time this syndrome occurs.

Supraspinatus Syndrome
See Painful Arc Syndrome

Sweet Syndrome (Acute Febrile Neutrophilic Dermatosis)

DES: Multiple tender red or purple skin plaques on neck and limbs, myalgia, fever, arthralgia, (joint effusions, acute myeloid leukaemia in 20%, ulcerative colitis in 3%).
TEST: B.neutrophils (H), skin plaque histology (excess mature neutrophils).
TRT: Prednisone.
COMM: More common in women. Heals spontaneously over 2 or more months. Recurrences common.

Syndrome of Inappropriate ADH (Vasopressin) Secretion [SIADH]

DES: Weight gain, weakness, lethargy, mental confusion and convulsions caused by hyponatraemia, water retention and high levels of antidiuretic hormone.
TEST: S.ADH (H), S.sodium (L), B.urea (L), S.creatinine (L), S.albumin (L), S.osmolality (L), U.osmolality > S.osmolality.
TRT: Restrict fluid intake, saline solution IV, frusemide for water overload.
COMM: May be caused by malignant neoplasms with autonomous ADH release (eg. oat cell carcinoma of lung, carcinoma of pancreas), nonmalignant pulmonary disease (eg. TB, pneumonia), CNS disorders (eg. skull fracture, intracranial haemorrhage, cerebrovascular thrombosis), hypothyroidism, positive pressure respiration or drugs (eg. SSRI, chlorpropamide, vincristine, narcotics).

Syndrome X

See Reaven Syndrome

Synovial Plica Syndrome

DES: Anterior knee pain caused by synovial fold of the medial patello-femoral joint being caught between patella and femur during knee exercise
TEST: Nil specific.
TRT: Rest, splinting, arthroscopic removal of excess synovium, NSAIDs, quadriceps physiotherapy

Tarsal Tunnel Syndrome

DES: Paraesthesia in toes and sole, weakness of foot intrinsic muscles.
TRT: Corticosteroid injection, surgery.
COMM: Due to compression of posterior tibial nerve at ankle.

Tethered Cord Syndrome

DES: Neurological deficits below level of spinal cord tether that slowly progress (eg. lower motor neurone lesion, muscle weakness, fallen arches, abnormal sensation, urinary incontinence)
TEST: CT and/or MRI of spine (AB), reflexes (AB)

TRT: Neurosurgery to remove cause of tethering in spinal canal
COMM: May be due to an elongated spinal cord attached to a thick filum or spina bifida occulta presenting in childhood (group one), or pressure from a lipoma or other benign spinal canal mass presenting in an adult (group two)

Tetralogy of Fallot

See Fallot's Tetralogy

Thalamic Pain Syndrome

See Déjerine-Roussy Syndrome

Thoracic Outlet Syndromes

See Cervical Rib Syndrome; Scapulocostal Syndrome; Subclavian Steal Syndrome

Thymic Dysplasia

See Nezelof Syndrome

Thymic Hypoplasia

See Di George Syndrome

Tibial Stress Syndrome (Shin Splints)

DES: Athletes and runners (particularly novices and unfit, and running on hard surfaces), pain and tenderness over distal posteromedial border of tibia.
TRT: Rest, NSAIDs.
COMM: Tendonitis and periostitis at insertion of tibialis posterior on the interosseous membrane.

Tietze's Syndrome(Costochondral Syndrome, Anterior Chest Wall Syndrome)

DES: Painful, tender swellings of costochondral junctions.
TEST: ESR (N). Nil specific.
TRT: Analgesics, NSAIDs, corticosteroid infiltration.
COMM: Self-limiting disease lasting 2 weeks to 6 months. 30-50 years of age. Only one attack normally.

Tolosa-Hunt Syndrome

DES: Painful paralysis of one eye, ptosis, mydriasis.
COMM: May be due to internal carotid artery aneurysm.

Tourette Syndrome

See Gilles de la Tourette Syndrome

Toxic Epidermal Necrolysis

See Scalded Skin Syndrome

Toxic Shock Syndrome

DES: Fever, vomiting, watery diarrhoea, (myalgia, hypotension, headache, rash, conjunctivitis, renal and cardiac failure).

TEST: Throat or vaginal swab M/C/S (*Staph. aureus* isolated).
TRT: Rehydration, antibiotics against *S.aureus*.
COMM: Mortality rate up to 5%. Majority occur in women during or immediately after menstruation and has been associated with tampon use.

Treacher-Collins Syndrome

DES: Mandibular hypoplasia, large mouth, absent frontonasal angle, antimongoloid eye slant, notched lower lids, sparse medial eyelashes, hairy cheeks, low set ears, deaf, middle ear abnormalities.
COMM: Transmitted by irregularly dominant gene.

Trisomy 13-15
See Patau Syndrome

Trisomy 18
See Edward Syndrome

Trisomy 21
See Down Syndrome

Trousseau Syndrome

DES: Thrombophlebitis migrans visceral carcinoma.
TRT: Treat underlying carcinoma.

Tumour Lysis Syndrome

DES: Weakness, malaise, ileus, cardiac arrhythmias, and acute renal failure in a patient receiving chemotherapy for a bulky, chemosensitive tumour.
TEST: S.potassium (VH), S.phosphate (H), S.urate (H), S.calcium (HL).
TRT: Prevent by good hydration, urinary alkalinisers and allopurinol. Treated by rehydration, monitoring electrolytes carefully.
COMM: Metabolic disturbance due to rapid release of intracellular metabolites from the tumour lysis by chemotherapy.

Turcot Syndrome

DES: Malignant brain tumours, polyposis coli.
COMM: Very rare.

Turner Syndrome (Gonadal Dysgenesis, XO Syndrome)

DES: Congenital absence of ovaries, genital hypoplasia, amenorrhoea, breast agenesis, short stature, scanty pubic and axillary hair, increased carrying angle of arms, neck webbing, (eye disorders, cardiovascular disorders, stocky chest, osteoporosis, naevi, diabetes).
TEST: U. and S.FSH (H), S.17-ketosteroids (L), bone

age X-ray (retarded development), chromosomes (XO).
TRT: Oestrogens and/or androgens cyclically, growth hormone, surgical correction of cardiovascular anomalies and webbing of neck.
COMM: Due to XO chromosome pattern. Rare disorder, whose sufferers can be made to function like females in all ways except fertility.

See also Blackfan-Diamond Syndrome, Noonan Syndrome

Twelfth Rib Syndrome

DES: Loin pain aggravated by movement and pressure on twelfth rib.
TEST: Exclude renal pathology.
TRT: NSAIDs, corticosteroid injection, surgery.
COMM: Entrapment of the lateral arcuate ligament under the twelfth rib.

Tyrisonaemia Type II
See Richner-Hanhart Syndrome

Ulysses Syndrome

DES: Patient taken through a long, costly and potentially hazardous series of investigations and procedures in order to explain one randomly abnormal pathology test result that has no clinical features. Iatrogenic condition.
TEST: Stop all investigations.
TRT: Reassure patient that abnormality is not significant.
COMM: The more tests that are performed, the greater the chance that one abnormality will be found. That abnormality should not be pursued unless clinically significant.

Unstable Angina
See Intermediate Coronary Syndrome

Uraemic Syndrome
See Haemolytic Uraemic Syndrome

Urethral Syndrome

DES: Dysuria, urinary frequency, sterile urine.
TEST: U.M/C/S (N), specific U.M/C/S for anaerobes and fastidious organisms (eg. *Ureaplasma urealyticum* (N or B), cystoscopy (N or AB).
TRT: Antibiotics, urinary alkalinisers, bladder irrigation with antiseptic solution. Prevent by post-intercourse micturition and/or antibiotics.
COMM: May be due to unidentified bacterial infection, interstitial cystitis, trigonitis, bladder tumours, or bladder prolapse.

Urge Syndrome

DES: Nocturia, urinary frequency, micturitional

urgency, urge incontinence, (enuresis).
TEST: Exclude diabetes, infection, bladder tumours and calculi, renal disease.
TRT: Avoid bladder stimulants (eg. coffee, colas, tea, alcohol). Fluid restriction, bladder training, fluid intake/output recording, oxybutynin, propantheline, amitriptyline, imipramine, temazepam (at night), psychiatric assessment, surgery (rarely).
COMM: 10% of adult population affected at some time. 80% women.

Usher Syndrome

DES: Deaf, retinitis pigmentosa.
COMM: Autosomal recessive trait.

Uveoparotid Syndrome

See Heerfordt Syndrome

Vasovagal Syndrome

DES: Recurrent syncope, hypotension, pallor, bradycardia, sensory or emotional trauma.
TEST: BP (L), pulse (L), ECG (AB during attack).
TRT: Avoid precipitating causes (eg. prolonged standing), lie down or bend forward with onset of symptoms, aromatic inhalations.

Velocardiofacial Syndrome (Shprintzen Syndrome)

DES: Small stature, abnormal facial features [downturned corners of the mouth, cleft palate, long midface, retrognathia, cylindrical nose], nasal speech pattern, heart abnormalities (ventriculoseptal or atrioseptal defect, Tetralogy of Fallot), (tortuous retinal vessels, strabismus, feeding difficulties, slender hands, emotional lability and learning disability).
TEST: Chromosomal analysis (AB)
TRT: Surgical correction of cardiac, palatal and facial abnormalities
COMM: Autosomal dominant abnormality of chromosome 22

Vogt-Koyanagi-Harada Syndrome

DES: Acute iridocyclitis, patchy choroiditis, retinal detachment, fever, headache, vertigo, dysacusis, (vitiligo, white patch of hair, deaf, tinnitus, meningitis). May occur in one or both eyes.
COMM: Anterior eye disease self-limiting, posterior changes indolent with visual impairment.

von Gierke Syndrome

DES: Neonate, hypoglycaemia, hepatosplenomegaly, failure to thrive, stunted growth, diarrhoea, neutropenia.
TEST: B.lactate (VH), WCC (L), B.glucose (L), S.urate (H), S.lipids (H).
TRT: High glucose diet, nocturnal glucose infusion.

COMM: Most die in infancy, very few progress to adult life, where disease remits. Glycogen storage disease caused by glucose-6-phosphatase deficiency.

von Hippel-Lindau Syndrome

DES: Young adult, visual disturbances, retinal hamartomatous tumour, (cerebellar hamartomatous tumour, neurological disturbances).
TEST: Ophthalmoscopy (AB), CT scan (AB or N).
TRT: Laser photocoagulation or surgical resection of retinal lesions, cerebellar surgery.
COMM: Autosomal dominant inheritance with variable penetrance. Tumours are capillary haemangiomas.

Vulvodynia

See Burning Vulva Syndrome

Waardenburg-Klein Syndrome

DES: Uni- or bilateral deafness, broad root of nose with lateral displacement of inner canthus, confluent eyebrows, white forelock, heterochroma iridium (ie. irises different colours).
TRT: Plastic surgery.
COMM: Autosomal dominant trait.

WAGR Syndrome

DES: Name an acroynm for the symptoms of Wilms' tumour, aniridia (no iris), gonadoblastoma, mental retardation.
TEST: Chromosomal analysis (AB).
TRT: Treatment of Wilms' tumour.
COMM: Congenital condition localised to chromosome 11p13.

Waterhouse-Friderichsen Syndrome (Fulminant Meningococcaemia)

DES: Prostration, petechiae, purpura, circumoral cyanosis, pallor, (coma, cardiac failure, circulatory collapse).
TEST: B.culture (meningococcus), metabolic abnormalities.
TRT: Appropriate antibiotics parenterally, control shock, hydrocortisone.
COMM: Due to bilateral adrenal haemorrhage and destruction causing an acute Addisonian crisis. Death may occur within a few hours.

Weil Syndrome

DES: Pharyngitis, myalgia, diarrhoea, coagulopathy, renal failure, hepatic failure, leptospirosis infection, exposure to rodents.
TEST: Serology for Leptospirosis (+), S.CK (H), B.culture (+).
TRT: Penicillin or tetracycline.
COMM: Significant morbidity, occasionally fatal.

Werdnig-Hoffman Syndrome

DES: Familial, progressive muscular dystrophy, neonate, proximal muscles affected more than distal, respiratory infections.
TEST: Muscle biopsy (AB).
TRT: Nil effective.
COMM: Recessive trait. Progressive loss of the motor neurones in the anterior horns of spinal cord. Usually fatal by 5 years of age.

Werner Syndrome (Multiple Endocrine Neoplasia Type 1)

DES: Neoplastic involvement of the pituitary, parathyroid and pancreatic islet cells, (intestinal carcinoid, phaeochromocytoma, atrophic skin, cataracts)
TEST: Regular endocrine screening
TRT: Surgery, chronic endocrine management
COMM: Familial. Genetic screening possible

Wernicke-Korsakoff Syndrome

DES: Ataxia, mental deterioration, disturbed ocular motility, (diplopia, polyneuropathy, ptosis, miosis).
TEST: S.thiamine (L).
TRT: Thiamine (vitamin B_1), good diet, no alcohol.
COMM: Due to alcoholism and its effect on cerebrum and brain stem. Prognosis reasonable.

Whistling Face Syndrome

See Freeman-Sheldon Syndrome

Williams Syndrome

DES: Blue irises, lacy irises, long philtrum, prominent epicanthic folds, prominent lips, pendular cheeks, slight mental deterioration, outgoing personality, (Neonatal hypercalcaemia, aortic stenosis).
TRT: Nil.
COMM: Sporadic inheritance.

Wiskott-Aldrich Syndrome

DES: Eczema, thrombocytopenia, recurrent severe infections, male.
TEST: S.IgM (L), S.IgE (H), S.IgG (N), S.IgA (N), reduced skin response, platelets (L), B.lymphocytes (L).
TRT: Aggressive treatment of infections, cortisone, blood transfusions, avoid allergens, bone marrow transplant, splenectomy.
COMM: Mean survival time 9 years. X-linked recessive disorder.

Wittmaack-Ekbom Syndrome

See Restless Legs Syndrome

Wolff-Parkinson-White Syndrome (Accelerated Conduction Syndrome)

DES: Paroxysmal arrhythmia, ECG shows short PR interval and wide QRS cmplex with slurred delta wave at QRS onset
TEST: ECG (AB)
TRT: See TREATMENT SECTION 5.
COMM: May be congenital or acquired. Due to abnormal short circuit pathway between atria and ventricles

Wolf-Hirschhorn Syndrome

DES: Mental retardation, growth retardation, abnormal nasal bridge ("Greek helmet" appearance), cleft lip, short philtrum.
TEST: Chromosomal analysis.
TRT: Plastic surgery.
COMM: Congenital conditional localised to chromosome 4p16.1.

Xiphoid Syndrome (Xiphoidalgia)

DES: Tender painful xiphoid sternum, nausea, vomiting.
TRT: NSAIDs, corticosteroid/local anaesthetic injection.

XO Syndrome

See Turner Syndrome

XXX Syndrome

DES: Chromosomal abnormality, normal phenotype, minor mental retardation, (psychoses).
TEST: Antenatal chorionic villus sampling (AB).
TRT: Nil.
COMM: Fertile and offspring genetically normal. Incidence 1/800.

XXY Syndrome

See Klinefelter Syndrome

XYY Syndrome

DES: Male, tall stature, aggressive, violent.
TEST: Chromosomes (47 XYY). Antenatal chorionic villus sampling (AB).
TRT: Behavioural therapy.
COMM: Incidence 1:500 males. Usually discovered accidentally on routine chromosome analysis.

Yellow Nail Syndrome

DES: Chronic lung disease and/or lymphoedema, nails stop growing, thick yellow nails, excessive side to side nail curvature, no cuticle, onycholysis, oedema and erythema of proximal nail fold
TEST: Treat underlying lung problem or lymphoedema, topical azelaic acid, vitamin E, zinc
COMM: Uncommon. Chronic bronchitis and bronchiectasis often responsible

Zellweger Syndrome (Cerebro-hepato-renal Syndrome)

DES: Flat long face, large fontanelle, hypotonia, birth asphyxia, hepatomegaly, hepatic failure, fits, (glaucoma, cataracts, joint contractures, skeletal abnormalities, cryptorchidism).

TEST: U.pH (L), LFT (AB), lateral X-ray patella (+ cardiac stippling).

TRT: Nil available.

COMM: Death at birth or within two months. Autosomal recessive inheritance.

Zollinger-Ellison Syndrome (Gastrinoma)

DES: Severe recurrent gastric ulcers, diarrhoea.

TEST: S.gastrin (VH), S.calcium (H), gastric hypersecretion, Ba meal or gastroscopy (peptic ulcer(s) and gastritis).

TRT: High dose H_2-antagnoists, proton pump inhibitors, gastrectomy, gastrinoma excision.

COMM: Due to gastrin secreting tumour (often in pancreas) that may be malignant. Haemorrhage and perforation of ulcers common.